Pathological Mechanisms in Diabetes

Pathological Mechanisms in Diabetes

Editor

Maria Grau

MDPI • Basel • Beijing • Wuhan • Barcelona • Belgrade • Manchester • Tokyo • Cluj • Tianjin

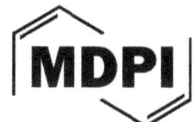

Editor
Maria Grau
University of Barcelona
Spain

Editorial Office
MDPI
St. Alban-Anlage 66
4052 Basel, Switzerland

This is a reprint of articles from the Special Issue published online in the open access journal *Biomedicines* (ISSN 2227-9059) (available at: https://www.mdpi.com/journal/biomedicines/special_issues/Diabetes_Pathological_Mechanisms).

For citation purposes, cite each article independently as indicated on the article page online and as indicated below:

LastName, A.A.; LastName, B.B.; LastName, C.C. Article Title. *Journal Name* **Year**, *Volume Number*, Page Range.

ISBN 978-3-0365-5801-1 (Hbk)
ISBN 978-3-0365-5802-8 (PDF)

Cover image courtesy of Nighthawk Shoots from Unsplash.com

© 2023 by the authors. Articles in this book are Open Access and distributed under the Creative Commons Attribution (CC BY) license, which allows users to download, copy and build upon published articles, as long as the author and publisher are properly credited, which ensures maximum dissemination and a wider impact of our publications.

The book as a whole is distributed by MDPI under the terms and conditions of the Creative Commons license CC BY-NC-ND.

Contents

About the Editor vii

María Grau and Carles Pericas
Diabetes: A Multifaceted Disorder
Reprinted from: *Biomedicines* **2022**, *10*, 1698, doi:10.3390/biomedicines10071698 1

Hideaki Kaneto, Tomohiko Kimura, Masashi Shimoda, Atsushi Obata, Junpei Sanada, Yoshiro Fushimi, et al.
Molecular Mechanism of Pancreatic β-Cell Failure in Type 2 Diabetes Mellitus
Reprinted from: *Biomedicines* **2022**, *10*, 818, doi:10.3390/biomedicines10040818 5

Judit Mohás-Cseh, Gergő Attila Molnár, Marianna Pap, Boglárka Laczy, Tibor Vas, Melinda Kertész, et al.
Incorporation of Oxidized Phenylalanine Derivatives into Insulin Signaling Relevant Proteins May Link Oxidative Stress to Signaling Conditions Underlying Chronic Insulin Resistance
Reprinted from: *Biomedicines* **2022**, *10*, 975, doi:10.3390/biomedicines10050975 19

Grace Chung, Ramkumar Mohan, Megan Beetch, Seokwon Jo and Emilyn Uy Alejandro
Placental Insulin Receptor Transiently Regulates Glucose Homeostasis in the Adult Mouse Offspring of Multiparous Dams
Reprinted from: *Biomedicines* **2022**, *10*, 575, doi:10.3390/biomedicines10030575 43

Adela-Viviana Sitar-Tăut, Angela Cozma, Adriana Fodor, Sorina-Cezara Coste, Olga Hilda Orasan, Vasile Negrean, et al.
New Insights on the Relationship between Leptin, Ghrelin, and Leptin/Ghrelin Ratio Enforced by Body Mass Index in Obesity and Diabetes
Reprinted from: *Biomedicines* **2021**, *9*, 1657, doi:10.3390/biomedicines9111657 57

Iris M. de Hoogh, Wilrike J. Pasman, André Boorsma, Ben van Ommen and Suzan Wopereis
Effects of a 13-Week Personalized Lifestyle Intervention Based on the Diabetes Subtype for People with Newly Diagnosed Type 2 Diabetes
Reprinted from: *Biomedicines* **2022**, *10*, 643, doi:10.3390/biomedicines10030643 73

Akira Matsumori
Novel Biomarkers of Inflammation for the Management of Diabetes: Immunoglobulin-Free Light Chains
Reprinted from: *Biomedicines* **2022**, *10*, 666, doi:10.3390/biomedicines10030666 87

Natsuki Eguchi, Arvin John Toribio, Michael Alexander, Ivana Xu, David Lee Whaley, Luis F. Hernandez, et al.
Dysregulation of β-Cell Proliferation in Diabetes: Possibilities of Combination Therapy in the Development of a Comprehensive Treatment
Reprinted from: *Biomedicines* **2022**, *10*, 472, doi:10.3390/biomedicines10020472 101

Eric Jankowski, Sophie Wulf, Nadja Ziller, Gunter Wolf and Ivonne Loeffler
MORG1—A Negative Modulator of Renal Lipid Metabolism in Murine Diabetes
Reprinted from: *Biomedicines* **2022**, *10*, 30, doi:10.3390/biomedicines10010030 119

Midori Fujishiro, Hisamitsu Ishihara, Katsuhiko Ogawa, Takayo Murase, Takashi Nakamura, Kentaro Watanabe, et al.
Impact of Plasma Xanthine Oxidoreductase Activity on the Mechanisms of Distal Symmetric Polyneuropathy Development in Patients with Type 2 Diabetes
Reprinted from: *Biomedicines* **2021**, *9*, 1052, doi:10.3390/biomedicines9081052 137

**Ana Boned-Murillo, Henar Albertos-Arranz, María Dolores Diaz-Barreda,
Elvira Orduna-Hospital, Ana Sánchez-Cano, Antonio Ferreras, et al.**
Optical Coherence Tomography Angiography in Diabetic Patients: A Systematic Review
Reprinted from: *Biomedicines* **2022**, *10*, 88, doi:10.3390/biomedicines10010088 . . . . **157**

**Cristina Rey-Reñones, Sara Martinez-Torres, Francisco M. Martín-Luján, Carles Pericas,
Ana Redondo, Carles Vilaplana-Carnerero, et al.**
Type 2 Diabetes Mellitus and COVID-19: A Narrative Review
Reprinted from: *Biomedicines* **2022**, *10*, 2089, doi:10.3390/biomedicines10092089 . . . . **183**

**Olivier Deckmyn, Thierry Poynard, Pierre Bedossa, Valérie Paradis, Valentina Peta,
Raluca Pais, et al.**
Clinical Interest of Serum Alpha-2 Macroglobulin, Apolipoprotein A1, and Haptoglobin in
Patients with Non-Alcoholic Fatty Liver Disease, with and without Type 2 Diabetes, before or
during COVID-19
Reprinted from: *Biomedicines* **2022**, *10*, 699, doi:10.3390/biomedicines10030699 . . . . **195**

Vladimir Grubelnik, Jan Zmazek, Matej Završnik and Marko Marhl
Lipotoxity in a Vicious Cycle of Pancreatic Beta Cell Exhaustion
Reprinted from: *Biomedicines* **2022**, *10*, 1627, doi:10.3390/biomedicines10071627 . . . . **233**

About the Editor

María Grau

María Grau, Serra Húnter Fellow, Department of Medicine, University of Barcelona, 08036 Barcelona, Spain; Biomedical Research Consortium in Epidemiology and Public Health (CIBERESP), 08036 Barcelona, Spain; August Pi i Sunyer Biomedical Research Institute (IDIBAPS), 08036 Barcelona, Spain

Professor Serra-Hunter at the University of Barcelona since 2021 and researcher at the August Pi i Sunyer Biomedical Research Institute (IDIBAPS), also in Barcelona. Professor Maria Grau was chosen in 2013 as one of the 25 most promising young researchers in Spain. Her scientific career can be summarized by three main characteristics: (1) A comprehensive view of public health; her research line is focused on the promotion of healthy aging as a way to prevent the most common causes of death in high-income countries with notable population aging; (2) the use of innovative methodologies to produce new scientific findings; and (3) the application of excellent scientific methodology. She has published as first author in top-ranked journals that also have high impact in the mass media. She has been recognized as a key opinion leader in innovation and citizen science. Since 2020, she is part of the Consortium for Biomedical Research in Epidemiology and Public Health funded by the Ministry of Science of the Spanish Government.

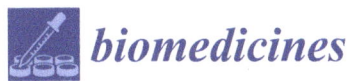

Editorial
Diabetes: A Multifaceted Disorder

María Grau [1,2,3,*] and Carles Pericas [1]

1. Serra Húnter Fellow, Department of Medicine, University of Barcelona, 08036 Barcelona, Spain; carlespericas@ub.edu
2. Biomedical Research Consortium in Epidemiology and Public Health (CIBERESP), 08036 Barcelona, Spain
3. August Pi i Sunyer Biomedical Research Institute (IDIBAPS), 08036 Barcelona, Spain
* Correspondence: mariagrau@ub.edu

Diabetes is a chronic disease associated with increased morbidity and mortality from cardiovascular diseases cancer, chronic obstructive pulmonary disease, and kidney or liver disease [1,2]. Despite the fact that aging is the main risk factor for the onset and progression of type 2 diabetes mellitus (the most common type of diabetes), in recent decades, age-standardized all-cause mortality in the population with type 2 diabetes has fallen more than in the general population [3]. However, age-specific data indicate that this trend in the total diabetes population is predominantly influenced by trends in those aged 80 or more years. The figures observed in those younger than 80 years indicate that improvements in the management of diabetes and its complications may not have translated into a direct prevention of premature deaths related to type 2 diabetes [4].

This Special Issue of *Biomedicines* presents a compilation of high-quality scientific evidence aimed at unraveling the molecular mechanisms involved in the association between diabetes and comorbidities and at describing their clinical and therapeutic implications. The issue has been structured accordingly and subdivided in three sections.

The first section focuses on diabetes mellitus itself; the second focuses on the complications of such a disorder—particularly nephropathy, polyneuropathy, and diabetic retinopathy—and the third one presents the consequences of COVID-19 in the population with diabetes.

The first section starts with a narrative review about the molecular mechanisms implied in the failure of pancreatic β-cell failure [5]. The review is followed by a computational model aimed to analyze the effects of hyperlipidemia, particularly free fatty acids, on pancreatic beta cells and insulin secretion [6]. After, two experimental studies, the first examines the role of tyrosine isoforms ortho- and meta-tyrosine in the development of insulin resistance [7]. The second, conducted in a mouse model, focuses on the impairment of the insulin signaling pathway in the placenta during pregnancies complicated by maternal obesity and gestational diabetes mellitus [8]. Additionally, four studies conducted in human samples have been included. The first one is a cross-sectional study, which assessed the relationship between adipokines, and their ratio with obesity and diabetes [9]. The second one is an intervention study, which evaluated a 13-week personalized lifestyle intervention in newly diagnosed type 2 diabetes mellitus. The results showed an improvement in type 2 diabetes mellitus parameters compared with patients who received usual care [10]. The final two studies are narrative reviews devoted to the treatment of diabetes mellitus. One suggests that the nuclear factor-kappa B could be a target for an anti-inflammatory strategy in preventing and treating diabetes when immunoglobulin-free light chain is modified [11]. The second focuses on the role of β-cell mass/proliferation pathways, dysregulated in diabetes, in treating and reversing diabetes as well as the current therapeutic agents studied to induce β-cell proliferation [12].

In the second section, three manuscripts show the broad spectrum of pathologies related with diabetes. First, an experimental study in a mouse model presents the detection of MORG1 expression, a scaffold protein, as a promising strategy to reduce lipid metabolic

Citation: Grau, M.; Pericas, C. Diabetes: A Multifaceted Disorder. *Biomedicines* **2022**, *10*, 1698. https://doi.org/10.3390/biomedicines10071698

Received: 6 July 2022
Accepted: 8 July 2022
Published: 14 July 2022

Publisher's Note: MDPI stays neutral with regard to jurisdictional claims in published maps and institutional affiliations.

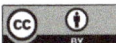

Copyright: © 2022 by the authors. Licensee MDPI, Basel, Switzerland. This article is an open access article distributed under the terms and conditions of the Creative Commons Attribution (CC BY) license (https://creativecommons.org/licenses/by/4.0/).

alterations in diabetic nephropathy [13]. Regarding the other studies, conducted in human samples, Fujishiro et al. evaluated the impact of plasma xanthine oxidoreductase activity on the mechanisms of distal symmetric polyneuropathy development [14], and Boned-Murillo et al. performed a systematic review to analyze the current applications of optical coherence tomography angiography and to provide an updated overview on its role in the evaluation of diabetic retinopathy [15].

Finally, COVID-19 also has a space in our Special Issue, with two scientific works. The first article is a narrative review, which provides an overview of the most recent studies that determine type 2 diabetes mellitus as a risk factor and link it to poor prognosis of COVID-19 [16]. The second one assessed how alpha-2 macroglobulin, apolipoprotein A1, and haptoglobin are associated with the risk of liver fibrosis, inflammation, and COVID-19 in patients with non-alcoholic fatty liver disease with or without type 2 diabetes mellitus [17].

The variety of updated topics included from different approaches shows the need for more efficient preventive activities to reduce the incidence of this disease and its related complications.

On one final note, it is important to point out that diabetes is a worldwide public health problem that can be explained by the classic model of the determinants of health. This model shows how individual lifestyles are embedded in social norms and networks and in living and working conditions, which in turn are related to the wider socioeconomic and cultural environment [18]. Therefore, success in preventing diabetes mellitus and its associated complications not only depends on the individual but also on social and community networks as well as general socioeconomic, cultural, and environmental conditions [19]. Indeed, the final aim is to create conditions that ensure good health and social care for an entire population through the development and implementation of preventive strategies, promotion of healthy lifestyles, protection from diseases, and the design of targeted screening strategies. This aligns with the United Nations Sustainable Development goal number 3, good health and well-being, which includes the achievement of universal health coverage and access to quality essential healthcare services. In addition, this also has a direct link to goal number 10, which focuses on reducing inequalities within and among countries [20].

Additionally, we have analyzed the gender balance and authors' nationalities in this Special Issue. Although 62% of the first authors are women, after analyzing the percentage of senior authors by gender, this figure dropped to 38%. The authors of the works included are from nine different countries, guaranteeing an international representation.

Author Contributions: Both authors (M.G. and C.P.) have significantly contributed to the manuscript writing and critical review. All authors have read and agreed to the published version of the manuscript.

Funding: This research received no external funding.

Conflicts of Interest: The authors declare no conflict of interest.

References

1. Baena-Díez, J.M.; Peñafiel, J.; Subirana, I.; Ramos, R.; Elosua, R.; Marín-Ibañez, A.; Guembe, M.J.; Rigo, F.; Tormo-Díaz, M.J.; Moreno-Iribas, C.; et al. Risk of Cause-Specific Death in Individuals with Diabetes: A Competing Risks Analysis. *Diabetes Care* **2016**, *39*, 1987–1995. [CrossRef] [PubMed]
2. Rey-Reñones, C.; Baena-Díez, J.M.; Aguilar-Palacio, I.; Miquel, C.; Grau, M. Type 2 Diabetes Mellitus and Cancer: Epidemiology, Physiopathology and Prevention. *Biomedicines* **2021**, *9*, 1429. [CrossRef] [PubMed]
3. *IDF Diabetes Atlas*, 9th ed.; 2019. Available online: https://www.diabetesatlas.org/en/ (accessed on 9 June 2022).
4. Sacre, J.W.; Harding, J.L.; Shaw, J.E.; Magliano, D.J. Declining mortality in older people with type 2 diabetes masks rising excess risks at younger ages: A population-based study of all-cause and cause-specific mortality over 13 years. *Int. J Epidemiol.* **2021**, *50*, 1362–1372. [CrossRef] [PubMed]
5. Kaneto, H.; Kimura, T.; Shimoda, M.; Obata, A.; Sanada, J.; Fushimi, Y.; Matsuoka, T.A.; Kaku, K. Molecular Mechanism of Pancreatic β-Cell Failure in Type 2 Diabetes Mellitus. *Biomedicines* **2022**, *10*, 818. [CrossRef] [PubMed]
6. Grubelnik, V.; Zmazek, J.; Završnik, M.; Marhl, M. Lipotoxicity in a Vicious Cycle of Pancreatic Beta Cell Exhaustion. *Biomedicines* **2022**, *10*, 1627. [CrossRef]

7. Mohás-Cseh, J.; Molnár, G.A.; Pap, M.; Laczy, B.; Vas, T.; Kertész, M.; Németh, K.; Hetényi, C.; Csikós, O.; Tóth, G.K.; et al. Incorporation of Oxidized Phenylalanine Derivatives into Insulin Signaling Relevant Proteins May Link Oxidative Stress to Signaling Conditions Underlying Chronic Insulin Resistance. *Biomedicines* **2022**, *10*, 975. [CrossRef] [PubMed]
8. Chung, G.; Mohan, R.; Beetch, M.; Jo, S.; Alejandro, E.U. Placental Insulin Receptor Transiently Regulates Glucose Homeostasis in the Adult Mouse Offspring of Multiparous Dams. *Biomedicines* **2022**, *10*, 575. [CrossRef] [PubMed]
9. Sitar-Tăut, A.V.; Cozma, A.; Fodor, A.; Coste, S.C.; Orasan, O.H.; Negrean, V.; Pop, D.; Sitar-Tăut, D.A. New Insights on the Relationship between Leptin, Ghrelin, and Leptin/Ghrelin Ratio Enforced by Body Mass Index in Obesity and Diabetes. *Biomedicines* **2021**, *9*, 1657. [CrossRef] [PubMed]
10. de Hoogh, I.M.; Pasman, W.J.; Boorsma, A.; van Ommen, B.; Wopereis, S. Effects of a 13-Week Personalized Lifestyle Intervention Based on the Diabetes Subtype for People with Newly Diagnosed Type 2 Diabetes. *Biomedicines* **2022**, *10*, 643. [CrossRef] [PubMed]
11. Matsumori, A. Novel Biomarkers of Inflammation for the Management of Diabetes: Immunoglobulin-Free Light Chains. *Biomedicines* **2022**, *10*, 666. [CrossRef] [PubMed]
12. Eguchi, N.; Toribio, A.J.; Alexander, M.; Xu, I.; Whaley, D.L.; Hernandez, L.F.; Dafoe, D.; Ichii, H. Dysregulation of β-Cell Proliferation in Diabetes: Possibilities of Combination Therapy in the Development of a Comprehensive Treatment. *Biomedicines* **2022**, *10*, 472. [CrossRef] [PubMed]
13. Jankowski, E.; Wulf, S.; Ziller, N.; Wolf, G.; Loeffler, I. MORG1-A Negative Modulator of Renal Lipid Metabolism in Murine Diabetes. *Biomedicines* **2021**, *10*, 30. [CrossRef] [PubMed]
14. Fujishiro, M.; Ishihara, H.; Ogawa, K.; Murase, T.; Nakamura, T.; Watanabe, K.; Sakoda, H.; Ono, H.; Yamamotoya, T.; Nakatsu, Y.; et al. Impact of Plasma Xanthine Oxidoreductase Activity on the Mechanisms of Distal Symmetric Polyneuropathy Development in Patients with Type 2 Diabetes. *Biomedicines* **2021**, *9*, 1052. [CrossRef] [PubMed]
15. Boned-Murillo, A.; Albertos-Arranz, H.; Diaz-Barreda, M.D.; Orduna-Hospital, E.; Sánchez-Cano, A.; Ferreras, A.; Cuenca, N.; Pinilla, I. Optical Coherence Tomography Angiography in Diabetic Patients: A Systematic Review. *Biomedicines* **2021**, *10*, 88. [CrossRef]
16. Rey-Reñones, C.; Martinez-Torres, S.; Martín-Luján, F.M.; Pericas, C.; Redondo, A.; Grau, M. Type 2 diabetes mellitus and COVID-19: A narrative review. *Biomedicines* **2022**, *12*, 609470.
17. Deckmyn, O.; Poynard, T.; Bedossa, P.; Paradis, V.; Peta, V.; Pais, R.; Ratziu, V.; Thabut, D.; Brzustowski, A.; Gautier, J.F.; et al. Clinical Interest of Serum Alpha-2 Macroglobulin, Apolipoprotein A1, and Haptoglobin in Patients with Non-Alcoholic Fatty Liver Disease, with and without Type 2 Diabetes, before or during COVID-19. *Biomedicines* **2022**, *10*, 699. [CrossRef] [PubMed]
18. Dahlgren, G.; Whitehead, M. European Strategies for Tackling Social Inequities in Health: Levelling up Part 2. Available online: http://www.euro.who.int/__data/assets/pdf_file/0018/103824/E89384.pdf (accessed on 13 June 2022).
19. Grant, P.J.; Cosentino, F. The 2019 ESC guidelines on diabetes, pre-diabetes, and cardiovascular diseases developed in collaboration with the EASD: New features and the 'ten command ments' of the 2019 guidelines are discussed by Professor Peter, J. Grant and Professor Francesco Cosentino, the task force chairmen. *Eur. Heart J.* **2019**, *40*, 3215–3217. [PubMed]
20. United Nations. Transforming Our World: The 2030 Agenda for Sustainable Development. Available online: https://sdgs.un.org/ (accessed on 18 June 2022).

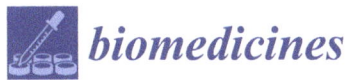

Review

Molecular Mechanism of Pancreatic β-Cell Failure in Type 2 Diabetes Mellitus

Hideaki Kaneto [1,*], Tomohiko Kimura [1], Masashi Shimoda [1], Atsushi Obata [1], Junpei Sanada [1], Yoshiro Fushimi [1], Taka-aki Matsuoka [2] and Kohei Kaku [1]

1. Department of Diabetes, Endocrinology and Metabolism, Kawasaki Medical School, 577 Matsushima, Kurashiki 701-0192, Japan; tomohiko@med.kawasaki-m.ac.jp (T.K.); masashi-s@med.kawasaki-m.ac.jp (M.S.); obata-tky@med.kawasaki-m.ac.jp (A.O.); gengorou@med.kawasaki-m.ac.jp (J.S.); fussy.k0113@med.kawasaki-m.ac.jp (Y.F.); kka@med.kawasaki-m.ac.jp (K.K.)
2. The First Department of Internal Medicine, Wakayama Medical University, 811-1 Kiimidera, Wakayama 641-8509, Japan; matsuoka@wakayama-med.ac.jp
* Correspondence: kaneto@med.kawasaki-m.ac.jp

Abstract: Various important transcription factors in the pancreas are involved in the process of pancreas development, the differentiation of endocrine progenitor cells into mature insulin-producing pancreatic β-cells and the preservation of mature β-cell function. However, when β-cells are continuously exposed to a high glucose concentration for a long period of time, the expression levels of several insulin gene transcription factors are substantially suppressed, which finally leads to pancreatic β-cell failure found in type 2 diabetes mellitus. Here we show the possible underlying pathway for β-cell failure. It is likely that reduced expression levels of MafA and PDX-1 and/or incretin receptor in β-cells are closely associated with β-cell failure in type 2 diabetes mellitus. Additionally, since incretin receptor expression is reduced in the advanced stage of diabetes mellitus, incretin-based medicines show more favorable effects against β-cell failure, especially in the early stage of diabetes mellitus compared to the advanced stage. On the other hand, many subjects have recently suffered from life-threatening coronavirus infection, and coronavirus infection has brought about a new and persistent pandemic. Additionally, the spread of coronavirus infection has led to various limitations on the activities of daily life and has restricted economic development worldwide. It has been reported recently that SARS-CoV-2 directly infects β-cells through neuropilin-1, leading to apoptotic β-cell death and a reduction in insulin secretion. In this review article, we feature a possible molecular mechanism for pancreatic β-cell failure, which is often observed in type 2 diabetes mellitus. Finally, we are hopeful that coronavirus infection will decline and normal daily life will soon resume all over the world.

Keywords: PDX-1; MafA; incretin receptor; GLP-1 receptor activator; coronavirus infection

Citation: Kaneto, H.; Kimura, T.; Shimoda, M.; Obata, A.; Sanada, J.; Fushimi, Y.; Matsuoka, T.-a.; Kaku, K. Molecular Mechanism of Pancreatic β-Cell Failure in Type 2 Diabetes Mellitus. *Biomedicines* **2022**, *10*, 818. https://doi.org/10.3390/biomedicines10040818

Academic Editor: Maria Grau

Received: 19 March 2022
Accepted: 29 March 2022
Published: 31 March 2022

Publisher's Note: MDPI stays neutral with regard to jurisdictional claims in published maps and institutional affiliations.

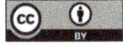

Copyright: © 2022 by the authors. Licensee MDPI, Basel, Switzerland. This article is an open access article distributed under the terms and conditions of the Creative Commons Attribution (CC BY) license (https:// creativecommons.org/licenses/by/ 4.0/).

1. A Variety of Pancreatic Transcription Factors Are Involved in the Development of the Pancreas and Differentiation of Endocrine Progenitor Cells into Mature Pancreatic β-Cells: Pancreas-Related Phenotype in Knockout Mice of Each Transcription Factor

Pancreatic islets are composed of α-, β-, δ-, ε-, and PP-cells, which secrete glucagon, insulin, somatostatin, ghrelin, and pancreatic polypeptide, respectively. A variety of pancreatic transcription factors are involved in the development of the pancreas and differentiation of endocrine progenitor cells into mature β-cells. Pancreatic and duodenal homeobox factor-1 (PDX-1) was identified by several independent research groups at around the same time. It is well known that PDX-1 plays a crucial role in the early stage of the development of the entire pancreas [1–12]. Hb9 plays an important role in the development of the dorsal pancreas [13,14] (Table 1). Arx, Isl-1, Pax4, Pax6, Nkx6.1 and Nkx2.2 are also involved in the development of the pancreas [15–26]. The phenotype in the pancreas in knockout mice of each transcription factor is as follows: Arx knockout mice, absence of α-cells and increase in β- and δ-cells [26]; Isl-1 knockout mice, absence of islet cells [15]; Pax4 knockout mice, absence of β-cells, decrease in δ-cells, and increase in α- and ε-cells [16,23]; Pax6 knockout mice, absence of α-cells, decrease in β-, δ- and PP-cells, increase in ε-cells [17,18,24]; Nkx6.1 knockout mice, decrease in β-cells; Nkx2.2 knockout mice, absence of β-cells, decrease in α- and PP-cells, and increase in ε-cells [19,20,23] (Table 1).

Table 1. Expression pattern in mature islets and phenotype in the pancreas in knockout mice of each pancreatic transcription factor.

Transcription Factor	Expression Site in Mature Islets	Pancreas-Related Phenotype in Each Knockout Mouse
PDX-1	β- and δ-cells	absence of the pancreas
Hb9	β-cells	absence of the dorsal pancreas
Isl-1	all islet cells	absence of islet cells and dorsal pancreatic mesoderm
Pax4	not detected	absence of β- and δ-cells increase in α- and ε-cells
Pax6	all islet cells	absence of α-cells decrease in β-, δ- and PP-cells increase in ε-cells
Nkx2.2	α-, β- and PP-cells	absence of β-cells decrease in α- and PP-cells
Nkx6.1	β-cells	decrease in β-cells
Ngn3	not detected	absence of endocrine cells
NeuroD	all islet cells	decrease in endocrine cells
MafA	β-cells	decrease in insulin biosynthesis and secretion

It is well known that PDX-1 plays a crucial role in the development of the whole pancreas [1–12], the differentiation of endocrine progenitor cells into mature β-cells [27–37], and maintenance of mature β-cell function [38–45]. PDX-1 is initially expressed in the gut region in the early stages of embryonic development. PDX-1 expression is preserved in endocrine progenitor cells during the development of the pancreas, but its expression is restricted to insulin-producing β-cells in the mature pancreas. In PDX-1 knockout mice, there was no pancreas [1], which clearly shows that PDX-1 plays a very important role during the process of pancreas formation (Table 1). Moreover, pancreatic agenesis is observed in subjects with loss of PDX-1 function [9]. In mature β-cells, PDX-1 transactivates several β-cell-related genes including insulin, GLUT2 and glucokinase [41,42]. Abnormal glucose metabolism, an increase in β-cell apoptosis and a decrease in islet mass were also observed in PDX-1 hetero-deficient mice [13,42].

NeuroD and neurogenin3 (Ngn3) function as transcription factors in the pancreas. NeuroD plays an important role in the development of the pancreas and in regulation as insulin gene transcription in mature β-cells [46–52]. It was reported that in NeuroD knockout mice, the β-cell number was markedly reduced, leading to severe diabetes mellitus and perinatal death [47] (Table 1). Neurogenin3 (Ngn3) is also involved in the differentiation of endocrine progenitor cells [51–60]. After bud formation, Ngn3 is transiently expressed in endocrine progenitor cells, and functions as a potential initiator of endocrine differentiation. It was reported that in transgenic mice overexpressing Ngn3, endocrine cell formation was markedly increased [52]. In contrast, it was reported that in Ngn3 knockout mice there were no endocrine cells. These findings clearly show that Ngn3 plays a crucial role in endocrine differentiation [53] (Table 1).

MafA was identified by several independent research groups around the same time. MafA transactivates insulin gene by binding the RIPE3b1 element, and its expression is observed only in β-cells [61–72]. Furthermore, abnormality of glucose metabolism was induced by MafA knockout [61]. In MafA knockout mice, insulin biosynthesis and glucose-stimulated insulin secretion were reduced (Table 1). These findings clearly show that MafA plays a crucial role in the maintenance of mature pancreatic β-cell function.

2. Reduced Expression Levels of Insulin Gene Transcription Factors Such as PDX-1 and MafA Are Involved in Pancreatic β-Cell Failure Found in Type 2 Diabetes Mellitus

Recently, obesity has markedly increased all over the world. Previously, it was thought that obesity was simple accumulation of fat tissues. However, it is now well known that obesity exerts different effects on our body, depending on the site of fat deposition. Obesity is the starting point of most metabolic diseases such as metabolic syndrome and type 2 diabetes mellitus. In subjects with obesity and/or metabolic syndrome, insulin resistance develops mainly due to overeating and/or lack of exercise, but sufficient insulin is secreted from intact β-cells to compensate for the insulin resistance. However, in subjects with insulin resistance, β-cells have no choice but to produce and secrete larger amounts of insulin, which finally leads to β-cell overwork. Additionally, β-cell function gradually deteriorates due to a large amount of free fatty acids and/or various inflammatory cytokines that are secreted from visceral fat tissues. This process is known as β-cell lipotoxicity. Such β-cell overwork and lipotoxicity finally lead to the development of type 2 diabetes mellitus in subjects with obesity and/or metabolic syndrome.

The major function of pancreatic β-cells is to secrete insulin when blood glucose levels are increased. However, when β-cells are exposed to chronic hyperglycemia after the onset of type 2 diabetes mellitus, β-cell function gradually deteriorates due to overwork for insulin biosynthesis and secretion. Once hyperglycemia becomes overt, β-cell function progressively deteriorates. Such β-cell failure is often observed in subjects with type 2 diabetes mellitus and is known as pancreatic β-cell glucose toxicity in clinical practice, as well as in the islet biology research area. In the diabetic state, hyperglycemia and the subsequently provoked oxidative stress suppress insulin biosynthesis and secretion and finally lead to apoptotic β-cell death [73–85]. This reduction in insulin biosynthesis and secretion is preserved by mitigating pancreatic β-cell failure with insulin preparation or SGLT2 inhibitors [86–90]. Additionally, an important concept regarding β-cell failure was recently proposed. It was shown that the reduction in β-cell mass was not only due to apoptotic β-cell death but also due to differentiation of insulin-producing mature β-cells into Ngn3-expressing endocrine progenitor cells [54,55]. Moreover, it was shown that insulin therapy facilitated re-differentiation of Ngn3-expressing endocrine progenitor cells into insulin-producing mature β-cells [55]. These findings clearly show that de-differentiation of insulin-producing mature β-cells into other cell types is involved in pancreatic β-cell failure in type 2 diabetes mellitus. Additionally, such findings show that insulin therapy protects β-cells not only through the suppression of apoptotic β-cell death, but also through the facilitation of re-differentiation of progenitor cells into insulin-producing mature β-cells.

Under diabetic conditions, oxidative stress is provoked through several pathways and is involved in pancreatic β-cell failure [76]. Since the expression levels of antioxidant enzymes in β-cells are very low compared to other tissues, it is thought that β-cells are more easily damaged by oxidative stress compared to other kinds of cells or tissues. Provoked oxidative stress reduces the expression levels of insulin and its transcription factors PDX-1 and MafA. Consequently, it is likely that chronic exposure of β-cells to a high glucose concentration finally leads to β-cell failure by inducing oxidative stress (Figure 1). Additionally, it has been shown that such a reduction in insulin biosynthesis and secretion together with a reduction in PDX-1 and MafA is preserved by mitigating pancreatic β-cell failure with insulin preparation or SGLT2 inhibitors, especially in the early stage of diabetes mellitus [86–90].

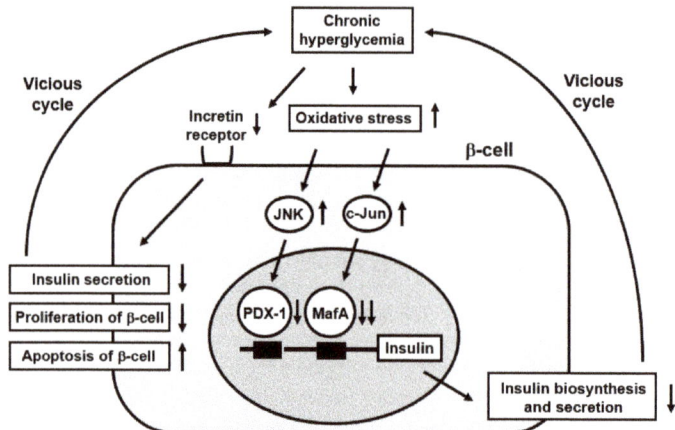

Figure 1. Possible underlying pathway of β-cell failure. Chronic hyperglycemia provokes oxidative stress and thus substantially reduces PDX-1 and MafA expression in nuclei, which finally reduces insulin biosynthesis and secretion. After chronic exposure to a high glucose concentration, incretin receptor expression level is also reduced, which leads to pancreatic β-cell failure.

It has been thought that the activated JNK pathway is, at least partially, associated with β-cell failure. It was reported that inhibition of this pathway protected β-cells from oxidative stress [91]. Additionally, it was shown that inhibition of the JNK pathway suppressed nucleo-cytoplasmic translocation of PDX-1 induced by oxidative stress [92]. On the other hand, it was reported that MafA expression was not clearly observed in almost all β-cells expressing c-Jun, and that c-Jun overexpression with c-Jun expressing adenovirus in β-cells significantly reduced MafA expression level [65]. Taken together, it is likely that the activated JNK pathway and induced c-Jun expression are closely associated with β-cell failure found in type 2 diabetes mellitus (Figure 1).

Moreover, it was clearly demonstrated that MafA overexpression in β-cells preserved β-cell mass and function and finally alleviated β-cell failure, which is often observed in type 2 diabetes mellitus [67]. In β-cell-specific MafA overexpressing transgenic mice, plasma insulin levels were increased, and plasma glucose levels were decreased. Additionally, β-cell mass was preserved, and insulin biosynthesis and secretion were preserved in the β-cell-specific MafA transgenic mice [67]. In conclusion, it is likely that down-regulation of MafA expression is closely associated with β-cell failure found in type 2 diabetes mellitus.

In addition, it is known that the transcription factor Nrf2 plays a crucial role in protecting β-cells from oxidative stress. The preservation of β-cell mass and function largely depends on the presence of Nrf2. Indeed, it was reported that activated Nrf2 alleviates inflammation and maintains β-cell mass by suppressing apoptotic β-cell death and promoting β-cell proliferation. [84]. Various kinds of Nrf2 activators have been examined in clinical trials for the treatment for the preservation of β-cell function and mass in addition to the prevention of diabetic complications. We think that modulating Nrf2 activity in β-cells would be a promising and useful therapeutic approach for the treatment of type 2 diabetes mellitus.

3. Alteration of Exosome microRNAs in Pancreatic β-Cells Is, at Least in Part, Involved in Pancreatic β-Cell Failure Found in Type 2 Diabetes Mellitus

It has been thought that exosomes are a useful tool for the diagnosis and treatment of various diseases in the early stage of the disease. It has been shown that various kinds of exosome-microRNAs such as miR-375 and miR-29 are associated with abnormality of glucose and lipid metabolism [93–95]. Among them, miR-375 is closely associated with pancreatic β-cell failure. First, a combination of inflammatory cytokines induces a significant change in miR-375 expression level [96]. Second, since miR-375 expression level is higher in subjects with diabetes mellitus compared to those without it, it is likely that miR-375 is an early marker of β-cell failure. Third, miR-375 is important for glucose-regulated insulin secretion. Indeed, when human embryonic stem cells differentiate into endodermal lineages, miR-375 expression level is substantially increased. Taken together, miR-375 plays an important role in the process of pancreas development, β-cell growth and proliferation, and insulin secretion, which could be regulated by the above-mentioned pancreatic transcription factors. Furthermore, since miR-375 plays a crucial role in β-cells, it may be a potential target to treat diabetes mellitus. In addition, microRNAs secreted from β-cells can be transferred to other tissues, which in turn regulates β-cell activity. For instance, when miR-26a is transferred to the liver, it enhances insulin sensitivity and alleviates the abnormal glucose metabolism [97]. In conclusion, the alteration of exosome microRNAs in β-cells is, at least in part, involved in pancreatic β-cell failure found in type 2 diabetes mellitus.

4. Impairment of Incretin Signaling in Pancreatic β-Cells Is, at Least in Part, Involved in Pancreatic β-cell Failure Found in Type 2 Diabetes Mellitus

Two kinds of incretins, GLP-1 and GIP bind to each receptor in β-cells and facilitate insulin secretion. Such insulin secretion is regulated through various pathways in β-cells. First, cyclic adenosine monophosphate (cAMP) facilitates insulin secretion through phosphorylation of protein kinase A (PKA). Second, cAMP has another target Epac in β-cells [98–101]. Third, a physiologically low concentration of GLP-1 activates protein kinase C (PKC) and enhances insulin secretion [102]. Taken together, it is likely that GLP-1 enhances glucose-stimulated insulin secretion through various pathways, depending on its concentration.

It has been reported, however, that expression levels of incretin receptors in β-cells are reduced under diabetic conditions, leading to the impairment of incretin effects [103,104] (Figure 1). It has also been shown that a reduction in transcription factor 7-like 2 (TCF7L2) expression level is involved in the reduced incretin receptor expression [105–107]. Taken together, down-regulation of incretin receptor expression after chronic exposure to a high glucose concentration is likely associated with the impairment of incretin effects and is involved in β-cell failure found in type 2 diabetes mellitus.

It has also been reported that TCF7L2 is closely associated with the maintenance of β-cell mass and function though activation of the AKT and mTOR pathway [108–111]. Indeed, inactivation of TCF7L2 impairs insulin secretion and abnormality of glucose metabolism. Additionally, it is known that common genetic variations of TCF7L2 are associated with type 2 diabetes mellitus and that subjects with its high-risk allele of TCF7L2 show impaired insulin secretion [112–116].

5. Incretin-Based Medicine Shows Protective Effects against Pancreatic β-Cell Failure Found in Type 2 Diabetes Mellitus

Incretin-based medicines such as the GLP-1 receptor activator and DPP-IV inhibitor ameliorate glycemic control and mitigate the deterioration in β-cell function in human subjects as well as animal models. It has been reported that the GLP-1 receptor activator preserves pancreatic β-cell function and mass in several types of type 2 diabetes animals [117–123]. For instance, it was shown that when type 2 diabetes db/db mice were treated with the GLP-1 receptor activator, liraglutide for 2 weeks, insulin biosynthesis and glucose-stimulated insulin secretion were increased [117]. Liraglutide enhanced the gene expression involved in cellular differentiation (Hb9, NeuroD and PDX-1) and proliferation (cyclin D and Erk-1) in pancreatic islets even in normoglycemic m/m mice, strongly suggesting the direct effect of GLP-1 on β-cell kinetics [117]. There have been several similar reports so far, indicating that the GLP-1 receptor activator exerts protective effects on β-cell mass and function in other kinds of diabetic model animals [120–123]. Indeed, in alloxan-induced diabetic mice, both β-cell mass and function were substantially preserved by liraglutide treatment, which led to amelioration of glycemic control [120]. It was also shown that β-cell mass was preserved by liraglutide treatment due to an increase in β-cell proliferation and a decrease in β-cell apoptosis. Moreover, the beneficial effects of liraglutide in these mice were preserved even 2 weeks after drug withdrawal [120]. In conclusion, incretin-based medicine shows protective effects against pancreatic β-cell failure in type 2 diabetes mellitus.

It has been shown that the GLP-1 receptor activator shows more beneficial effects in the early stages of diabetes mellitus [118,119]. Obese type 2 diabetic db/db mice were treated with GLP-1 receptor activator liraglutide and/or insulin sensitizer pioglitazone for 2 weeks at 7 weeks old as the early stage and at 16 weeks old as the advanced stage. Insulin biosynthesis and glucose-stimulated insulin secretion were markedly enhanced by the treatment only in the early stage. [119]. We assume that reduced GLP-1 receptor expression after chronic exposure to a high glucose concentration explains why the GLP-1 receptor activator did not show beneficial effects in the advanced stage [119]. Taken together, we should use incretin-based medicine in the early stages without hesitation or clinical inertia in order to maintain β-cell mass and function and ameliorate glycemic control.

In addition, it was shown that DPP-IV inhibitor together with SGLT2 inhibitor exerted more favorable effects on β-cell function and mass, especially in the early stage of diabetes mellitus compared to the advanced stage in type 2 diabetic db/db mice [90]. In the study, 7-week-old and 16-week-old db/db mice were used as an early and advanced stage of diabetes mellitus, respectively, and all mice were treated for 2 weeks with DPP-IV inhibitor, linagliptin and/or SGLT2 inhibitor, empagliflozin. In the combination group, β-cell mass and function were significantly preserved compared to those without treatment only at the early stage, together with enhanced β-cell proliferation [90]. Taken together, such combination therapy shows beneficial effects on β-cells, particularly in the early stages.

6. GLP-1 Receptor Activator Shows Protective Effects against Pancreatic β-Cell Failure for a Long Period of Time without Down-Regulating GLP-1 Receptor Expression Level in β-Cells

In general, chronic exposure to a large amount of ligand leads to down-regulation of its receptor. Additionally, it is known that the serum GLP-1 concentration becomes extremely and non-physiologically high after usage of GLP-1 receptor activator. It remained unknown, however, whether the long-time usage of GLP-1 receptor activator down-regulates its receptor. However, it was reported that GLP-1 receptor expression was not reduced, even after treatment with the GLP-1 receptor activator, dulaglutide for as long as 17 weeks in type 2 diabetic db/db mice [124]. Treatment with dulaglutide ameliorated glycemic control for 17 weeks in the mice compared to those without treatment. In addition, treatment with dulaglutide enhanced insulin biosynthesis and glucose-stimulated insulin secretion [124]. Taken together, the GLP-1 receptor activator protects β-cells against glucose toxicity for a long time due to preservation of GLP-1 receptor expression level in β-cells.

GLP-1 binds to its receptor in various kinds of cells, and the complex of GLP-1 ligand and its receptor is internalized in the cells. It is thought that receptors that are internalized in cells preserve their expression level compared to those without internalization. Consequently, although speculative, we think that such characteristics of the GLP-1 receptor could explain, at least in part, why GLP-1 receptor expression in β-cells was not down-regulated even after long-term exposure to GLP-1 ligand. Moreover, a strategy for the use of some drugs has been developed based on such phenomena [125–128].

7. SARS-CoV-2 Directly Infects Pancreatic β-Cells through Neuropilin-1, Leading to Pancreatic β-Cell Failure such as Apoptotic β-Cell Death and Reduction in Insulin Secretion

Many subjects have recently suffered from life-threatening coronavirus infection, especially coronavirus-mediated pneumonia, all over the world, and coronavirus infection has brought about a new and persistent pandemic. The mortality in subjects with coronavirus infection is extremely high, and the main reason for this is coronavirus-mediated pneumonia [129]. It seems that in subjects with a coronavirus infection, various kinds of inflammatory cytokines are produced and are likely associated with the aggravation of infection. The defense mechanism against the inflammation is substantially weakened, especially in elderly subjects with comorbidities such as diabetes mellitus. Indeed, it was shown that the mortality rate due to coronavirus infection was quite high in subjects with diabetes mellitus [130,131]. Additionally, the spread of coronavirus infection has led to various limitations on the activities of daily life and the obstruction of economic development all over the world. However, we are hopeful that coronavirus infection will decline and normal daily life will soon resume all over the world

It is thought that there is some association between diabetes mellitus and coronavirus infection. Although it remains unclear, subjects with diabetes mellitus are more easily infected with coronavirus compared to healthy subjects, and it is likely that coronavirus infection becomes severe more easily in subjects with poor glycemic control compared to healthy subjects. In addition, although it has been thought that the deterioration of β-cell function is a key factor in the pathogenesis of diabetes mellitus due to coronavirus infection, it remains controversial as to whether β-cells are directly damaged by coronavirus or not. Indeed, it is thought that the coronavirus does not directly infect β-cells because of the low expression level of angiotensin-converting enzyme 2 (ACE2), which allows the coronavirus to go into cells [132,133]. Very recently, however, it has been reported that SARS-CoV-2 directly infects β-cells through neuropilin-1, leading to apoptotic β-cell death and a reduction in insulin secretion [134–139] (Figure 2). It was reported that there was SARS-CoV-2-containing nucleocapsid protein in β-cells after infection with SARS-CoV-2. It was also shown that such phenomena were suppressed by a neuropilin-1 antagonist. These data clearly indicate that neuropilin-1 is important for SARS-CoV-2 to go into β-cells. Furthermore, it was shown that neuropilin-1 expression was high in β-cells with SARS-CoV-2 infection compared to those without the infection. Infection with SARS-CoV-2 increases TUNEL-positive apoptotic β-cell death. Indeed, it was reported that infection with SARS-CoV-2 stimulated p21-activated kinase (PAK) and c-Jun N-terminal kinase (JNK) pathways in β-cells (Figure 2). Activation of the JNK pathway finally increases apoptotic β-cell death and reduces insulin secretion. In addition, as described above, it has been shown that activation of the JNK pathway reduces the expression level and activity of insulin gene transcription factor PDX-1, which we assume also leads to a reduction in insulin biosynthesis and secretion. It was also shown that the expression of α-cell markers and acinar cell markers was increased in β-cells after SARS-CoV-2 infection. Therefore, it is possible that β-cells undergo trans-differentiation to α-cells or acinar cells after the infection. It was also reported that eIF2-mediated response was closely associated with the pathology of β-cell failure induced by SARS-CoV-2 infection. (Figure 2). In conclusion, it is likely that SARS-CoV-2 directly infects pancreatic β-cells through neuropilin-1, and various pathways are activated in β-cells, and finally, apoptotic β-cell death, a reduction in insulin secretion, and trans-differentiation of β-cells into other cell types are brought about by the activation of various pathways in β-cells (Figure 2).

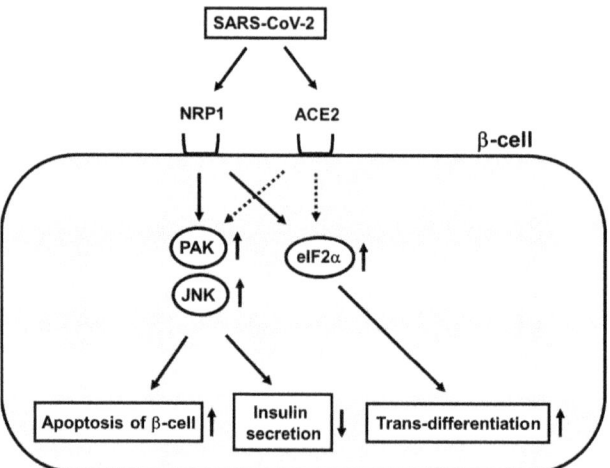

Figure 2. Pancreatic β-cell failure induced by coronavirus infection. SARS-CoV-2 directly binds to NRF1 and ACE2 in pancreatic β-cell membrane. Then, PAK, JNK and eIF2α are activated within pancreatic β-cells, which finally leads to increase in apoptotic β-cell death, reduction in insulin biosynthesis, and trans-differentiation of β-cells to other cell types.

8. Conclusions

Various transcription factors play crucial roles in the differentiation of endocrine progenitor cells into mature insulin-producing β-cells and preservation of adult β-cell function. However, after the exposure of β-cells to a high glucose concentration for a long period of time under diabetic conditions, the expression levels and activities of PDX-1 and MafA are reduced, which leads to β-cell failure. Additionally, the expression levels of incretin receptors in β-cells are reduced after the onset of diabetes mellitus. It is likely that the reduced expression level of insulin gene transcription factors and incretin receptors explains, at least in part, the molecular mechanism for β-cell failure found in type 2 diabetes mellitus. Additionally, since incretin receptor expression is reduced in the advanced stage of diabetes mellitus, incretin-based medicine shows more favorable effects against β-cell glucose toxicity, especially in the early stage of diabetes mellitus compared to the advanced stage. On the other hand, many subjects have recently suffered from life-threatening coronavirus infection and coronavirus infection has brought about a new and persistent pandemic. Additionally, coronavirus infection has led to various limitations on daily activities and restricted economic development worldwide. It has been reported recently that SARS-CoV-2 directly infects β-cells through neuropilin-1, leading to apoptotic β-cell death and reduction in insulin secretion. Additionally, it was shown that there was SARS-CoV-2-containing nucleocapsid protein in β-cells after coronavirus infection. In this review article, we featured a possible molecular mechanism for pancreatic β-cell failure, which is often observed in type 2 diabetes mellitus. Finally, we are hopeful that coronavirus infection will be cleared up and normal daily life will soon resume all over the world.

Author Contributions: H.K. wrote this manuscript. T.K., M.S., A.O., J.S., Y.F., T.-a.M. and K.K. participated in discussion. All authors have read and agreed to the published version of the manuscript.

Funding: This research received no external funding.

Conflicts of Interest: H.K. has received honoraria for lectures, received scholarship grants, and received research grant from Novo Nordisk Pharma, Sanofi, Eli Lilly, Boehringer Ingelheim, Taisho Pharma, Sumitomo Dainippon Pharma, Takeda Pharma, Ono Pharma, Daiichi Sankyo, Mitsubishi Tanabe Pharma, Kissei Pharma, MSD, AstraZeneca, Astellas, Novartis, Kowa, Abbott. K.K. has been an advisor to, received honoraria for lectures from, and received scholarship grants from Novo Nordisk

Pharma, Sanwa Kagaku, Takeda, Taisho Pharma, MSD, Kowa, Sumitomo Dainippon Pharma, Novartis, Mitsubishi Tanabe Pharma, AstraZeneca, Boehringer Ingelheim, Chugai, Daiichi Sankyo, Sanofi.

References

1. Jonsson, J.; Carlsson, L.; Edlund, T.; Edlund, H. Insulin-promoter-factor 1 is required for pancreas development in mice. *Nature* **1993**, *37*, 606–609. [CrossRef]
2. Stoffers, D.A.; Zinkin, N.T.; Stanojevic, V.; Clarke, W.L.; Habener, J.F. Pancreatic agenesis attributable to a single nucleotide deletion in the human IPF1 gene coding sequence. *Nat. Genet.* **1997**, *15*, 106–110. [CrossRef]
3. Dutta, S.; Bonner-Weir, S.; Montminy, M.; Wright, C. Regulatory factor linked to late-onset diabetes? *Nature* **1998**, *392*, 560. [CrossRef]
4. Holland, A.M.; Hale, M.A.; Kagami, H.; Hammer, R.E.; MacDonald, R.J. Experimental control of pancreatic development and maintenance. *Proc. Natl. Acad. Sci. USA* **2002**, *99*, 12236–12241. [CrossRef]
5. Hayes, H.L.; Zhang, L.; Becker, T.C.; Haldeman, J.M.; Stephens, S.B.; Arlotto, M.; Moss, L.G.; Newgard, C.B.; Hohmeier, H.E. A pdx-1-regulated soluble factor activates rat and human islet cell proliferation. *Mol. Cell. Biol.* **2016**, *36*, 2918–2930. [CrossRef]
6. Spaeth, J.M.; Walker, E.; Stein, R. Impact of Pdx1-associated chromatin modifiers on islet beta-cells. *Diabetes Obes. Metab.* **2016**, *18* (Suppl. 1), 123–127. [CrossRef]
7. Zhu, Y.; Liu, Q.; Zhou, Z.; Ikeda, Y. PDX1, Neurogenin-3, and MAFA: Critical transcription regulators for beta cell development and regeneration. *Stem Cell Res. Ther.* **2017**, *8*, 240. [CrossRef]
8. Swisa, A.; Glaser, B.; Dor, Y. Metabolic stress and compromised identity of pancreatic beta cells. *Front. Genet.* **2017**, *8*, 21. [CrossRef]
9. Wang, X.; Sterr, M.; Ansarullah; Burtscher, I.; Bottcher, A.; Beckenbauer, J.; Siehler, J.; Meitinger, T.; Haring, H.U.; Staiger, H.; et al. Point mutations in the PDX1 transactivation domain impair human beta-cell development and function. *Mol. Metab.* **2019**, *24*, 80–97. [CrossRef]
10. Jennings, R.E.; Scharfmann, R.; Staels, W. Transcription factors that shape the mammalian pancreas. *Diabetologia* **2020**, *63*, 1974–1980. [CrossRef]
11. Aigha, I.I.; Abdelalim, E.M. NKX6. 1 transcription factor: A crucial regulator of pancreatic β cell development, identity, and proliferation. *Stem Cell Res. Ther.* **2020**, *11*, 459. [CrossRef] [PubMed]
12. Zhu, X.; Oguh, A.; Gingerich, M.A.; Soleimanpour, S.A.; Stoffers, D.A.; Gannon, M. Cell cycle regulation of the pdx1 transcription factor in developing pancreas and insulin-producing beta-cells. *Diabetes* **2021**, *70*, 903–916. [CrossRef] [PubMed]
13. Harrison, K.A.; Thaler, J.; Pfaff, S.L.; Gu, H.; Kehrl, J.H. Pancreas dorsal lobe agenesis and abnormal islets of Langerhans in Hlxb9-deficient mice. *Nat. Genet.* **1999**, *23*, 71–75. [CrossRef]
14. Li, H.; Arber, S.; Jessell, T.M.; Edlund, H. Selective agenesis of the dorsal pancreas in mice lacking homeobox gene Hlxb9. *Nat. Genet.* **1999**, *23*, 67–70. [CrossRef]
15. Ahlgren, U.; Pfaff, S.L.; Jessell, T.M.; Edlund, T.; Edlund, H. Independent requirement for ISL1 in formation of pancreatic mesenchyme and islet cells. *Nature* **1997**, *385*, 257–260. [CrossRef]
16. Sosa-Pineda, B.; Chowdhury, K.; Torres, M.; Oliver, G.; Gruss, P. The Pax4 gene is essential for differentiation of insulin-producing beta cells in the mammalian pancreas. *Nature* **1997**, *386*, 399–402. [CrossRef]
17. St-Onge, L.; Sosa-Pineda, B.; Chowdhury, K.; Mansouri, A.; Gruss, P. Pax6 is required for differentiation of glucagon-producing alpha-cells in mouse pancreas. *Nature* **1997**, *387*, 406–409. [CrossRef]
18. Sander, M.; Neubuser, A.; Kalamaras, J.; Ee, H.C.; Martin, G.R.; German, M.S. Genetic analysis reveals that PAX6 is required for normal transcription of pancreatic hormone genes and islet development. *Genes Dev.* **1997**, *11*, 1662–1673. [CrossRef]
19. Sander, M.; Sussel, L.; Conners, J.; Scheel, D.; Kalamaras, J.; Dela Cruz, F.; Schwitzgebel, V.; Hayes-Jordan, A.; German, M. Homeobox gene Nkx6.1 lies downstream of Nkx2.2 in the major pathway of beta-cell formation in the pancreas. *Development* **2000**, *127*, 5533–5540. [CrossRef]
20. Sussel, L.; Kalamaras, J.; Hartigan-O'Connor, D.J.; Meneses, J.J.; Pedersen, R.A.; Rubenstein, J.L.; German, M.S. Mice lacking the homeodomain transcription factor Nkx2.2 have diabetes due to arrested differentiation of pancreatic beta cells. *Development* **1998**, *125*, 2213–2221. [CrossRef]
21. Panneerselvam, A.; Kannan, A.; Mariajoseph-Antony, L.F.; Prahalathan, C. PAX proteins and their role in pancreas. *Diabetes Res. Clin. Pract.* **2019**, *155*, 107792. [CrossRef] [PubMed]
22. Smith, S.B.; Ee, H.C.; Conners, J.R.; German, M.S. Paired-homeodomain transcription factor PAX4 acts as a transcriptional repressor in early pancreatic development. *Mol. Cell. Biol.* **1999**, *19*, 8272–8280. [CrossRef] [PubMed]
23. Prado, C.L.; Pugh-Bernard, A.E.; Elghazi, L.; Sosa-Pineda, B.; Sussel, L. Ghrelin cells replace insulin-producing β cells in two mouse model of pancreas development. *Proc. Natl. Acad. Sci. USA* **2004**, *101*, 2924–2929. [CrossRef]
24. Heller, R.S.; Jenny, M.; Collombat, P.; Mansouri, A.; Tomasetto, C.; Madsen, O.D.; Mellitzer, G.; Gradwohl, G.; Serup, P. Genetic determinants of pancreatic β-cell development. *Dev. Biol.* **2005**, *286*, 217–224. [CrossRef] [PubMed]
25. Pedersen, J.K.; Nelson, S.B.; Jorgensen, M.C.; Henseleit, K.D.; Fujitani, Y.; Wright, C.V.; Sander, M.; Serup, P. Endodermal expression of Nkx6 genes depends differentially on Pdx1. *Dev. Biol.* **2005**, *288*, 487–501. [CrossRef]
26. Collombat, P.; Mansouri, A.; Hecksher-Sorensen, J.; Serup, P.; Krull, J.; Gradwohl, G.; Gruss, P. Opposing actions of Arx and Pax4 in endocrine pancreas development. *Genes Dev.* **2003**, *17*, 2591–2603. [CrossRef]

27. Pedica, F.; Beccari, S.; Pedron, S.; Montagna, L.; Piccoli, P.; Doglioni, C.; Chilosi, M. PDX-1 (pancreatic/duodenal homeobox-1 protein 1). *Pathologica* **2014**, *106*, 315–321.
28. Vinogradova, T.V.; Sverdlov, E.D. PDX1: A unique pancreatic master regulator constantly changes its functions during embryonic development and progression of pancreatic cancer. *Biochemistry* **2017**, *82*, 887–893. [CrossRef]
29. Liu, J.; Lang, G.; Shi, J. Epigenetic Regulation of PDX-1 in type 2 diabetes mellitus. *Diabetes Metab. Syndr. Obes.* **2021**, *14*, 431–442. [CrossRef]
30. Assouline-Thomas, B.; Ellis, D.; Petropavlovskaia, M.; Makhlin, J.; Ding, J.; Rosenberg, L. Islet Neogenesis Associated Protein (INGAP) induces the differentiation of an adult human pancreatic ductal cell line into insulin-expressing cells through stepwise activation of key transcription factors for embryonic beta cell development. *Differentiation* **2015**, *90*, 77–90. [CrossRef]
31. Bahrebar, M.; Soleimani, M.; Karimi, M.H.; Vahdati, A.; Yaghobi, R. Generation of islet-like cell aggregates from human adipose tissue-derived stem cells by lentiviral overexpression of PDX-1. *Int. J. Organ Transplant. Med.* **2015**, *6*, 61–76. [PubMed]
32. Hunter, C.S.; Stein, R.W. Evidence for loss in identity, de-differentiation, and trans-differentiation of islet β-cells in type 2 diabetes. *Front. Genet.* **2017**, *8*, 35. [CrossRef] [PubMed]
33. Kassem, D.H.; Kamal, M.M.; El-Kholy, A.-L.; El-Mesallamy, H.O. Exendin-4 enhances the differentiation of Wharton's jelly mesenchymal stem cells into insulin-producing cells through activation of various beta-cell markers. *Stem Cell Res. Ther.* **2016**, *7*, 1–11. [CrossRef] [PubMed]
34. Hwang, Y.; Cha, S.H.; Hong, Y.; Jung, A.R.; Jun, H.S. Direct differentiation of insulin-producing cells from human urine-derived stem cells. *Int. J. Med. Sci.* **2019**, *16*, 1668–1676. [CrossRef] [PubMed]
35. Kim, M.J.; Lee, E.Y.; You, Y.H.; Yang, H.K.; Yoon, K.H.; Kim, J.W. Generation of iPSC-derived insulin-producing cells from patients with type 1 and type 2 diabetes compared with healthy control. *Stem Cell Res.* **2020**, *48*, 101958. [CrossRef] [PubMed]
36. Abazari, M.F.; Zare Karizi, S.; Hajati-Birgani, N.; Norouzi, S.; Khazeni, Z.; Hashemi, J.; Shafaghi, L.; Soleimanifar, F.; Mansour, R.N.; Enderami, S.E. PHBV nanofibers promotes insulin-producing cells differentiation of human induced pluripotent stem cells. *Gene* **2021**, *768*, 145333. [CrossRef]
37. Eydian, Z.; Mohammad Ghasemi, A.; Ansari, S.; Kamali, A.N.; Khosravi, M.; Momtaz, S.; Riki, S.; Rafighdoost, L.; Entezari Heravi, R. Differentiation of multipotent stem cells to insulin-producing cells for treatment of diabetes mellitus: Bone marrow- and adipose tissue-derived cells comparison. *Mol. Biol. Rep.* **2022**. [CrossRef]
38. Ahlgren, U.; Jonsson, J.; Jonsson, L.; Simu, K.; Edlund, H. β-cell-specific inactivation of the mouse *Ipf1/Pdx1* gene results in loss of the β-cell phenotype and maturity onset diabetes. *Genes Dev.* **1998**, *12*, 1763–1768. [CrossRef]
39. Wang, H.; Maechler, P.; Ritz-Laser, B.; Hagenfeldt, K.A.; Ishihara, H.; Philippe, J.; Wollheim, C.B. Pdx1 level defines pancreatic gene expression pattern and cell lineage differentiation. *J. Biol. Chem.* **2001**, *276*, 25279–25286. [CrossRef]
40. Brissova, M.; Shiota, M.; Nicholson, W.E.; Gannon, M.; Knobel, S.M.; Piston, D.W.; Wright, C.V.; Powers, A.C. Reduction in pancreatic transcription factor PDX-1 impairs glucose-stimulated insulin secretion. *J. Biol. Chem.* **2002**, *277*, 1125–1132. [CrossRef]
41. Kulkarni, R.N.; Jhala, U.S.; Winnay, J.N.; Krajewski, S.; Montminy, M.; Kahn, C.R. PDX-1 haploinsufficiency limits the compensatory islet hyperplasia that occurs in response to insulin resistance. *J. Clin. Investig.* **2004**, *114*, 828–836. [CrossRef] [PubMed]
42. Holland, A.M.; Gonez, L.J.; Naselli, G.; MacDonald, R.J.; Harrison, L.C. Conditional expression demonstrates the role of the homeodomain transcription factor Pdx1 in maintenance and regeneration of beta-cells in the adult pancreas. *Diabetes* **2005**, *54*, 2586–2595. [CrossRef] [PubMed]
43. Yamamoto, Y.; Miyatsuka, T.; Sasaki, S.; Miyashita, K.; Kubo, N.; Shimo, N.; Takebe, S.; Watada, H.; Kaneto, H.; Matsuoka, T.; et al. Recovered expression of Pdx1 improves β-cell failure in diabetic mice. *Biochem. Biophys. Res. Commun.* **2017**, *483*, 418–424. [CrossRef] [PubMed]
44. Zhang, M.; Yang, C.; Zhu, M.; Qian, L.; Luo, Y.; Cheng, H.; Geng, R.; Xu, X.; Qian, C.; Liu, Y. Saturated fatty acids entrap PDX1 in stress granules and impede islet beta cell function. *Diabetologia* **2021**, *64*, 1144–1157. [CrossRef] [PubMed]
45. Cao, G.; Gonzalez, J.; Oritz Fragola, J.P.; Muller, A.; Tumarkin, M.; Moriondo, M.; Azzato, F.; Blanco, M.V.; Milei, J. Structural changes in endocrine pancreas of male Wistar rats due to chronic cola drink consumption. Role of PDX-1. *PLoS ONE* **2021**, *11*, e0243340. [CrossRef]
46. Naya, F.J.; Stellrecht, C.M.M.; Tsai, M.-J. Tissue-specific regulation of the insulin gene by a novel basic helix-loop-helix transcription factor. *Genes Dev.* **1995**, *9*, 1009–1019. [CrossRef]
47. Naya, F.J.; Huang, H.; Qiu, Y.; Mutoh, H.; DeMayo, F.; Leiter, A.B.; Tsai, M.-J. Diabetes, defective pancreatic morphogenesis, and abnormal enteroendocrine differentiation in BETA2/neuroD-deficient mice. *Genes Dev.* **1997**, *11*, 323–334. [CrossRef]
48. Kojima, H.; Fujimiya, M.; Matsumura, K.; Younan, P.; Imaeda, H.; Maeda, M.; Chan, L. NeuroD-betacellulin gene therapy induces islet neogenesis in the liver and reverses diabetes in mice. *Nat. Med.* **2003**, *9*, 595–603. [CrossRef]
49. Noguchi, H.; Bonner-Weir, S.; Wei, F.-Y.; Matsushita, M.; Matsumoto, S. BETA2/NeuroD protein can be transduced into cells due to an arginine- and lysine-rich sequence. *Diabetes* **2005**, *54*, 2859–2866. [CrossRef]
50. Han, S.I.; Tsunekage, Y.; Kataoka, K. Phosphorylation of MafA enhances interaction with Beta2/NeuroD1. *Acta Diabetol.* **2016**, *53*, 651–660. [CrossRef]
51. Apelqvist, A.; Li, H.; Sommer, L.; Beatus, P.; Anderson, D.J.; Honjo, T.; de Angelis, M.H.; Lendahl, U.; Edlund, H. Notch signaling controls pancreatic cell differentiation. *Nature* **1999**, *400*, 877–881. [CrossRef] [PubMed]

52. Schwitzgebel, V.M.; Scheel, D.W.; Conners, J.R.; Kalamaras, J.; Lee, J.E.; Anderson, D.J.; Sussel, L.; Johnson, J.D.; German, M.S. Expression of neurogenin3 reveals an islet cell precursor population in the pancreas. *Development* **2000**, *127*, 3533–3542. [CrossRef] [PubMed]
53. Gradwohl, G.; Dierich, A.; LeMeur, M.; Guillemot, F. neurogenin3 is required for the development of the four endocrine cell lineages of the pancreas. *Proc. Natl. Acad. Sci. USA* **2000**, *97*, 1607–1611. [CrossRef] [PubMed]
54. Talchai, C.; Xuan, S.; Lin, H.V.; Sussel, L.; Accili, D. Pancreatic β cell dedifferentiation as a mechanism of diabetic β cell failure. *Cell* **2012**, *150*, 1223–1234. [CrossRef] [PubMed]
55. Wang, Z.; York, N.W.; Nichols, C.G.; Remedi, M.S. Pancreatic β cell dedifferentiation in diabetes and redifferentiation following insulin therapy. *Cell Metab.* **2014**, *19*, 872–882. [CrossRef] [PubMed]
56. McGrath, P.S.; Watson, C.L.; Ingram, C.; Helmrath, M.A.; Wells, J.M. The basic helix-loop-helix transcription factor NEUROG3 is required for development of the human endocrine pancreas. *Diabetes* **2015**, *64*, 2497–2505. [CrossRef] [PubMed]
57. Cavelti-Weder, C.; Li, W.; Zumsteg, A.; Stemann-Andersen, M.; Zhang, Y.; Yamada, T.; Wang, M.; Lu, J.; Jermendy, A.; Bee, Y.M.; et al. Hyperglycaemia attenuates in vivo reprogramming of pancreatic exocrine cells to beta cells in mice. *Diabetologia* **2016**, *59*, 522–532. [CrossRef]
58. Azzarelli, R.; Hurley, C.; Sznurkowska, M.K.; Rulands, S.; Hardwick, L.; Gamper, I.; Ali, F.; McCracken, L.; Hindley, C.; McDuff, F.; et al. Multi-site Neurogenin3 Phosphorylation Controls Pancreatic Endocrine Differentiation. *Dev. Cell* **2017**, *41*, 274–286. [CrossRef]
59. Azzarelli, R.; Rulands, S.; Nestorowa, S.; Davies, J.; Campinoti, S.; Gillotin, S.; Bonfanti, P.; Gottgens, B.; Huch, M.; Simons, B.; et al. Neurogenin3 phosphorylation controls reprogramming efficiency of pancreatic ductal organoids into endocrine cells. *Sci. Rep.* **2018**, *8*, 1–12. [CrossRef]
60. Kimura-Nakajima, C.; Sakaguchi, K.; Hatano, Y.; Matsumoto, M.; Okazaki, Y.; Tanaka, K.; Yamane, T.; Oishi, Y.; Kamimoto, K.; Iwatsuki, K. Ngn3-positive cells arise from pancreatic duct cells. *Int. J. Mol. Sci.* **2021**, *22*, 8548. [CrossRef]
61. Zhang, C.; Moriguchi, T.; Kajihara, M.; Esaki, R.; Harada, A.; Shimohata, H.; Oishi, H.; Hamada, M.; Morito, N.; Hasegawa, K.; et al. MafA is a key regulator of glucose-stimulated insulin secretion. *Mol. Cell. Biol.* **2005**, *25*, 4969–4976. [CrossRef] [PubMed]
62. Wang, H.; Brun, T.; Kataoka, K.; Sharma, A.J.; Wollheim, C.B. MAFA controls genes implicated in insulin biosynthesis and secretion. *Diabetologia* **2007**, *50*, 348–358. [CrossRef] [PubMed]
63. Hang, Y.; Stein, R. MafA and MafB activity in pancreatic beta cells. *Trends Endocrinol. Metab.* **2011**, *22*, 364–373. [CrossRef] [PubMed]
64. Hang, Y.; Yamamoto, T.; Benniger, R.K.; Brissova, M.; Guo, M.; Bush, W.; Piston, D.W.; Powers, A.C.; Magnuson, M.; Thurmond, D.C.; et al. The MafA transcription factor becomes essential to islet β-cells soon after birth. *Diabetes* **2014**, *63*, 1994–2005. [CrossRef]
65. Matsuoka, T.; Kaneto, H.; Miyatsuka, T.; Yamamoto, T.; Yamamoto, K.; Kato, K.; Shimomura, I.; Stein, R.; Matsuhisa, M. Regulation of MafA expression in pancreatic β-cells in db/db mice with diabetes. *Diabetes* **2010**, *59*, 1709–1720. [CrossRef]
66. Ganic, E.; Singh, T.; Luan, C.; Fadista, J.; Johansson, J.K.; Cyphert, H.A.; Bennet, H.; Storm, P.; Prost, G.; Ahlenius, H.; et al. MafA-controlled nicotinic receptor expression is essential for insulin secretion and is impaired in patients with type 2 diabetes. *Cell Rep.* **2016**, *14*, 1991–2002. [CrossRef]
67. Matsuoka, T.; Kaneto, H.; Kawashima, S.; Miyatsuka, T.; Tochino, Y.; Yoshikawa, A.; Imagawa, A.; Miyazaki, J.; Gannon, M.; Stein, R.; et al. Preserving MafA expression in diabetic islet β-cells improves glycemic control in vivo. *J. Biol. Chem.* **2015**, *290*, 7647–7657. [CrossRef]
68. Luan, C.; Ye, Y.; Singh, T.; Barghouth, M.; Eliasson, L.; Artner, I.; Zhang, E.; Renstrom, E. The calcium channel subunit gamma-4 is regulated by MafA and necessary for pancreatic beta-cell specification. *Commun. Biol.* **2019**, *2*, 1–14. [CrossRef]
69. Singh, T.; Colberg, J.K.; Sarmiento, L.; Chaves, P.; Hansen, L.; Bsharat, S.; Cataldo, L.R.; Dudenhoffer-Pfeifer, M.; Fex, M.; Bryder, D.; et al. Loss of MafA and MafB expression promotes islet inflammation. *Sci. Rep.* **2019**, *9*, 9074. [CrossRef]
70. Deng, Z.; Matsumoto, Y.; Kuno, A.; Ojima, M.; Xiafukaiti, G.; Takahashi, S. An inducible diabetes mellitus murine model based on MafB conditional knockout under MafA-deficient condition. *Int. J. Mol. Sci.* **2020**, *21*, 5606. [CrossRef]
71. Ono, Y.; Kataoka, K. MafA, NeuroD1, and HNF1beta synergistically activate the Slc2a2 (Glut2) gene in beta-cells. *J. Mol. Endocrinol.* **2021**, *67*, 71–82. [CrossRef] [PubMed]
72. Nasteska, D.; Fine, N.H.F.; Ashford, F.B.; Cuozzo, F.; Viloria, K.; Smith, G.; Dahir, A.; Dawson, P.W.J.; Lai, Y.C.; Bastidas-Ponce, A.; et al. PDX1(LOW) MAFA(LOW) beta-cells contribute to islet function and insulin release. *Nat. Commun.* **2021**, *12*, 674. [CrossRef]
73. Halban, P.A.; Polonsky, K.S.; Bowden, D.W.; Hawkins, M.A.; Ling, C.; Mather, K.J.; Powers, A.C.; Rhodes, C.J.; Sussel, L.; Weir, G.C. β-Cell failure in type 2 diabetes: Postulated mechanisms and prospects for prevention and treatment. *Diabetes Care* **2014**, *37*, 1751–1758. [CrossRef] [PubMed]
74. Weir, G.C.; Butler, P.C.; Bonner-Weir, S. The beta-cell glucose toxicity hypothesis: Attractive but difficult to prove. *Metabolism* **2021**, *124*, 154870. [CrossRef] [PubMed]
75. Alarcon, C.; Boland, B.B.; Uchizono, Y.; Moore, P.C.; Peterson, B.; Rajan, S.; Rhodes, O.S.; Noske, A.B.; Haataja, L.; Arvan, P.; et al. Pancreatic β-cell adaptive plasticity in obesity increases insulin production but adversely affects secretory function. *Diabetes* **2016**, *65*, 438–450. [CrossRef] [PubMed]

76. Boland, B.B.; Brown, C., Jr.; Boland, M.L.; Cann, J.; Sulikowski, M.; Hansen, G.; Grønlund, R.V.; King, W.; Rondinone, C.; Trevaskis, J.; et al. Pancreatic beta-cell rest replenishes insulin secretory capacity and attenuates diabetes in an extreme model of obese type 2 diabetes. *Diabetes* **2019**, *68*, 131–140. [CrossRef]
77. Hall, E.; Jonsson, J.; Ofori, J.K.; Volkov, P.; Perfilyev, A.; Dekker Nitert, M.; Eliasson, L.; Ling, C.; Bacos, K. Glucolipotoxicity alters insulin secretion via epigenetic changes in human islets. *Diabetes* **2019**, *68*, 1965–1974. [CrossRef]
78. Lytrivi, M.; Castell, A.L.; Poitout, V.; Cnop, M. Recent insights into mechanisms of beta-cell lipo- and glucolipotoxicity in Type 2 Diabetes. *J. Mol. Biol.* **2020**, *432*, 1514–1534. [CrossRef]
79. Roma, L.P.; Jonas, J.C. Nutrient metabolism, subcellular redox state, and oxidative stress in pancreatic islets and beta-cells. *J. Mol. Biol.* **2020**, *432*, 1461–1493. [CrossRef]
80. Benito-Vicente, A.; Jebari-Benslaiman, S.; Galicia-Garcia, U.; Larrea-Sebal, A.; Uribe, K.B.; Martin, S. Molecular mechanisms of lipotoxicity-induced pancreatic beta-cell dysfunction. *Int. Rev. Cell Mol. Biol.* **2021**, *359*, 357–402.
81. Hong, J.H.; Kim, D.H.; Lee, M.K. Glucolipotoxicity and GLP-1 secretion. *BMJ Open Diabetes Res. Care* **2021**, *9*, e001905. [CrossRef] [PubMed]
82. Hwang, Y.J.; Jung, G.S.; Jeon, W.; Lee, K.M. Lin28a ameliorates glucotoxicity-induced β-cell dysfunction and apoptosis. *BMB Rep.* **2021**, *54*, 215–220. [CrossRef] [PubMed]
83. Nagai, Y.; Matsuoka, T.A.; Shimo, N.; Miyatsuka, T.; Miyazaki, S.; Tashiro, F.; Miyazaki, J.I.; Katakami, N.; Shimomura, I. Glucotoxicity-induced suppression of Cox6a2 expression provokes β-cell dysfunction via augmented ROS production. *Biochem. Biophys. Res. Commun.* **2021**, *556*, 134–141. [CrossRef] [PubMed]
84. Baumel-Alterzon, S.; Katz, L.S.; Brill, G.; Garcia-Ocana, A.; Scott, D.K. Nrf2: The master and captain of beta cell fate. *Trends Endocrinol. Metab.* **2021**, *32*, 7–19. [CrossRef] [PubMed]
85. Wu, T.; Zhang, S.; Xu, J.; Zhang, Y.; Sun, T.; Shao, Y.; Wang, J.; Tang, W.; Chen, F.; Han, X. HRD1, an important player in pancreatic β-cell failure and therapeutic target for type 2 diabetic mice. *Diabetes* **2020**, *69*, 940–953. [CrossRef]
86. Takahashi, K.; Nakamura, A.; Miyoshi, H.; Nomoto, H.; Kitao, N.; Omori, K.; Yamamoto, K.; Cho, K.Y.; Terauchi, Y.; Atsumi, T. Effect of the sodium-glucose cotransporter 2 inhibitor luseogliflozin on pancreatic beta cell mass in db/db mice of different ages. *Sci. Rep.* **2018**, *8*, 6864. [CrossRef]
87. Omori, K.; Nakamura, A.; Miyoshi, H.; Takahashi, K.; Kitao, N.; Nomoto, H.; Kameda, H.; Cho, K.Y.; Takagi, R.; Hatanaka, K.C.; et al. Effects of dapagliflozin and/or insulin glargine on beta cell mass and hepatic steatosis in db/db mice. *Metabolism* **2019**, *98*, 27–36. [CrossRef]
88. Shyr, Z.A.; Yan, Z.; Ustione, A.; Egan, E.M.; Remedi, M.S. SGLT2 inhibitors therapy protects glucotoxicity-induced beta-cell failure in a mouse model of human KATP-induced diabetes through mitigation of oxidative and ER stress. *PLoS ONE* **2022**, *17*, e0258054. [CrossRef]
89. Kimura, T.; Obata, A.; Shimoda, M.; Okauchi, S.; Kanda-Kimura, Y.; Nogami, Y.; Hirukawa, H.; Kohara, K.; Nakanishi, S.; Mune, T.; et al. Protective effects of SGLT2 inhibitor luseogliflozin on pancreatic β-cells in obese diabetic db/db mice: The earlier and longer, the better. *Diabetes Obes. Metab.* **2018**, *20*, 2442–2457. [CrossRef]
90. Fushimi, Y.; Obata, A.; Sanada, J.; Nogami, Y.; Ikeda, T.; Yamasaki, Y.; Obata, Y.; Shimoda, M.; Nakanishi, S.; Mune, T.; et al. Combination of dipeptidyl peptidase 4 (DPP-4) inhibitor and sodium glucose cotransporter 2 (SGLT2) inhibitor substantially protects pancreatic β-cells especially in early phase of diabetes rather than advanced phase. *Sci. Rep.* **2021**, *11*, 16120. [CrossRef]
91. Kaneto, H.; Xu, G.; Fujii, N.; Kim, S.; Bonner-Weir, S.; Weir, G.C. Involvement of c-Jun N-terminal kinase in oxidative stress-mediated suppression of insulin gene expression. *J. Biol. Chem.* **2002**, *277*, 30010–30018. [CrossRef] [PubMed]
92. Kawamori, D.; Kajimoto, Y.; Kaneto, H.; Umayahara, Y.; Fujitani, Y.; Miyatsuka, T.; Watada, H.; Leibiger, I.B.; Yamasaki, Y.; Hori, M. Oxidative stress induces nucleo-cytoplasmic translocation of pancreatic transcription factor PDX-1 through activation of c-Jun N-terminal kinase. *Diabetes* **2003**, *52*, 2896–2904. [CrossRef] [PubMed]
93. Li, X. MiR-375, a microRNA related to diabetes. *Gene* **2014**, *533*, 1–4. [CrossRef] [PubMed]
94. Massart, J.; Sjogren, R.; Lundell, L.S.; Mudry, J.M.; Franck, N.; O'Gorman, D.J.; Egan, B.; Zierath, J.R.; Krook, A. Altered miR-29 expression in type 2 diabetes influences glu-cose and lipid metabolism in skeletal muscle. *Diabetes* **2017**, *66*, 1807–1818. [CrossRef] [PubMed]
95. Cione, E.; Cannataro, R.; Gallelli, L.; Sarro, G.D.; Caroleo, M.C. Exosome microRNAs in metabolic syndrome as tools for the early monitoring of diabetes and possible therapeutic options. *Pharmaceuticals* **2021**, *14*, 1257. [CrossRef] [PubMed]
96. Fu, Q.; Jiang, H.; Wang, Z.; Wang, X.; Chen, H.; Shen, Z.; Xiao, L.; Guo, X.; Yang, T. Injury factors alter miRNAs profiles of exosomes derived from islets and circulation. *Aging* **2018**, *10*, 3986–3999. [CrossRef]
97. Xu, H.; Du, X.; Xu, J.; Zhang, Y.; Tian, Y.; Liu, G.; Wang, X.; Ma, M.; Du, W.; Liu, Y.; et al. Pancreatic beta-cell microRNA-26a alleviates type 2 diabetes by improving pe-ripheral insulin sensitivity and preserving beta cell function. *PLoS Biol.* **2020**, *18*, e3000603. [CrossRef]
98. Seino, S.; Takahashi, H.; Fujimoto, W.; Shibasaki, T. Roles of cAMP signalling in insulin granule exocytosis. *Diabetes Obes. Metab.* **2009**, *11*, 180–188. [CrossRef]
99. Yu, Y.; Jin, T. New insights into the role of cAMP in the production and function of the incretin hormone glucagon-like peptide-1 (GLP-1). *Cell. Signal.* **2010**, *22*, 1–8. [CrossRef]
100. Tengholm, A.; Gylfe, E. cAMP signalling in insulin and glucagon secretion. *Diabetes Obes. Metab.* **2017**, *19*, 42–53. [CrossRef]

101. Alhosaini, K.; Azhar, A.; Alonazi, A.; Al-Zoghaibi, F. GPCRs: The most promiscuous druggable receptor of the mankind. *Saudi Pharm. J.* **2021**, *29*, 539–551. [CrossRef] [PubMed]
102. Shigeto, M.; Ramracheya, R.; Tarasov, A.I.; Cha, C.Y.; Chibalina, M.V.; Hastoy, B.; Philippaert, K.; Reinbothe, T.; Rorsman, N.; Salehi, A.; et al. GLP-1 stimulates insulin secretion by PKC-dependent TRPM4 and TRPM5 activation. *J. Clin. Investig.* **2015**, *125*, 4714–4728. [CrossRef] [PubMed]
103. Shu, L.; Matveyenko, A.V.; Kerr-Conte, J.; Cho, J.H.; McIntosh, C.H.; Maedler, K. Decreased TCF7L2 protein levels in type 2 diabetes mellitus correlate with downregulation of GIP- and GLP-1 receptors and impaired beta-cell function. *Hum. Mol. Genet.* **2009**, *18*, 2388–2399. [CrossRef] [PubMed]
104. Xu, G.; Kaneto, H.; Laybutt, D.R.; Duvivier-Kali, V.; Trivedi, N.; Suzuma, K.; King, G.L.; Weir, G.C.; Bonner-Weir, S. Downregulation of GLP-1 and GIP receptor expression by hyperglycemia: Possible contribution to the impaired incretin effects in diabetes. *Diabetes* **2007**, *56*, 1551–1558. [CrossRef]
105. Liu, Z.; Habener, J.F. Glucagon-like peptide-1 activation of TCF7L2-dependent Wnt signaling enhances pancreatic beta cell proliferation. *J. Biol. Chem.* **2008**, *283*, 8723–8735. [CrossRef]
106. Takamoto, I.; Kubota, N.; Nakaya, K.; Kumagai, K.; Hashimoto, S.; Kubota, T.; Inoue, M.; Kajiwara, E.; Katsuyama, H.; Obata, A.; et al. TCF7L2 in mouse pancreatic beta cells plays a crucial role in glucose homeostasis by regulating beta cell mass. *Diabetologia* **2014**, *57*, 542–553. [CrossRef]
107. Mitchell, R.K.; Mondragon, A.; Chen, L.; McGinty, J.A.; French, P.M.; Ferrer, J.; Thorens, B.; Hodson, D.J.; Rutter, G.A.; Xavier, G.D. Selective disruption of Tcf7l2 in the pancreatic β cell impairs secretory function and lowers β cell mass. *Hum. Mol. Genet.* **2015**, *24*, 1390–1399. [CrossRef]
108. Jainandunsing, S.; Koole, H.R.; van Miert, J.N.I.; Rietveld, T.; Wattimena, J.L.D.; Sijbrands, E.J.G.; de Rooij, F.W.M. Transcription factor 7-like 2 gene links increased in vivo insulin synthesis to type 2 diabetes. *EBioMedicine* **2018**, *30*, 295–302. [CrossRef]
109. Nguyen-Tu, M.S.; da Silva Xavier, G.; Leclerc, I.; Rutter, G.A. Transcription factor-7-like 2 (TCF7L2) gene acts downstream of the Lkb1/Stk11 kinase to control mTOR signaling, beta cell growth, and insulin secretion. *J. Biol. Chem.* **2018**, *293*, 14178–14189. [CrossRef]
110. Wu, H.H.; Li, Y.L.; Liu, N.J.; Yang, Z.; Tao, X.M.; Du, Y.P.; Wang, X.C.; Lu, B.; Zhang, Z.Y.; Hu, R.M.; et al. TCF7L2 regulates pancreatic beta-cell function through PI3K/AKT signal pathway. *Diabetol. Metab. Syndr.* **2019**, *11*, 55. [CrossRef]
111. Zhang, Z.; Xu, L.; Xu, X. The role of transcription factor 7-like 2 in metabolic disorders. *Obes. Rev.* **2021**, *22*, e13166. [CrossRef] [PubMed]
112. Vinuela, A.; Varshney, A.; van de Bunt, M.; Prasad, R.B.; Asplund, O.; Bennett, A.; Boehnke, M.; Brown, A.A.; Erdos, M.R.; Fadista, J.; et al. Genetic variant effects on gene expression in human pancreatic islets and their implications for T2D. *Nat. Commun.* **2020**, *11*, 4912. [CrossRef] [PubMed]
113. Galderisi, A.; Trico, D.; Pierpont, B.; Shabanova, V.; Samuels, S.; Dalla Man, C.; Galuppo, B.; Santoro, N.; Caprio, S. A reduced incretin effect mediated by the rs7903146 variant in the TCF7L2 gene is an early marker of beta-cell dysfunction in obese youth. *Diabetes Care* **2020**, *43*, 2553–2563. [CrossRef] [PubMed]
114. Juttada, U.; Kumpatla, S.; Parveen, R.; Viswanathan, V. TCF7L2 polymorphism a prominent marker among subjects with Type-2-Diabetes with a positive family history of diabetes. *Int. J. Biol. Macromol.* **2020**, *159*, 402–405. [CrossRef] [PubMed]
115. Del Bosque-Plata, L.; Martinez-Martinez, E.; Espinoza-Camacho, M.A.; Gragnoli, C. The role of TCF7L2 in type 2 diabetes. *Diabetes* **2021**, *70*, 1220–1228. [CrossRef]
116. Aboelkhair, N.T.; Kasem, H.E.; Abdelmoaty, A.A.; El-Edel, R.H. TCF7L2 gene polymorphism as a risk for type 2 diabetes mellitus and diabetic microvascular complications. *Mol. Biol. Rep.* **2021**, *48*, 5283–5290. [CrossRef]
117. Shimoda, M.; Kanda, Y.; Hamamoto, S.; Tawaramoto, K.; Hashiramoto, M.; Matsuki, M.; Kaku, K. The human glucagon-like peptide-1 analogue liraglutide preserves pancreatic beta cells via regulation of cell kinetics and suppression of oxidative and endoplasmic reticulum stress in a mouse model of diabetes. *Diabetologia* **2011**, *54*, 10598–11108. [CrossRef]
118. Cernea, S.; Raz, I. Therapy in the early stage: Incretins. *Diabetes Care* **2011**, *34*, S264–S271. [CrossRef]
119. Kimura, T.; Kaneto, H.; Shimoda, M.; Hirukawa, H.; Hamamoto, S.; Tawaramoto, K.; Hashiramoto, M.; Kaku, K. Protective effects of pioglitazone and/or liraglutide on pancreatic β-cells: Comparison of their effects between in an early and advanced stage of diabetes. *Mol. Cell. Endocrinol.* **2015**, *400*, 78–89. [CrossRef]
120. Tamura, K.; Minami, K.; Kudo, M.; Iemoto, K.; Takahashi, H.; Seino, S. Liraglutide improves pancreatic beta cell mass and function in Alloxan-induced diabetic mice. *PLoS ONE* **2015**, *10*, e0126003. [CrossRef]
121. Zheng, J.; Chen, T.; Zhu, Y.; Li, H.-Q.; Deng, X.-L.; Wang, Q.-H.; Zhang, J.-Y.; Chen, L.-L. Liraglutide prevents fast weight gain and β-cell dysfunction in male catch-up growth rats. *Exp. Biol. Med.* **2015**, *240*, 1165–1176. [CrossRef] [PubMed]
122. Kapodistria, K.; Tsilibary, E.-P.; Kotsopoulou, E.; Moustardas, P.; Kitsiou, P. Liraglutide, a human glucagon-like peptide-1 analogue, stimulates AKT-dependent survival signalling and inhibits pancreatic β-cell apoptosis. *J. Cell. Mol. Med.* **2018**, *22*, 2970–2980. [CrossRef] [PubMed]
123. Gao, M.; Deng, X.-L.; Liu, Z.-H.; Song, H.-J.; Zheng, J.; Cui, Z.-H.; Xiao, K.-L.; Chen, L.-L.; Li, H.-Q. Liraglutide protects β-cell function by reversing histone modification of Pdx-1 proximal promoter in catch-up growth male rats. *J. Diabetes Complicat.* **2018**, *32*, 985–994. [CrossRef] [PubMed]

124. Kimura, T.; Obata, A.; Shimoda, M.; Hirukawa, H.; Kanda-Kimura, Y.; Nogami, Y.; Kohara, K.; Nakanishi, S.; Mune, T.; Kaku, K.; et al. Durability of protective effect of dulaglutide on pancreatic β-cells in diabetic mice: GLP-1 receptor expression is not reduced at all even after long-term exposure to dulaglutide. *Diabetes Metab.* **2018**, *44*, 250–260. [CrossRef]
125. Abu Hashim, H. Gonadotrophin-releasing hormone analogues and endometriosis: Current strategies and new insights. *Gynecol. Endocrinol.* **2012**, *28*, 314–321. [CrossRef]
126. Yamamura, T.; Wakabayashi, Y.; Sakamoto, K.; Matsui, H.; Kusaka, M.; Tanaka, T.; Ohkura, S.; Okamura, H. The effects of chronic subcutaneous administration of an investigational kisspeptin analog, TAK-683, on gonadotropin-releasing hormone pulse generator activity in goats. *Neuroendocrinology* **2014**, *100*, 250–264. [CrossRef]
127. Hough, D.; Bellingham, M.; Haraldsen, I.R.; McLaughlin, M.; Robinson, J.E.; Solbakk, A.K.; Evans, N.P. A reduction in long-term spatial memory persists after discontinuation of peripubertal GnRH agonist treatment in sheep. *Psychoneuroendocrinology* **2017**, *77*, 1–8. [CrossRef]
128. Stalewski, J.; Hargrove, D.M.; Wolfe, M.; Kohout, T.A.; Kamal, A. Additive effect of simultaneous continuous administration of degarelix and TAK-448 on LH suppression in a castrated rat model. *Eur. J. Pharmacol.* **2018**, *824*, 24–29. [CrossRef]
129. Zhu, N.; Zhang, D.; Wang, W.; Li, X.; Yang, B.; Song, J.; Zhao, X.; Huang, B.; Shi, W.; Lu, R.; et al. A novel coronavirus from patients with pneumonia in China, 2019. *N. Engl. J. Med.* **2020**, *382*, 727–733. [CrossRef]
130. Guan, W.J.; Ni, Z.Y.; Hu, Y.; Liang, W.H.; Ou, C.Q.; He, J.X.; Liu, L.; Shan, H.; Lei, C.L.; Hui, D.S.C.; et al. Clinical characteristics of coronavirus disease 2019 in China. *N. Engl. J. Med.* **2020**, *382*, 1708–1720. [CrossRef]
131. Huang, I.; Lim, M.A.; Pranata, R. Diabetes mellitus is associated with increased mortality and severity of disease in COVID-19 pneumoniae: A systematic review, meta-analysis, and meta-regression. *Diabetes Metab. Syndr. Clin. Res. Rev.* **2020**, *14*, 395–403. [CrossRef] [PubMed]
132. Coate, K.C.; Cha, J.; Shrestha, S.; Wang, W.; Gonçalves, L.M.; Almaça, J.; Kapp, M.E.; Fasolino, M.; Morgan, A.; Dai, C.; et al. SARS-CoV-2 cell entry factors ACE2 and TMPRSS2 are expressed in the microvasculature and ducts of human pancreas but are not enriched in beta cells. *Cell Metab.* **2020**, *32*, 1028–1040. [CrossRef] [PubMed]
133. Kusmartseva, I.; Wu, W.; Syed, F.; Van Der Heide, V.; Jorgensen, M.; Joseph, P.; Tang, X.; Candelario-Jalil, E.; Yang, C.; Nick, H.; et al. Expression of SARS-CoV-2 entry factors in the pancreas of normal organ donors and individuals with COVID-19. *Cell Metab.* **2020**, *32*, 1041–1051. [CrossRef] [PubMed]
134. Daly, J.L.; Simonetti, B.; Klein, K.; Chen, K.E.; Williamson, M.K.; Anton-Plagaro, C.; Shoemark, D.K.; Simon-Gracia, L.; Bauer, M.; Hollandi, R.; et al. Neuropilin-1 is a host factor for SARS-CoV-2 infection. *Science* **2020**, *370*, 861–865. [CrossRef] [PubMed]
135. Cantuti-Castelvetri, L.; Ojha, R.; Pedro, L.D.; Djannatian, M.; Franz, J.; Kuivanen, S.; van der Meer, F.; Kallio, K.; Kaya, T.; Anastasina, M.; et al. Neuropilin-1 facilitates SARS-CoV-2 cell entry and infectivity. *Science* **2020**, *370*, 856–860. [CrossRef]
136. Muller, J.A.; Groß, R.; Conzelmann, C.; Kruger, J.; Merle, U.; Steinhart, J.; Weil, T.; Koepke, L.; Bozzo, C.P.; Read, C.; et al. SARS-CoV-2 infects and replicates in cells of the human endocrine and exocrine pancreas. *Nat. Metab.* **2021**, *3*, 149–165. [CrossRef]
137. Tang, X.; Uhl, S.; Zhang, T.; Xue, D.; Li, B.; Vandana, J.J.; Acklin, J.A.; Bonnycastle, L.L.; Narisu, N.; Erdos, M.R.; et al. SARS-CoV-2 infection induces beta cell transdifferentiation. *Cell Metab.* **2021**, *33*, 1577–1591. [CrossRef]
138. Wu, C.T.; Lidsky, P.V.; Xiao, Y.; Lee, I.T.; Cheng, R.; Nakayama, T.; Jiang, S.; Demeter, J.; Bevacqua, R.J.; Chang, C.A.; et al. SARS-CoV-2 infects human pancreatic beta cells and elicits beta cell impairment. *Cell Metab.* **2021**, *33*, 1565–1576. [CrossRef]
139. Steenblock, C.; Richter, S.; Berger, I.; Barovic, M.; Schmid, J.; Schubert, U.; Jarzebska, N.; von Massenhausen, A.; Linkermann, A.; Schurmann, A.; et al. Viral infiltration of pancreatic islets in patients with COVID-19. *Nat. Commun.* **2021**, *12*, 3534. [CrossRef]

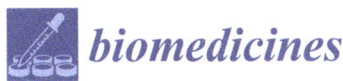

Article

Incorporation of Oxidized Phenylalanine Derivatives into Insulin Signaling Relevant Proteins May Link Oxidative Stress to Signaling Conditions Underlying Chronic Insulin Resistance

Judit Mohás-Cseh [1], Gergő Attila Molnár [1], Marianna Pap [2,3], Boglárka Laczy [1], Tibor Vas [1], Melinda Kertész [1], Krisztina Németh [4], Csaba Hetényi [5], Orsolya Csikós [6], Gábor K. Tóth [6], Attila Reményi [4] and István Wittmann [1,*]

[1] 2nd Department of Medicine and Nephrology-Diabetes Center, University of Pécs Medical School, 7624 Pécs, Hungary; mohas-cseh.judit@pte.hu (J.M.-C.); molnar.gergo@pte.hu (G.A.M.); laczy.boglarka@pte.hu (B.L.); vas.tibor2@pte.hu (T.V.); meli871106@gmail.com (M.K.)
[2] Department of Medical Biology and Central Electron Microscopic Laboratory, University of Pécs Medical School, 7643 Pécs, Hungary; pap.marianna@pte.hu
[3] Signal Transduction Research Group, Szentágothai Research Centre, University of Pécs, 7624 Pécs, Hungary
[4] Institute of Organic Chemistry, Research Centre for Natural Sciences, 1117 Budapest, Hungary; nemeth.krisztina@ttk.hu (K.N.); remenyi.attila@ttk.mta.hu (A.R.)
[5] Department of Pharmacology and Pharmacotherapy, University of Pécs Medical School, 7643 Pécs, Hungary; hetenyi.csaba@pte.hu
[6] Department of Medical Chemistry, Albert Szent-Györgyi Medical School, University of Szeged, 6725 Szeged, Hungary; csikos.orsolya@icloud.com (O.C.); toth.gabor@med.u-szeged.hu (G.K.T.)
* Correspondence: wittmann.istvan@pte.hu; Tel.: +36-72-536-050; Fax: +36-72-536-051

Abstract: A link between oxidative stress and insulin resistance has been suggested. Hydroxyl free radicals are known to be able to convert phenylalanine (Phe) into the non-physiological tyrosine isoforms ortho- and meta-tyrosine (o-Tyr, m-Tyr). The aim of our study was to examine the role of o-Tyr and m-Tyr in the development of insulin resistance. We found that insulin-induced uptake of glucose was blunted in cultures of 3T3-L1 grown on media containing o- or m-Tyr. We show that these modified amino acids are incorporated into cellular proteins. We focused on insulin receptor substrate 1 (IRS-1), which plays a role in insulin signaling. The activating phosphorylation of IRS-1 was increased by insulin, the effect of which was abolished in cells grown in m-Tyr or o-Tyr media. We found that phosphorylation of m- or o-Tyr containing IRS-1 segments by insulin receptor (IR) kinase was greatly reduced, PTP-1B phosphatase was incapable of dephosphorylating phosphorylated m- or o-Tyr IRS-1 peptides, and the SH2 domains of phosphoinositide 3-kinase (PI3K) bound the o-Tyr IRS-1 peptides with greatly reduced affinity. According to our data, m- or o-Tyr incorporation into IRS-1 modifies its protein–protein interactions with regulating enzymes and effectors, thus IRS-1 eventually loses its capacity to play its role in insulin signaling, leading to insulin resistance.

Keywords: insulin resistance; oxidative stress; hydroxyl free radical; ortho-tyrosine; meta-tyrosine; IRS-1; phosphorylation; dephosphorylation

1. Introduction

1.1. Pathogenesis of Insulin Resistance

The pathogenesis of type 2 diabetes is complex [1,2], but one of the hallmarks of the development of type 2 diabetes—at least in obese patients with type 2 diabetes—is peripheral chronic insulin resistance, with a reduced uptake of glucose into adipose tissue [3]. The triggering factor for insulin resistance is oxidative stress due to systemic subclinical inflammation and hormonal interactions which all induce oxidative stress by the activation of nicotinamide nucleotide (NAD(P)H) oxidase enzyme [4]. In obesity, overfeeding may lead to glycotoxicity and lipotoxicity. This is especially the case for the liver, as non-alcoholic fatty liver disease is a frequent companion to obesity. The affected tissues may face serious damage, and with time, exhaustion of the mitochondria. The strong beta-oxidation and uncoupling of the production of adenosine triphosphate (ATP) and terminal oxidation may lead to a higher rate of the formation of reactive oxygen species (ROS), contributing to the development of insulin resistance [5].

1.2. Acute Insulin Resistance

Acute insulin resistance induced by tumor necrosis factor alpha (TNFα) or dexamethasone could be ameliorated by the antioxidants N-acetylcysteine, manganese (III) tetrakis (4-benzoicacid) porphyrin (MnTBAP), or by induction of antioxidant enzymes such as superoxide dismutase or catalase [6]. These data suggest a strong connection between oxidative stress and the development of acute insulin resistance.

1.3. Chronic Insulin Resistance

In clinical settings, chronic antioxidant therapy of patients (e.g., in the case of diabetic neuropathy using alpha-lipoic acid) is able to improve chronic insulin resistance [7]. Moreover, using the so-called "breakthrough" therapy, a 2–4 week decrease in glucotoxicity is able to normalize glycemia by decreasing insulin resistance for months or years [8,9]. Because clinical insulin resistance can be reverted, it is not an alteration of the DNA, but rather some type of protein abnormality; this can be hypothesized given the background of this oxidative stress-induced clinical condition.

This theory is further augmented by the observation that a low advanced glycation end products (AGE) diet, which is associated with a state of increased oxidative stress and subclinical inflammation, ameliorated insulin resistance in obese people with the metabolic syndrome [10].

Oxidative stress may develop in type 2 diabetes mellitus because of the activation of the polyol pathway leading to a depletion in the glutathione pool, non-enzymatic glycation, and interaction of the resulting AGEs with their receptors (receptor for AGE, RAGE), which in turn may augment the same pro-oxidant NAD(P)H oxidase (NOX) via protein kinase C signaling and the hexosamine pathway. Moreover, superoxide overproduction in the mitochondria due to hyperglycemia may activate all of these pathways, resulting in a vicious cycle [11] (Figure 1).

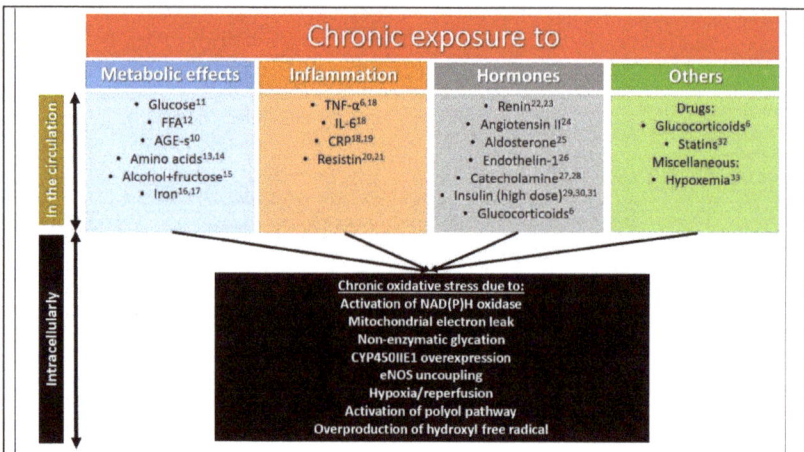

Figure 1. Chronic exposure leading to oxidative stress and insulin resistance [6,10–33]. Those factors are listed which cause oxidative stress and insulin resistance at the same time in a chronic setting. The arrows indicate a causal relationship between alterations in the circulation leading to intracellular abnormalities.

1.4. Tyrosine Isomers and Hydroxyl Free Radical

Reactive oxygen species (ROS) that arise from oxidative stress processes are highly reactive and may attack macromolecules, such as lipids, nucleic acids, proteins, and amino acids [34]. Stable products of ROS-derived macromolecular damage may be used as markers of oxidative stress.

Phenylalanine (Phe) is an essential amino acid that is further used for the production of para-tyrosine, dihydroxy-phenylalanine (DOPA), catecholamines, melanine, and thyroid hormones [35]. Beyond these important enzymatic reactions, Phe, due to the vulnerability of its aromatic ring, may also be a subject of non-enzymatic oxidation processes, i.e., the attack of ROS [36]. The isomers of the physiological para-tyrosine (p-Tyr), namely meta- and ortho-tyrosine (m-Tyr and o-Tyr), are formed this way [36] (Figure 2).

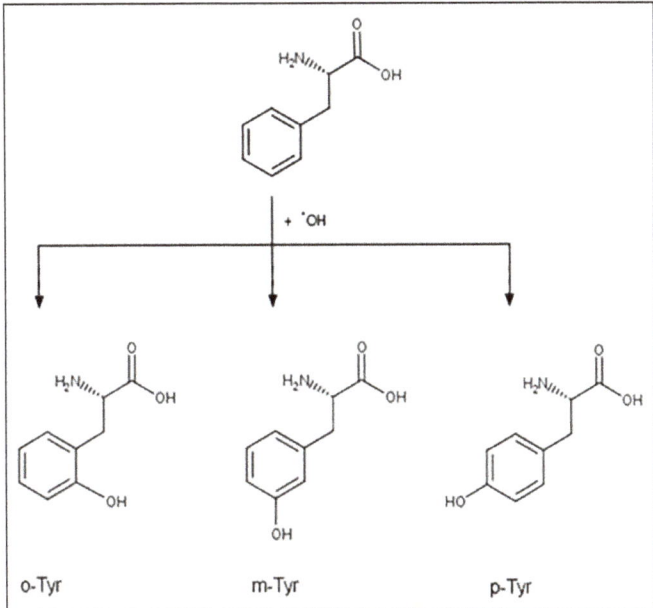

Figure 2. Hydroxyl free radical induced production of tyrosine isomers.

1.5. Non-Physiological Tyrosine Isomers as Markers

Elevated levels of m- and/or o-Tyr have been described in the vascular wall of cynomolgus monkeys [37] as well as in cataract lenses [38]. In previous studies by our group, the non-physiological Tyr isomers (m- and o-Tyr) have been shown to be oxidative stress markers in patients with type 2 diabetes with or without chronic kidney disease [39] in patients with end-stage renal disease or patients with severe sepsis. We have also shown that type 2 diabetic patients treated with resveratrol showed a decrease in urinary excretion of o-Tyr, and a concomitant improvement in insulin resistance [40]. These data suggest that m- and o-Tyr may be used as markers of oxidative stress.

1.6. Non-Physiological Tyrosine Isomers as "Makers"

Furthermore, m- and o-Tyr may have a role beyond being markers ROS attack. Namely, m-Tyr has been shown to act as a natural herbicide and inhibit the growth of plants [41]. Additionally, m-Tyr seems to be involved in the inhibition of concomitant tumor growth [42]. These data suggest that m-Tyr is more than just a marker, but it also plays a pathogenetic role under some circumstances. For example, we have described that patients on renal replacement therapy show a connection between plasma levels of o-Tyr and erythropoietin

(EPO) resistance. In a further set of experiments, m- and o-Tyr inhibited the EPO-dependent proliferation of erythroblasts, in a time- and dose-dependent manner [43].

With all of the above-mentioned data taken into account, we hypothesized that m- and o-Tyr—on the basis of their potential role in EPO-resistance—are able to induce chronic insulin resistance in fat cells, HEK cells, podocytes, and macrophages, and that intracellular signaling of insulin may be disrupted this way.

Thus, proof-of-concept experiments were designed to address this question. Our results suggest that oxidative stress-induced o- and m-Tyr could incorporate into cellular proteins, interfere with insulin signaling, inhibit glucose uptake, and thus induce chronic insulin resistance.

2. Materials and Methods

2.1. Cell Culture

Early passages of mouse embryo fibroblast (3T3-L1) (ATCC, Manassas, VA, US) were cultured in Dulbecco's modified Eagle medium (DMEM, Sigma Aldrich, Budapest, Hungary, CAT number: D6046; Invitrogen, Waltham, MA, USA, CAT number: 41966-029) supplemented with 100 U/mL penicillin, 0.1 mg/mL streptomycin (Gibco, Budapest, Hungary, CAT number: 15070-063) and 10% heat-inactivated Fetal Bovine Serum (FBS, Gibco, CAT number: 16170-078), supplemented with 398 nM p-, m-, or o-Tyr (equimolar to the original p-Tyr content of the medium) purchased from Sigma (CAT number: para-Tyr: T8566, m-Tyr: T3629, o-Tyr: 93851). Media contained 25 or 5 mmol/L glucose (experiment dependent) pyruvate and L-glutamine. Cells were grown at 37 °C and 5% CO_2. Adipocyte differentiation was achieved by DMEM supplemented with 10% FBS (Gibco, Csertex, Budapest, Hungary, CAT number: 10106-169) (FBS) and a 0.17 nmol/L insulin (Sigma Aldrich, Budapest, Hungary, CAT number: I 9278), 0.5 nmol/L isobuthylmethylxanthine (Sigma Aldrich, Budapest, Hungary, CAT number: I 5879), and 250 nmol/L dexamethasone (Sigma Aldrich, Budapest, Hungary, CAT number: 861871) containing cocktail. From day 4 onward, cultures were maintained in DMEM containing 1.5 µg/mL insulin and 10% FBS with a medium change every other day until experimental treatments were started. After 90% of the cell population reached the adipocyte phenotype, prior to all treatments, cells were incubated overnight in serum-deprived medium. Experimental treatment was performed in serum-deprived medium containing 200 or 400 nmol/L insulin, for 5 min.

The conditionally immortalized human podocyte cell line (provided by Moin Saleem, University of Bristol, UK) was cultured in RPMI1640 medium (R8756, Sigma Aldrich, Budapest, Hungary) supplemented with 10% heat-inactivated FBS (16170-078, Gibco, Budapest, Hungary), insulin-transferrin-selenium supplement (41400-045, Gibco), 100 U/mL penicillin, 0.1 mg/mL streptomycin (P4333, Sigma), and 112.5 nM (equimolar to the original p-Tyr content of the medium) para-, meta-, or ortho-Tyr. The cells were grown at 33 °C 5% CO_2, and when they reached 40–60% confluency they were transferred to 37 °C to differentiate. Following the thermoswitching, cells were kept on RPMI1640 medium containing 2% FBS, antibiotics, and different tyrosines. Before every treatment, cells were incubated in serum-deprived medium overnight.

HEK-293 immortalized cell line (ATCC, Manassas, VA, USA) of epithelial morphology and the J774A.1 mouse BALB/C monocyte-macrophage cell lines (91051511-1VL, Sigma Aldrich, Budapest, Hungary) were cultured in Petri dishes with a medium composed of Dulbecco's modified Eagle's medium (DMEM, Sigma Aldrich, Budapest, Hungary, CAT number: D6046, Invitrogen, CAT number: 41966-029), with a 10% heat-inactivated FBS supplementation (16170-078, Gibco), insulin-transferrin-selenium supplement (41400-045, Gibco, Budapest, Hungary,), 100 U/mL penicillin and 0.1 mg/mL streptomycin (P4333, Sigma) and 398 nM para (5 and 25 mmol/L), meta-, or ortho-Tyr (T8566, T3629, 93851, Sigma). Before treatment, cells were incubated in serum-deprived medium overnight as well. After the treatment, cells were washed twice with saline (4 °C) and then exposed to 80 µL lysis buffer/plate, containing 1 mol/L Trisbase, pH 7.4, 1.15% Triton X, 0.2 mol/L EGTA, pH 7, 0.5 mol/L EDTA, pH 8, 5 mg/mL phenylmethylsulfonyl fluoride (PMSF),

0.1 mol/L dithiothreitol (DTT), 0.1 mol/L Na$_3$VO$_4$, 5 mg/mL aprotinin, 5 mg/mL leupeptin, and phosphatase inhibitor cocktails 1 and 2 (Sigma Aldrich, Budapest, Hungary, CAT number: P5726 and P2850). Cells were scraped off mechanically and then were frozen at −70 °C.

2.2. Isotope Glucose Uptake

Initially, cells were kept in glucose-free DMEM (Gibco, Csertex, Budapest, Hungary) for 30 min and then were treated with 2, 20, 200, or 400 nmol/L insulin for 100 min. Concurrently, 1 µCi/mL deoxy-D-glucose 2-[1 2-3H(N)] (3.7 × 10^4 Bq/mL) (Izotóp Intézet, Budapest, Hungary) was added to the plates for 100 min. After scraping the cells into the medium, they were centrifuged for 5 min at 1000 rpm. We dissolved the sediment in 70 µL of lysis buffer, then glucose uptake was determined by scintillation counting by measuring 30 µL of the sample, using a Beckman LS 5000 TD counter, in counts per minute (CPM), for five minutes each, with average activity was used as the outcome. Following freezing overnight at −70 °C, protein concentration was measured with a Hitachi spectrophotometer. Results were normalized for protein content [44].

2.3. HPLC Analysis

The type of tyrosine aimed to be measured determined the sample preparation. Methods were based on earlier publications with minor modifications [39].

To measure the total intracellular non-protein-bound tyrosine concentration, prior to the freezing of samples overnight at −70 °C to achieve cell lysis, 200 µL distilled water was added to each. After melting up, samples were centrifuged for 15 min at 15,000 rpm. A total of 200 µL of the supernatant was mixed with 200 µL of 60% trichloroacetic acid. After 30 min incubation on ice, samples were centrifuged again at 15,000 rpm for 15 min. Then, the supernatant was filtered and was diluted 5-fold and then 160 µL distilled water was added to 40 µL of filtrate, followed by the injection of the mixture onto the HPLC column.

The total protein-bound cellular tyrosine content was measured by adding 200 µL of distilled water to the samples, followed by freezing overnight at −70 °C to achieve cell lysis. After melting and centrifugation for 10 min at 4000 rpm, 200 µL supernatant was mixed with 200 µL 60% trichloroacetic followed by incubation on ice for 30 min to precipitate proteins. After the second centrifugation for 10 min at 4000 rpm, the sediment was resuspended in 1% trichloroacetic acid and 4 µL of 400 mmol/L desferrioxamine. A total of 40 µL of 500 mmol/L butylated hydroxytoluene was added to the samples to avoid possible free radical formation during hydrolysis. Then, 200 µL of 6 N hydrochloric acid was added in order to hydrolyze the proteins at 120 °C overnight. The hydrolysate was then filtered through a 0.2 µm filter (Millipore Co., Billerica, MA, USA) and 20 µL of the filtrate was injected onto the HPLC column of a Shimadzu Class LC-10 ADVP HPLC system (Shimadzu USA Manufacturing Inc., Canby, OR, USA) using a Rheodyne manual injector.

The amounts of p-, o-, m-Tyr and Phe in the samples were determined by measuring their autofluorescence. Thus, no derivatization or staining was needed. Samples were measured on a Shimadzu Class 10 HPLC system equipped with an RF-10 AXL fluorescent detector (Shimadzu USA Manufacturing Inc., Canby, OR, USA). The mobile phase consisted of 1% sodium acetate and 1% acetic acid dissolved in water. The separation took place on a LiChroCHART 250-4 column (Merck KGaA, Darmstadt 64271, Germany) in an isocratic run. Wavelengths of 275 nm for excitation and 305 nm for emission were used to assess p-, o- and m-Tyr, while Phe was detected at 258 nm excitation and 288 nm emission wavelengths. Determination of the area under the curve (AUC) plus external standard calibration was used to calculate the precise concentrations of the amino acids.

2.4. Western Blot Analysis

The samples of lysates were vortexed and centrifuged (10 min, 13,000 rpm, at 4 °C). Protein content of the samples was determined by the Lowry method using bovine serum albumin as a standard. Samples were solubilized in 100 mmol/L Tris-HCl (pH 6.8), 4.0%

sodium dodecyl sulphate (SDS), 20% glycerol, 200 mmol/L DTT, and 0.2% bromophenol blue containing buffer. Samples (80 to 120 µg protein) were electrophoretically resolved on 7.5% polyacrylamide gels and transferred to PVDF membranes (Amersham-Biotech, AP Hungary, Budapest, Hungary). Membranes were stained with Ponceau dye to ensure successful transfer. The non-specific antibody binding sites were blocked in 5% BSA in TBS-T solution at room temperature for one hour. Membranes were incubated in the primary antibodies anti-phospho-(Ser473)-Akt (Cell Signaling Technology, #7074, Beverly, CA, USA), to detect p-Akt in a final dilution of 1:2000, or anti-phospho-(Tyr612)-IRS-1 (1:2000 I2658 Sigma, Budapest Hungary) and they were used overnight at 4 °C. Membranes were washed three times for 5 min with TBS-T and incubated with HRP-conjugated anti-rabbit IgG secondary antibody (#7074, Cell Signaling) diluted in the blocking solution (1:4000) for one hour at room temperature. Membranes were washed three times for 5 min with TBS-T.

To re-probe Western blots with alternative primary antibodies, the stripping of membranes took place as follows: they were washed in 0.1% TBS-T for 10 min, the membranes were merged in stripping buffer containing 0.1% SDS, 1.5% glycine, and 1% Tween-20 at pH 2.2, twice for 10 min, then were washed in PBS twice for 5 min, and then in TBS-T 0.1% twice for 5 min. The membranes were blocked in 5% BSA in TBS-T solution at room temperature for one hour and then incubated with the following antibodies: total PKB/Akt in 1:1000 final dilution (#9272, Cell Signaling Technology, Beverly, MA USA) and total IRS-1 in 1:1000 final dilution (I7153 Sigma) overnight at 4 °C. The membranes were washed three times for 5 min with TBS-T and incubated with HRP-conjugated secondary antibody (#7074 Cell Signaling Technology, Beverly, MA USA) diluted in the blocking solution (1:2000) for one hour at room temperature. Membranes were washed three times for 5 min with TBS-T. Afterwards, membranes were incubated in enhanced chemiluminescence HRP substrate (ECL; Pierce Biotech, Bio-Rad, Budapest, Hungary) according to the manufacturer's instructions. Computerized densitometry (integrated optical density) of the specific bands was analyzed using Scion Image for Windows software. Protein signals were corrected for total Akt or total IRS-1 protein levels and adjusted to controls.

2.5. Protein Expression

The cDNA segment encoding the human PTP1B catalytic domain (1–299 aa) was PCR amplified from a HEK293T cDNA pool and inserted into the pBH4 vector with BamHI and NotI restriction sites. This construct is only missing the C-terminal flexible region and the membrane binding segment of PTP1B. The protein was expressed with an N-terminal hexa-histidine tag. Recombinant active PTP1B was expressed in the Escherichia coli BL21 (DE3) bacterial strain. Briefly, cells were grown in an ampicillin-containing LB medium at 37 °C to OD = 0.6 and then cooled down to 18 °C and induced by the addition of 0.05 mM isopropyl-beta-D-thiogalactoside (IPTG). After an overnight expression at 18 °C, the pellet was harvested and washed with phosphate buffered saline (PBS). Following freezing at −80 °C, cells were lysed in an appropriate buffer (300 mM NaCl, 50 mM phosphate, 10 mM imidazole, 2 mM beta-mercapto-ethanol, 0.1% IGEPAL with pH = 8.0, and 0.5 mM benzamidine with 0.5 mM PMSF protease inhibitors added) with the help of sonification. The lysate was centrifuged at 20,000 rpm for 30 min and the supernatant (~30 mL) was mixed with 1 mL Ni-NTA resin slurry (50%). After 45 min incubation at 4 °C, the mixture was transferred to gravity columns and washed with 10-10 mL of imidazole (40 mM imidazole, 300 mM NaCl, 50 mM phosphate, pH = 8.0 with 2 mM beta-mercapto-ethanol) and high salt (1000 mM NaCl, 20 mM imidazole, 20 mM TRIS, pH = 8.0 with 2 mM beta-mercapto-ethanol) containing wash buffers, each. PTP1B was eluted by applying 5 mL elution buffer (400 mM imidazole, 200 mM NaCl, 10% glycerol, 20 mM TRIS, pH = 8.0, with 0.1% IGEPAL). The eluted protein was supplemented with tricarboxy-ethyl-phosphine (TCEP) reducing agent at 2 mM concentration.

The Ni-NTA purified PTP1B protein was further purified by anion exchange chromatography. After an overnight dialysis against 1 L buffer with low salt (5 mM NaCl, 10%

glycerol, 20 mM TRIS, pH = 8.0 with 1 mM dithiothreitol reducing agent), it was loaded on a resource Q anion exchange column and subjected to a gradient from 5 mM to 1 M NaCl. The protein practically eluted in a single peak, which was then pooled, supplemented with a reducing agent (TCEP), and frozen on liquid nitrogen. Final protein samples checked by SDS-PAGE were found to have a purity over 95%.

The N- and C-terminal SH2 domains (regions 321–433 and 614–724, respectively) of the PI3K regulatory subunit were subcloned into a bacterial expression vector by PCR and then similarly expressed and purified as described above.

Enzymatically active IR kinase (989–1382, fused to GST and produced in SF9 cells) was ordered from SinoBiological (catalog number 11081-H20B1). The stock solution was aliquoted and frozen separately to preserve activity. Prior to comparative measurements, the activity of recombinant IR kinase was tested on internal control peptides and found to be suitable for kinase assays.

2.6. Peptide Synthesis

Peptides conferring to one of the YxxM motif regions (626-GRKGSGDYMPMSPKV-639) of human IRS-1 were chemically synthesized. The Y abbreviation denotes normal, ortho, and meta tyrosine. The solid-phase peptide syntheses were performed using a Liberty Microwave Peptide Synthesiser (CEM Corporation, Matthews, NC, USA) applying the Fmoc/tBu strategy. The resin used was PL-Rink-Amide MBHA. The Fmoc group was removed by 4.5 equiv. piperazine/HOBtxH$_2$O in DMF. The coupling steps were performed with 4 equiv. of Fmoc amino acids in DMF, 4.5 equiv. of HOBt/HBTU in DMF and 10 equiv. DIPEA in NMP, using a microwave power of 25 W for 2 × 300 s. All couplings were performed at standard double coupling conditions at a maximum temperature of 75 °C, except for the following amino acids: 2-Fmoc-amino-3-(3-hydroxyphenyl)-propanoic acid, 2-Fmoc-amino-3-(2-hydroxyphenyl)-propanoic acid, and 2-Fmoc-amino-3-(4-hydroxyphenyl)-propanoic acid (Fmoc-tyrosine), which were double coupled using a 25 min coupling followed by a 5 min period at 25 W. The phenolic hydroxyls were unprotected. Cleavage of the peptides from the solid support was carried out using a TFA containing cocktail with TFA 90%, water 5%, TIS 2.5%, and DTT 2.5%. Conditions: 10 mL cocktail, 3.5 h reaction time, RT. The resulted crude peptides were filtered, and the filtrates were lyophilized. The peptides were analyzed on an Agilent 1200/Waters SQD RP-HPLC/MS instrument, applying Phenomenex Proteo 4µm C18 90 Å column (4.6 × 250 mm) at 1 mL/min flow using a liner gradient of 5% to 85% B over 25 min. The solvent system used was A (0.1% TFA in H$_2$O) and B (0.1% TFA in MeCN). The crude peptides were purified on a semipreparative RP-HPLC Shimadzu instrument applying a Phenomenex Luna 10 µm C18 100 Å 10 × 250 mm column.

For the synthesis of the phosphorylated derivatives, first, the C-terminal octapeptides were prepared in a manner similar to the previous ones. After the incorporation of the tyrosine moiety, the phosphorylation was made on-line, so the elongation of the peptide chains was stopped. The phosphorylation of the hydroxyl unprotected tyrosines was carried out on solid-phase using 10 equiv. di-tert-butylN,N-diethylphosphoramidite, 20 equiv. 1H-tetrazole, THF, followed by oxidation using 14% tert-butyl hydroperoxide/water. After the formation of the appropriately protected phosphotyrosine-containing peptides, the elongation of the peptide chains was continued and the remaining 7 amino acids were incorporated as described previously. Cleavage from the solid support and the processing of the crude peptide was performed using the above-mentioned methodology.

The two methionines in the sequence during the oxidation of the phosphite to phosphate were converted to methionine sulfoxide. Therefore, an additional step was necessary to transform the sulfoxides back to thioether. The reduction of the sulfoxides was performed in the solution phase using 20 equivalents of NH$_4$I in TFA/H$_2$O (1:1 v/v%) at 0 °C. It was particularly fast, with 100% conversion to the desired peptides after 30 min. The resulting phosphopeptides were purified as mentioned above. The HPLC characterization is in Table 1.

Table 1. HPLC characterization of the peptides.

Peptide	t_R (min)
GRKGSGDF(4-hydroxy)MPMSPKV	t_R = 9.96
GRKGSGDF(3-hydroxy)MPMSPKV	t_R = 9.19
GRKGSGDF(2-hydroxy)MPMSPKV	t_R = 12.08
GRKGSGDF(4-PO$_4$H$_2$)MPMSPKV	t_R = 9.06
GRKGSGDF(3-PO$_4$H$_2$)MPMSPKV	t_R = 8.24
GRKGSGDF(2-PO$_4$H$_2$)MPMSPKV	t_R = 8.59

Gradient 20–35 % (B) in 15 min, flow 1.0 mL/min.

Mass spectrometry: calculated Mw 1608.89, measured Mw 1608.6 (nonphosphorylated peptides); calculated Mw 1688.89, measured Mw 1689.0 (phosphorylated peptides).

2.7. Phosphorylation and Dephosphorylation Assays—Capillary Electrophoresis

The kinase assay mixture contained 200 μM peptide (GRKGSGDYMPMSPKV) and 875 nM IR kinase in kinase buffer (20 mM potassium phosphate (monobasic), 15 mM sodium phosphate (dibasic), 103 mM NaCl, 5 mM MgCl$_2$, 5% glycerol, 0.05% Igepal; pH 7.5). The reaction was initialized by addition of 1 mM ATP. The phosphatase reaction mixture contained 80 μM peptide (GRKGSGD(phosphoY)MPMSPKV) in buffer (50 mM TRIS, 150 mM NaCl, 1 mM EDTA and 2 mM DTT; pH 7.4). The reaction was initialized by addition of 25 nM PTP1B enzyme. Equal aliquots of the kinase or the phosphatase reaction mixture were subjected to capillary electrophoresis analysis at the indicated time points after the start the reaction.

Background electrolyte (BGE) components phosphoric acid and triethylamine were purchased from Sigma (St. Louis, MO, USA) and from Merck GmbH (Darmstadt, Germany), respectively. Capillary electrophoresis was performed with an Agilent Capillary Electrophoresis 3DCE system (Agilent Technologies, Waldbronn, Germany) applying DB-WAX coated capillary having a 33.5 cm total and 25 cm effective length with 50 μm I.D. (Agilent Technologies, Santa Clara, CA, USA). On-line absorption at 200 nm was monitored by DAD UV-Vis detector. The capillary was thermostated at 25 °C. Before measurements, the capillary was rinsed subsequently with distilled water for 15 min and between measurements with BGE (100 mM trimethylamine-phosphate buffer; pH 2.5) for 3 min. Samples were injected by 5×10^3 Pa pressure for 6 s. Runs were performed in the positive-polarity mode with 20 kV.

2.8. Protein-Peptide Binding Assays

For in vitro fluorescence polarization (FP)-based affinity measurements, a peptide containing the phosphorylated tyrosine residue 632 of human IRS1 was labelled by lys-carboxyfluorescenine at its C-terminal end (GRKGSGD(pY)MPMSPKS(K-FITC). Synthesis of the labelled peptide was done by GenScript Inc. For competitive FP measurements, unlabeled peptides with either natural (para-phospho-Tyr) or unnatural (ortho-phospho-Tyr and meta-phospho-Tyr) phosphorylated amino acids (core sequence GRKGSGD(pY)MPMSPKV in all three cases) were used. Direct titration with the labelled peptide was done by generating a dilution series of the protein (N-terminal and C-terminal SH2 domains of PI3K regulatory subunit 1), with a constant (100 nM) peptide concentration in a standard buffer (100 mM NaCl, 20 mM TRIS pH = 8.0, 0.05% Brij-35 detergent). Competitive titrations were done by keeping the concentration of the protein-labelled peptide mixture constant (150 nM and 1500 nM C-terminal and N-terminal domain, respectively, with 100 nM labelled peptide) and varying the concentration of the unlabeled competitor peptide instead. Measurements were done in a Cytation C3 (BioTek Instruments) plate reader in black 384-well plates, using three parallels for all points. The resulting curves were fitted with OriginPro 7 (Origin Labs Inc., Wellesley, MA, USA).

2.9. Immunofluorescence

In a 6-well plate, 10⁴ cells were cultured on glass coverslips washed with alcohol and dried under UV light. The podocyte cells were grown in RPMI1640 medium supplemented with 10% heat-inactivated FBS at 33 °C, 5% CO_2. When they reached 60% confluence, the medium was changed to RPMI1640 medium containing 2% FBS and 112.05 nM of the different tyrosine isoforms, then the plates were transferred to 37 °C, 5% CO_2 to allow the cells to differentiate. The different tyrosine isoforms were added to the maintenance medium. The cells were serum deprived overnight, then incubated with 400 nmol/l insulin for 10 min. After removal of the medium, the coverslips were washed twice with PBS. The cells were fixed at room temperature in 2% paraformaldehyde and 4% sucrose for 8 min, then permeabilized using 0.3% Trion X-100 in 1xPBS for 20 min and blocked in 2.5% BSA for 45 min [45]. The primary antibody was diluted in 1xPBS, and the cells were incubated in it for 60 min in humid conditions. The antibodies we used were mouse anti-WT1 antibody (H-1) (1:100, Santa Cruz Biotechnology, Dallas, TX, USA), chicken anti-vimentin antibody (1:100, Abcam), rabbit anti-glucose transporter GLUT4 antibody (1:100, Abcam, Cambridge, UK), mouse Insulin Receptor Substrate-1 antibody (1:100, Invitrogen, Waltham, MA, USA), and rabbit anti-phospho-Insulin Receptor Substrate-1 (pTyr612) antibody (1:10, Sigma). Coverslips were washed in PBS three times for 5 min in PBS and incubated in the fluorophore-conjugated secondary antibodies anti-goat, anti-chicken, secondary antibody Alexa fluor 647, anti-rabbit Alexa fluor 350, and anti-mouse Alexa Fluor 488 (1:10, Invitrogen) for 60 min. Samples were then washed in PBS three times for 5 min and mounted in Vectashield (Vector Laboratories). Images were taken with a Nikon Eclipse Ti2 microscope.

2.10. Statistical Analysis

Statistical analysis was carried out using the SPSS Statistics 27 (IBM Company, Chicago, IL, USA) and GraphPad Prism vs 8 software (GraphPad Software, San Diego, CA, USA) packages. Experiments were carried out in replications up to n = 5–10 for certain experiments. The data obtained were checked for normality of distribution using the Kolmogorov–Smirnov test. Data with normal distribution were analyzed using parametric tests, while non-parametric tests were used for non-normally distributed data. For multiple comparisons, analysis of variance (ANOVA) with post-hoc analysis was performed for normally distributed data. For non-normally distributed data, the Kruskal–Wallis test, and, upon significance, pairwise comparison with the Mann–Whitney U tests were carried out. Pairwise comparisons of normally distributed data were carried out using independent samples *t*-tests. If the control was set to 100% and different experimental setting were compared to that (e.g., Figures 3–5), a one-sample *t*-test was used.

3. Results

3.1. Ortho- and Meta-Tyrosine Inhibit Insulin-Induced Glucose Uptake

We first tested the glucose uptake of differentiated 3T3-L1 cells in the absence and presence of o-Tyr and m-Tyr in culture media containing normal or high concentrations of glucose. In cells grown on p-Tyr containing cell culture media, increasing concentrations of insulin led to a marked increase in glucose uptake in 5 mmol/L glucose, but not in 25 mmol/L glucose. Similarly to the high glucose environment, in cells grown in media supplemented with o- and m-Tyr increasing concentrations of insulin failed to induce the glucose uptake under normal (5 mmol/L) glucose concentrations (Figure 3).

The inhibitory effect of o- and m-Tyr was also tested for zero time-dependence (Figure 4). While in cells grown on p-Tyr insulin led to an approximately two-fold increase in glucose uptake, cells grown in media supplemented with o- and m-Tyr insulin showed no significant effect, and even non-stimulated (basal) glucose uptake was lower than that of the p-Tyr control. Importantly, cells grown on o- and m-Tyr displayed similar deficiency in response to insulin under low and high glucose conditions alike, after one day or up to as long as twelve days (Figure 4).

The inhibitory effect of o-, and m-Tyr on the glucose uptake was ameliorated by increasing concentrations of p-Tyr (Figure 5).

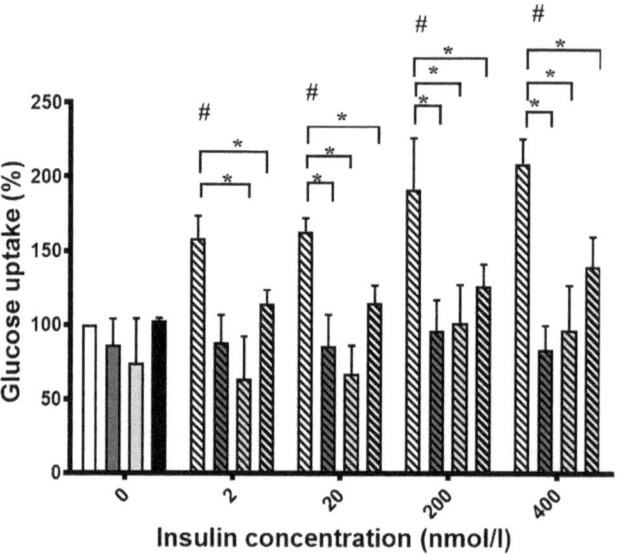

Figure 3. Insulin-dependent uptake of deoxy-D-glucose 2-[1 2-3H(N)] into differentiated 3T3-L1 adipocytes was assessed in media containing (i) para-tyrosine with 5 mmol/L glucose content (white column and first striated column in each block), (ii) meta-tyrosine with 5 mmol/L glucose (dark grey column and second striated column in each block), (iii) ortho-tyrosine with 5 mmol/L glucose (light grey column and third striated column in each block), and (iv) para-tyrosine with 25 mmol/L glucose content (black column and fourth striated column in each block). Cells were treated with 2, 20, 200, and 400 nmol/L insulin as shown (#, $p < 0.05$ vs. control para-tyrosine using one-sample t-test, *, $p < 0.05$ vs. 5 mmol/L glucose para-tyrosine using independent samples t-tests). Glucose uptake of untreated cells grown on para-tyrosine and 5 mmol/L glucose containing medium was set to 100%. Results are shown as a mean ± SEM for n = 5–10 individual measurements.

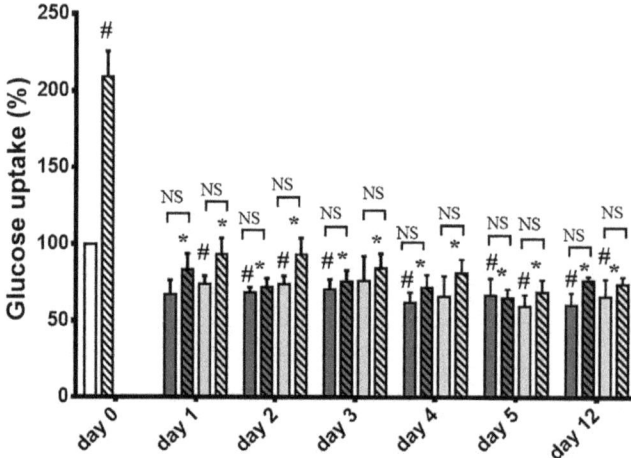

Figure 4. Insulin-dependent uptake of deoxy-D-glucose 2-[1 2-3H(N)] into 3T3-L1 adipocytes after cells were grown in media containing para-tyrosine meta-tyrosine or ortho-tyrosine for 1, 2, 3, 4, 5,

or 12 days, with or without insulin treatment (200 nmol/L). The glucose uptake of untreated adipocytes grown on 5 mmol/L glucose medium containing para-tyrosine was set to 100%. Results are shown as a mean ± SEM for n = 5–8 individual measurements. #, $p < 0.05$ vs. para-tyrosine control (one-sample t-test); *, $p < 0.05$ vs. para-tyrosine + insulin (independent samples t-test), NS: non-significant. Bars indicate para-tyrosine (white column), meta-tyrosine (dark grey columns), ortho-tyrosine (light grey columns), control (simple columns), and insulin-treated (striated columns).

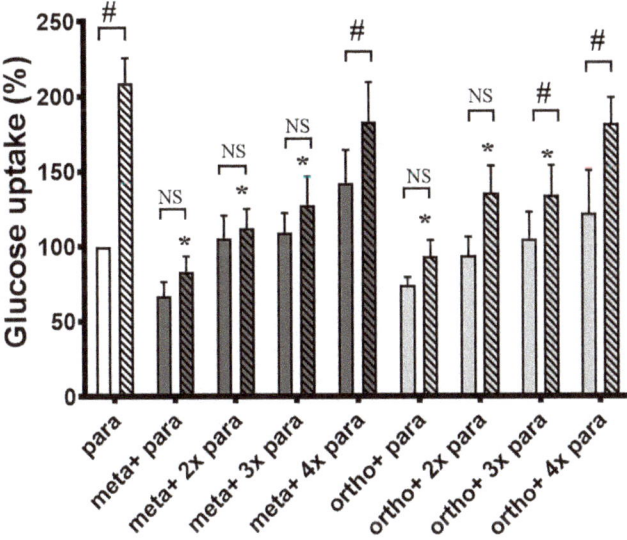

Figure 5. para-Tyr reverses the inhibitory effects of o- and m-Tyr. Examination of deoxy-D-glucose 2-[1 2-3H(N)] uptake of 3T3-L1 adipocytes depending on the ortho- and meta-tyrosine content of the medium in the absence of insulin (non-striated bars) or in the presence of 400 nmol/L insulin (corresponding striated bars). The basal glucose uptake of the cells, grown on the original 0.39 mmol/L para-tyrosine containing medium was considered to be 100%. Results are shown as mean ± SEM after n = 10 individual measurements. *, $p < 0.05$ vs. para-tyrosine + insulin (independent samples t-test), #, $p < 0.05$ vs. identical control (one sample t-test or independent samples t-test accordingly), NS: non-significant.

3.1.1. Both o- and m-Tyr Can Be Taken Up by Fat Cells within Several Minutes and Are Incorporated into Cellular Proteins

Abnormal amino acids may alter insulin signaling by incorporation into proteins, which requires the cellular uptake of these amino acids. Therefore, we tested if the abnormal amino acids could be taken up by the cells. For that reason, non-protein-bound intracellular p-Tyr content, as well as the o-Tyr/p-Tyr and m-Tyr/p-Tyr ratios were measured. We found a continuous uptake of amino acids which was independent of glucose concentration (5 or 25 mmol/L) and the presence of insulin in the medium (Figure 6).

In a long-term experiment, we tested whether o- and m-Tyr are incorporated into cellular proteins. In cells grown on o-Tyr or m-Tyr, the p-Tyr/Phe ratio showed either a decrease or remained unchanged (Figure 7A,D,G,J), while protein-bound o-Tyr/p-Tyr and m-Tyr/p-Tyr increased (Figure 7B,C,E,F,H,I,K,L).

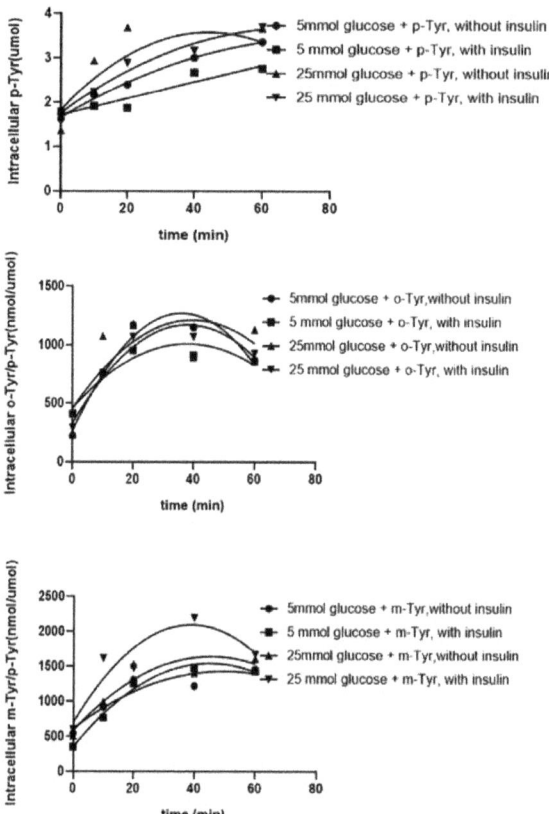

Figure 6. HPLC measurement of non-protein-bound, cytosolic, intracellular para- (upper panel), meta- (middle panel), and ortho-tyrosine (lower panel) content of 3T3-L1 adipocytes after time-dependent incubation with different tyrosines, without insulin, and after grown either in 5 mmol/L glucose containing medium or in 25 mmol/L glucose containing medium, or with insulin treatment (400 nmol/L), either in 5 mmol/L glucose containing medium or in 25 mmol/L glucose containing medium. Note that p-Tyr is shown as an absolute concentration, while o- and m-Tyr are depicted as their ratios to p-Tyr. There was no significant difference between the measurements (ANOVA).

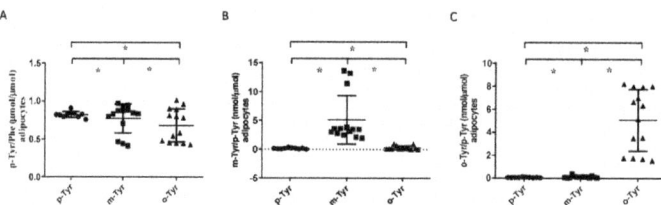

Figure 7. *Cont.*

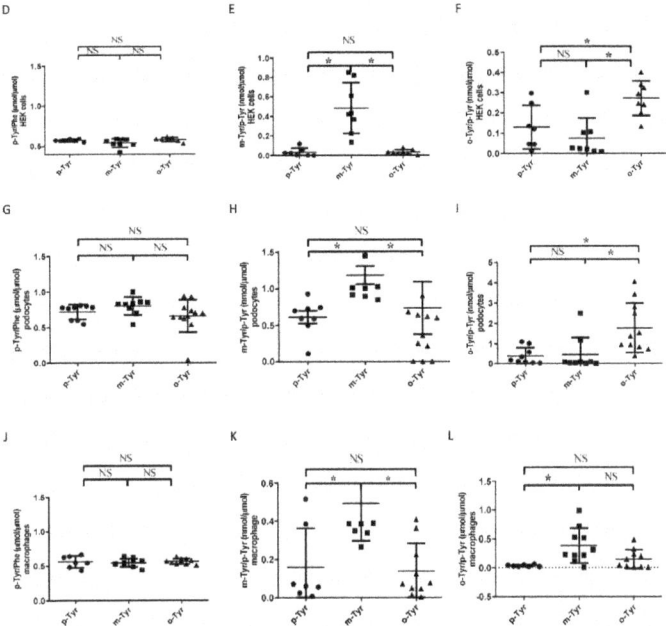

Figure 7. p-, m-, and o-Tyr content of the total proteins of cells grown in different Tyr media. HPLC measurement of protein-bound different tyrosine isomeres in cell lysates, grown in media containing para-, ortho-, or meta-tyrosine.* $p < 0.05$, NS: non-significant (using Kruskal–Wallis test for multiple comparisons and subsequently Mann–Whitney U test for pairwise comparison, as data were non-normally distributed). Results are mean ± SEM for n = 5–10 individual measurements. Note that the amount of p-Tyr is shown as p-Tyr/Phe ratio and is expressed in μmol/μmol units (panel **A,D,G,J**), while o- and m-Tyr are depicted as their ratio to p-Tyr (i.e., o-Tyr/p-Tyr and m-Tyr/p-Tyr, respectively) and the units are nmol/μmol (m-Tyr, panel **B,E,H,K**; o-Tyr, panel **C,F,I,L**).

3.1.2. Phosphorylation of IRS-1 in Cells Grown on o- or m-Tyr

In order to elucidate the mechanism underlying the inhibitory effect of o- and m-Tyr on insulin-induced glucose uptake, the phosphorylation levels of the insulin-receptor substrate-1 (IRS-1) and Akt (protein kinase B) steps of insulin signaling responsible for glucose uptake were studied. We found that in p-Tyr containing media, insulin treatment led to an approximately two-fold increase in the activating phosphorylation of IRS-1 and Akt. Interestingly, in cells grown on o- and m-Tyr containing media, the basal levels of IRS 1 and Akt phosphorylation were either unchanged or higher, which, however, could not be further raised by insulin treatment (Figure 8).

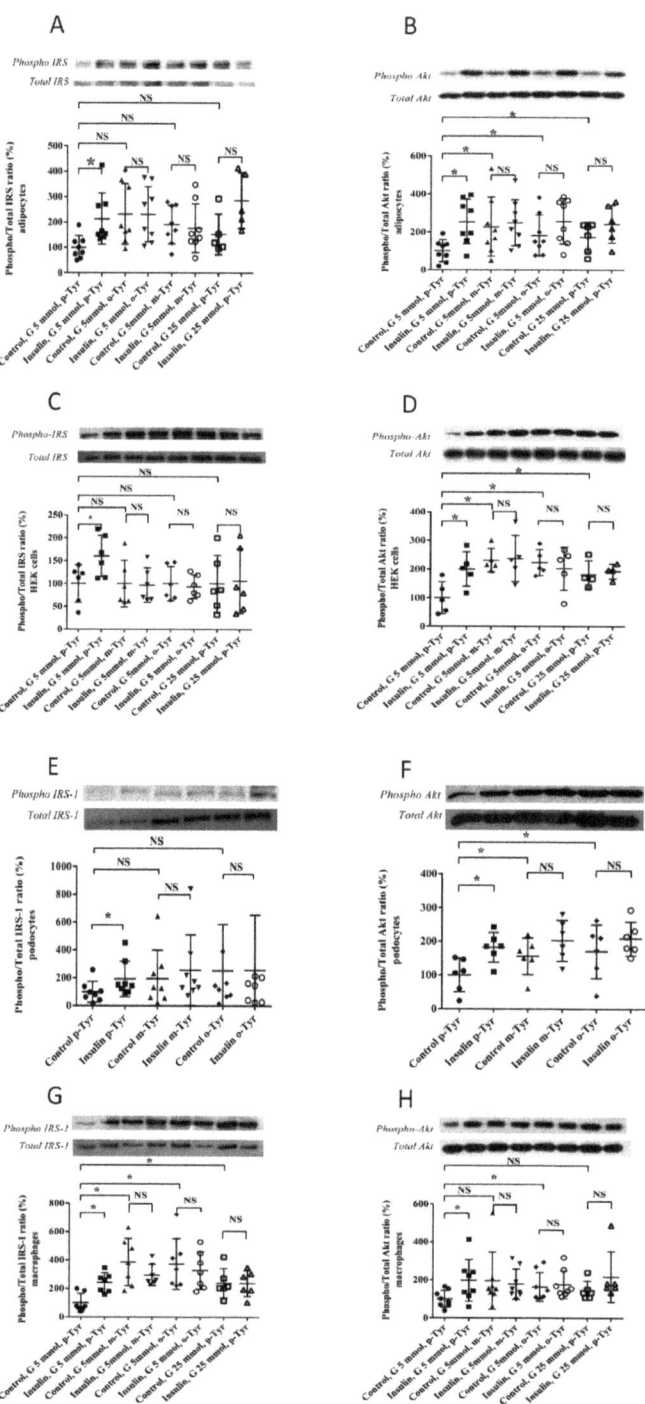

Figure 8. Western blot analysis of activating phosphorylation of IRS-1 (Tyr612, panel **A,C,E,G**) and Akt (Ser473, panel **B,D,F,H**) in the four cell lines (adipocytes, panel **A,B**; HEK cells panel **C,D**; podocytes,

E,F; macrophages, panel **G,H**). Insulin-induced phosphorylation of IRS-1 (insulin receptor substrate-1) at the tyrosine of the first YXXM motif (Tyr612) in cells grown in media containing para-, meta-, or ortho-tyrosine with and without insulin treatment (400 nmol/L). Results are mean ± SEM for n= 4–8 individual measurements. * $p < 0.05$ (for non-normally distributed data, a Kruskal–Wallis test and, upon significance, pairwise comparisons with Mann–Whitney U test were carried out. Pairwise comparisons of normally distributed data were carried out using independent samples *t*-tests).

3.2. Biochemical Characterization of IRS Peptides Containing Different Forms of Tyrosine

Insulin receptor (IR) kinase phosphorylates multiple tyrosine residues in IRS-1 and its phosphorylation plays a central role in mediating signals towards downstream targets [46]. IRS-1 binds to activated IR kinase by its phospho-tyrosine binding (PTB) domain, and its plekstrin homology (PH) domain is instrumental to its cell membrane binding. In addition, this adapter protein contains a long, disordered C-terminal tail containing six YXXM motifs phosphorylated by the IR kinase, and thus provides a versatile contact for tyrosine phosphorylation dependent recognition of multiple regulator and effector proteins involved in the insulin pathway (Figure 9A). In addition to being the major substrate sites for the IR kinase, phosphorylated YXXM motifs are dephosphorylated by protein tyrosine phosphatase 1B (PTP1B) [47]. Furthermore, phosphoinositide 3-kinase (PI3K) is recruited to the IR kinase signaling complex at the cell membrane via the Src homology 2 (SH2) domains of its p85 regulatory subunit [48].

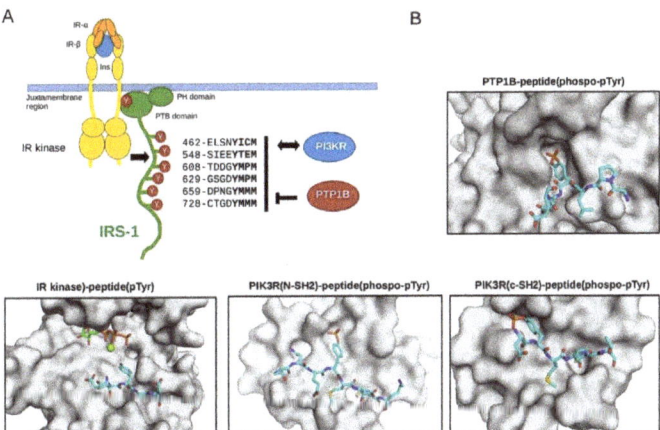

Figure 9. The role of IRS YXXM motifs in insulin mediated signaling. (**A**) Schematic of IR kinase mediated signaling: IR kinase, IRS-1 (PTB, PH domains and C-tail with YXXM motif positions and sequences indicated), PTP1B and PI3K regulatory subunits with SH2 domains. IRS-1 contains six YxxM motifs that play a central role in downstream signaling from the insulin receptor. The insulin receptor (IR)—comprised of two subunits—is dimerized upon binding to insulin (Ins). This activates the IR kinase which then creates a recruitment site in its juxtamembrane region for the PTB domain of IRS-1 by tyrosine phosphorylation. The PH domain helps recruiting IRS-1 to the cell membrane. (**B**) Crystallographic models of p-Tyr containing peptides binding to the deep substrate binding pocket of PTP1B, to the shallow substrate binding pocket of the IR kinase, and to the N-terminal SH2 domain of PI3K regulatory subunit (from left to right). IRS-1 partners are shown in surface representation, while substrate or ligand peptides from various proteins are shown with sticks. Structural figures were made by using the following protein–peptide PDB structures: 4zrt, PTP1B–Nephrin substrate phospho-peptide [49]; 3bu5, IR kinase IRS2–KRLB region peptide [50]; 2iuh, PI3KR-(N)SH2–c-Kit phospho-peptide [51]; 5aul, PI3KR-(C)SH2–CDC28 phospho-peptide [52].

In order to address the putative roles of o- and m-tyrosine incorporated into IRS-1, we studied the phosphorylation and the dephosphorylation of IRS-1 YxxM motif containing peptides by IR kinase and PTB1B, respectively. Peptides, corresponding to a fifteen amino acid long YXXM motif containing IRS1 (region 626–639) fragment, were chemically synthesized with unphosphorylated or phosphorylated p-, o- or m-tyrosines. The phosphorylation state of these peptides was examined by capillary electrophoresis in an in vitro kinetic experiment. In this assay, the electrophoretic mobility of peptides changed according to the tyrosine phosphorylation state. We found that neither o- nor m-tyrosine containing peptides are substrates for the IR kinase, while the enzyme efficiently phosphorylated the p-Tyr containing "natural" peptide (Figure 10A). Similarly, apart from the p-Tyr peptide, none of the modified Tyr containing peptides could be dephosphorylated by PTP1B (Figure 10B).

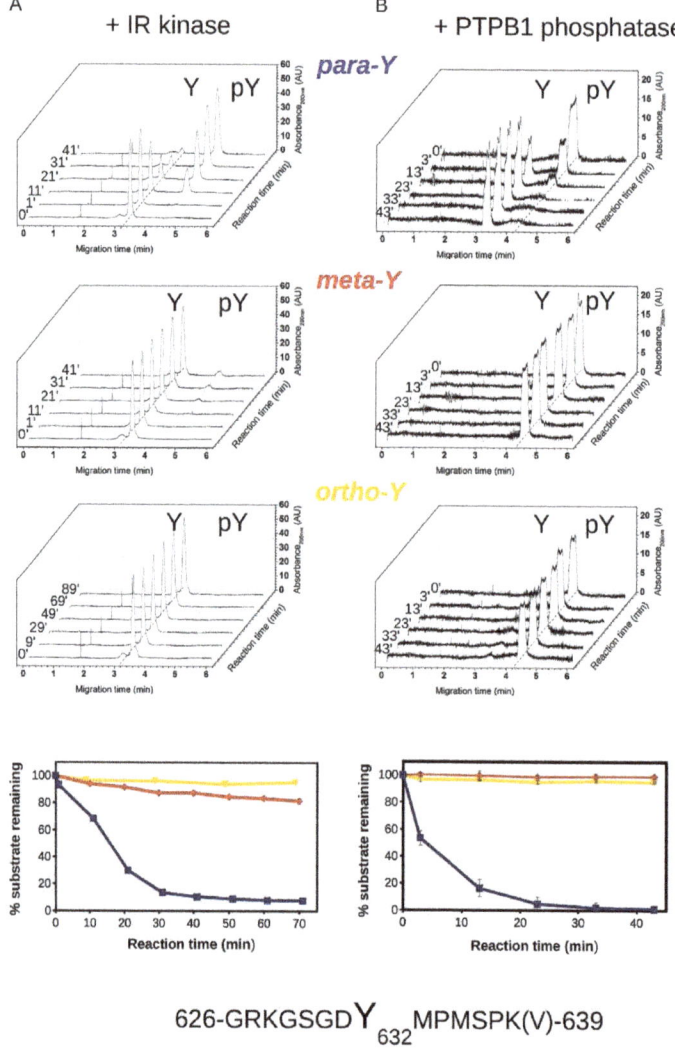

Figure 10. Phosphorylation and dephosphorylation of p-, m-, and o-Tyr containing IRS-1 peptides. (**A**) Results of in vitro kinase assays using recombinant IR kinase. Phosphorylation of IRS1 YXXM

motif containing peptides with para-, meta-, and ortho-tyrosines was analyzed by capillary electrophoresis. After starting the reactions, sample aliquots were injected to the capillary at the indicated time points. Characteristic migration times for the unphosphorylated peptide are indicated by a dashed line (~3.2 min). Notice the appearance of a slower migrating peak (at ~4.2 min) corresponding to the phosphorylated peptide in the case of the peptide with para-tyrosine. (**B**) Results of PTP1B dephosphorylation assays. Experiments were performed similarly to kinase reactions, but the substrate peptides were previously phosphorylated. Characteristic migration times for the phosphorylated peptide are indicated by a dashed line (~4.2 min). Notice the appearance of a faster migrating peak (at ~3.2 min) corresponding to the dephosphorylated peptide in the case of the peptide with para-tyrosine.

In order to study the role of o- and m-Tyr amino acid incorporation regarding other IRS-1 partner proteins relaying insulin signals, the binding capacity of para-, ortho-, and meta-tyrosine containing IRS-1 peptides to PI3K SH2 domains were also investigated (the regulatory subunit contains an N- and C-terminal SH2 domain). Using an in vitro protein-peptide binding assay, we found that o- and m-Tyr containing peptides had greatly reduced binding affinity to these SH2 domains (Figure 11). These in vitro protein–peptide binding and enzyme activity results can be structurally explained by observing the crystal structures of known protein–peptide complexes containing natural, p-Tyr, or phospho-p-Tyr possessing peptides: the topology of the binding surface on the interacting protein is only compatible with p-Tyr or phospho-p-Tyr for IR kinase or PTB1B and SH2 domains of PI3K, respectively (Figure 9B).

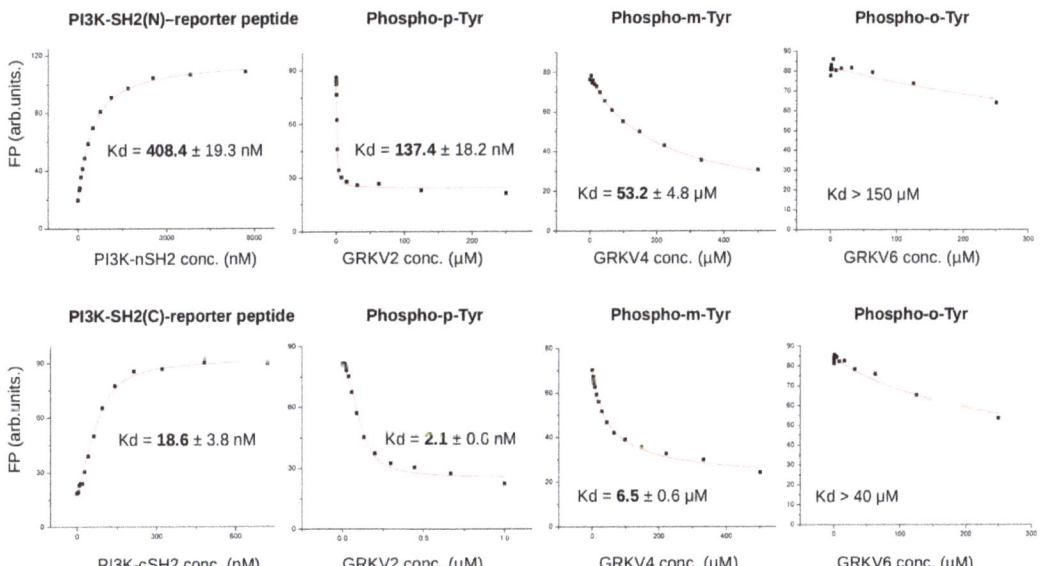

Figure 11. Binding of m- and o-Tyr IRS1 peptides to the SH2 domains of PI3K regulatory subunit. The error in the Kd values show the uncertainty of the numerical fit to the direct (**top**) and competitive (**bottom**) binding curves plotted as the mean of three technical replicates. For the GRKV6 peptide, the binding was so weak that its binding affinity could only be estimated. Please also take note that the binding affinity of the para-Tyr peptide is nanomolar (nM), while for the meta- and ortho-Tyr peptides this value is micromolar (μM), making statistical comparison unnecessary.

The panels below show that para-tyrosine containing peptides are efficiently phosphorylated and dephosphorylated by IR kinase and PTP1B, respectively, while meta- and ortho-tyrosine peptides are very poor substrates of these enzymes.

Results of the fluorescence polarization (FP)-based binding assays. To the left, the panels show the direct titration of the fluorescently labelled para-tyrosine containing phosphorylated IRS-1 peptide with the isolated N-terminal and C-terminal SH2 domains of the PI3K regulatory subunit (top and bottom, respectively). The next three panels on the right show the competitive binding curves with increasing amounts of phospho-para- (GRKV2), phospho-meta- (GRKV4), and phospho-ortho-Tyr (GRKV6) containing peptides. Notice that both modified phospho-tyrosine containing peptides (GRKV4 and 6) have greatly reduced binding affinity to the SH2 domains compared to the phospho-para-Tyr containing peptide (GRKV2). Note the change from nanomolar to micromolar binding affinity.

3.3. Microscopical Analysis

Visualization of insulin signaling is shown in Figures 12 and 13. IRS-1 phosphorylation leads to membrane translocation of this signaling protein, which is clearly demonstrated by Figure 12 in p-Tyr containing medium, but this translocation is absent in the presence of m- and o-Ty. Moreover, the intensity of p-IRS-1 is also lower in the case of m- and o-Tyr. The same membrane translocation on insulin treatment is also characteristic of GLUT-4, which is responsible for insulin dependent glucose transport. Figure 13 shows this characteristic localization of GLUT-4 positivity in the presence of p-Tyr, which is absent in samples treated with m- and o-Tyr.

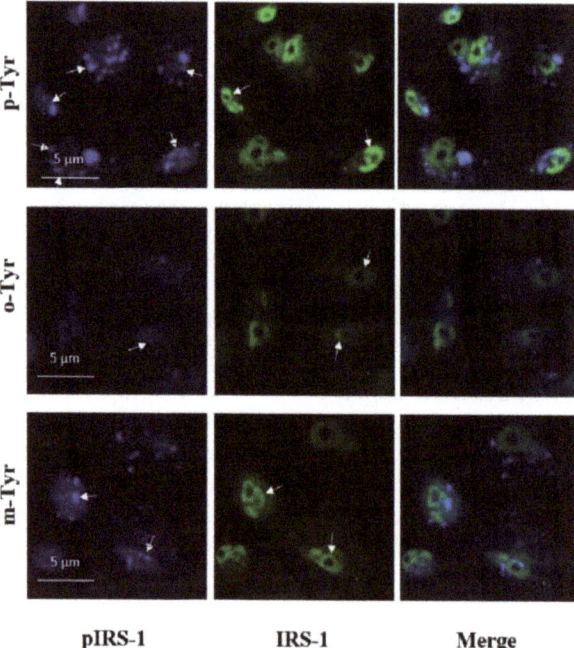

Figure 12. Immunofluorescence staining of insulin-treated podocytes for p-IRS-1 (blue) and total IRS-1 (green). p-IRS-1 (indicated by the white arrows) is located in the membrane when cells cultured in the presence of p-Tyr, which is not characteristic in cell treated with o- and m-Tyr. Moreover, p-IRS-1 is more intense in cells cultured in medium containing p-Tyr and the signal almost disappears in cells treated with o-Tyr. Total IRS-1 localization is mainly perinuclear.

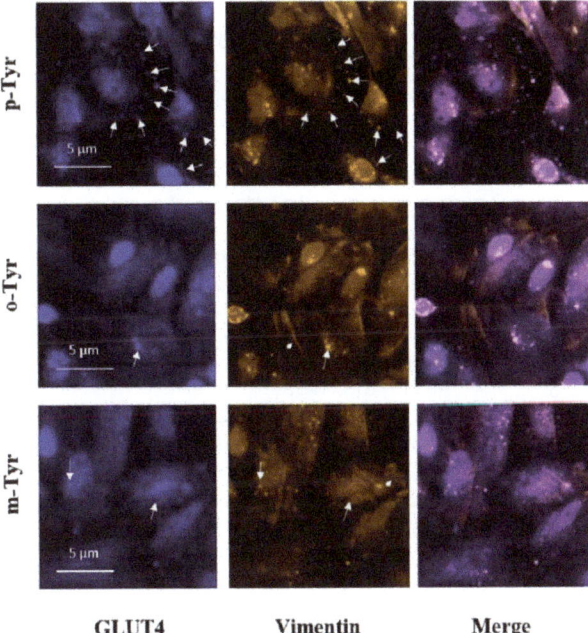

Figure 13. Immunofluorescence staining of insulin-treated podocytes for GLUT4 (blue) and vimentin (yellow). In p-Tyr-treated cells, GLUT4 aggregates are transported to the membrane. This localization is slightly visible in cells treated with m-Tyr, but it is not characteristic in o-Tyr treated cells, which shows rather a perinuclear localization. Typical localization of GLUT4 and vimentin is highlighted by the white arrows. Vimentin shows a colocalization with GLUT4. The arrowhead indicates the thicker vimentin filaments appearing in cells treated with m- and o-Tyr.

4. Discussion

In this study, we report for the first time, that the abnormal amino acids, o- and m-Tyr inhibit glucose uptake of fat cells. Furthermore, we provide evidence that insulin signaling may be altered in cells grown on media containing o- or m-Tyr. We also observed that o- and m-Tyr can be taken up by the cells and incorporates into cellular proteins.

It is suggested that there is a causal connection between oxidative stress and insulin resistance, e.g., oxidized LDL, as well as isoprostanes correlated with insulin resistance as measured by the homeostasis model assessment index (HOMAIR) [53]. On the other hand, oxidative stress has been shown to activate serine protein kinases that would interfere with insulin signaling [23]. Oxidative stress is believed to lead to the activation of inflammatory processes that could further contribute to the development of insulin resistance through inflammatory cells [4] or via activation of stress-kinases (e.g., JNK), which could lead to the serine/threonine (Ser/Thr) phosphorylation of IRS-1 and IRS-2 and in this way impair insulin signaling [54].

The abnormal amino acids o- and m-Tyr are results of the attack of hydroxyl radicals on Phe molecules or the Phe residues of proteins [55]. o- and m-Tyr are regarded as specific, stable markers of hydroxyl radicals [56], and have been detected in increasing amounts in cataract lenses [38], in urine of preterm infants [57], in Fabry's disease [58], and in cardiopulmonary bypass [59], among others. The abnormal tyrosine isomers offer the advantage of fluorescent detection without derivatization upon their autofluorescence [60].

Our data suggest that while in cells grown on p-Tyr containing culture medium, insulin is able to induce glucose uptake to approximately two-fold; in cells grown on media enriched with glucose, o-, or m-Tyr, glucose uptake is similarly blunted. The effects can already be observed after a single day, and last at for least up to 12 days. These observations prompt for a direct role of o- and m-Tyr, and not the role of oxidative stress itself, as in this setting o- and m-Tyr were applied in the absence of an obvious oxidative stress.

Our present data suggest that supplementation of four different cell lines with o- or m-Tyr leads to insulin resistance in the cells, similarly to a high glucose environment. In the o- and m-Tyr grown cells, insulin failed to increase IRS-1 phosphorylation.

While insulin was able to stimulate Akt phosphorylation in p-Tyr grown cells in normal glucose media, in the presence of o- and m-Tyr, insulin was unable to exert any effect, similar to the high glucose environment.

From the insulin receptor substrate proteins, only IRS-1, but not IRS-2, was studied, and both would have an impact on Akt phosphorylation [61,62]. Furthermore, only one phosphorylation site of IRS-1 was investigated, although numerous Tyr phosphorylation sites exist [63]. Furthermore, incorporation of o- or m-Tyr into cellular proteins such as IRS-1 might alter immunologic recognition by antibodies, especially directed against phosphorylated tyrosine residues.

Moreover, other protein kinases, e.g., stress kinases (e.g., JNK) may influence insulin signaling at different levels [54,62], and hypothetically, these kinases could also be altered by the addition of o- or m-Tyr to the culture media.

Additionally, constant stimulation of insulin signaling has been shown to alter kinetics and extent of phosphorylation of IRS-1 and Akt and cause seeming disparities between them [64]. Nevertheless, the results of Akt phosphorylation and glucose uptake match each other well, indicating the development of insulin resistance at both levels upon o- or m-Tyr supplementation.

Biochemical characterization of a YXXM motif containing IRS1 peptide demonstrated that the position of the phosphorylatable hydroxyl group greatly affects its binding capacity to several IRS1 interactors (IR, PTP1B and PI3K-SH2). These interactors have binding grooves with distinct binding surface topographies varying from shallow (IR) to deep (PTP1B), but o- and m-Tyr were deleterious for binding in each case. This indicates that incorporation of these phenylalanine oxidization by-products into signaling proteins will greatly perturb network output and behavior because of the fundamentally altered protein–protein binding capacity of their components.

Altogether, we present a rather indirect connection between the incorporation of o-and m-Tyr into proteins and their effect on insulin signaling. Unfortunately, to date, there are no commercially available antibodies raised against o- and m-Tyr or o- and m-Tyr containing proteins. Moreover, the lack of isotope-labelled o- or m-Tyr precluded providing a more direct link. For the same reason, the incorporation of o- or m-Tyr into specific proteins, such as the insulin receptor IRS-1 or other signaling molecules, cannot be demonstrated. Furthermore, 3T3-L1 cells are not real fat cells, but fat cell-like cells; however, they provide a widely accepted model to study insulin signaling in fatty tissue.

In spite of these shortcomings, our study does suggest that o- and m-Tyr would be able to incorporate into cellular proteins in fat cells. Moreover, our results are consistent with a model in which these incorporated amino acids interfere with insulin signaling and inhibit insulin-stimulated glucose uptake, i.e., they induce metabolic insulin resistance in the cells, just like under hyperglycemic circumstances (Figure 14).

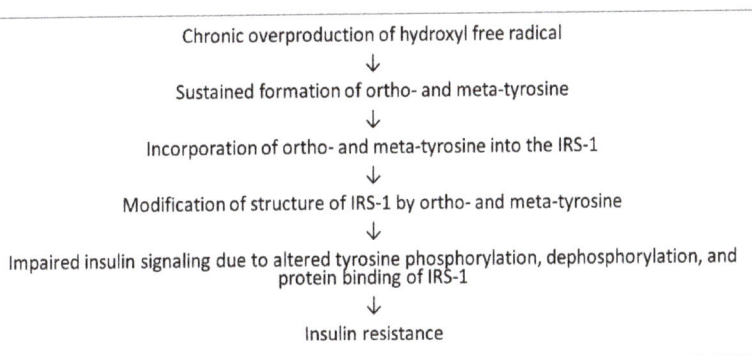

Figure 14. Suggested role of o- and m-Tyr in the development of insulin resistance.

These results are in line with our previous observations regarding vascular insulin resistance [65], vascular liraglutide resistance [66], and EPO resistance [43], and suggest a potentially more universal role of o- and m-Tyr in the development of hormone resistances in conditions with high oxidative stress.

Author Contributions: Conceptualization: I.W., methodology: M.P., B.L., T.V., K.N. and O.C.; software: M.K. and G.A.M.; validation: I.W., G.K.T., A.R. and C.H.; formal analysis: J.M.-C., M.K., K.N. and O.C.; investigation: J.M.-C., M.K., M.P., K.N. and O.C.; resources: I.W.; data curation: J.M.-C., G.K.T., A.R. and I.W. writing—original draft preparation: J.M.-C., G.A.M., G.K.T., A.R. and I.W.; writing—review and editing: G.K.T., A.R. and I.W.; visualization: J.M.-C., T.V. and M.K.; supervision: B.L., G.K.T., A.R. and I.W.; project administration: J.M.-C.; funding acquisition: I.W., A.R. and G.K.T. All authors have read and agreed to the published version of the manuscript.

Funding: This work was supported by the National Research Development and Innovation Office (NKFIH) grant (KKP 126963 awarded to AR) and VEKOP-2.3.3-15-2016-00011 and TKP2021-EGA-32 (GKT).

Institutional Review Board Statement: Not applicable.

Informed Consent Statement: Not applicable.

Data Availability Statement: Data presented in this study are available on request from the corresponding author.

Acknowledgments: The authors would like to thank József Andor for revision of language and style, András Perczel for his scientific suggestions, Enikő Bodor for technical assistance, and András Zeke for his help in protein production and purification.

Conflicts of Interest: The authors declare no conflict of interest. The funders had no role in the design of the study; in the collection, analyses, or interpretation of data; in the writing of the manuscript, or in the decision to publish the results.

References

1. De Fronzo, R.A. From the triumvirate to the ominous octet: A new paradigm for the treatment of type 2 diabetes mellitus. *Diabetes* **2009**, *58*, 773–795. [CrossRef] [PubMed]
2. Schwartz, S.S.; Epstein, S.; Corkey, B.E.; Grant, S.F.A.; Gavin, J.R.; Aguilar, R.B. The time is right for a new classification system for diabetes: Rationale and implications of the beta-cell-centric classification schema. *Diabetes Care* **2016**, *39*, 179–186. [CrossRef] [PubMed]
3. Khan, A.H.; Pessin, J.E. Insulin regulation of glucose uptake: A complex interplay of intracellular signalling pathways. *Diabetologia* **2002**, *45*, 1475–1483. [CrossRef] [PubMed]
4. Tangvarasittichai, S. Oxidative stress, insulin resistance, dyslipidemia and type 2 diabetes mellitus. *World J. Diabetes* **2015**, *6*, 456–480. [CrossRef] [PubMed]
5. Galiero, R.; Caturano, A.; Vetrano, E.; Cesaro, A.; Rinaldi, L.; Salvatore, T.; Marfella, R.; Sardu, C.; Moscarella, E.; Gragnano, F.; et al. Pathophysiological mechanisms and clinical evidence of relationship between Nonalcoholic fatty liver disease (NAFLD) and cardiovascular disease. *Rev. Cardiovasc. Med.* **2021**, *22*, 755–768. [CrossRef]

6. Houstis, N.; Rosen, E.D.; Lander, E.S. Reactive oxygen species have a causal role in multiple forms of insulin resistance. *Nature* **2006**, *440*, 944–948. [CrossRef]
7. Akbari, M.; Ostadmohammadi, V.; Lankarani, K.B.; Tabrizi, R.; Kolahdooz, F.; Khatibi, S.R.; Asemi, Z. The effects of alpha-lipoic acid supplementation on glucose control and lipid profiles among patients with metabolic diseases: A systematic review and meta-analysis of randomized controlled trials. *Metabolism* **2018**, *87*, 56–69. [CrossRef]
8. Garvey, W.T.; Olefsky, J.M.; Griffin, J.; Hamman, R.F.; Kolterman, O.G. The effect of insulin treatment on insulin secretion and insulin action in type, I.I.; diabetes mellitus. *Diabetes* **1985**, *34*, 222–234. [CrossRef]
9. Weng, J.; Li, Y.; Xu, W.; Shi, L.; Zhang, Q.; Zhu, D.; Hu, Y.; Zhou, Z.; Yan, X.; Tian, H.; et al. Effect of intensive insulin therapy on beta-cell function and glycaemic control in patients with newly diagnosed type 2 diabetes: A multicentre randomised parallel-group trial. *Lancet* **2008**, *371*, 1753–1760. [CrossRef]
10. Vlassara, H.; Cai, W.; Tripp, E.; Pyzik, R.; Yee, K.; Goldberg, L.; Tansman, L.; Chen, X.; Mani, V.; Fayad, Z.A.; et al. Oral AGE restriction ameliorates insulin resistance in obese individuals with the metabolic syndrome: A randomised controlled trial. *Diabetologia* **2016**, *59*, 2181–2192. [CrossRef]
11. Brownlee, M. Biochemistry and molecular cell biology of diabetic complications. *Nature* **2001**, *414*, 813–820. [CrossRef]
12. Pereira, S.; Park, E.; Mori, Y.; Haber, C.A.; Han, P.; Uchida, T.; Stavar, L.; Oprescu, A.I.; Koulajian, K.; Ivovic, A.; et al. FFA-induced hepatic insulin resistance in vivo is mediated by, P.K.;Cδ, NADPH oxidase, and oxidative stress. *Am. J. Physiol. Endocrinol. Metab.* **2014**, *307*, E34–E46. [CrossRef]
13. Li, H.; Lee, J.; He, C.; Zou, M.-H.; Xie, Z. Suppression of the mTORC1/STAT3/Notch1 pathway by activated, A.M.;PK prevents hepatic insulin resistance induced by excess amino acids. *Am. J. Physiol. Metab.* **2014**, *306*, E197–E209. [CrossRef]
14. Gu, C.; Shi, Y.; Le, G. Effect of dietary protein level and origin on the redox status in the digestive tract of mice. *Int. J. Mol. Sci.* **2008**, *9*, 464–475. [CrossRef]
15. Alwahsh, S.M.; Xu, M.; Schultze, F.C.; Wilting, J.; Mihm, S.; Raddatz, D.; Ramadori, G. Combination of alcohol and fructose exacerbates metabolic imbalance in terms of hepatic damage, dyslipidemia, and insulin resistance in rats. *PLoS ONE* **2014**, *9*, e104220. [CrossRef]
16. Wlazlo, N.; van Greevenbroek, M.M.; Ferreira, I.; Jansen, E.H.; Feskens, E.J.; van der Kallen, C.J.; Schalkwijk, C.G.; Bravenboer, B.; Stehouwer, C.D. Iron metabolism is associated with adipocyte insulin resistance and plasma adiponectin: The Cohort on Diabetes and Atherosclerosis Maastricht (CODAM) study. *Diabetes Care* **2013**, *36*, 309–315. [CrossRef] [PubMed]
17. Messner, D.J.; Rhieu, B.H.; Kowdley, K.V. Iron Overload Causes Oxidative Stress and Impaired Insulin Signaling in AML-12 Hepatocytes. *Am. J. Dig. Dis.* **2013**, *58*, 1899–1908. [CrossRef]
18. Bastard, J.P.; Maachi, M.; Lagathu, C.; Kim, M.J.; Caron, M.; Vidal, H.; Capeau, J.; Feve, B. Recent advances in the relationship between obesity, inflammation, and insulin resistance. *Eur. Cytokine Netw.* **2006**, *17*, 4–12.
19. Qamirani, E.; Ren, Y.; Kuo, L.; Hein, T.W. C-reactive protein inhibits endothelium-dependent, N.O.;-mediated dilation in coronary arterioles by activating p38 kinase and, N.A.;D(P)H oxidase. *Arter. Thromb. Vasc. Biol.* **2005**, *25*, 995–1001. [CrossRef] [PubMed]
20. Piya, M.K.; McTernan, P.G.; Kumar, S. Adipokine inflammation and insulin resistance: The role of glucose, lipids and endotoxin. *J. Endocrinol.* **2013**, *216*, T1–T15. [CrossRef]
21. Raghuraman, G.; Zuniga, M.C.; Yuan, H.; Zhou, W. PKCε mediates resistin-induced, N.A.;DPH oxidase activation and inflammation leading to smooth muscle cell dysfunction and intimal hyperplasia. *Atherosclerosis* **2016**, *253*, 29–37. [CrossRef] [PubMed]
22. Peng, H.; Li, W.; Seth, D.M.; Nair, A.R.; Francis, J.; Feng, Y. (Pro)renin receptor mediates both angiotensin, I.I.;-dependent and -independent oxidative stress in neuronal cells. *PLoS ONE* **2013**, *8*, e58339. [CrossRef]
23. Habibi, J.; Whaley-Connell, A.; Hayden, M.R.; DeMarco, V.; Schneider, R.; Sowers, S.D.; Karuparthi, P.; Ferrario, C.M.; Sowers, J.R. Renin inhibition attenuates insulin resistance, oxidative stress, and pancreatic remodeling in the transgenic Ren2 rat. *Endocrinology* **2008**, *149*, 5643–5653. [CrossRef] [PubMed]
24. Henriksen, E.J.; Diamond-Stanic, M.K.; Marchionne, E.M. Oxidative stress and the etiology of insulin resistance and type 2 diabetes. *Free Radic. Biol. Med.* **2011**, *51*, 993–999. [CrossRef] [PubMed]
25. Whaley-Connell, A.; Sowers, J.R. Oxidative stress in the cardiorenal metabolic syndrome. *Curr. Hypertens. Rep.* **2012**, *14*, 360–365. [CrossRef]
26. Ishibashi, K.I.; Imamura, T.; Sharma, P.M.; Huang, J.; Ugi, S.; Olefsky, J.M. Chronic endothelin-1 treatment leads to heterologous desensitization of insulin signaling in 3T3-L1 adipocytes. *J. Clin. Investig.* **2001**, *107*, 1193–1202. [CrossRef]
27. Häring, H.; Kirsch, D.; Obermaier, B.; Ermel, B.; Machicao, F. Decreased tyrosine kinase activity of insulin receptor isolated from rat adipocytes rendered insulin-resistant by catecholamine treatment in vitro. *Biochem. J.* **1986**, *234*, 59–66. [CrossRef] [PubMed]
28. Bleeke, T.; Zhang, H.; Madamanchi, N.; Patterson, C.; Faber, J.E. Catecholamine-induced vascular wall growth is dependent on generation of reactive oxygen species. *Circ. Res.* **2004**, *94*, 37–45. [CrossRef] [PubMed]
29. Chen, G.; Raman, P.; Bhonagiri, P.; Strawbridge, A.B.; Pattar, G.R.; Elmendorf, J.S. Protective Effect of Phosphatidylinositol 4,5-Bisphosphate against Cortical Filamentous Actin Loss and Insulin Resistance Induced by Sustained Exposure of 3T3-L1 Adipocytes to Insulin. *J. Biol. Chem.* **2004**, *279*, 39705–39709. [CrossRef] [PubMed]
30. Catalano, K.J.; Maddux, B.A.; Szary, J.; Youngren, J.F.; Goldfine, I.D.; Schaufele, F. Insulin resistance induced by hyperinsulinemia coincides with a persistent alteration at the insulin receptor tyrosine kinase domain. *PLoS ONE* **2014**, *9*, e108693. [CrossRef] [PubMed]

31. Goldstein, B.J.; Mahadev, K.; Wu, X.; Zhu, L.; Motoshima, H. Role of Insulin-Induced Reactive Oxygen Species in the Insulin Signaling Pathway. *Antioxidants Redox Signal.* **2005**, *7*, 1021–1031. [CrossRef]
32. Kain, V.; Kapadia, B.; Misra, P.; Saxena, U. Simvastatin may induce insulin resistance through a novel fatty acid mediated cholesterol independent mechanism. *Sci. Rep.* **2015**, *5*, srep13823. [CrossRef] [PubMed]
33. Olea, E.; Agapito, M.T.; Gallego-Martin, T.; Rocher, A.; Gomez-Niño, A.; Obeso, A.; Gonzalez, C.; Yubero, S. Intermittent hypoxia and diet-induced obesity: Effects on oxidative status, sympathetic tone, plasma glucose and insulin levels, and arterial pressure. *J. Appl. Physiol.* **2014**, *117*, 706–719. [CrossRef] [PubMed]
34. Thannickal, V.J.; Fanburg, B.L. Reactive oxygen species in cell signaling. *Am. J. Physiol. Cell. Mol. Physiol.* **2000**, *279*, L1005–L1028. [CrossRef] [PubMed]
35. Lerner, A.B. On the metabolism of phenylalanine and tyrosine. *J. Biol. Chem.* **1949**, *181*, 281–294. [CrossRef]
36. Molnár, G.A.; Kun, S.; Sélley, E.; Kertész, M.; Szélig, L.; Csontos, C.; Böddi, K.; Bogár, L.; Miseta, A. Role of tyrosine isomers in acute and chronic diseases leading to oxidative stress-A Review. *Curr. Med. Chem.* **2016**, *23*, 667–685. [CrossRef]
37. Pennathur, S.; Wagner, J.D.; Leeuwenburgh, C.; Litwak, K.N.; Heinecke, J.W. A hydroxyl radical-like species oxidizes cynomolgus monkey artery wall proteins in early diabetic vascular disease. *J. Clin. Investig.* **2001**, *107*, 853–860. [CrossRef] [PubMed]
38. Fu, S.; Dean, R.T.; Southan, M.; Truscott, R. The hydroxyl radical in lens nuclear cataractogenesis. *J. Biol. Chem.* **1998**, *273*, 28603–28609. [CrossRef] [PubMed]
39. Molnár, G.A.; Wagner, Z.; Markó, L.; Kőszegi, T.; Mohás, M.; Kocsis, B.; Matus, Z.; Wagner, L.; Tamaskó, M.; Mazák, I.; et al. Urinary ortho-tyrosine excretion in diabetes mellitus and renal failure: Evidence for hydroxyl radical production. *Kidney Int.* **2005**, *68*, 2281–2287. [CrossRef]
40. Brasnyó, P.; Molnar, G.A.; Mohás, M.; Markó, L.; Laczy, B.; Cseh, J.; Mikolás, E.; Szijártó, I.A.; Mérei, A.; Halmai, R.; et al. Resveratrol improves insulin sensitivity, reduces oxidative stress and activates the Akt pathway in type 2 diabetic patients. *Br. J. Nutr.* **2011**, *106*, 383–389. [CrossRef] [PubMed]
41. Duke, S.O. The emergence of grass root chemical ecology. *Proc. Natl. Acad. Sci. USA* **2007**, *104*, 16729–16730. [CrossRef] [PubMed]
42. Ruggiero, R.A.; Bruzzo, J.; Chiarella, P.; Di Gianni, P.; Isturiz, M.A.; Linskens, S.; Speziale, N.; Meiss, R.P.; Bustuoabad, O.D.; Pasqualini, C.D. Tyrosine isomers mediate the classical phenomenon of concomitant tumor resistance. *Cancer Res.* **2011**, *71*, 7113–7124. [CrossRef] [PubMed]
43. Mikolás, E.; Kun, S.; Laczy, B.; Molnár, G.A.; Sélley, E.; Wittmann, I.; Koszegi, T. Incorporation of ortho- and meta-tyrosine into cellular proteins leads to erythropoietin-resistance in an erythroid cell line. *Kidney Blood Press. Res.* **2013**, *38*, 217–225. [CrossRef] [PubMed]
44. Kaddai, V.; Gonzalez, T.; Keslair, F.; Grémeaux, T.; Bonnafous, S.; Gugenheim, J.; Tran, A.; Gual, P.; Le Marchand-Brustel, Y.; Cormont, M. Rab4b is a small, G.T.;Pase involved in the control of the glucose transporter, G.L.;UT4 localization in adipocyte. *PLoS ONE* **2009**, *4*, e5257. [CrossRef] [PubMed]
45. Schiwek, D.; Endlich, N.; Holzman, L.; Holthöfer, H.; Kriz, W.; Endlich, K. Stable expression of nephrin and localization to cell-cell contacts in novel murine podocyte cell lines. *Kidney Int.* **2004**, *66*, 91–101. [CrossRef]
46. Shoelson, S.E.; Chatterjee, S.; Chaudhuri, M.; White, M.F. YMXM motifs of, I.R.;S-1 define substrate specificity of the insulin receptor kinase. *Proc. Natl. Acad. Sci. USA* **1992**, *89*, 2027–2031. [CrossRef] [PubMed]
47. Goldstein, B.J.; Bittner-Kowalczyk, A.; White, M.F.; Harbeck, M. Tyrosine dephosphorylation and deactivation of insulin receptor substrate-1 by protein-tyrosine phosphatase 1B. Possible facilitation by the formation of a ternary complex with the Grb2 adaptor protein. *J. Biol. Chem.* **2000**, *275*, 4283–4289. [CrossRef]
48. Sánchez-Margalet, V.; Goldfine, I.D.; Truitt, K.; Imboden, J.; Sung, C.K. Role of p85 subunit of phosphatidylinositol-3-kinase as an adaptor molecule linking the insulin receptor to insulin receptor substrate 1. *Mol. Endocrinol.* **1995**, *9*, 435–442. [CrossRef]
49. Selner, N.G.; Luechapanichkul, R.; Chen, X.; Neel, B.G.; Zhang, Z.Y.; Knapp, S.; Bell, C.E.; Pei, D. Diverse levels of sequence selectivity and catalytic efficiency of protein-tyrosine phosphatases. *Biochemistry* **2014**, *53*, 397–412. [CrossRef] [PubMed]
50. Wu, J.; Tseng, Y.D.; Xu, C.F.; Neubert, T.A.; White, M.F.; Hubbard, S.R. Structural and biochemical characterization of the KRLB region in insulin receptor substrate-2. *Nat. Struct. Mol. Biol.* **2008**, *15*, 251–258. [CrossRef] [PubMed]
51. Nolte, R.T.; Eck, M.J.; Schlessinger, J.; Shoelson, S.E.; Harrison, S.C. Crystal structure of the, P.I.; 3-kinase p85 amino-terminal, S.H.;2 domain and its phosphopeptide complexes. *Nat. Struct. Mol. Biol.* **1996**, *3*, 364–374. [CrossRef] [PubMed]
52. Inaba, S.; Numoto, N.; Ogawa, S.; Morii, H.; Ikura, T.; Abe, R.; Ito, N.; Oda, M. Crystal Structures and Thermodynamic Analysis Reveal Distinct Mechanisms of CD28 Phosphopeptide Binding to the Src Homology 2 (SH2) Domains of Three Adaptor Proteins. *J. Biol. Chem.* **2017**, *292*, 1052–1060. [CrossRef] [PubMed]
53. Park, K.; Gross, M.; Lee, D.H.; Holvoet, P.; Himes, J.H.; Shikany, J.M.; Jacobs, D.R. Oxidative stress and insulin resistance: The coronary artery risk development in young adults study. *Diabetes Care* **2009**, *32*, 1302–1307. [CrossRef] [PubMed]
54. Solinas, G.; Karin, M. JNK1 and IKKβ: Molecular links between obesity and metabolic dysfunction. *FASEB J.* **2010**, *24*, 2596–2611. [CrossRef] [PubMed]
55. Sitte, N. Oxidative damage to proteins. In *Ageing at the Molecular Level*; von Thomas, Z., Ed.; Springer: Dordrecht, The Netherlands, 2003; pp. 27–45.
56. Torres-Cuevas, I.; Kuligowski, J.; Escobar, J.; Vento, M. Determination of biomarkers of protein oxidation in tissue and plasma. *Free Radic. Biol. Med.* **2014**, *75* (Suppl. S1), S51. [CrossRef]

57. Ledo, A.; Arduini, A.; A Asensi, M.; Sastre, J.; Escrig, R.; Brugada, M.; Aguar, M.; Saenz, P.; Vento, M. Human milk enhances antioxidant defenses against hydroxyl radical aggression in preterm infants. *Am. J. Clin. Nutr.* **2008**, *89*, 210–215. [CrossRef] [PubMed]
58. Shu, L.; Park, J.L.; Byun, J.; Pennathur, S.; Kollmeyer, J.; Shayman, J.A. Decreased Nitric Oxide Bioavailability in a Mouse Model of Fabry Disease. *J. Am. Soc. Nephrol.* **2009**, *20*, 1975–1985. [CrossRef] [PubMed]
59. Schultz, S.; Creed, J.; Schears, G.; Zaitseva, T.; Greeley, W.; Wilson, D.F.; Pastuszko, A. Comparison of low-flow cardiopulmonary bypass and circulatory arrest on brain oxygen and metabolism. *Ann. Thorac. Surg.* **2004**, *77*, 2138–2143. [CrossRef] [PubMed]
60. Ishimitsu, S.; Fujimoto, S.; Ohara, A. High-performance liquid chromatographic determination of m-tyrosine and o-tyrosine in rat urine. *J. Chromatogr. B Biomed. Sci. Appl.* **1989**, *489*, 377–383. [CrossRef]
61. Huang, C.; Wu, M.; Du, J.; Liu, D.; Chan, C. Systematic modeling for the insulin signaling network mediated by IRS1 and IRS2. *J. Theor. Biol.* **2014**, *355*, 40–52. [CrossRef] [PubMed]
62. Wu, M.; Yang, X.; Chan, C. A Dynamic Analysis of IRS-PKR Signaling in Liver Cells: A Discrete Modeling Approach. *PLoS ONE* **2009**, *4*, e8040. [CrossRef] [PubMed]
63. Hubbard, S.R. The insulin receptor: Both a prototypical and atypical receptor tyrosine kinase. *Cold Spring Harb. Perspect. Biol.* **2013**, *5*. [CrossRef] [PubMed]
64. Matveyenko, A.V.; Liuwantara, D.; Gurlo, T.; Kirakossian, D.; Man, C.D.; Cobelli, C.; White, M.F.; Copps, K.D.; Volpi, E.; Fujita, S.; et al. Pulsatile Portal Vein Insulin Delivery Enhances Hepatic Insulin Action and Signaling. *Diabetes* **2012**, *61*, 2269–2279. [CrossRef] [PubMed]
65. Szijártó, I.A.; Molnár, G.A.; Mikolás, E.; Fisi, V.; Cseh, J.; Laczy, B.; Kovács, T.; Böddi, K.; Takátsy, A.; Gollasch, M.; et al. Elevated Vascular Level of ortho-Tyrosine Contributes to the Impairment of Insulin-Induced Arterial Relaxation. *Horm. Metab. Res.* **2014**, *46*, 749–752. [CrossRef] [PubMed]
66. Selley, E.; Kun, S.; Kürthy, M.; Kovacs, T.; Wittmann, I.; Molnar, G. Para-Tyrosine Supplementation Improves Insulin- and Liraglutide- Induced Vasorelaxation in Cholesterol-Fed Rats. *Protein Pept. Lett.* **2015**, *22*, 736–742. [CrossRef] [PubMed]

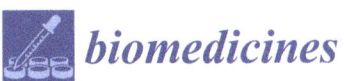

Article

Placental Insulin Receptor Transiently Regulates Glucose Homeostasis in the Adult Mouse Offspring of Multiparous Dams

Grace Chung, Ramkumar Mohan, Megan Beetch, Seokwon Jo and Emilyn Uy Alejandro *

Department of Integrative Biology and Physiology, University of Minnesota Medical School, University of Minnesota, Minneapolis, MN 55455, USA; chung491@umn.edu (G.C.); rammohan@med.umich.edu (R.M.); beet0013@umn.edu (M.B.); joxxx057@umn.edu (S.J.)
* Correspondence: ealejand@umn.edu

Abstract: In pregnancies complicated by maternal obesity and gestational diabetes mellitus, there is strong evidence to suggest that the insulin signaling pathway in the placenta may be impaired. This may have potential effects on the programming of the metabolic health in the offspring; however, a direct link between the placental insulin signaling pathway and the offspring health remains unknown. Here, we aimed to understand whether specific placental loss of the insulin receptor (InsR) has a lasting effect on the offspring health in mice. Obesity and glucose homeostasis were assessed in the adult mouse offspring on a normal chow diet (NCD) followed by a high-fat diet (HFD) challenge. Compared to their littermate controls, InsR KO^{placenta} offspring were born with normal body weight and pancreatic β-cell mass. Adult InsR KO^{placenta} mice exhibited normal glucose homeostasis on an NCD. Interestingly, under a HFD challenge, adult male InsR KO^{placenta} offspring demonstrated lower body weight and a mildly improved glucose homeostasis associated with parity. Together, our data show that placenta-specific insulin receptor deletion does not adversely affect offspring glucose homeostasis during adulthood. Rather, there may potentially be a mild and transient protective effect in the mouse offspring of multiparous dams under the condition of a diet-induced obesogenic challenge.

Keywords: placental insulin receptor; gestational diabetes; fetal programming; multiparity; obesity; type 2 diabetes

Citation: Chung, G.; Mohan, R.; Beetch, M.; Jo, S.; Alejandro, E.U. Placental Insulin Receptor Transiently Regulates Glucose Homeostasis in the Adult Mouse Offspring of Multiparous Dams. *Biomedicines* 2022, 10, 575. https://doi.org/10.3390/biomedicines10030575

Academic Editor: Maria Grau

Received: 3 February 2022
Accepted: 27 February 2022
Published: 1 March 2022

Publisher's Note: MDPI stays neutral with regard to jurisdictional claims in published maps and institutional affiliations.

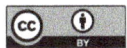

Copyright: © 2022 by the authors. Licensee MDPI, Basel, Switzerland. This article is an open access article distributed under the terms and conditions of the Creative Commons Attribution (CC BY) license (https://creativecommons.org/licenses/by/4.0/).

1. Introduction

The growing prevalence of obesity and diabetes in pregnant women and women of reproductive age have become major concerns in women's health, with over 60% of women of reproductive age being obese or overweight and an increasing number of pregnancies complicated by gestational diabetes mellitus (GDM) [1–4]. Maternal obesity and diabetes during pregnancy are associated with short- and long-term adverse pregnancy complications for both the mother and the baby [5–10]. Exposure to maternal obesity or diabetes in utero is associated with an increased risk for child and adult obesity, type 2 diabetes (T2D), cardiovascular disease, and neurodevelopmental disorders in the offspring [7,11–15]. Thus, maternal obesity and diabetes during pregnancy are important considerations in the programming of the metabolic health in the offspring and may have intergenerational effects, further perpetuating the vicious cycle of obesity and diabetes [9,16]. An important risk factor of maternal obesity is multiparity, which exacerbates gestational weight gain, inflammation, and risk of adverse metabolic outcomes in the offspring [17–19].

The placenta is critical for the development and growth of the fetus, and evidence suggests that the placenta plays an important role in the long-term health of the offspring [20–25]. Insulin is an important growth factor and regulates placental and fetal growth, nutrient transfer, and hormone secretion [26–28]. In early pregnancy, maternal insulin response has been associated with placental weight at birth, which has been associated with neonatal birth weight and adiposity at term [27]. In pregnancies complicated by maternal obesity and GDM, there is evidence to suggest that the insulin signaling pathway in the placenta may be impaired and may contribute to changes in the metabolic programming of the offspring [26,28–32]. However, a direct link between the placental insulin signaling pathway and the metabolic health of the offspring remains unknown.

Despite strict glycemic control in the modern clinical management of pregnant women with prediabetes and GDM, fetal overgrowth remains an important clinical problem [33]. Further, insulin therapy during pregnancy is potentially associated with a risk of developing T2D in the offspring later in life, but it has not been investigated directly. Jansson et al. highlights the importance of placental function and the possible role of maternal insulin [34]. Therefore, a greater understanding of the programming impact of maternal insulin on the metabolic health of the offspring will be significant in illuminating the effects of insulin therapy on the children of women with GDM, T1D, or T2D during pregnancy.

Due to the limitations of human clinical studies (i.e., ethical issues), preclinical models lend feasibility to assess how specific features of maternal health such as hyperinsulinemia contribute to the programming of the metabolic health in the offspring. Therefore, there is a need for preclinical studies to specifically assess the role of the placental insulin receptor in the metabolic health trajectory of the adult offspring.

The placental insulin receptor (InsR) impacts the nutrient flux from the mother to the fetus and may affect the developing insulin-producing β-cells, which are highly sensitive to changes in the nutrient flux in utero [35]. Moreover, the roles for maternal insulin and placental InsR in the metabolic health of the offspring are untested, and we have the state-of-the art preclinical model to address this gap in knowledge. Therefore, in the present study, we aimed to understand whether specific placental loss of the insulin receptor has a lasting effect on the fetus, altering the birthweight and the long-term metabolic health trajectory of the mouse offspring. Mice with a genetic specific deletion of the insulin receptor in the placental trophoblast (Cyp19-cre; InsR$^{f/f}$ hereinafter, referred to as InsR KO^{placenta}) were generated using the cre/loxP system described further in the Methods section [23,36–38]. Fetal and newborn body weight and pancreatic β-cell mass were assessed in littermate male and female offspring. Obesity and glucose homeostasis were assessed in the adult offspring from multiparous and non-multiparous dams on a normal chow diet (NCD), followed by a high-fat diet (HFD) challenge.

2. Materials and Methods

2.1. Generation of the Animal Mouse Model and Diet

The cre/loxP system is a novel and powerful tool to generate mice with a tissue-specific knockout of a specific gene. Under the control of the human *Cyp19* promoter, Cyp19-cre is a placenta-specific cre recombinase active in the mouse spongiotrophoblast and syncytiotrophoblast cells [38]. Cyp19-cre mice were generated and gifted by Dr. Gustavo Leone (Medical College of Wisconsin) [38]. In this present study, conditional deletion of the LoxP-flanked InsR gene in the placental trophoblast cells may allow for better understanding of how the insulin signaling pathway can affect placental and fetal development. To generate placental trophoblast-specific insulin receptor knockout mice (Cyp19-cre; InsR$^{f/f}$) and their littermate controls (InsR$^{f/f}$), floxed InsR male mice (InsR$^{f/f}$) (purchased from Jackson Laboratory, stock No. 006955) were bred with floxed InsR female mice expressing the placenta-specific Cre recombinase (Cyp19-cre; InsR$^{f/f}$). For mating, one male was placed in a cage with two females. The male was then separated while the dams were pregnant. For multiparous females, pups were born and allowed to suckle. The pups were weaned at 21–28 days postpartum, and the females were remated within 5 days of weaning, and the process repeated. The dams were allowed to give birth to up to four litters.

The placenta and the associated extraembryonic membranes are formed from the zygote at the start of each pregnancy and thus have the same genetic composition as the fetus. Therefore, the placental genotypes were determined by the offspring genotypes (whether they are control or KO), and this was done prior to weaning using standard PCR on the tissue collected on postnatal (P) day 6–8. The primers used are listed below: CYP19cre forward: GACCTTGCTGAGATTAGATC; CYP19cre reverse: GACGATGAAG-CATGTTTAGCT GGCC; InsR tm1Khn forward: GGG GCA GTG AGT ATT TTG GA; and InsR tm1Khn reverse: TGG CCGTGA AAGTTAAGAGG. Validation of the efficiency of Cre was assessed by our group and others [23,37]. All the mice were group-housed under a 14:10 light–dark cycle with ad libitum access to food. At 13 weeks of age, the mice were switched to a high-fat rodent diet with 60 kcal% fat (Research Diets, Inc., D12492) until the time of harvest. The adult offspring under a normal chow diet and a high-fat diet were from 2–3 dams. All the animal studies were performed in accordance with the University of Minnesota Institutional Animal Care and Use Committee (protocol #2106-39213A).

2.2. Newborn Pancreas Collection

The pregnant dams were allowed to deliver spontaneously, with the morning of the vaginal plug denoting E0.5. The newborns were separated out from the cage and euthanized by decapitation. Blood was collected and centrifuged at $10,000 \times g$ for 10 min at room temperature. The supernatant serum was collected and stored at $-80\ ^\circ C$ to be run for serum insulin concentration using an ALPCO ELISA kit as per the kit's instructions (ALPCO Mouse Ultrasensitive Insulin ELISA; ALPCO Rat High Range Insulin ELISA, ALPCO Diagnostic, Salem, NH, USA). A five-parameter logistic fit was used for analysis through the MyAssays software. Newborn pancreata were harvested, weighed, fixed in 3.7% formalin for 4–6 h, and stored in 70% EtOH (diluted with $1\times$ PBS) at $4\ ^\circ C$ until tissue processing. The tissues were processed under the normal tissue processing settings and embedded in paraffin. The paraffin-embedded pancreata were sectioned 5 microns apart from top to bottom. Tails from the newborn mice were collected separately during harvesting for genotyping by standard PCR (see the information about the primers above). The pups for embryonic data were collected from three dams. The newborn data were collected from six dams.

2.3. Glucose Tolerance Test

The mice were fasted overnight for 14 h, after which fasting body weight and fasting blood glucose were measured. A dosage of 2 g/kg of 50% dextrose solution (Hospira, Inc., Lake Forest, IL, USA) was administered intraperitoneally. Blood glucose levels were recorded through a small tail clip at 30, 60, and 120 min after the initial injection. Blood glucose was measured using a Bayer Contour Blood Glucose Monitoring System. The adult offspring under a normal chow diet and a high-fat diet were from 2–3 dams.

2.4. Insulin Tolerance Test

The mice were fasted for 6 h, beginning in the morning, after which fasted body weight and fasted blood glucose were measured. A dosage of 0.75 U/kg insulin (Humalog, Eli Lilly, Indianapolis, IN, USA) in 0.9% sterile saline was administered intraperitoneally, and blood glucose levels were recorded through a small tail clip at 30, 60, and 120 min after the initial injection. Blood glucose was measured using a Bayer Contour Blood Glucose Monitoring System. The data are presented as the baseline percentage (%) corrected to the blood glucose level taken at $T = 0$ min after a 6 h fast.

2.5. Body Composition and Indirect Calorimetry

Body composition (EchoMRI, Echo Medical Systems LLC, Houston, TX, USA) and indirect calorimetry (Oxymax/CLAMS Lab Animal Monitoring System, Columbus Instruments) were performed by the Integrative Biology and Physiology (IBP) Core at the University of Minnesota.

2.6. Immunofluorescence and H&E Staining

For immunofluorescence imaging, paraffin-embedded tissue sections were deparaffinized and rehydrated, followed by antigen retrieval in citric buffer by boiling. The sections were incubated with primary antibodies against guinea pig or mouse insulin (guinea pig insulin primary antibody (1:400; DAKO, Agilent, Santa Clara, CA, USA); mouse insulin primary antibody (1:400; Abcam, Waltham, MA, USA)) at 4 °C overnight. The sections were subsequently washed with 1× PBS + 0.01% Tween 20 (1× PBST) with mild shaking and incubated with secondary antibodies conjugated to FITC (fluorescein isothiocyanate, Jackson ImmunoResearch, West Grove, PA, USA), a bright green fluorophore, for 1.5 h at 37 °C. Following incubation, the sections were subsequently washed with 1× PBST and counterstained for nuclei using a DAPI (4′,6-diamidino-2-phenylindole, Fisher Scientific, Hampton, NH) dip, a blue fluorescent stain with a high affinity for DNA. The sections were then cover-slipped with a mounting media and imaged on a motorized microscope (Nikon Eclipse NI-E; Nikon, Melville, NY, USA). H&E was used to assess macroscopic observation of the mouse placenta. Sagittal cuts were performed on the middle section of mouse placenta paraffin-embedded cut side down. The standard Citri Solv (Thermo Fisher Scientific, Waltham, MA, USA) deparaffinization and dehydration procedure was performed on the mouse placenta tissue. H&E staining was performed as per the manufacturer's protocol. Placental tissues were visualized using a Nikon ECLIPSE NI-E microscope.

2.7. Beta Cell Mass Analysis

The newborn paraffin-embedded pancreata were sectioned 5 microns apart from top to bottom per animal. The sections stained for insulin were selected incrementally at 100 μM apart, covering the whole pancreas. The sections were incubated with the insulin primary antibody overnight at 4 °C (see the dilution information above). The area of insulin-positive cells divided by the total pancreas area was quantified using FIJI ImageJ (NIH, Bethesda, MD, USA) to give the β-cell area/total pancreas area ratio per animal. The ratio was then multiplied by the matching pancreas weight (β-cell area/pancreatic area × pancreas weight) and averaged to give an average β-cell mass, as previously described [39]. The stained newborn tissue sections were imaged at 10× magnification using a Nikon Eclipse NI-E (Nikon Instruments) microscope. Individual islets were imaged at 20× magnification.

2.8. Statistical Analysis

All the reported values are expressed as the mean ± standard error of mean (SEM). Analyses of repeated data measures were performed using repeated measures two-way ANOVA with tests for sphericity. Individual offspring were the repeated measures subjects without regard to dams. An unpaired t-test was performed to analyze data where only two groups were compared. The area under the curve (AUC) values were calculated with zero as the baseline value. All the statistical analyses were completed using GraphPad Prism (San Diego, CA, USA) version 8 with a significance threshold of $p \leq 0.05$.

3. Results

3.1. Newborn Offspring with Placenta-Specific InsR Ablation Presenting with Normal Body Weight and Pancreatic β-Cell Mass

Using the Cyp19-cre recombinase, InsR was deleted genetically specifically in the placental trophoblast cells to generate InsR KO^{placenta} offspring and their littermate InsR floxed (InsR$^{f/f}$) controls, as presented in the timeline of our study in Figure 1A. The efficiency of using the Cyp19-cre promoter to target specific genes within the placental trophoblast cell lineage was previously validated within our laboratory as well as by others [23,37,40]. In this study, we show that a cre reporter transgene expressing the green fluorescence protein (GFP) is expressed in the placental trophoblast cells where the Cyp19-cre recombinase is expected to be active and not in the control placenta (Figure 1B).

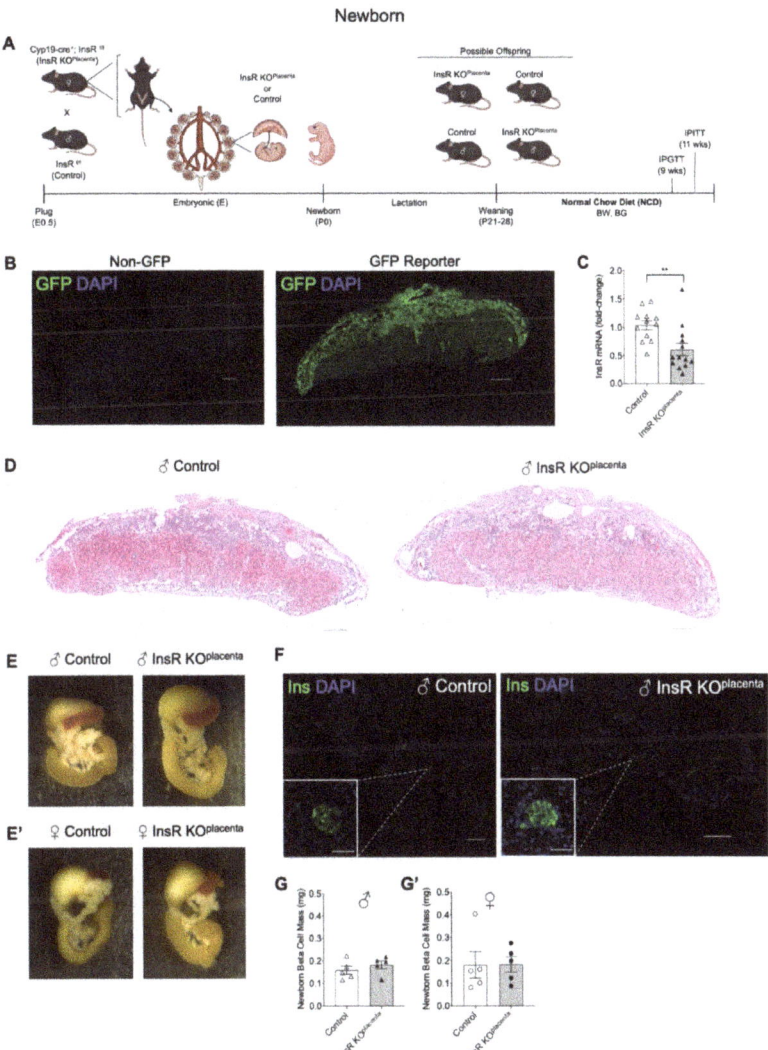

Figure 1. Newborn offspring with placenta-specific InsR ablation presented with normal body weight and pancreatic β-cell mass. (**A**) Experimental schematic for generating InsR KO^{placenta} and littermate controls. (**B**) GFP reporter (Cyp19-cre; CAG$^{+/+}$) expressing endogenous green fluorescence (GFP) in a mouse embryonic E17.5 placenta section compared to the non-GFP control (CAG$^{+/+}$) (scale bars: 500 μm). (**C**) InsR mRNA expression in the E17.5 InsR KO^{placenta} compared to controls by quantitative reverse transcription polymerase chain reaction (qPCR) (n = 12, 13). (**D**) Histology of the E17.5 male control placentas (left) compared to InsR KO^{placenta} (right) (scale bars: 500 μm). Background of images was subtracted post-imaging. (**E**) Gross morphology of the male and (**E′**) female control (left) and the InsR KO^{placenta} (right) newborn pancreata. (**F**) Whole pancreatic sections (scale bars: 500 μm) of the male newborn control (left) and the InsR KO^{placenta} (right) mice immunostained for insulin-positive islets (green) and DAPI (blue). Single islet β-cells (scale bars: 50 μm) shown as insets. Single islet images were cropped post-imaging to highlight the single islet. (**G**) Beta cell mass for the male (n = 5) and (**G′**) female (n = 5) newborns. The values are reported as the means ± SEM, ** p <0.01. E: embryonic; P: postnatal; BW: body weight; BG: blood glucose; IPGTT: intraperitoneal glucose tolerance test; IPITT; intraperitoneal insulin tolerance test; NCD: normal chow diet.

Quantitative reverse transcription polymerase chain reaction (qPCR) was performed on embryonic (E) 17.5 placentas to demonstrate effective reduction of InsR mRNA levels in the InsR KO^{placenta} placentas compared to their controls (p = 0.0055, Figure 1C). To assess alteration of InsR levels in the offspring (non-placental tissue), we measured InsR mRNA in the liver and adipose tissues of the adult offspring. The levels of the InsR transcript were comparable between InsR KO^{placenta} and their controls (data not shown), suggesting a placental specificity of Cyp19-cre in the placenta.

Placentas harvested on E17.5 did not differ in total weight between the InsR KO^{placenta} and their littermate controls (Figure S1A). Preliminary assessment of the gross placental morphology at E17.5 appears to be comparable between the littermate controls and the InsR KO^{placenta} placenta (Figure 1D), suggesting that placental IR is not required for the development of the placenta. Fetal body weight and pancreas weight at E17.5 also revealed no differences between the two genotypes (Figure S1B,C). The male and female InsR KO^{placenta} newborns presented with normal body weight compared to their respective controls (Table 1). There were also no differences in non-fasting blood glucose levels or serum insulin levels at birth among the groups (Table 1). Examination of the gross pancreas morphology, pancreas weight, and liver weight showed no apparent differences between genotypes for either male or female mice (Figure 1E, Table 1). Assessment of the basal pancreatic β-cell mass at birth demonstrated no differences between the InsR KO^{placenta} and their controls (Figure 1F,G,G′).

Table 1. Male and female offspring characteristics in newborns (P0) and adults (parity ≥ 3) on a normal chow diet. Newborn characteristics in terms of body weight, non-fasting blood glucose, non-fasting serum insulin, pancreas weight, and liver weight. Adult offspring characteristics in terms of fasting and non-fasting blood glucose levels measured at 9 and 10 weeks of age, respectively. The data are presented as the means ± SEM.

	Male Offspring		Female Offspring	
Newborn (P0)	Control	InsR KO^{placenta}	Control	InsR KO^{placenta}
Body weight	1.226 ± 0.03039	1.318 ± 0.03808	1.242 ± 0.02603	1.251 ± 0.03923
Non-fasting blood glucose	39.67 ± 6.888	36.50 ± 3.833	33.17 ± 5.183	34.90 ± 3.093
Non-fasting serum insulin	0.3919 ± 0.1794	0.4409 ± 0.1791	0.4676 ± 0.1500	0.4622 ± 0.1129
Pancreas weight	7.514 ± 0.3269	8.079 ± 0.4086	8.093 ± 0.6240	8.207 ± 0.6032
Liver weight	46.33 ± 3.449	49.26 ± 2.904	47.92 ± 2.351	49.58 ± 3.411
Adult (Parity ≥ 3) Normal Chow Diet	Control	InsR KO^{placenta}	Control	InsR KO^{placenta}
Fasting blood glucose (9 weeks old)	61.25 ± 1.652	57.25 ± 4.029	60.25 ± 2.175	56.25 ± 2.810
Non-fasting blood glucose (10 weeks old)	132.5 ± 13.85	135.0 ± 5.212	138.3 ± 18.03	126.8 ± 13.81

3.2. Adult InsR KO^{placenta} Mice Displayed Normal Glucose Homeostasis on a Normal Chow Diet

The InsR KO^{placenta} mice and their littermate controls were weaned onto a normal chow diet (NCD) at 4 weeks of age. There were no differences in the post-weaning body weight, measured from 4 to 13 weeks of age in male and female offspring, independent of parity (defined as the number of pregnancies the dam carried) (Figure 2A,A′). Fasting and non-fasting blood glucose levels, measured at 9 and 10 weeks of age, respectively, demonstrated no differences in either male or female mice from multiparous dams, which we defined as parity ≥ three pregnancies (Table 1). Glucose homeostasis in the adult offspring was assessed via an intraperitoneal (IP) glucose tolerance test (GTT) and an insulin tolerance test (ITT) performed at 9 weeks and 11 weeks of age, respectively. The male InsR KO^{placenta} mice from multiparous dams exhibited normal glucose and insulin tolerance

(Figure 2B,C). The female InsR KO^{placenta} mice similarly demonstrated normal glucose tolerance but did show a significant change during the IPITT at timepoint T = 120 min (p = 0.0231) (Figure 2B′,C′). Analysis of the overall response (area under the curve, AUC), however, showed no significant differences in the female InsR KO^{placenta} mice compared to their controls (Figure 2C′). To assess whether the genotype of the dam (InsR$^{f/f}$ vs. Cyp19-Cre; InsR$^{f/f}$) impacts the glucose homeostasis of the adult offspring, glucose homeostasis measurements were performed on the InsR KO^{placenta} and control mice with either the dam or the sire as the carrier of the Cyp19-cre recombinase. Glucose and insulin tolerance remained unchanged (Figure S2). IPGTT and IPITT were performed on a separate cohort of offspring from parity ≤ 2, similarly demonstrating normal glucose and insulin tolerance (Figure S3A,A′,B,B′). Using a subset of mice from this group, IPGTT was performed at 20 weeks of age, which revealed that glucose tolerance did not differ between the two genotypes in either sex with age (Figure S3C,C′). We also generated heterozygous InsR Het^{placenta} (Cyp19-Cre; InsR$^{f/+}$) and a respective control (InsR$^{f/+}$) to assess a dosage effect of the InsR gene. There were no differences in glucose tolerance between the two genotypes in males and females (Figure S4).

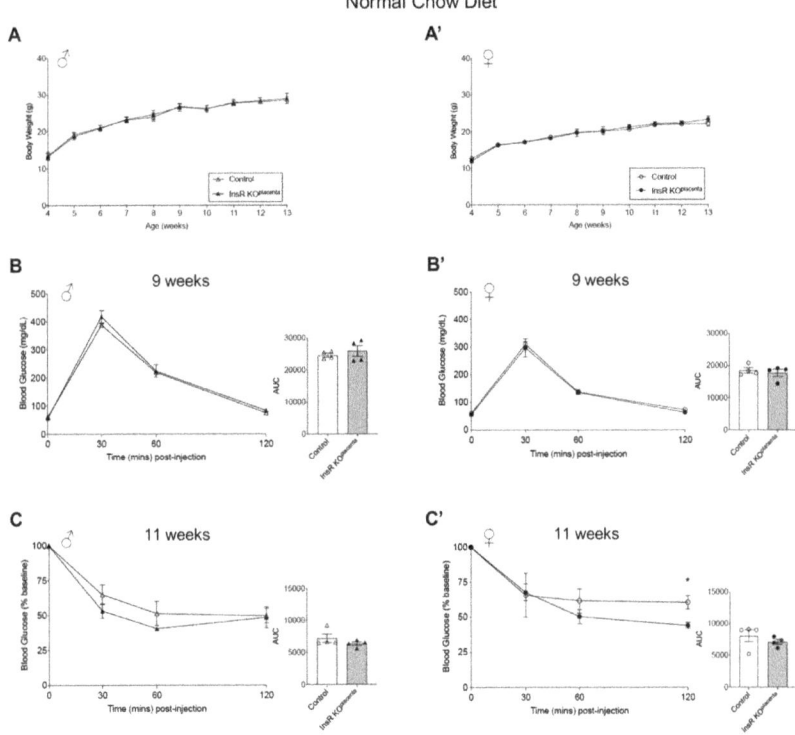

Figure 2. Adult InsR KO^{placenta} mice displayed normal glucose homeostasis on a normal chow diet. (**A**) Body weight in all the males (n = 9, 10) and (**A′**) the female (n = 13) InsR KO^{placenta} and control mice on a normal chow diet. Body weight for the offspring presented as combined data from parity ≥ 3 and ≤2 litters. (**B**) IPGTT and AUC analysis (right) for the male (n = 4) and (**B′**) female (n = 4) mice from parity ≥ 3 on a normal chow diet at 9 weeks of age. (**C**) IPITT and AUC analysis (right) for the males (n = 4) and (**C′**) females (n = 4) from parity ≥ 3 at 11 weeks of age. Blood glucose values for IPITT are expressed as the baseline percentage of blood glucose. The values are reported as the means ± SEM, * p < 0.05.

3.3. Adult Male InsR KO^{placenta} Offspring Demonstrated a Lower Body Weight on a High-Fat Diet Challenge

Since we observed normal glucose tolerance under an NCD, we then tested whether placental InsR reduction increased the risk of obesity and metabolic dysfunction in the offspring under a diet-induced obesogenic challenge. Beginning at 13 weeks of age, the male and female InsR KO^{placenta} mice and their littermate controls were challenged with a high-fat diet (HFD, 60% energy by fat) to examine their response to an obesogenic challenge (Figure 3A). As expected, both the male and female mice, regardless of the genotype, increased in body weight over the 17 weeks on HFD treatment (Figure 3B,B'). Interestingly, when all the data from parity 1–4 were combined, the male InsR KO^{placenta} mice exhibited a significantly reduced body weight gain compared to their controls ($p = 0.0112$, Figure 3B). However, when parity ≤ 2 and ≥ 3 were considered separately, there were no differences (Figures S5A and S6A). In contrast, the female InsR KO^{placenta} mice did not differ in body weight compared to their controls over the 17 weeks on a HFD regardless of parity (Figure 3B', Figures S5A' and S6A'). Weekly non-fasted blood glucose measurements showed no notable differences between the InsR KO^{placenta} mice and their controls for either sex (Figure 3C,C', Figures S5B,B' and S6B,B'). Fasting blood glucose levels were measured after a 14 h fast at 4, 8, and 10 weeks on a HFD. No differences were observed in fasting blood glucose levels between the genotypes at any point in either sex regardless of parity (Figure 3D,D'). Body composition assessed by EchoMRI revealed no differences in fat mass or lean mass for either male or female mice after 18–19 weeks on a HFD (Figure 3E,E',F,F'). Pancreas tissue harvested after 19–20 weeks on a HFD did not show weight differences between the genotypes for either the male or female mice regardless of parity (Figure 3G,G').

3.4. Adult Male InsR KO^{placenta} Offspring from Multiparous Dams Presented with a Mild and Transient Improved Glucose Homeostasis on a High-Fat Diet Challenge

In the male InsR KO^{placenta} mice on a HFD, the mild reduction in weight gain suggested a potential effect of reduced placental InsR on glucose homeostasis. IPGTT was conducted on the male and female InsR KO^{placenta} mice and their controls from either parity ≥ 3 or ≤ 2 at 4, 8, and 10 weeks on a HFD. At 4 weeks of a HFD, IPGTT results demonstrated no differences in glucose tolerance in either the male or female groups (Figure S5C,C'). Interestingly, at 8 weeks on a HFD, the male InsR KO^{placenta} mice from parity ≥ 3 demonstrated significantly improved glucose tolerance compared to their controls ($p = 0.0332$, Figure 4A). In contrast, there were no differences in the female group from parity ≥ 3 (Figure 4A'). IPGTT performed at 10 weeks on a HFD in the same group demonstrated a sustained improvement in glucose tolerance in the male InsR KO^{placenta} mice, but the effect was mild and did not reach statistical significance ($p = 0.0899$, Figure S5D). Glucose tolerance in the female group showed no difference at this time (Figure S5D'). Consistent with the mild improvement in glucose tolerance, IPITT conducted at 14 weeks on a HFD revealed a mild improvement in insulin tolerance in the male InsR KO^{placenta} mice from parity ≥ 3 compared to their controls ($p = 0.0867$, Figure 4B). There were no changes in insulin tolerance in the female group (Figure 4B'). IPITT was repeated at 18 weeks on a HFD to see if the improvement was sustained in the male InsR KO^{placenta} mice, but the results revealed no differences in insulin tolerance in the male or female mice at this time (Figure S5E,E'). IPGTT and IPITT were performed on a separate group of mice on a HFD from parity ≤ 2, but interestingly, the transient improvement in glucose homeostasis was not observed in this group (Figure S6C,C',D,D',E,E'). Within a subset of males from this group, activity levels and energy utilization were assessed using indirect calorimetry over a 48 h period. Both O_2 consumption (day $p = 0.0213$; night $p = 0.0272$) and CO_2 (day $p = 0.0142$; night $p = 0.0165$) production were significantly reduced in the InsR KO^{placenta} mice compared to the controls (Figure S7A,B). However, the respiratory exchange ratio (RER) and energy expenditure were comparable between the two groups (Figure S7C,D). Activity levels from day and night were significantly different within each genotype in the males (control $p = 0.0003$; InsR KO^{placenta} $p = 0.0005$), but between the two groups, the activity level was comparable (Figure S7E).

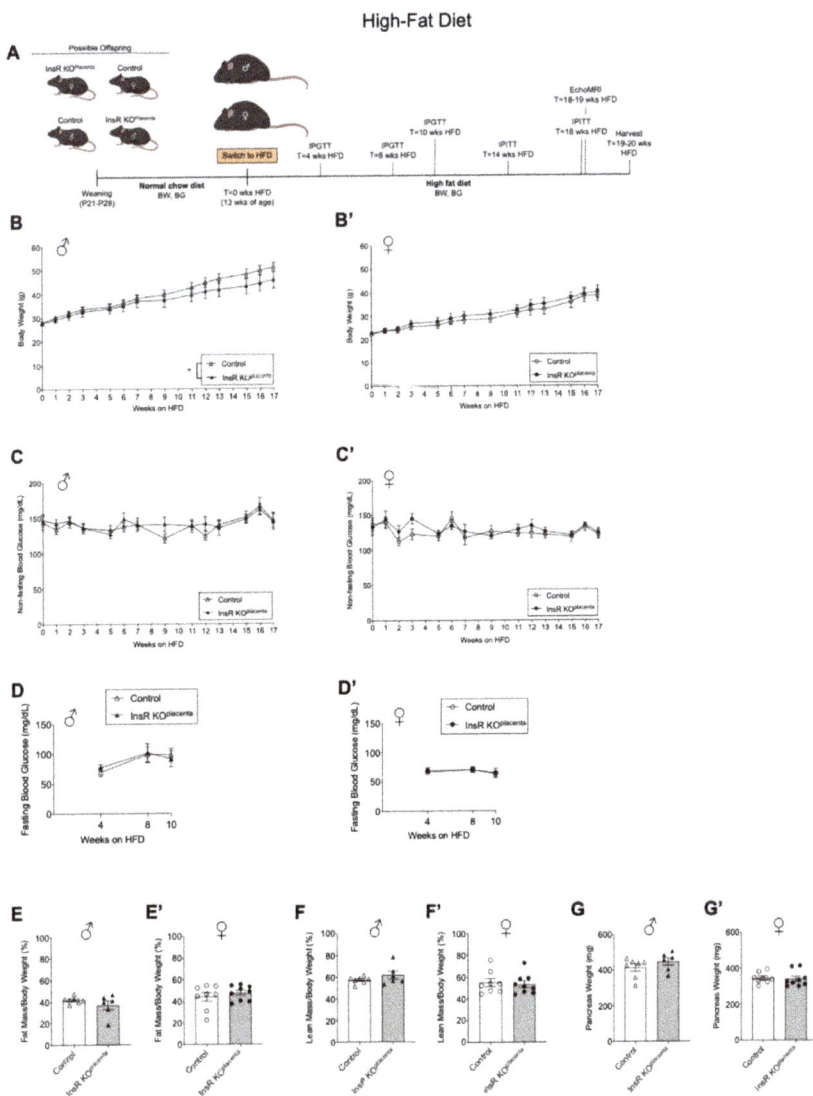

Figure 3. Adult male InsR KO^{placenta} offspring demonstrated lower body weight under a high-fat diet challenge. (**A**) Schematic of experimental design for a high-fat diet (HFD). (**B**) Body weight monitored in all the males ($n = 6, 7$) and (**B′**) females ($n = 8, 9$) from parity ≥ 3 and ≤ 2 across 17 weeks on a HFD. (**C**) Non-fasting blood glucose levels for all the males ($n = 6, 7$) and (**C′**) females ($n = 8, 9$) from parity was ≥ 3 and ≤ 2 (measured across 17 weeks on a HFD). Measurements not included for T = 4, 8, 10, 14, and 18 weeks on a HFD due to phenotyping performed on these weeks. (**D**) Fasting blood glucose measured for the males ($n = 4, 7$) and (**D′**) females ($n = 4, 9$) from parity ≥ 3 and ≤ 2 at 4, 8, and 10 weeks on a HFD. (**E**) Fat mass for the males ($n = 6, 7$) and (**E′**) females ($n = 8, 9$) from parity ≥ 3 and ≤ 2 as assessed by EchoMRI at 18–19 weeks on a HFD. (**F**) Lean mass for the males ($n = 6, 7$) and (**F′**) females ($n = 8, 9$) from parity ≥ 3 and ≤ 2 as assessed by EchoMRI at 18–19 weeks on a HFD. (**G**) Pancreas weight for the males ($n = 6, 7$) and (**G′**) females ($n = 8, 9$) from parity ≥ 3 and ≤ 2 upon harvest at 19–20 weeks on a HFD. The values are reported as the means $\pm$ SEM, * $p < 0.05$. P: postnatal; BW: body weight; BG: blood glucose; IPGTT: intraperitoneal glucose tolerance test; IPITT; intraperitoneal insulin tolerance test; HFD: high-fat diet.

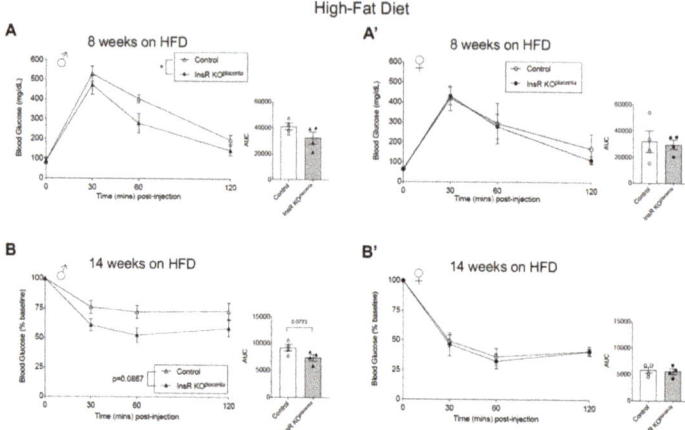

Figure 4. Adult male InsR KO^placenta mice from multiparous dams presented with a mild and transient improved glucose homeostasis on a high-fat diet challenge. (**A**) IPGTT and AUC analysis (right) for the male ($n = 4$) and (**A′**) female ($n = 4$) mice from parity ≥ 3 at 8 weeks on a HFD. Repeated measures two-way ANOVA revealed significant differences ($p = 0.0332$) between the InsR KO^placenta and control males at 8 weeks on a HFD. A separate unpaired t-test performed specifically for T = 60 min revealed $p = 0.0593$. (**B**) IPITT and AUC analysis (right) for the males ($n = 4$) and (**B′**) females ($n = 4$) from parity ≥ 3 at 14 weeks on a HFD. Blood glucose values for IPITT are expressed as the baseline percentage of blood glucose. Repeated measures two-way ANOVA analysis revealed a p-value of 0.0867 in the males at 14 weeks on a HFD. A separate unpaired t-test performed specifically for T = 30 and T = 60 min revealed $p = 0.0843$ and $p = 0.0600$, respectively. The values are reported as the means ± SEM, * $p < 0.05$.

4. Discussion

Maternal obesity and diabetes during pregnancy continue to be serious public health concerns and are associated with adverse pregnancy complications for both the mother and the child [5–15]. In our present study, we aimed to understand the effect of altered insulin receptor availability in the placenta on the metabolic health of the mouse offspring. We uncovered that placenta-specific insulin receptor deficiency in a normal mouse pregnancy condition does not adversely affect glucose homeostasis in the male or female offspring at birth and during adulthood. Under a diet-induced obesogenic challenge, however, adult male offspring with a placental insulin receptor deletion displayed transient protection from glucose homeostasis dysfunction, which appears to be dependent on the number of pregnancies the dam has experienced.

Placental trophoblast-specific loss of the insulin receptor did not affect placental weight, fetal and newborn weight, or β-cell mass in the male or female newborns. These results were consistent with findings that placental trophoblast-specific deletion of InsR alone does not adversely impact offspring growth in mice [40]. Another study looking at the effects of a total body insulin receptor knockout also found normal fetal development with normal or slightly reduced body weight at birth [41,42]. The minimal impact on body weight is likely attributable to the effects of insulin-like growth factor 1 receptor (IGF1R) in normal fetal growth and development [41,42]. The insulin receptor and the IGF1 receptor (IGF1R) share high homology in their ligand-binding and intracellular tyrosine kinase domains, and thus insulin can activate both receptors (not IGF2R) albeit with lower affinity to IGF1R [43–45]. Thus, future studies into the independent role of IGF1R and the combined role of InsR and IGF1R in the placenta may reveal new insights regarding the full effect of placental insulin signaling, which will better inform us of the full effects of maternal insulin on birthweight and β-cell mass at birth.

Glucose and insulin tolerances of the adult InsR KO^{placenta} offspring on a normal chow diet were unaffected and suggest that placental InsR on its own is not sufficient to induce lasting effects on glucose homeostasis of the offspring. Normal glucose tolerance in the adult offspring was also observed by Bronson et al. [40]. However, when challenged with a HFD, male InsR KO^{placenta} mice demonstrated lower body weight gain compared to their littermate controls. Male InsR KO^{placenta} offspring also demonstrated improved glucose and insulin tolerance, although this was a mild and transient effect dependent on maternal parity. The improved glucose and insulin tolerance was demonstrated in the cohort from multiparous dams, which we defined as having ≥ three pregnancies. We observed no changes in glucose homeostasis parameters in different cohorts of offspring from dams with parity ≤ 2. While we are careful in the interpretation of this analysis, deletion of the placental insulin receptor may potentially be associated with a mild protective effect against diet-induced obesity and glucose homeostasis dysfunction in male InsR KO^{placenta} offspring when challenged with a HFD. This phenotype appears to be dependent on the number of pregnancies the dam has experienced. Thus, ablation of the placental InsR may have health beneficial effects in the male offspring of multiparous dams, where they often present higher obesity [46,47] and hyperinsulinemia [48]. Indeed, epidemiological and experimental studies have shown that increased parity may be associated with an increased risk of maternal diabetes, glucose homeostasis dysfunction, and placental inflammation [17,33,49,50]. In a preclinical model, there is also evidence demonstrating that male offspring from multiparous dams have increased adiposity and metabolic dysfunction [17]. We are uncertain what factors may be mediating this effect in multiparous dams, but repeated pregnancies may adversely change the intrauterine environment through changes related to pregnancy-induced obesity, maternal and placental inflammation, maternal hyperinsulinemia, and placental nutrient transport [17]. Interestingly, placental insulin receptor ablation was also shown to significantly increase hypothalamic-pituitary–adrenal axis stress response and impair sensorimotor gating in males [40]. Thus, sex-specific neurodevelopmental and metabolic risk programming should be investigated in the future.

5. Conclusions and Future Directions

In the present study, we explored the role of the placental insulin receptor in a normal mouse pregnancy using a preclinical model, and our results suggest that placental InsR may contribute to the long-term offspring health when metabolically challenged with diet-induced obesity. This study suggests that reduction of placental insulin in dams with hyper-nutrient conditions such as obesity and hyperinsulinemia (i.e., PCOS) may improve metabolic health of the offspring. Our data highlights the need for a greater understanding of the role of insulin signaling in placental biology and the mechanisms of developmental programming of the metabolic health in the offspring. This study also highlights that multiple pregnancies may have heritable and independent consequences in the offspring and warrants further investigation using preclinical models and in human studies.

Future studies should be directed toward exploring more closely the impact of parity on the metabolic health of the dams and the offspring by characterizing glucose homeostasis of multiparous wild type or InsR KO dams to define how their metabolic health may be altered with an increasing number of pregnancies. With a more robust amount of dams, confounding variables such as the dams' age, weight gain between pregnancies, and litter effects within dams corrected, a more thorough study may shed some insight into why male offspring with a placental deletion of the insulin receptor may present with a mildly protective phenotype. Assessment of the offspring's metabolic health if the sire is a Cre carrier should also be considered. Fetal sex has been shown to play a role in sex-specific responses to changes in the in utero environment and may partially explain the sexual dimorphic differences observed in our study and others [23,40,51–53]. Thus, an important future study should also investigate the role of the insulin receptor in placental nutrient-sensing and placental vascularization. Moreover, future interventions may be targeted to break the obesity cycle that could occur between mothers and their offspring.

Supplementary Materials: The following supporting information can be downloaded at: https://www.mdpi.com/article/10.3390/biomedicines10030575/s1, Figure S1. Normal placental and fetal weight in InsR KOplacenta offspring. Figure S2. Normal glucose homeostasis in InsR KOplacenta offspring from sire Cyp19-cre carrier. Figure S3. A separate cohort of adult InsR KOplacenta mice from parity ≤ 2 demonstrated normal glucose homeostasis on normal chow diet. Figure S4. Placental InsR heterozygous mice demonstrated normal glucose homeostasis on normal chow diet. Figure S5. Adult male InsR KOplacenta mice from multiparous dams presented with a mild and transient improved glucose homeostasis on a high-fat diet challenge. Figure S6. Adult male InsR KOplacenta mice from parity ≤ 2 exhibited normal glucose homeostasis on a high-fat diet challenge. Figure S7. Adult male InsR KOplacenta mice displayed normal energy expenditure on a high-fat diet challenge.

Author Contributions: Conceptualization, E.U.A.; methodology, E.U.A. and G.C.; software, G.C.; validation, G.C.; formal analysis, G.C., R.M., M.B. and S.J.; investigation, G.C.; resources, E.U.A.; data curation, G.C., R.M., M.B. and S.J.; writing—original draft preparation, G.C.; writing—review and editing, G.C. and E.U.A.; visualization, G.C.; supervision, E.U.A.; funding acquisition, E.U.A. All authors have read and agreed to the published version of the manuscript.

Funding: This work was supported by National Institutes of Health grant (NIDDK R21HD100840 and R01DK115720), Regenerative Medicine of Minnesota, and the McKnight Foundation.

Institutional Review Board Statement: All the animal studies were performed in accordance with the University of Minnesota Institutional Animal Care and Use Committee (protocol #2106-39213A).

Informed Consent Statement: Not applicable.

Data Availability Statement: Not applicable.

Acknowledgments: We thank Gustavo W. Leone (Medical College of Wisconsin) for providing us the Cyp19Cre animals. We thank Ronald Regal (Department of Mathematics, University of Minnesota, Duluth, MN, USA) for assistance with data analysis and editing of the final manuscript. We thank the IBP Physiology Core for their assistance in the body composition and indirect calorimetry analysis. We also thank Briana Clifton for technical assistance.

Conflicts of Interest: The authors declare no conflict of interest.

References

1. Singh, G.K.; DiBari, J.N. Marked disparities in pre-pregnancy obesity and overweight prevalence among US women by race/ethnicity, nativity/immigrant status, and sociodemographic characteristics, 2012–2014. *J. Obes.* **2019**, *2019*, 2419263. [CrossRef] [PubMed]
2. DeSisto, C.L.; Kim, S.Y.; Sharma, A.J. Prevalence estimates of gestational diabetes mellitus in the United States, pregnancy risk assessment monitoring system (PRAMS), 2007–2010. *Prev. Chronic Dis.* **2014**, *11*, E104. [CrossRef]
3. Zhu, Y.; Zhang, C. Prevalence of Gestational Diabetes and Risk of Progression to Type 2 Diabetes: A Global Perspective. *Curr. Diabetes Rep.* **2016**, *16*, 7. [CrossRef] [PubMed]
4. Friedman, J.E. Developmental Programming of Obesity and Diabetes in Mouse, Monkey, and Man in 2018: Where Are We Headed? *Diabetes* **2018**, *67*, 2137–2151. [CrossRef] [PubMed]
5. Harmon, H.M.; Hannon, T.S. Maternal obesity: A serious pediatric health crisis. *Pediatr. Res.* **2018**, *83*, 1087–1089. [CrossRef] [PubMed]
6. Godfrey, K.M.; Reynolds, R.M.; Prescott, S.L.; Nyirenda, M.; Jaddoe, V.W.; Eriksson, J.G.; Broekman, B.F. Influence of maternal obesity on the long-term health of offspring. *Lancet Diabetes Endocrinol.* **2017**, *5*, 53–64. [CrossRef]
7. Catalano, P.M.; Shankar, K. Obesity and pregnancy: Mechanisms of short term and long term adverse consequences for mother and child. *BMJ* **2017**, *356*, j1. [CrossRef] [PubMed]
8. Catalano, P.M. The impact of gestational diabetes and maternal obesity on the mother and her offspring. *J. Dev. Orig. Health Dis.* **2010**, *1*, 208–215. [CrossRef]
9. Poston, L.; Caleyachetty, R.; Cnattingius, S.; Corvalán, C.; Uauy, R.; Herring, S.; Gillman, M.W. Preconceptional and maternal obesity: Epidemiology and health consequences. *Lancet Diabetes Endocrinol.* **2016**, *4*, 1025–1036. [CrossRef]
10. Poston, L.; Harthoorn, L.F.; Van Der Beek, E.M.; Workshop, C.I.E. Obesity in pregnancy: Implications for the mother and lifelong health of the child. A consensus statement. *Pediatr. Res.* **2011**, *69*, 175–180. [CrossRef] [PubMed]

11. Gaillard, R.; Santos, S.; Duijts, L.; Felix, J.F. Childhood Health Consequences of Maternal Obesity during Pregnancy: A Narrative Review. *Ann. Nutr. Metab.* **2016**, *69*, 171–180. [CrossRef] [PubMed]
12. Catalano, P.M.; Ehrenberg, H.M. The short- and long-term implications of maternal obesity on the mother and her offspring. *BJOG* **2006**, *113*, 1126–1133. [CrossRef]
13. Kong, L.; Chen, X.; Gissler, M.; Lavebratt, C. Relationship of prenatal maternal obesity and diabetes to offspring neurodevelopmental and psychiatric disorders: A narrative review. *Int. J. Obes. (Lond.)* **2020**, *44*, 1981–2000. [CrossRef]
14. Metzger, B.E. Long-term outcomes in mothers diagnosed with gestational diabetes mellitus and their offspring. *Clin. Obstet. Gynecol.* **2007**, *50*, 972–979. [CrossRef]
15. Bianco, M.E.; Josefson, J.L. Hyperglycemia During Pregnancy and Long-Term Offspring Outcomes. *Curr. Diabetes Rep.* **2019**, *19*, 143. [CrossRef]
16. Gillman, M.W. Interrupting Intergenerational Cycles of Maternal Obesity. *Nestle Nutr. Inst. Workshop Ser.* **2016**, *85*, 59–69. [CrossRef]
17. Rebholz, S.L.; Jones, T.; Burke, K.T.; Jaeschke, A.; Tso, P.; D'Alessio, D.A.; Woollett, L.A. Multiparity leads to obesity and inflammation in mothers and obesity in male offspring. *Am. J. Physiol. Endocrinol. Metab.* **2012**, *302*, E449–E457. [CrossRef]
18. Davis, E.M.; Zyzanski, S.J.; Olson, C.M.; Stange, K.C.; Horwitz, R.I. Racial, ethnic, and socioeconomic differences in the incidence of obesity related to childbirth. *Am. J. Public Health* **2009**, *99*, 294–299. [CrossRef]
19. Gunderson, E.P.; Jacobs, D.R., Jr.; Chiang, V.; Lewis, C.E.; Tsai, A.; Quesenberry, C.P., Jr.; Sidney, S. Childbearing is associated with higher incidence of the metabolic syndrome among women of reproductive age controlling for measurements before pregnancy: The CARDIA study. *Am. J. Obs. Gynecol.* **2009**, *201*, 177.e1–177.e9. [CrossRef] [PubMed]
20. Dimasuay, K.G.; Boeuf, P.; Powell, T.L.; Jansson, T. Placental Responses to Changes in the Maternal Environment Determine Fetal Growth. *Front. Physiol.* **2016**, *7*, 12. [CrossRef] [PubMed]
21. Castillo-Castrejon, M.; Yamaguchi, K.; Rodel, R.L.; Erickson, K.; Kramer, A.; Hirsch, N.M.; Rolloff, K.; Jansson, T.; Barbour, L.A.; Powell, T.L. Effect of type 2 diabetes mellitus on placental expression and activity of nutrient transporters and their association with birth weight and neonatal adiposity. *Mol. Cell. Endocrinol.* **2021**, *532*, 111319. [CrossRef]
22. Mohan, R.; Baumann, D.; Alejandro, E.U. Fetal undernutrition, placental insufficiency, and pancreatic β-cell development programming in utero. *Am. J. Physiol. Regul. Integr. Comp. Physiol.* **2018**, *315*, R867–R878. [CrossRef] [PubMed]
23. Akhaphong, B.; Baumann, D.C.; Beetch, M.; Lockridge, A.D.; Jo, S.; Wong, A.; Zemanovic, T.; Mohan, R.; Fondevilla, D.L.; Sia, M.; et al. Placental mTOR complex 1 regulates fetal programming of obesity and insulin resistance in mice. *JCI Insight* **2021**, *6*, e149271. [CrossRef] [PubMed]
24. Hart, B.; Morgan, E.; Alejandro, E.U. Nutrient sensor signaling pathways and cellular stress in fetal growth restriction. *J. Mol. Endocrinol.* **2019**, *62*, R155–R165. [CrossRef] [PubMed]
25. Jansson, T.; Powell, T.L. Role of placental nutrient sensing in developmental programming. *Clin. Obs. Gynecol.* **2013**, *56*, 591–601. [CrossRef] [PubMed]
26. Ruiz-Palacios, M.; Ruiz-Alcaraz, A.J.; Sanchez-Campillo, M.; Larqué, E. Role of Insulin in Placental Transport of Nutrients in Gestational Diabetes Mellitus. *Ann. Nutr. Metab.* **2017**, *70*, 16–25. [CrossRef] [PubMed]
27. O'Tierney-Ginn, P.; Presley, L.; Myers, S.; Catalano, P. Placental growth response to maternal insulin in early pregnancy. *J. Clin. Endocrinol. Metab.* **2015**, *100*, 159–165. [CrossRef] [PubMed]
28. Hiden, U.; Glitzner, E.; Hartmann, M.; Desoye, G. Insulin and the IGF system in the human placenta of normal and diabetic pregnancies. *J. Anat.* **2009**, *215*, 60–68. [CrossRef]
29. Colomiere, M.; Permezel, M.; Riley, C.; Desoye, G.; Lappas, M. Defective insulin signaling in placenta from pregnancies complicated by gestational diabetes mellitus. *Eur. J. Endocrinol.* **2009**, *160*, 567–578. [CrossRef]
30. Desoye, G.; Hauguel-de Mouzon, S. The human placenta in gestational diabetes mellitus. The insulin and cytokine network. *Diabetes Care* **2007**, *30* (Suppl. 2), S120–S126. [CrossRef]
31. Desoye, G.; Hofmann, H.H.; Weiss, P.A. Insulin binding to trophoblast plasma membranes and placental glycogen content in well-controlled gestational diabetic women treated with diet or insulin, in well-controlled overt diabetic patients and in healthy control subjects. *Diabetologia* **1992**, *35*, 45–55. [CrossRef]
32. Catalano, P.M. Trying to understand gestational diabetes. *Diabet. Med.* **2014**, *31*, 273–281. [CrossRef]
33. Alejandro, E.U.; Mamerto, T.P.; Chung, G.; Villavieja, A.; Gaus, N.L.; Morgan, E.; Pineda-Cortel, M.R.B. Gestational Diabetes Mellitus: A Harbinger of the Vicious Cycle of Diabetes. *Int. J. Mol. Sci.* **2020**, *21*, 5003. [CrossRef]
34. Jansson, T.; Cetin, I.; Powell, T.L.; Desoye, G.; Radaelli, T.; Ericsson, A.; Sibley, C.P. Placental transport and metabolism in fetal overgrowth—A workshop report. *Placenta* **2006**, *27* (Suppl. A), S109–S113. [CrossRef] [PubMed]
35. Alejandro, E.U.; Jo, S.; Akhaphong, B.; Llacer, P.R.; Gianchandani, M.; Gregg, B.; Parlee, S.D.; MacDougald, O.A.; Bernal-Mizrachi, E. Maternal low-protein diet on the last week of pregnancy contributes to insulin resistance and β-cell dysfunction in the mouse offspring. *Am. J. Physiol. Regul. Integr. Comp. Physiol.* **2020**, *319*, R485–R496. [CrossRef] [PubMed]
36. Moore, M.; Avula, N.; Jo, S.; Beetch, M.; Alejandro, E.U. Disruption of O-Linked N-Acetylglucosamine Signaling in Placenta Induces Insulin Sensitivity in Female Offspring. *Int. J. Mol. Sci.* **2021**, *22*, 6918. [CrossRef] [PubMed]
37. López-Tello, J.; Pérez-García, V.; Khaira, J.; Kusinski, L.C.; Cooper, W.N.; Andreani, A.; Grant, I.; Fernández de Liger, E.; Lam, B.Y.; Hemberger, M.; et al. Fetal and trophoblast PI3K p110α have distinct roles in regulating resource supply to the growing fetus in mice. *Elife* **2019**, *8*, e45282. [CrossRef] [PubMed]

38. Wenzel, P.L.; Leone, G. Expression of Cre recombinase in early diploid trophoblast cells of the mouse placenta. *Genesis* **2007**, *45*, 129–134. [CrossRef] [PubMed]
39. Baumann, D.; Wong, A.; Akhaphong, B.; Jo, S.; Pritchard, S.; Mohan, R.; Chung, G.; Zhang, Y.; Alejandro, E.U. Role of nutrient-driven O-GlcNAc-post-translational modification in pancreatic exocrine and endocrine islet development. *Development* **2020**, *147*, dev186643. [CrossRef]
40. Bronson, S.L.; Chan, J.C.; Bale, T.L. Sex-Specific Neurodevelopmental Programming by Placental Insulin Receptors on Stress Reactivity and Sensorimotor Gating. *Biol. Psychiatry* **2017**, *82*, 127–138. [CrossRef] [PubMed]
41. Louvi, A.; Accili, D.; Efstratiadis, A. Growth-promoting interaction of IGF-II with the insulin receptor during mouse embryonic development. *Dev. Biol.* **1997**, *189*, 33–48. [CrossRef]
42. Kitamura, T.; Kahn, C.R.; Accili, D. Insulin receptor knockout mice. *Annu. Rev. Physiol.* **2003**, *65*, 313–332. [CrossRef]
43. Cai, W.; Sakaguchi, M.; Kleinridders, A.; Gonzalez-Del Pino, G.; Dreyfuss, J.M.; O'Neill, B.T.; Ramirez, A.K.; Pan, H.; Winnay, J.N.; Boucher, J.; et al. Domain-dependent effects of insulin and IGF-1 receptors on signalling and gene expression. *Nat. Commun.* **2017**, *8*, 14892. [CrossRef]
44. Boucher, J.; Tseng, Y.H.; Kahn, C.R. Insulin and insulin-like growth factor-1 receptors act as ligand-specific amplitude modulators of a common pathway regulating gene transcription. *J. Biol. Chem.* **2010**, *285*, 17235–17245. [CrossRef]
45. Hawkes, C.P.; Lorraine, L.K. Growth Factor Regulation of Fetal Growth. In *Fetal and Neonatal Physiology*, 5th ed.; Elsevier Health Sciences: Amsterdam, The Netherlands, 2017; Volume 2, pp. 1461–1470.
46. Huayanay-Espinoza, C.A.; Quispe, R.; Poterico, J.A.; Carrillo-Larco, R.M.; Bazo-Alvarez, J.C.; Miranda, J.J. Parity and Overweight/Obesity in Peruvian Women. *Prev. Chronic Dis.* **2017**, *14*, E102. [CrossRef]
47. Wu, J.; Xu, G.; Shen, L.; Zhang, Y.; Song, L.; Yang, S.; Yang, H.; Yuan, J.; Liang, Y.; Wang, Y.; et al. Parity and risk of metabolic syndrome among Chinese women. *J. Womens Health (Larchmt)* **2015**, *24*, 602–607. [CrossRef] [PubMed]
48. Eldin Ahmed Abdelsalam, K.; Alobeid, M.E.A. Influence of Grand Multiparity on the Levels of Insulin, Glucose and HOMA-IR in Comparison with Nulliparity and Primiparity. *Pak. J. Biol. Sci.* **2017**, *20*, 42–46. [CrossRef] [PubMed]
49. Khan, R.; Ali, K.; Khan, Z. Socio-demographic Risk Factors of Gestational Diabetes Mellitus. *Pak. J. Med. Sci.* **2013**, *29*, 843–846. [CrossRef]
50. Abu-Heija, A.T.; Al-Bash, M.R.; Al-Kalbani, M.A. Effects of maternal age, parity and pre-pregnancy body mass index on the glucose challenge test and gestational diabetes mellitus. *J. Taibah Univ. Med. Sci.* **2017**, *12*, 338–342. [CrossRef]
51. Rosenfeld, C.S. Sex-Specific Placental Responses in Fetal Development. *Endocrinology* **2015**, *156*, 3422–3434. [CrossRef]
52. Gabory, A.; Roseboom, T.J.; Moore, T.; Moore, L.G.; Junien, C. Placental contribution to the origins of sexual dimorphism in health and diseases: Sex chromosomes and epigenetics. *Biol. Sex Differ.* **2013**, *4*, 5. [CrossRef]
53. Jiang, S.; Teague, A.M.; Tryggestad, J.B.; Aston, C.E.; Lyons, T.; Chernausek, S.D. Effects of maternal diabetes and fetal sex on human placenta mitochondrial biogenesis. *Placenta* **2017**, *57*, 26–32. [CrossRef]

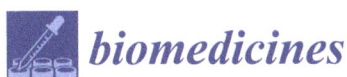

Article

New Insights on the Relationship between Leptin, Ghrelin, and Leptin/Ghrelin Ratio Enforced by Body Mass Index in Obesity and Diabetes

Adela-Viviana Sitar-Tăut [1,*], Angela Cozma [1], Adriana Fodor [2], Sorina-Cezara Coste [1], Olga Hilda Orasan [1], Vasile Negrean [1], Dana Pop [3] and Dan-Andrei Sitar-Tăut [4]

1. Internal Medicine Department, 4th Medical Clinic, Faculty of Medicine, "Iuliu Hațieganu" University of Medicine and Pharmacy, 400012 Cluj-Napoca, Romania; angelacozma@yahoo.com (A.C.); secara.sorina@yahoo.com (S.-C.C.); olgaorasan@yahoo.com (O.H.O.); vasile.negrean@umfcluj.ro (V.N.)
2. Clinical Center of Diabetes, Nutrition, Metabolic Diseases, Faculty of Medicine, "Iuliu Hațieganu" University of Medicine and Pharmacy, 400012 Cluj-Napoca, Romania; adifodor@yahoo.com
3. Department of Cardiology, Clinical Rehabilitation Hospital, Faculty of Medicine, "Iuliu Hațieganu" University of Medicine and Pharmacy, 400012 Cluj-Napoca, Romania; pop67dana@gmail.com
4. Business Information Systems Department, Faculty of Economics and Business Administration 58-60 Theodor Mihaly Street, "Babeș-Bolyai" University, 400591 Cluj-Napoca, Romania; dan.sitar@econ.ubbcluj.ro
* Correspondence: adelasitar@yahoo.com

Abstract: Currently, adipose tissue is considered an endocrine organ, however, there are still many questions regarding the roles of adipokines—leptin and ghrelin being two adipokines. The purpose of the study was to assess the relationship between the adipokines and their ratio with obesity and diabetes. Methods: Sixty patients (mean age 61.88 ± 10.08) were evaluated. Cardiovascular risk factors, leptin, ghrelin, and insulin resistance score values were assessed. The patients were classified according to their body mass index (BMI) as normal weight, overweight, and obese. Results: 20% normal weight, 51.7% overweight, 28.3% obese, and 23.3% diabetic. Obese patients had higher leptin values (in obese 34,360 pg/mL vs. overweight 18,000 pg/mL vs. normal weight 14,350 pg/mL, $p = 0.0049$) and leptin/ghrelin ratio (1055 ± 641 vs. 771.36 ± 921 vs. 370.7 ± 257, $p = 0.0228$). Stratifying the analyses according to the presence of obesity and patients' gender, differences were found for leptin ($p = 0.0020$ in women, $p = 0.0055$ in men) and leptin/ghrelin ratio ($p = 0.048$ in women, $p = 0.004$ in men). Mean leptin/BMI and leptin/ghrelin/BMI ratios were significantly higher, and the ghrelin/BMI ratio was significantly lower in obese and diabetic patients. In conclusion, obesity and diabetes are associated with changes not only in the total amount but also in the level of adipokines/kg/m². Changes appear even in overweight subjects, offering a basis for early intervention in diabetic and obese patients.

Keywords: obesity; body mass index; diabetes; leptin; ghrelin

Citation: Sitar-Tăut, A.-V.; Cozma, A.; Fodor, A.; Coste, S.-C.; Orasan, O.H.; Negrean, V.; Pop, D.; Sitar-Tăut, D.-A. New Insights on the Relationship between Leptin, Ghrelin, and Leptin/Ghrelin Ratio Enforced by Body Mass Index in Obesity and Diabetes. *Biomedicines* **2021**, *9*, 1657. https://doi.org/10.3390/biomedicines9111657

Academic Editors: Maria Grau and Jun Lu

Received: 22 September 2021
Accepted: 8 November 2021
Published: 10 November 2021

Publisher's Note: MDPI stays neutral with regard to jurisdictional claims in published maps and institutional affiliations.

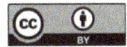

Copyright: © 2021 by the authors. Licensee MDPI, Basel, Switzerland. This article is an open access article distributed under the terms and conditions of the Creative Commons Attribution (CC BY) license (https://creativecommons.org/licenses/by/4.0/).

1. Introduction

It is well known that in last 50 years diet (with an excessive supply of energy delivered with food), lower energy expenditure and lifestyle changes are responsible for increasing prevalence of obesity (2.5 billion adults being reported as overweight or obese in 2016 [1]) and diabetes mellitus (more than 400 million adults diagnosed in 2019) [2–4]. Obesity and diabetes are both considered at this time public health issues [5–9]. Hundreds of millions of people, all over the world [4,10,11], are confronting their effects, literature suggesting a strong association between them [12].

Currently, obesity is considered a heterogeneous syndrome [13], the same fat mass excess being associated with various types of metabolic profile and risk [3,14]. Various types of intervention for obesity prevention and treatment have been proposed (diets, pharmacological interventions, or bariatric surgery). It is very important to make an accurate selection of obese patients gaining the most benefits, but also identify those with developing high-risk complications.

Taking into consideration the previously mentioned data, in recent years, the focus has shifted from adipose tissue as a fat storage organ [15] to an endocrine and immune organ [7,10,16–23], secreting various types of molecules [7,11,15,22]. The last decade has witnessed an increase in the number of discovered adipokines, with more than 600 adipokines being secreted by adipose tissue, and with an increasing need to identify their roles and clinical relevance [18]. Adipokines are involved in appetite regulation [22], energy balance, glucose homeostasis, lipid metabolism, in the pathogenesis of insulin resistance [18,20], diabetes mellitus, atherosclerosis, hypertension, metabolic syndrome, cardiovascular disease, and cancer [21,24–27]. Currently, inadequate adipokines' secretion can emphasize adipose tissue dysfunction [15,18,21], linking obesity to other comorbidities (including diabetes) [15,18–20,22,23,28,29].

Despite this great interest in the implied mechanism in obesity and diabetes, there are still many questions in the debate on the role of adipokines. Most research on this topic has focused on the individual adipokines' roles and values in diabetes or obesity. To the best of our knowledge, their relationship and the influence of body mass index over them have rarely been evaluated.

Knowledge of the possible interactions and pathological implications is needed for personalized prevention [18], early diagnosis, estimation of the risk of complications, and early intervention to reduce morbidity and mortality.

Leptin and ghrelin appear to be involved in glucose and lipid metabolism, eating behavior [7,11,22,30] and energy balance [1,23], playing important roles in hormonal regulation of food intake [17,30], being potent appetite influencers in the opposite direction [1,7,26]. Due to their interaction, they are considered in a "ghrelin-leptin tango" [17].

The aim of this work is to extend our knowledge on the relationship between adipokine (leptin, ghrelin) and their ratio enforced by body mass index, obesity, diabetes, and metabolic syndrome. Moreover, we have intended to evaluate a possible subtle relationship between adipokines and body mass index (their ratio)—a possible substrate for framing the same BMI patient category in different risk classes.

2. Materials and Methods

The current study was conducted in the Department of Cardiology of the Rehabilitation Hospital in Cluj-Napoca, a total number of 60 consecutively recruited hospital-admitted patients (44 women) were enrolled in this study. The mean age was 61.88 ± 10.08 years. Subjects who did not consent in writing to participate were excluded from the present study; also, those who present systemic or inflammatory diseases. At the same time, taking into account recently published papers with controversial data on the interaction between lipid-lowering therapy (depending on dose, duration, and type of treatment) and adipokines levels [31–37], patients with no data related to this topic have also been excluded.

A complete clinical examination was performed by a physician (according to the current European Society of Cardiology guidelines). Bodyweight, height, body mass index (BMI, calculated as weight divided by squared height, expressed as kg/m^2), waist circumference (in centimeters), present or past smoking, obesity, presence of dyslipidemia (total cholesterol $\geq$ 200 mg/dL or serum triglycerides $\geq$ 150 mg/dL), hypertension (blood pressure $\geq$ 140/90 mmHg or under hypotensive treatment), and diabetes were recorded.

For each patient, a blood sample was collected in the morning (between 7:00 a.m. and 9:00 a.m.); lipid fractions, glycemia were determined. The insulin resistance score was assessed as homeostatic model assessment (HOMA index) = insulin ($\mu U/mL$) $\times$ glycemia (mg/dL)/405.

Using the commercially available ELISA kits method (enzyme-linked immunosorbent assay, R&D Systems Inc., Minneapolis, MN, USA) serum total ghrelin (pg/mL) and serum leptin (pg/mL) levels were determined for each patient.

Patients were classified according to their body mass index in normal weight (body mass index BMI 18.5–24.9 kg/m^2), overweight (BMI 25–29.9 kg/m^2), and obese (BMI $\geq$ 30 kg/m^2). The classification of metabolic syndrome (MetS) was based on International Diabetes Federation (IDF) guidelines (central obesity plus any two of the following: triglycerides $\geq$ 150 mg/dL, low HDL-cholesterol, increased blood pressure, elevated fasting plasma glucose, or diabetes) [38].

The local University Ethics Committee (following the Declaration of Helsinki) approved the study protocol.

The statistical packages MedCalc version 10.3.0.0 (MedCalc Software, Ostend, Belgium) and SPSS for Windows version 16.0 (IBM Corporation, Armonk, New York, NY, USA) were used for processing statistical analysis. For all quantitative variables, distribution's normality was tested using the Kolmogorov–Smirnov and D'Agostino–Pearson tests; quantitative data were presented as the mean ± standard deviation, median values, respectively; qualitative data as numbers and percentages. Independent sample t-test, Mann–Whitney, χ2 test, ANOVA (analysis of variance), or Kruskal–Wallis test were used to analyze differences between variables or groups; relationships were assessed using Spearman and Pearson correlation coefficients. Univariate and multivariate regression were used to identify independent prognostic factors. A p-value < 0.05 was considered statistically significant.

3. Results

Twelve (20%) patients presented as normal weight, 31 (51.7%) overweight and 17 (28.3%) were obese; 23.3% were diabetics (type 2 DM—all of them), 47 (78.3%) hypertensive, 11 (18.3%) current smokers, 41 (68.3%) with dyslipidemia, and 71.7% with MetS. Moreover, 53.3% were diagnosed with cardiovascular disease (ischemic heart disease, heart failure, peripheral artery disease, previous stroke).

The mean age of the evaluated patients was 61.88 ± 10.08; no noteworthy differences (regarding age) were found between the groups (normal weight vs. overweight vs. obese ones). The tests revealed significant differences between the three groups in relationship with abdominal circumference ($p < 0.001$), body mass index ($p < 0.001$), glycemia ($p = 0.016$), presence of diabetes ($p = 0.0099$).

The overall mean ± SD (median) values were for ghrelin—39.55 ± 18.90 (34.25) pg/mL, for HOMA-index—2.07 ± 1.19 (1.72), and for leptin/ghrelin ratio—771.68 ± 791.43 (508.61). The characteristics of the studied group are presented extensively in Table 1.

When absolute values were compared, obese patients presented higher values of leptin (p trend = 0.0049), leptin/ghrelin ratio (p trend = 0.0228) and HOMA index (p trend = 0.003)—complete data are presented in Figure 1. Significant differences were found between obese patients and overweight (for leptin $p < 0.05$, for leptin/ghrelin ratio $p < 0.05$) and between obese and normal weight patients (for leptin $p < 0.05$, for leptin/ghrelin ratio $p < 0.05$). No relationship was found between ghrelin level and ponderal status (p = NS).

Stratifying the analyzes according to the presence of obesity and patients' gender, significant differences were found for leptin in both sexes. Obese female presented greater values (16,930 pg/mL in normal weight vs. 32,227 pg/mL in overweight vs. 39,270 pg/mL in obese, p trend = 0.0020); same results were found for men (1560 pg/mL in normal weight vs. 3480 pg/mL in overweight vs. 20,240 pg/mL in obese, p trend = 0.0055).

For the leptin/ghrelin ratio, significant differences were found between groups for both sexes—for women (437.93 ± 225.87 vs. 1019.48 ± 992.11 vs. 1295.81 ± 669, p trend = 0.048) and for men (34.55 ± 4.29 vs. 164.84 ± 140.84 vs. 478.11 ± 189.65, p trend = 0.004).

HOMA index was significantly higher in obese women (p trend = 0.008), but not in obese men (p trend = 0.11).

Table 1. Subjects' characteristics.

		Normal Weight	Overweight	Obese	p-Value	MetS−	MetS+	p*-Value
Patients		12 (20)	31 (51.7)	17 (28.3)		17 (28.3)	43 (71.7)	
Age		64.58 ± 8.09	63.29 ± 10.79	57.41 ± 9.01	p = 0.08	59.88 ± 9.17	62.67 ± 10.42	p = 0.33
Gender	Female	10 (83.33)	22 (70.96)	12 (70.58)	p = 0.48	14 (82.35)	30 (69.76)	p = 0.50
	Male	2 (16.66)	9 (29.03)	5 (29.41)		3 (17.64)	13 (30.23)	
WC		85.16 ± 9.59	97.48 ± 7.16	107.70 ± 6.88	p < 0.001	91.76 ± 11.73	100.34 ± 9.5	p = 0.0046
BMI (kg/m^2)		23.22 ± 1.89	27.68 ± 1.52	33.59 ± 2.35	p < 0.001	25.98 ± 3.99	29.44 ± 3.75	p = 0.0025
Systolic blood pressure		126.25 ± 17.46 (120)	133.22 ± 16.66 (130)	134.41 ± 17.84 130)	p = 0.40	120.58 ± 14.45	136.74 ± 16.03	p = 0.0006
Diastolic blood pressure *		75.41 ± 5.82 (80)	86.45 ± 20.46 (80)	84.41 ± 13.67 (80)	p = 0.049	77.94 ± 10.16 (80)	85.93 ± 18.62 (80)	p = 0.072
Diabetes	Yes	1(8.33)	5 (16.12)	8 (47.05)	p = 0.0099	0 (0)	14 (32.55)	p = 0.0189
	No	11 (91.66)	26 (83.87)	9(52.94)		17 (100)	29 (67.44)	
Hypertension	Yes	7 (58.33)	25 (80.64)	15 (88.23)	p = 0.06	8 (47.05)	39 (90.69)	p = 0.0008
	No	5(41.66)	6 (19.35)	2 (11.76)		9 (52.94)	4 (9.3)	
Current smokers	Yes	2 (16.66)	5 (16.12)	4 (23.52)	p = 0.60	3 (17.64)	8 (18.60)	p = 0.77
	No	10 (83.33)	26 (83.87)	13 (76.47)		14 (82.35)	35 (81.39)	
Glycemia * (mg/dL)		86.50 ± 6.54 (86)	101.12 ± 45.77 (91)	110.76 ± 30.31 (105)	p = 0.016	85.94 ± 8.09 (86)	106.86 ± 42.48 (97)	p = 0.005
Dyslipidemia	Yes	9 (75)	20 (64.51)	12 (70.58)	p = 0.86	12 (70.58)	29 (67.44)	p = 0.94
	No	3 (25)	11 (35.48)	5 (29.41)		5 (29.41)	14 (32.55)	
Total-C (mg/dL)		224.5 ± 51.60	207.83 ± 40.86	210.82 ± 61	p = 0.60	220.94 ± 41.63	208.48 ± 51.58	p = 0.37
LDL-C (mg/dL)		146 ± 42.13	134.67 ± 30.87	129.58 ± 47.03	p = 0.52	143.76 ± 35.84	132.23 ± 38.81	p = 0.29
Triglycerides (mg/dL)		165.08 ± 68.23	149.77 ± 67.05	171.70 ± 89.11	p = 0.59	122.76 ± 47.64	173.39 ± 77.37	p = 0.003
HDL-C (mg/dL)		45.50 ± 8.67	43.22 ± 10.42	40.82 ± 9.37	p = 0.44	52.70 ± 8.32	39.16 ± 7.41	p < 0.0001
Leptin * (pg/mL)		13,004 ± 8955 (14,350)	24,134 ± 23,769 (18,000)	39,284 ± 26,063 (34,360)	p = 0.0049	19,132 ± 19,904 (13,640)	28,995 ± 25,027 (21,500)	p = 0.11
Insulin (µU/mL) *		7.19 ± 0.28 (7.05)	7.97 ± 1.35 (7.4)	9.02 ± 3.43 (7.5)	p = 0.008	7.35 ± 0.41 (7.3)	8.41 ± 2.45 (7.4)	p = 0.08
HOMA index *		1.53 ± 0.15 (1.51)	2.06 ± 1.41 (1.73)	2.46 ± 1.07 (2.18)	p = 0.003	1.56 ± 0.19 (1.57)	2.27 ± 1.36 (1.83)	p = 0.0040
Ghrelin * (pg/mL)		37.16 ± 9.49 (36)	39.11 ± 21.81 (33)	42.02 ± 18.76 (36)	p = 0.70	42.91 ± 25.07 (36)	38.22 ± 15.99 (33)	p = 0.37
Leptin/ghrelin ratio		370.70 ± 257 (448)	771.36 ± 921 (396.46)	1055.31 ± 681.64 (985)	p = 0.0228	525.03 ± 584.30 (368)	869.19 ± 845 (564)	p = 0.0797

BMI = body mass index; Total-C = total cholesterol; LDL-C = LDL cholesterol = low-density lipoprotein; HDL-C = HDL cholesterol = high-density lipoprotein cholesterol; WC = waist circumference; HOMA index = homeostatic model assessment; * does not present the normal distribution; data are presented as mean ± standard deviation (median value); for categorical data as number (percentage); p was calculated with Student's test, Mann–Whitney test, or χ2 test; for p trend ANOVA (analysis of variance) or Kruskal-Wallis test were used; p = p trend normal weight vs. overweight vs. obese; p* = p between MetS+ vs. Mets−; NS (not statistically significant) p > 0.05.

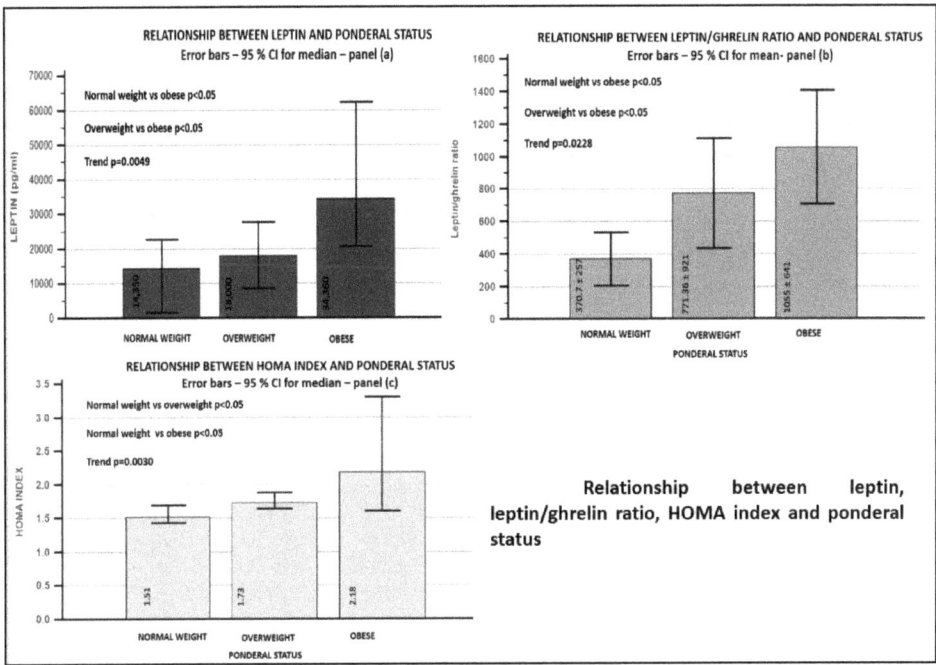

Figure 1. Relationship between adipokines, insulin resistance score and ponderal status. Panel (**a**)—relationship between leptin and ponderal status; panel (**b**)—relationship between leptin/ghrelin ratio and ponderal status; panel (**c**)—relationship between HOMA index and ponderal status.

Globally, significant correlations were found between leptin and BMI (rho = 0.402, $p = 0.001$), insulin (rho = 0.271, $p = 0.036$), ponderal status (rho = 0.420, $p = 0.0012$) and patients' sex (rho = -0.57, $p < 0.001$). Significant relationships were found between ghrelin and age (rho = -0.344, $p = 0.007$), diabetes presence (rho = -0.266, $p = 0.04$). The leptin/ghrelin ratio correlated with BMI (r = 0.304, $p = 0.018$), ponderal status (r = 0.29, $p = 0.021$), diabetes presence (r = 0.318, $p = 0.013$), insulin (r = 0.287, $p = 0.026$), and patients' sex (r = -0.404, $p = 0.001$). Data are presented in Figure 2. No associations were found between leptin, ghrelin, or leptin/ghrelin ratio and glycemia, HOMA index, lipid fractions, abdominal circumference, systolic or diastolic blood pressure.

In women, leptin correlates with weight (rho = 0.496, $p = 0.001$), BMI (rho = 0.577, $p < 0.001$), abdominal circumference (rho = 0.505, $p < 0.001$), diabetes (rho = 0.408, $p = 0.006$) and ponderal status (rho = 0.537, $p < 0.001$) ghrelin with age (rho = -0.434, $p = 0.003$), weight (rho = 0.304 $p = 0.004$), and the leptin/ghrelin ratio with age (r = 0.363, $p = 0.015$), BMI (r = 0.387, $p = 0.009$), abdominal circumference (r = 0.338, $p = 0.018$), diabetes (r = 0.477, $p = 0.001$), and ponderal status (r = 0.359, $p = 0.017$). In men, leptin correlates with age (rho = -0.510, $p = 0.043$), weight (rho = 0.576, $p = 0.02$), BMI (rho = 0.697, $p = 0.025$), ponderal status (rho = 0.819, $p < 0.001$), and the leptin/ghrelin ratio with BMI (r = 0.603, $p = 0.013$) and ponderal status (r = 0.735, $p = 0.001$).

The predictors of leptin, ghrelin, and the leptin/ghrelin ratio were studied using univariate and multivariate analysis. For leptin in the univariate analysis, independent predictors were body mass index ($R^2 = 0.125$, $p = 0.003$), insulin ($R^2 = 0.128$, $p = 0.005$), ponderal status ($R^2 = 0.150$, $p = 0.002$), and patient sex ($R^2 = 0.210$, $p < 0.001$). In the multivariate analysis (stepwise method), independent factors were ponderal status and patient sex.

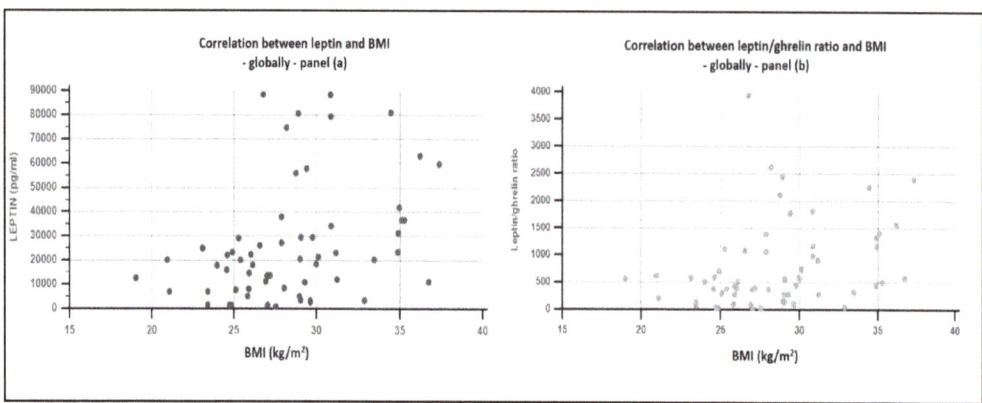

Figure 2. Correlation between leptin, leptin/ghrelin ratio, and body mass index. Panel (**a**)—correlation between leptin value and body mass index; panel (**b**)—correlation between leptin/ghrelin ratio and body mass index.

In the univariate analysis, for ghrelin age ($R^2 = 0.166$, $p = 0.001$) and for the leptin/ghrelin ratio BMI ($R^2 = 0.093$, $p = 0.018$), ponderal status ($R^2 = 0.088$, $p = 0.021$), diabetes ($R^2 = 0.101$, $p = 0.013$), insulin ($R^2 = 0.082$, $p = 0.026$), and patient sex ($R^2 = 0.163$, $p = 0.001$) were independent predictive factors. In the multivariate analysis, for the leptin/ghrelin ratio, patients 'gender, diabetes, and body mass index were independent factors.

No significant differences were found in the values of leptin and ghrelin between patients with MetS vs. those without MetS. Patients with MetS presented higher values of leptin/ghrelin (869.19 ± 845 vs. 525.03 ± 584, $p = 0.07$) and the HOMA index (1.83 vs. 1.57, $p = 0.004$).

Considering diabetic patients, as highlighted in Table 2, globally significant differences were found regarding insulin, HOMA index, ghrelin ($p = 0.0409$), and the leptin/ghrelin ratio ($p = 0.0131$). Differences were also present in women, in men registered p being non-significant.

Diabetic and obese patients (vs diabetic and nonobese patients) presented greater leptin values (32,810 pg/mL vs. 14,505 pg/mL), lower ghrelin levels (25.75 pg/mL vs. 29 pg/mL); no difference in relationship with the leptin/ghrelin ratio (1242.42 ± 663 pg/mL vs. 1201.10 ± 1616 pg/mL, $p =$ NS) was found. Detailed data regarding the relationship between BMI category and diabetes are presented in Figure 3.

After calculating the adipokines/BMI ratio (data presented in Table 3), we should mention that no statistical significance was achieved, mean ghrelin/BMI was the lowest in obese subjects (1.59 ± 0.35 in normal weight vs. 1.41 ± 0.8 in overweight vs. 1.26 ± 0.58 in obese). The mean leptin/BMI ratio and leptin/ghrelin/BMI ratio were highest in obese patients (data in Table 3 and graphic representation in Figure 4).

In metabolic syndrome, respectively, in diabetic patients, a lower ghrelin/BMI ratio and a higher leptin/ghrelin/BMI ratio were also found.

Globally, the determined area under the ROC curve for MetS identification was 0.687 (Se = 44.2%, Sp = 82.4%, criterion > 600.54) for the leptin/ghrelin ratio. For the HOMA index, the AUROC was 0.740 (Se = 48.8%, Sp = 100%, criterion > 1.83).

In men, the leptin/ghrelin ratio had a better capacity to identify patients with metabolic syndrome (AUROC = 0.923, Se = 76.9%, Sp = 100%) compared to leptin (AUROC = 0.821), ghrelin (AUROC = 0.718), or the HOMA index (AUROC = 0.654); $p = 0.09$ between the leptin/ghrelin ratio AUROC vs. AUROC-HOMA.

In women, no significant differences were found between AUROCs (AUROC-HOMA = 0.752 vs. AUROC-leptin = 0.706 vs. AUROC-ghrelin = 0.536 vs. AUROC-leptin/ghrelin ratio = 0.690). Data are presented in Table 4.

Table 2. Relationship between adipokines and diabetes' presence.

	DM+			DM−			p Global	p Women	p Men
	Global	Women	Men	Global	Women	Men			
	14 (23.3%) patients	9	5	46 (76.7%) patients	35	11			
Leptin * (pg/mL)	36,309 ± 30,848 (27,190)	51,488 ± 28,158 (36,650)	8986 ± 7366 (8500)	23,124 ± 20,867 (18,270)	27,942 ± 21,395 (22,200)	7797.27 ± 7971 (5150)	p = 0.13	p = 0.0074	p = 0.58
Insulin (μU/mL) *	9.2 ± 3.28 (7.75)	10.17 ± 3.79 (9.3)	7.44 ± 0.35 (7.5)	7.78 ± 1.55 (7.4)	7.93 ± 1.75 (7.4)	7.32 ± 0.40 (7.2)	p = 0.0253	p = 0.0118	p = 0.58
HOMA index *	3.06 ± 2.04 (2.39)	3.62 ± 2.26 (2.69)	2.04 ± 0.58 (2.12)	1.77 ± 0.53 (1.64)	1.79 ± 0.59 (1.64)	1.71 ± 0.29 (1.67)	p = 0.0002	p = 0.0002	p = 0.26
Ghrelin * (pg/mL)	34.14 ± 16.54 (25.7)	34.16 ± 16.92 (26)	34.10 ± 17.79 (25)	41.19 ± 19.42 (35.5)	42.67 ± 21.35 (36)	36.50 ± 10.79 (33)	p = 0.0409	p = 0.0626	p = 0.44
Leptin/ghrelin ratio	1224.71 ± 1114 (1035)	1742.93 ± 1072 (1405)	291.93 ± 213 (326.45)	633.80 ± 615.7 (450.99)	762.04 ± 644 (564)	225.79 ± 228 (110)	p = 0.0131	p = 0.0055	p = 0.58

HOMA index = homeostatic model assessment; DM = diabetes mellitus; * does not respect the normal distribution; data are presented as the mean ± standard deviation (median value); p was calculated with Student's test, Mann–Whitney test; p global—p between diabetic vs. non-diabetic patients; p women = p between diabetic women vs. non-diabetic women; p men = p between diabetic men vs. non-diabetic men.

Table 3. The relationship between adipokines/BMI ratio and ponderal status, metabolic syndrome, and diabetes.

	Global	Normal Weight	Overweight	Obese	p	MetS−	MetS+	p*	DM−	DM+	p⁺
L/BMI ratio *	894.15 ± 781 (710)	564.48 ± 381 (660.24)	868.03 ± 845 (618.61)	1174.49 ± 803 (1039.12)	p = 0.0717	687.47 ± 589 (570.82)	975.86 ± 837 (741.97)	p = 0.25	808.3 ± 661 (680)	1176 ± 1070 (818.96)	p=0.33
G/BMI ratio	1.41 ± 0.68	1.59 ± 0.35	1.41 ± 0.8	1.26 ± 0.58	p = 0.44	1.66 ± 0.92	1.31 ± 0.53	p = 0.07	1.49 ± 0.68	1.12 ± 0.57	p = 0.06
L/G/BMI ratio	26.47 ± 26.83	16.28 ± 11.48	27.82 ± 33.3	31.20 ± 19.47	p = 0.31	18.98 ± 17.84	29.43 ± 29.29	p = 0.09	22.47 ± 20.5	39.62 ± 39.58	p = 0.03

BMI = body mass index; L/BMI ratio = leptin/BMI ratio; G/BMI ratio = ghrelin/BMI ratio; L/G/BMI ratio = leptin/ghrelin/BMI ratio; DM = diabetes mellitus; * does not respect the normal distribution; data are presented as the mean ± standard deviation (median value); p was calculated with Student's test, Mann–Whitney test; for p trend ANOVA (analysis of variance) or Kruskal–Wallis test were used; p = p trend normal weight vs. overweight vs. obese; p* = p between MetS+ vs. MetS−; p⁺ = p between DM+ vs. DM−.

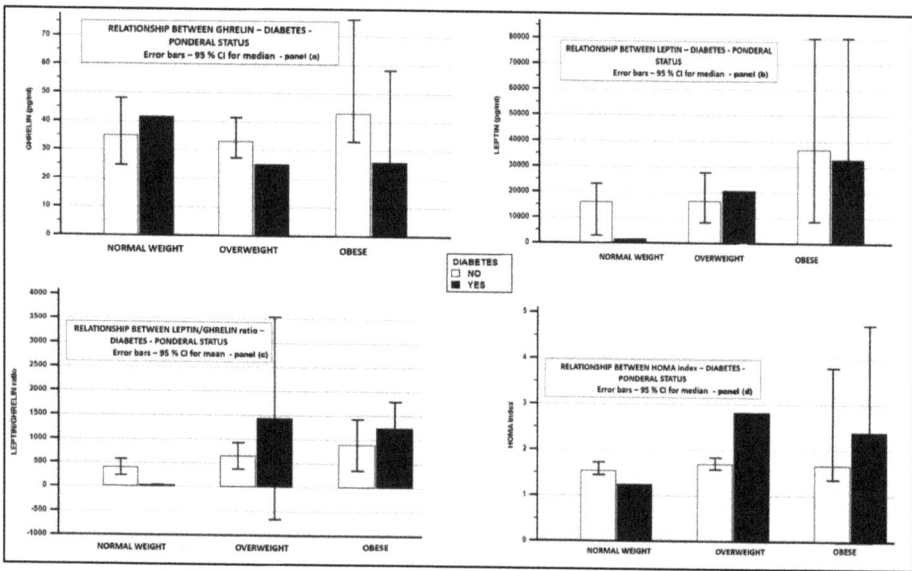

Figure 3. Relationship between adipokines—obesity—diabetes. Panel (**a**)—relationship between ghrelin—diabetes—ponderal status; panel (**b**)—relationship between leptin—diabetes—ponderal status; panel (**c**)—relationship between leptin/ghrelin ratio—diabetes—ponderal status; panel (**d**)—relationship between HOMA index—diabetes—ponderal status.

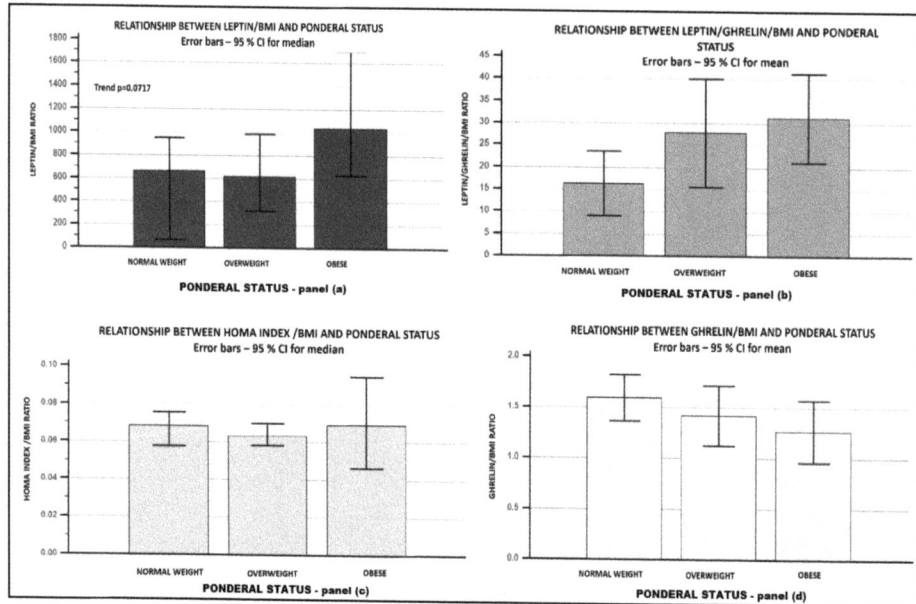

Figure 4. Relationship between leptin/BMI ratio, leptin/ghrelin/BMI ratio, Ghrelin/BMI ratio, HOMA index/BMI ratio and ponderal status. Panel (**a**)—relationship between leptin/BMI ratio—ponderal status; panel (**b**)—relationship between leptin/ghrelin/BMI ratio—ponderal status; panel (**c**)—relationship between HOMA index/BMI ratio—ponderal status; panel (**d**)—relationship between ghrelin/BMI ratio—ponderal status.

Table 4. AUROCs for adipokines and the HOMA index—for metabolic syndrome identification.

	Women				Men			
	AUROC	Se	Sp	Criterion	AUROC	Se	Sp	Criterion
L/G ratio	0.690	60	78.6	>600.54	0.923	76.9	100	>101.98
L	0.706	83.3	57.1	>17,910	0.821	53.8	100	>5150
G	0.536	53.3	71.4	≤33	0.718	84.6	66.7	≤43
HOMA	0.752	53.33	100	1.83	0.654	38.46	100	1.83

L/G = leptin/ghrelin ratio, L = leptin, G = ghrelin, HOMA index = homeostatic model assessment, AUROC = area under the ROC curve; Se = sensibility, Sp = specificity.

The presence of diabetes was better identified by the HOMA index (AUROC leptin/ghrelin ratio = 0.658, AUROC leptin = 0.632, AUROC ghrelin = 0.682, AUROC HOMA index = 0.831); the results were similar in both sexes.

4. Discussion

The increase in obesity and diabetes prevalence has important consequences on population health, the financial burden on the health system [18], and the impact on all body systems [3,7,8,39–43].

The body mass index (BMI) represents the most used tool to assess the degree of obesity. Although early studies believed that it is all about increasing in size and number of adipocytes, recent studies pointed to metabolism dysregulation, insulin resistance, systemic inflammation [18,44], responsible being the adipokines, cytokines, extracellular matrix proteins, vasoactive substances, and the release of hormone-like action proteins [7,45–47]. New data have suggested the idea that this variability in adipose tissue composition, distribution, and substance release is a substrate for people in the same BMI category being framed in various risk levels [3,7,13,21], and a key factor in obesity-related metabolic disorders [12]. Substances secreted by dysfunctional adiposity have pro-inflammatory, pro-thrombotic, and pro-atherogenic effects, but also affect vascular tone and motricity, endothelial function [7], promoting cardiac fibrosis appearance [7].

On the other hand, it is well known that a large proportion of type 2 diabetics are obese and, inversely, type 2 diabetes is more frequently met in obese people [21,48], a clear connection between those being already established. Over the last 10 years, the focus has shifted from two separate entities (obesity and diabetes) to an interwoven perspective.

Despite great interest in a complex relationship between adipokines–obesity–diabetics, many aspects are still unclear. Today, many theories and techniques have evolved to understand and prevent, to highlight the already appeared related complication of type 2 diabetes and obesity [49–52], to create estimative risk models [53].

On the other hand, the underlined mechanisms are not, at this moment, fully explained, and adipokines secretion dysregulation is considered as a possible missing chain between two entities.

Leptin and ghrelin are the main hormones that, working together, but in an opposite manner [26,27], regulating reciprocally [54], influence appetite and hunger sensations [17,26].

Leptin (from the Greek word leptos, which means thin [11]) is secreted by adipose tissue (in proportion with fat stores [29,55]), but also by the stomach and mammary gland [29]. It influences dietary intake, regulates food intake [7,15,17,22,23,29,55], energy consumption [15,29], induces the satiety sensation—"a satiety hormone" [21–23,26,47], and, consequently, determines the number of adipose deposits [25,56]. At the same time, it is considered a pro-inflammatory adipokine [15], being involved in low inflammation associated with an increased amount of fat tissue [22]. Most forms of obesity are associated even with leptin resistance [15,23]. Different mechanisms are responsible, including the fact that chronic high leptin level leads to leptin insensitivity [57]. Our results are in line with previous ones [11,17,18,22,28,55,58–62], showing higher levels in obese or diabetic patients and a positive correlation with body mass index (as reported in [15,28]).

Ghrelin, a stomach-derived hormone [30] secreted by P/D1 cells [17,63] also has an important role in short-term appetite regulation [11,17,30,64,65] and stimulation [11,26,27,60,63,66,67], but also involved in lipogenesis [67], insulin sensitivity, having anti-inflammatory properties [65], blocking the renin-angiotensin system [7,67], decreasing sympathetic activity [67,68], influencing blood pressure and heart rate [67,68], and finally being involved in cardiovascular disease development (low values being associated with increase global cardiovascular risk [54,69,70]). Previously reported data suggested the idea that a low ghrelin level could be one of the pathogenetic pathways of type 2 diabetes development [70,71].

The results presented in the current study are not in line with those previously published by [17,64,72–75], who found low ghrelin levels in obese patients, but in accordance with a 2021 published study finding no significant differences between obese and normal-weight patients regarding ghrelin levels [1]. We do not have a clear explanation for these discrepancies; probably, ghrelin levels are elevated due to 12 h fasting or food restriction [11,26,63], starvation [63]—knowing that its concentration increases before meal intake [17,66] and is influenced by low meal frequency, diet composition, exercise, and lifestyle [66]. There have also been published studies reporting the nocturnal increase in ghrelin levels [76,77]. At the same time, the literature describes the "obesity paradox"—obese subjects appear to have heterogeneous phenotypes [13]—from Metabolically UnHealthy Obesity (MuHOB) to Metabolically Obese Normal Weight (MONW or metabolically unhealthy normal BMI—normal BMI associated with obesity-related metabolic complications—more than 20% in US adults [3]) and Metabolically Healthy Obesity (MHOB—10–30% in European obese, more frequently met in women [13], 10% of US adults [3]). Just the simple use of the body mass index does not allow us to accurately discriminate between lean and fat mass, between MuHOB-MONW-MHOB [3,13].

However, our results support other published theories [65,70,71,78], theories founding lower ghrelin levels in diabetic patients.

Due to the discrepancy between the previous results, new parameters have been evaluated such as the leptin/ghrelin ratio, leptin/BMI ratio, ghrelin/BMI ratio, and leptin/ghrelin/BMI ratio.

The leptin/ghrelin ratio appears to be a hunger regulator [17], a higher ratio being associated with hunger and decreased appetite [17]. The previous hypothesis enunciated suggested the fact that leptin/ghrelin ratio can be used to identify subjects with an unfavorable evolution after obesity weight-loss therapeutic treatment [54,79], with weight regain after successful weight loss [54]. To our best knowledge, only a few studies have explored its relationship with obesity—metabolic syndrome—diabetes. Our results reinforce the data reported by [17,26,54], the leptin/ghrelin ratio being significantly higher in overweight/obese patients or diabetic or metabolic syndrome patients.

Furthermore, we should mention the fact that, in men, the leptin/ghrelin ratio had a very good discriminatory capacity for metabolic syndrome (AUROC = 0.923). Compared to previous studies that evaluated other parameters (such as the leptin/adiponectin ratio, HOMA index, QUICKI index, McAuley index, triglycerides/HDL-cholesterol ratio, cholesterol/HDL-cholesterol ratio, different measurement in abdominal CT—[80–83]) for the prediction of metabolic syndrome, leptin/ghrelin appears to have at least as good, if not a better (in men) prediction capacity.

Early findings suggest a different influence of fat amount on health status—the classification (according to BMI) in normal-weight vs. overweight vs. obese being too large, masking the differences in relationship with body mass index [3]. Metabolically obese normal-weight patients present hyperinsulinemia, insulin resistance, dyslipidemia, and an increased risk of cardiovascular diseases [3]. Therefore, we need more accurate instruments to differentiate between MuHOB-MONW-MHOB, such as the adipokines/BMI ratio.

The most striking observation that emerged from the analysis was the relationship between obesity, diabetes, and the adipokines/BMI ratio. The leptin/BMI ratio increased with the degree of obesity, the presence of metabolic syndrome, or diabetes. Although we did not find a decrease in the ghrelin level in obese subjects when we took into consideration the ghrelin/BMI ratio, a decrescendo trend was obvious. A positive parallel trend with the ponderal status of the leptin/ghrelin/BMI ratio was also revealed. Not achieving statistical significance was probably due to the small number of evaluated subjects. The results are consistent with (to our best knowledge) the only published study [27] that evaluated the adipokines/BMI ratio.

From this point of view, it seems important that not only the total adipokines' levels but also the idea that obesity and diabetes mellitus are associated with changes in adipokines' level/kg/m^2 (bringing a detailed look, a finesse one about a new possible involved mechanism).

Considering the small number of participants and discrepancy between the numbers of men/women due to consecutively admitted hospital patients (both of them being important limitations of the study), further research is needed to fully assess the relationship between adipokines, obesity, diabetes, and their pathophysiological involvement. Another serious limitation of the study is the incapacity to deepen the analysis according to the obesity degree. However, we should mention the fact that, even in a small sample, significant and interesting relationships involving leptin/ghrelin, leptin/BMI, ghrelin/BMI, and leptin/ghrelin/BMI ratios have been found.

This work provides new insights into the relationship between adipokines, diabetes, and obesity, opening new research directions to identify the changes responsible for the appearance and unfavorable disease evolution.

5. Conclusions

In conclusion, this study provides the backbone for future studies. There are still many unanswered questions surrounding the release, role, and prognostic value of adipokines. The results of this study suggest that obese and diabetic patients present both an alteration of total adipokines' level, but also changes in the relationship with body mass index. These changes seem to appear even in overweight subjects offering a base for early intervention in diabetic and obese patients.

Author Contributions: Conceptualization, A.-V.S.-T., D.-A.S.-T.; methodology, A.-V.S.-T., A.C., A.F. and D.-A.S.-T.; software, A.-V.S.-T.; validation, A.C., S.-C.C. and O.H.O.; formal analysis, A.-V.S.-T.; investigation, A.-V.S.-T. and A.C.; data curation, A.F., S.-C.C. and O.H.O.; writing—original draft preparation, A.-V.S.-T., D.-A.S.-T. and A.F.; writing—review and editing, A.-V.S.-T. and D.-A.S.-T.; visualization, A.-V.S.-T., A.C., O.H.O., V.N. and D.P.; supervision, A.-V.S.-T. and D.-A.S.-T.; project administration, A.-V.S.-T. and D.-A.S.-T. All authors have read and agreed to the published version of the manuscript.

Funding: This research received no external funding.

Institutional Review Board Statement: The study was conducted according to the guidelines of the Declaration of Helsinki, and approved by the Institutional Ethics Committee of "Iuliu Hațieganu" University of Medicine and Pharmacy, Cluj-Napoca, Romania.

Informed Consent Statement: Informed consent was obtained from all subjects involved in the study.

Conflicts of Interest: The authors declare no conflict of interest.

Abbreviations

BMI	Body mass index
WC	Waist circumference
IDF	International Diabetes Federation
HOMA index	Homeostatic model assessment index
MetS	Metabolic syndrome
HDL-cholesterol	HDL-C = high-density lipoprotein cholesterol
LDL-cholesterol	LDL-C = low-density lipoprotein cholesterol
Total-C	Total cholesterol
DM	Diabetes mellitus
AUROC	Area under the receiver operating characteristic
MuHOB	Metabolically UnHealthy Obesity
MONW	Metabolically Obese Normal Weight (MONW
MHOB	Metabolically Healthy Obesity
SD	Standard deviation

References

1. Atas, U.; Erin, N.; Tazegul, G.; Elpek, G.O.; Yildirim, B. Changes in ghrelin, substance P and vasoactive intestinal peptide levels in the gastroduodenal mucosa of patients with morbid obesity. *Neuropeptides* **2021**, *89*, 2–7. [CrossRef] [PubMed]
2. Cozma, A.; Sitar-Taut, A.; Urian, L.; Fodor, A.; Suharoschi, R.; Muresan, C.; Negrean, V.; Sampelean, D.; Zdrenghea, D.; Pop, D.; et al. Unhealthy lifestyle and the risk of metabolic syndrome—The Romanian experience. *JMMS* **2018**, *5*, 218–229. [CrossRef]
3. Ahima, R.S.; Lazar, M.A. The health risk of obesity—Better metrics imperative. *Science* **2013**, *341*, 856–858. [CrossRef] [PubMed]
4. Internation Diabetes Federation. IDF Diabetes Atlas Ninth. In *Atlas de la Diabetes de la FID 2019*; Internation Diabetes Federation: Bruselas, Belgium, 2019; ISBN 9782930229874.
5. Romacho, T.; Elsen, M.; Röhrborn, D.; Eckel, J. Adipose tissue and its role in organ crosstalk. *Acta Physiol.* **2014**, *210*, 733–753. [CrossRef] [PubMed]
6. Poher, A.L.; Tschöp, M.H.; Müller, T.D. Ghrelin regulation of glucose metabolism. *Peptides* **2018**, *100*, 236–242. [CrossRef]
7. Landecho, M.F.; Tuero, C.; Valentí, V.; Bilbao, I.; de la Higuera, M.; Frühbeck, G. Relevance of leptin and other adipokines in obesity-associated cardiovascular risk. *Nutrients* **2019**, *11*, 2664. [CrossRef]
8. Frühbeck, G.; Toplak, H.; Woodward, E.; Yumuk, V.; Maislos, M.; Oppert, J.M. Obesity: The gateway to ill health—An EASO position statement on a rising public health, clinical and scientific challenge in Europe. *Obes. Facts* **2013**, *6*, 117–120. [CrossRef]
9. Fodor, A.; Cozma, A.; Suharoschi, R.; Sitar-Taut, A.; Roman, G. Clinical and genetic predictors of diabetes drug's response. *Drug Metab. Rev.* **2019**, *51*, 408–427. [CrossRef]
10. Chait, A.; den Hartigh, L.J. Adipose Tissue Distribution, Inflammation and Its Metabolic Consequences, Including Diabetes and Cardiovascular Disease. *Front. Cardiovasc. Med.* **2020**, *7*, 22. [CrossRef]
11. Budak, E.; Fernández Sánchez, M.; Bellver, J.; Cerveró, A.; Simón, C.; Pellicer, A. Interactions of the hormones leptin, ghrelin, adiponectin, resistin, and PYY3-36 with the reproductive system. *Fertil. Steril.* **2006**, *85*, 1563–1581. [CrossRef]
12. Derosa, G.; Catena, G.; Gaudio, G.; D'Angelo, A.; Maffioli, P. Adipose tissue dysfunction and metabolic disorders: Is it possible to predict who will develop type 2 diabetes mellitus? Role of markers in the progression of dIabetes in obese patients (The RESISTIN trial). *Cytokine* **2020**, *127*, 154947. [CrossRef]
13. Vecchié, A.; Dallegri, F.; Carbone, F.; Bonaventura, A.; Liberale, L.; Portincasa, P.; Frühbeck, G.; Montecucco, F. Obesity phenotypes and their paradoxical association with cardiovascular diseases. *Eur. J. Intern. Med.* **2018**, *48*, 6–17. [CrossRef] [PubMed]
14. Catoi, A.; Parvu, A.; Andreicut, A.; Mironiuc, A.; Craciun, A.; Catoi, C.; Pop, I. Metabolically Healthy versus Unhealthy Morbidly Obese: Chronic Inflammation, Nitro-Oxidative Stress, and Insulin Resistance. *Nutrients* **2018**, *10*, 1199. [CrossRef]
15. Kyrou, I.; Mattu, H.S.; Chatha, K.; Randeva, H.S. Fat Hormones, Adipokines. In *Endocrinology of the Heart in Health and Disease*; Academic Press: Cambridge, MA, USA, 2017; ISBN 9780128031117.
16. Unamuno, X.; Gómez-Ambrosi, J.; Rodríguez, A.; Becerril, S.; Frühbeck, G.; Catalán, V. Adipokine dysregulation and adipose tissue inflammation in human obesity. *Eur. J. Clin. Investig.* **2018**, *48*, 1–11. [CrossRef]
17. Adamska-Patruno, E.; Ostrowska, L.; Goscik, J.; Pietraszewska, B.; Kretowski, A.; Gorska, M. The relationship between the leptin/ghrelin ratio and meals with various macronutrient contents in men with different nutritional status: A randomized crossover study. *Nutr. J.* **2018**, *17*, 1–7. [CrossRef] [PubMed]
18. Flehmig, G.; Scholz, M.; Kloting, N.; Fasshauer, M.; Tonjes, A.; Stumvoll, M.; Youn, B.S.; Bluher, M. Identification of adipokine clusters related to the parameters of fat mass, insulin sensitivity and inflammation. *PLoS ONE* **2014**, *9*, e99785.
19. Abd El-Kader, S.M.; Al-Jiffri, O.H. Impact of weight reduction on insulin resistance, adhesive molecules and adipokines dysregulation among obese type 2 diabetic patients. *Afr. Health Sci.* **2018**, *18*, 873–883. [CrossRef]
20. Alzaim, I.; Hammoud, S.H.; Al-Koussa, H.; Ghazi, A.; Eid, A.H.; El-Yazbi, A.F. Adipose tissue immunomodulation: A novel therapeutic approach in cardiovascular and metabolic diseases. *Front. Cardiovasc. Med.* **2020**, *7*, 1–40. [CrossRef]
21. Feijóo-Bandín, S.; Aragón-Herrera, A.; Moraña-Fernández, S.; Anido-Varela, L.; Tarazón, E.; Roselló-Lletí, E.; Portolés, M.; Moscoso, I.; Gualillo, O.; González-Juanatey, J.R.; et al. Adipokines and inflammation: Focus on cardiovascular diseases. *Int. J. Mol. Sci.* **2020**, *21*, 7711. [CrossRef]
22. Recinella, L.; Orlando, G.; Ferrante, C.; Chiavaroli, A.; Brunetti, L.; Leone, S. Adipokines: New Potential Therapeutic Target for Obesity and Metabolic, Rheumatic, and Cardiovascular Diseases. *Front. Physiol.* **2020**, *11*, 578966. [CrossRef]
23. Collazo, P.; Martínez-Sánchez, N.; Milbank, E.; Contreras, C. Incendiary leptin. *Nutrients* **2020**, *12*, 472. [CrossRef]
24. Kim, W.K.; Bae, K.-H.; Lee, S.C.; Oh, K.-J. The Latest Insights into Adipokines in Diabetes. *J. Clin. Med.* **2019**, *8*, 1874. [CrossRef]
25. Kojta, I.; Chacińska, M.; Błachnio-Zabielska, A. Obesity, Bioactive Lipids, and Adipose Tissue Inflammation in Insulin Resistance. *Nutrients* **2020**, *12*, 1305. [CrossRef] [PubMed]
26. Arabi, Y.M.; Jawdat, D.; Al-Dorzi, H.M.; Tamim, H.; Tamimi, W.; Bouchama, A.; Sadat, M.; Afesh, L.; Abdullah, M.L.; Mashaqbeh, W.; et al. Leptin, ghrelin, and leptin/ghrelin ratio in critically ill patients. *Nutrients* **2020**, *12*, 36. [CrossRef]
27. Miljković, M.; Šaranac, L.; Bašić, J.; Ilić, M.; Djindjić, B.; Stojiljković, M.; Kocić, G.; Cvetanović, G.; Dimitrijević, N. Evaluation of ghrelin and leptin levels in obese, lean and undernourished children. *Vojnosanit. Pregl.* **2017**, *74*, 963–969. [CrossRef]
28. Al-Amodi, H.S.; Abdelbasit, N.A.; Fatani, S.H.; Babakr, A.T.; Mukhtar, M.M. The effect of obesity and components of metabolic syndrome on leptin levels in Saudi women. *Diabetes Metab. Syndr. Clin. Res. Rev.* **2018**, *12*, 357–364. [CrossRef]
29. Pico, C.; Palou, M.; Pomar, C.; Rodriguez, A.; Palou, A. Leptin as a key regulator of the adipose organ. *Rev. Endocr. Metab. Disord.* **2021**. online ahead of print. [CrossRef] [PubMed]

30. Ouerghi, N.; Feki, M.; Bragazzi, N.L.; Knechtle, B.; Hill, L.; Nikolaidis, P.T.; Bouassida, A. Ghrelin Response to Acute and Chronic Exercise: Insights and Implications from a Systematic Review of the Literature. *Sport. Med.* **2021**, *51*, 2389–2410. [CrossRef] [PubMed]
31. Singh, P.; Zhang, Y.; Sharma, P.; Covassin, N.; Soucek, F. Statins decrease leptin expression in human white adipocytes. *Physiological reports* **2018**, *6*, 1–8. [CrossRef] [PubMed]
32. Takahash, Y.; Satoh, M.; Tabuchi, T.; Nakamura, M. Prospective, randomized, single-blind comparison of effects of 6 months' treatment with atorvastatin versus pravastatin on leptin and angiogenic factors in patients with coronary artery disease. *Heart Vessel.* **2012**, *27*, 337–343. [CrossRef] [PubMed]
33. Al-Azzam, S.I.; Alkhateeb, A.M.; Alzoubi, K.H.; Alzayadeen, R.N.; Ababneh, M.A.; Khabour, O.F. Atorvastatin treatment modulates the interaction between leptin and adiponectin, and the clinical parameters in patients with type II diabetes. *Exp. Ther. Med.* **2013**, *6*, 1565–1569. [CrossRef] [PubMed]
34. Szotowska, M.; Czerwienska, B.; Adamczak, M.; Chudek, J.; Wiecek, A. Effect of low-dose atorvastatin on plasma concentrations of adipokines in patients with metabolic syndrome. *Kidney Blood Press. Res.* **2012**, *35*, 226–232. [CrossRef] [PubMed]
35. Sahebkar, A.; Giua, R.; Pedone, C. Impact of Statin Therapy on Plasma Leptin Concentrations: A Systematic Review and Meta-Analysis of Randomized Placebo-Controlled Trials. *Br. J. Clin. Pharmacol.* **2016**, *82*, 1674–1684. [CrossRef]
36. Yorulmaz, H.; Ozkok, E.; Erguven, M.; Ates, G.; Aydın, I.; Tamer, S. Effect of simvastatin on mitochondrial enzyme activities, ghrelin, hypoxia-inducible factor 1α in hepatic tissue during early phase of sepsis. *Int. J. Clin. Exp. Med.* **2015**, *8*, 3640–3650. [PubMed]
37. Gruzdeva, O.; Uchasova, E.; Dyleva, Y.; Akbasheva, O.; Karetnikova, V.; Shilov, A.; Barbarash, O. Effect of different doses of statins on the development of type 2 diabetes mellitus in patients with myocardial infarction. *Diabetes Metab. Syndr. Obes. Targets Ther.* **2017**, *10*, 481–489. [CrossRef] [PubMed]
38. Pothiwala, P.; Jain, S.K.; Subhashini, Y. Metabolic syndrome and cancer. *Metab. Syndr. Relat. Disord.* **2009**, *7*, 279–287. [CrossRef]
39. Catalán, V.; Gómez-Ambrosi, J.; Rodríguez, A.; Frühbeck, G. Adipose tissue immunity and cancer. *Front. Physiol.* **2013**, *4*, 1–13. [CrossRef]
40. Alexescu, T.G.; Cozma, A.; Sitar-Tăut, A.; Negrean, V.; Handru, M.I.; Motocu, M.; Tohănean, N.; Lencu, C.; Para, I. Cardiac Changes in Overweight and Obese Patients. *Rom. J. Intern. Med.* **2016**, *54*, 161–172. [CrossRef] [PubMed]
41. Cooper, I.; Brookler, K.; Crofts, C. Rethinking Fragility Fractures in Type 2 Diabetes: The Link between Hyperinsulinaemia and Osteofragilitas. *Biomedicines* **2021**, *9*, 1165. [CrossRef]
42. Sitar Taut, A.V.; Pop, D.; Zdrenghea, D.T. NT-proBNP values in elderly heart failure patients with atrial fibrillation and diabetes. *J. Diabetes Complicat.* **2015**, *29*, 1119–1123. [CrossRef]
43. Dadarlat-Pop, A.; Sitar-Taut, A.-V.; Zdrenghea, D.; Caloian, B.; Tomoaia, R.; Pop, D.; Buzoianu, A. Profile of Obesity and Comorbidities in Elderly Patients with Heart Failure. *Clin. Interv. Aging* **2020**, *15*, 547–556. [CrossRef] [PubMed]
44. Ernst, M.C.; Sinal, C.J. Chemerin: At the crossroads of inflammation and obesity. *Trends Endocrinol. Metab.* **2010**, *21*, 660–667. [CrossRef] [PubMed]
45. Gateva, A.; Assyov, Y.; Tsakova, A.; Kamenov, Z. Classical (adiponectin, leptin, resistin) and new (chemerin, vaspin, omentin) adipocytokines in patients with prediabetes. *Horm. Mol. Biol. Clin. Investig.* **2018**, *34*, 1–9. [CrossRef] [PubMed]
46. Calabrò, P.; Golia, E.; Maddaloni, V.; Malvezzi, M.; Casillo, B.; Marotta, C.; Calabrò, R.; Golino, P. Adipose tissue-mediated inflammation: The missing link between obesity and cardiovascular disease? *Intern. Emerg. Med.* **2009**, *4*, 25–34. [CrossRef] [PubMed]
47. Reddy, P.; Lent-Schochet, D.; Ramakrishnan, N.; McLaughlin, M.; Jialal, I. Metabolic syndrome is an inflammatory disorder: A conspiracy between adipose tissue and phagocytes. *Clin. Chim. Acta* **2019**, *496*, 35–44. [CrossRef]
48. Weinstein, A.R.; Sesso, H.D.; Lee, I.M.; Cook, N.R.; Manson, J.A.E.; Buring, J.E.; Gaziano, J.M. Relationship of physical activity vs body mass index with type 2 diabetes in women. *J. Am. Med. Assoc.* **2004**, *292*, 1188–1194. [CrossRef] [PubMed]
49. Minciună, I.A.; Orășan, O.H.; Minciună, I.; Lazar, A.L.; Sitar-Tăut, A.V.; Oltean, M.; Tomoaia, R.; Pulu, M.; Sitar-Tăut, D.A.; Pop, D.; et al. Assessment of subclinical diabetic cardiomyopathy by speckle-tracking imaging. *Eur. J. Clin. Investig.* **2021**, *51*, e13475. [CrossRef] [PubMed]
50. Capparelli, R.; Iannelli, D. Role of epigenetics in type 2 diabetes and obesity. *Biomedicines* **2021**, *9*, 977. [CrossRef]
51. Kim, K.S.; Lee, J.S.; Park, J.H.; Lee, E.Y.; Moon, J.S.; Lee, S.K.; Lee, J.S.; Kim, J.H.; Kim, H.S. Identification of novel biomarker for early detection of diabetic nephropathy. *Biomedicines* **2021**, *9*, 457. [CrossRef]
52. Fringu, F.; Sitar-Taut, A.; Caloian, B.; Zdrenghea, D.; Comsa, D.; Gusetu, G.; Pop, D. The role of NT pro-BNP in the evaluation of diabetic patients with heart failure. *Endocr. Care* **2020**, *XVI*, 183–191. [CrossRef]
53. Sitar-Taut, D.-A.; Mocean, L.; Sitar-Taut, A.-V. Research about implementing E-PROCORD—New medical and modeling approaches in IT & C age applied on cardiovascular profile evaluation at molecular level. *J. Appl. Quant. Methods* **2009**, *4*, 175–189.
54. Crujeiras, A.B.; Díaz-Lagares, A.; Abete, I.; Goyenechea, E.; Amil, M.; Martínez, J.A.; Casanueva, F.F. Pre-treatment circulating leptin/ghrelin ratio as a non-invasive marker to identify patients likely to regain the lost weight after an energy restriction treatment. *J. Endocrinol. Investig.* **2014**, *37*, 119–126. [CrossRef]
55. Perakakis, N.; Farr, O.M.; Mantzoros, C.S. Leptin in Leanness and Obesity. *J. Am. Coll. Cardiol.* **2021**, *77*, 745–760. [CrossRef] [PubMed]

56. Lee, M.-W.; Lee, M.; Oh, K.-J. Adipose Tissue-Derived Signatures for Obesity and Type 2 Diabetes: Adipokines, Batokines and MicroRNAs. *J. Clin. Med.* **2019**, *8*, 854. [CrossRef] [PubMed]
57. Friedman, J.M. Leptin and the endocrine control of energy balance. *Nat. Metab.* **2019**, *1*, 754–764. [CrossRef] [PubMed]
58. Dadarlat-Pop, A.; Pop, D.; Procopciuc, L.; Sitar-Taut, A.; Zdrenghea, D.; Bodizs, G.; Tomoaia, R.; Gurzau, D.; Fringu, F.; Susca-Hojda, S.; et al. Leptin, galectin-3 and angiotensin II type 1 receptor polymorphism in overweight and obese patients with heart failure—Role and functional interplay. *Int. J. Gen. Med.* **2021**, *14*, 1727–1737. [CrossRef] [PubMed]
59. Wozniak, S.E.; Gee, L.L.; Wachtel, M.S.; Frezza, E.E. Adipose tissue: The new endocrine organ? A review article. *Dig. Dis. Sci.* **2009**, *54*, 1847–1856. [CrossRef]
60. Hajimohammadi, M.; Shab-Bidar, S.; Neyestani, T.R. Consumption of vitamin D-fortified yogurt drink increased leptin and ghrelin levels but reduced leptin to ghrelin ratio in type 2 diabetes patients: A single blind randomized controlled trial. *Eur. J. Nutr.* **2017**, *56*, 2029–2036. [CrossRef]
61. Daghestani, M.H.; Daghestani, M.; Daghistani, M.; El-Mazny, A.; Bjørklund, G.; Chirumbolo, S.; Al Saggaf, S.H.; Warsy, A. A study of ghrelin and leptin levels and their relationship to metabolic profiles in obese and lean Saudi women with polycystic ovary syndrome (PCOS). *Lipids Health Dis.* **2018**, *17*, 1–9. [CrossRef]
62. Sitar-Taut, A.-V.; Coste, S.C.; Tarmure, S.; Orasan, O.H.; Fodor, A.; Negrean, V.; Pop, D.; Zdrenghea, D.; Login, C.; Tiperciuc, B.; et al. Diabetes and Obesity-Cumulative or Complementary Effects On Adipokines, Inflammation, and Insulin Resistance. *J. Clin. Med.* **2020**, *9*, 2767. [CrossRef]
63. Yamada, C. Relationship between orexigenic peptide ghrelin signal, gender difference and disease. *Int. J. Mol. Sci.* **2021**, *22*, 3763. [CrossRef] [PubMed]
64. Alamri, B.N.; Shin, K.; Chappe, V.; Anini, Y. The role of ghrelin in the regulation of glucose homeostasis. *Horm. Mol. Biol. Clin. Investig.* **2016**, *26*, 3–11. [CrossRef] [PubMed]
65. Kadoglou, N.P.E.; Lampropoulos, S.; Kapelouzou, A.; Gkontopoulos, A.; Theofilogiannakos, E.K.; Fotiadis, G.; Kottas, G. Serum levels of apelin and ghrelin in patients with acute coronary syndromes and established coronary artery disease-KOZANI STUDY. *Transl. Res.* **2010**, *155*, 238–246. [CrossRef] [PubMed]
66. Lv, Y.; Liang, T.; Wang, G.; Li, Z. Ghrelin, a gastrointestinal hormone, regulates energy balance and lipid metabolism. *Biosci. Rep.* **2018**, *38*, BSR20181061. [CrossRef]
67. Tuero, C.; Valenti, V.; Rotellar, F.; Landecho, M.F.; Cienfuegos, J.A.; Frühbeck, G. Revisiting the Ghrelin Changes Following Bariatric and Metabolic Surgery. *Obes. Surg.* **2020**, *30*, 2763–2780. [CrossRef]
68. Rodríguez, A. Novel molecular aspects of ghrelin and leptin in the control of adipobiology and the cardiovascular system. *Obes. Facts* **2014**, *7*, 82–95. [CrossRef]
69. Pop, D.; Peter, P.; Dădârlat, A.; Sitar-Tăut, A.; Zdrenghea, D. Serum ghrelin level is associated with cardiovascular risk score. *Rom. J. Intern. Med.* **2015**, *53*, 140–145. [CrossRef] [PubMed]
70. Poykko, S. *Ghrelin, Metabolic Risk Factors and Carotid Artery Atherosclerosis*; University of Oulu: Oulu, Finland, 2005; ISBN 9514276558.
71. Poykko, S.; Kellokoski, E.; Horkko, S.; Kauma, H.; Kesaniemi, Y.; Ukkola, O. Low plasma ghrelin is associated with insulin resistance, hypertension and the prevalence of type 2 diabetes. *Diabetes* **2003**, *52*, 2546–2553. [CrossRef]
72. Razzaghy-Azar, M.; Nourbakhsh, M.; Pourmoteabed, A.; Nourbakhsh, M.; Ilbeigi, D.; Khosravi, M. An Evaluation of Acylated Ghrelin and Obestatin Levels in Childhood Obesity and Their Association with Insulin Resistance, Metabolic Syndrome, and Oxidative Stress. *J. Clin. Med.* **2016**, *5*, 61. [CrossRef]
73. Verdeș, G.; Duță, C.C.; Popescu, R.; Mitulețu, M.; Ursoniu, S.; Lazăr, O.F. Correlation between leptin and ghrelin expression in adipose visceral tissue and clinical-biological features in malignant obesity. *Rom. J. Morphol. Embryol.* **2017**, *58*, 923–929.
74. Korek, E.; Krauss, H.; Gibas-Dorna, M.; Kupsz, J.; Piątek, M.; Piątek, J. Fasting and postprandial levels of ghrelin, leptin and insulin in lean, obese and anorexic subjects. *Prz. Gastroenterol.* **2013**, *8*, 383–389. [CrossRef] [PubMed]
75. Mohamed, W.S.; Hassanien, M.; Abokhosheim, K. Role of Ghrelin, Leptin and Insulin Resistance in Development of Metabolic Syndrome in Obese Patients. *Endocrinol. Metab. Syndr.* **2014**, *3*, 1–6. [CrossRef]
76. Dzaja, A.; Dalal, M.A.; Himmerich, H.; Uhr, M.; Pollmächer, T.; Schuld, A. Sleep enhances nocturnal plasma ghrelin levels in healthy subjects. *Am. J. Physiol. Endocrinol. Metab.* **2004**, *286*, 963–967. [CrossRef]
77. Motivala, S.J.; Tomiyama, A.J.; Ziegler, M.; Khandrika, S.; Irwin, M.R. Nocturnal levels of ghrelin and leptin and sleep in chronic insomnia. *Psychoneuroendocrinology* **2009**, *34*, 540–545. [CrossRef] [PubMed]
78. Lindqvist, A.; Shcherbina, L.; Prasad, R.B.; Miskelly, M.G.; Abels, M.; Martínez-Lopéz, J.A.; Fred, R.G.; Nergård, B.J.; Hedenbro, J.; Groop, L.; et al. Ghrelin suppresses insulin secretion in human islets and type 2 diabetes patients have diminished islet ghrelin cell number and lower plasma ghrelin levels. *Mol. Cell. Endocrinol.* **2020**, *511*, 110835. [CrossRef] [PubMed]
79. Labayen, I.; Ortega, F.B.; Ruiz, J.R.; Lasa, A.; Simón, E.; Margareto, J. Role of baseline leptin and ghrelin levels on body weight and fat mass changes after an energy-restricted diet intervention in obese women: Effects on energy metabolism. *J. Clin. Endocrinol. Metab.* **2011**, *96*, 996–1000. [CrossRef] [PubMed]
80. Pickhardt, P.J.; Graffy, P.M.; Zea, R.; Lee, S.J.; Liu, J.; Sandfort, V.; Summers, R.M. Utilizing fully automated abdominal CT-based biomarkers for opportunistic screening for metabolic syndrome in adults without symptoms. *Am. J. Roentgenol.* **2021**, *216*, 85–92. [CrossRef] [PubMed]

81. Yoon, J.H.; Park, J.K.; Oh, S.S.; Lee, K.H.; Kim, S.K.; Cho, I.J.; Kim, J.K.; Kang, H.T.; Ahn, S.G.; Lee, J.W.; et al. The ratio of serum leptin to adiponectin provides adjunctive information to the risk of metabolic syndrome beyond the homeostasis model assessment insulin resistance: The Korean Genomic Rural Cohort Study. *Clin. Chim. Acta* **2011**, *412*, 2199–2205. [CrossRef]
82. Cozma, A.; Fodor, A.; Orăsan, O.H.; Suharoschi, R.; Muresan, C.; Vulturar, R.; Sampelean, D.; Negrean, V.; Pop, D.; Sitar-Tăut, A. A comparison between insulin resistance scores parameters in identifying patients with metabolic syndrome. *Stud. Univ. Babes-Bolyai Chem.* **2019**, *64*, 147–159. [CrossRef]
83. Blum, M.R.; Popat, R.A.; Nagy, A.; Cataldo, N.A.; McLaughlin, T.L. Using metabolic markers to identify insulin resistance in premenopausal women with and without polycystic ovary syndrome. *J. Endocrinol. Investig.* **2021**, *44*, 2123–2130. [CrossRef]

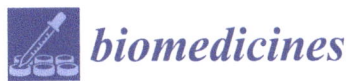

Article

Effects of a 13-Week Personalized Lifestyle Intervention Based on the Diabetes Subtype for People with Newly Diagnosed Type 2 Diabetes

Iris M. de Hoogh *, Wilrike J. Pasman, André Boorsma, Ben van Ommen and Suzan Wopereis

Research Group Microbiology & Systems Biology, TNO, Netherlands Organization for Applied Scientific Research, 3704 HE Zeist, The Netherlands; wilrike.pasman@tno.nl (W.J.P.); andre.boorsma@tno.nl (A.B.); ben.vanommen@tno.nl (B.v.O.); suzan.wopereis@tno.nl (S.W.)
* Correspondence: iris.dehoogh@tno.nl; Tel.: +31-088-8660911

Abstract: A type 2 diabetes mellitus (T2DM) subtyping method that determines the T2DM phenotype based on an extended oral glucose tolerance test is proposed. It assigns participants to one of seven subtypes according to their β-cell function and the presence of hepatic and/or muscle insulin resistance. The effectiveness of this subtyping approach and subsequent personalized lifestyle treatment in ameliorating T2DM was assessed in a primary care setting. Sixty participants, newly diagnosed with (pre)diabetes type 2 and not taking diabetes medication, completed the intervention. Retrospectively collected data of 60 people with T2DM from usual care were used as controls. Bodyweight ($p < 0.01$) and HbA1c ($p < 0.01$) were significantly reduced after 13 weeks in the intervention group, but not in the usual care group. The intervention group achieved 75.0% diabetes remission after 13 weeks (fasting glucose ≤ 6.9 mmol/L and HbA1c < 6.5% (48 mmol/mol)); for the usual care group, this was 22.0%. Lasting (two years) remission was especially achieved in subgroups with isolated hepatic insulin resistance. Our study shows that a personalized diagnosis and lifestyle intervention for T2DM in a primary care setting may be more effective in improving T2DM-related parameters than usual care, with long-term effects seen especially in subgroups with hepatic insulin resistance.

Keywords: type 2 diabetes; remission; lifestyle intervention; diet; subtypes; primary care

Citation: de Hoogh, I.M.; Pasman, W.J.; Boorsma, A.; van Ommen, B.; Wopereis, S. Effects of a 13-Week Personalized Lifestyle Intervention Based on the Diabetes Subtype for People with Newly Diagnosed Type 2 Diabetes. *Biomedicines* 2022, 10, 643. https://doi.org/10.3390/biomedicines10030643

Academic Editor: Myunggon Ko

Received: 20 January 2022
Accepted: 7 March 2022
Published: 10 March 2022

Publisher's Note: MDPI stays neutral with regard to jurisdictional claims in published maps and institutional affiliations.

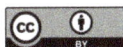

Copyright: © 2022 by the authors. Licensee MDPI, Basel, Switzerland. This article is an open access article distributed under the terms and conditions of the Creative Commons Attribution (CC BY) license (https://creativecommons.org/licenses/by/4.0/).

1. Introduction

The main pathophysiological defects in type 2 diabetes mellitus (T2DM) are insulin resistance (IR) of the liver, muscle, and adipose tissue, and reduced β-cell function (BCF) [1]. Current treatment primarily focuses on lowering blood glucose concentrations and glycated hemoglobin (HbA1c) levels instead of addressing the underlying pathophysiology. Therefore, limited effectiveness may be achieved in diabetes treatment, especially in the longer term [2–4]. Several studies have shown that lifestyle interventions have beneficial effects on glycemic control [5–7], and may even induce disease remission [8,9]. In the DiRECT trial, a primary-care-led weight management program for T2DM, 46% of the intervention participants achieved disease remission [3,4]. The remission rate appeared related to β-cell capacity [6], indicating that not all persons react similarly to such interventions. As T2DM is a multi-factorial disease affecting multiple organs, and because people differ in their genetics, phenotype, lifestyle, and environment, different mechanisms may underlie T2DM pathophysiology [10,11]. Impaired glucose tolerance (IGT) and impaired fasting glucose (IFG), which are both pre-stages of T2DM, can occur both separately and simultaneously, and differ in prevalence [12]. Moreover, plasma insulin levels in response to an oral glucose tolerance test (OGTT) differ [13]. A greater impairment in first-phase insulin secretion, indicative of hepatic insulin resistance (HIR), can be found in individuals with isolated IFG. People with IGT show higher two-hour insulin and glucose concentrations, indicative of muscle insulin resistance (MIR) [14]. The cardiometabolic T2DM etiologies of systemic low-grade inflammation and lipid dysmetabolism differ between people with MIR and people with HIR [15]. These differences in underlying T2DM pathophysiology may explain the differences in the effectiveness of lifestyle interventions. Indeed, it has been shown that in people with prediabetes with relatively high fasting insulin, a low-fat diet is most effective for weight loss, whereas for people with prediabetes with relatively low fasting insulin, a low-carbohydrate diet is most effective [16]. Another study comparing the two-year effects of both a low-fat and a Mediterranean diet showed a larger improvement in BCF on a low-fat diet in people with HIR, whilst people with MIR or a combination of muscle and liver IR (CIR) benefitted more from a Mediterranean diet [17]. Moreover, it is known that MIR is best counteracted by physical exercise [18], whereas caloric restriction seems to be effective in reducing HIR [19]. Thus, the diabetic subtype can be used to personalize—and potentially increase—the efficacy of and adherence to lifestyle treatment for T2DM.

Herein, we propose a subtyping method that determines an individual's diabetic phenotype and establishes the underlying pathophysiology [20]. T2DM subtyping was conducted by performing a five-timepoint OGTT, quantifying plasma glucose and insulin concentrations at baseline and 30 min intervals up to two hours. The resulting data were used to determine indices indicative of pancreatic insulin secretion and muscle and liver insulin resistance.

Based on the T2DM subtype, a personalized diagnosis and subsequent tailored treatment were determined. Next, we assessed the effectiveness of this T2DM subtyping approach in ameliorating T2DM by the evaluation of HbA1c and fasting plasma glucose (FPG), as well as the associated risk factors, including body weight, in comparison to usual care. Additionally, we elucidated whether personalized interventions improved the diabetic phenotype and induced diabetes remission. This study took place in a primary care setting to assess the feasibility of this more personalized approach in a real-life setting. The intervention lasted 13 weeks, with a two-year follow-up.

2. Materials and Methods

2.1. Study Population

Eighty-two participants with prediabetes or newly diagnosed T2DM (within the last 12 months), according to the Dutch general practitioners' standards, were recruited from eight primary care centers in Hillegom, The Netherlands. In The Netherlands, T2DM diagnosis is determined based on glucose values with two FPG of ≥ 7.0 mmol/L or one FPG of ≥ 7.0 mmol/L combined with non-FPG of ≥ 11.1 mmol/L on two different days, whereas prediabetes is defined as an FPG of ≥ 6.1 and <7.0 mmol/L and/or a non-FPG of ≥ 7.8 and <11.1 mmol/L. Participants were eligible for study participation if they were aged 30–80 years, and had a stable body mass index (BMI) between 25 and 35 kg/m^2. The exclusion criteria were the use of plasma glucose-lowering medication within the past year, the use of systemic corticosteroids and β-blockers in the past month, pancreatic or (late-onset) type 1 diabetes, and other medical conditions, including gastrointestinal dysfunction, psychiatric disorders, severe hypertension, and renal insufficiency. Of the 82 participants initially enrolled in the study, 16 were excluded after the baseline OGTT because of either very poor BCF (n = 8) or normal glucose metabolism (neither reduced BCF nor IR) (n = 8).

From the same primary care center, the data of 60 people with prediabetes or newly diagnosed T2DM in usual care, meeting the above-stated inclusion and exclusion criteria, i.e., aged 30–80 years, BMI between 25 and 35 kg/m^2, and no use of plasma glucose-lowering medication, were collected retrospectively as controls. The historic data included fewer people with prediabetes because there is no official monitoring protocol for prediabetes according to the Dutch general practitioners' standards [21], as a result of which registration and monitoring occurs less frequently.

All participants gave written informed consent. The study protocol was approved by the Medical Ethics Committee Brabant (NL48742.028.14). The study was performed in accordance with the Declaration of Helsinki and good clinical practice and was registered at ClinicalTrails.gov (NCT02196350).

2.2. Study Design

This study was exploratory. At baseline, clinical chemistry, blood pressure, and anthropometric measurements (length, body weight, waist circumference, and fat percentage) were performed. Based on the T2DM subtype, participants were allocated to one of seven personalized lifestyle treatments. The 13-week intervention was supervised by a dietician and/or physiotherapist. All participants visited the general practitioner's assistant at baseline and in weeks 4, 8, and 13, and participants visited the dietician at baseline and in weeks 1, 2, 6, 10, and 13 for (personalized) dietary advice. Those participants allocated to a treatment including exercise visited the physiotherapist for supervised personalized exercise training three times a week for 13 weeks. After the 13-week intervention, the measurements were repeated, including an OGTT to determine changes in glucose metabolism and the T2DM subtype. After the 13-week intervention, the participants returned to standard primary care. Anthropometry and clinical chemistry were repeated one and two years after baseline. Healthcare providers were instructed to be reluctant in prescribing oral diabetes medication or insulin therapy during the study. The intervention group was compared with historic data from a control group that received usual care according to the Dutch general practitioners' standards [21]. This states to start with prescribing oral diabetes medication when the HbA1c target level of 7.0% (53 mmol/mol) is not reached with a non-drug treatment. For this study, diabetes remission was defined as: (a) Fasting glucose $\leq$ 6.9 mmol/L, (b) HbA1c < 6.5% (48 mmol/mol), (c) no use of glucose-lowering medication, and (d) meeting these targets at the 12- and 24-month follow-up [2]. Figure 1 provides an overview of the study design.

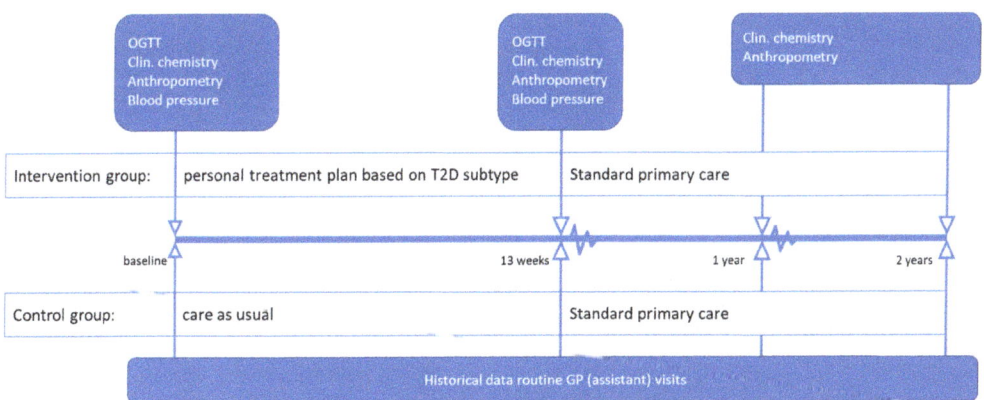

Figure 1. Study design. GP = general practitioner; OGTT = oral glucose tolerance test; clin. chemistry = clinical chemistry (HbA1c, triglycerides and HDL, LDL, and total cholesterol). Anthropometry includes body height (only at baseline), body weight, waist circumference, and fat percentage.

2.3. Clinical Chemistry and OGTT

After an overnight fast, blood samples were taken before (0 min) and at four time points after drinking a 75 g glucose solution (t = 30, 60, 90, and 120 min) to determine plasma glucose and insulin concentrations. HbA1c and lipids were assessed at baseline, 13 weeks, and at the one- and two-year follow-up. OGTT and blood sampling were performed at the service center Elsbroek by AtalMedial in Hillegom, The Netherlands. Lab analyses were performed by AtalMedials' lab located in Spaarne Gasthuis Hospital, The Netherlands.

2.4. Subtyping Rationale

Glucose and insulin response to the OGTT was used to calculate the following indices: Disposition Index (DI) [22–24], Matsuda Index, Hepatic Insulin Resistance Index (HIRI) [25], and Muscle Insulin Sensitivity Index (MISI) [26]. Cut-off values for these indices, to distinguish between healthy and diabetic scores, were determined using data from ~1100 participants [27–29]. These cut-offs were calculated and validated using different subsets of healthy participants, participants with prediabetes (IFG, IGT, or both), and people with undiagnosed and clinically diagnosed T2DM.

After calculating the indices, participants were assigned to one of seven subtypes according to BCF (moderate or low) and the presence of hepatic IR and/or muscle IR (Supplemental Table S1). Individuals with no IR and no BCF were excluded at baseline. If, after the intervention, participants reverted to no IR and no BCF, these participants were assigned to the "healthy" subtype.

2.5. Interventions

The HIR and CIR subgroup received a very-low-calorie diet (VLCD) for one week, using meal replacements (Modifast) three times a day (500 kcal/day), followed by a 12-week low-calorie diet (LCD; 1000 kcal/day) based on a personal meal plan provided by a dietician. Participants could opt for meal replacements for a maximum of one meal per day. Groups with poor BCF (PB), PB-HIR, or PB-CIR received 13 weeks of LCD, similar to the LCD of the HIR and CIR subgroups. Groups with MIR or PB-MIR followed an isocaloric diet (ICD), comprising normal food products.

In addition to the dietary intervention, participants in the HIR, PB, and PB-HIR subgroup were stimulated to adhere to the Dutch Norm for Healthy Physical Activity for overweight people (moderate exercise of 60 min/day). The CIR and PB-CIR subgroup were stimulated to adhere to the Dutch Norm for Physical Activity for one week, followed by 12 weeks of strength and endurance training (thrice a week for 60 min), supervised by a physiotherapist. The MIR and PB-MIR subgroups performed supervised strength and endurance training for 13 weeks.

2.6. Statistical Analysis

Complete case analysis was performed using only paired data at baseline and after 13 weeks. Two weighted linear mixed models were created, from which all statistical results were subsequently derived, using the "lmer" package [30]. One model included subtype as the main effect, whereas the other contained group. Both models included time as the main effect and the interaction of time with either group and subtype. Furthermore, both models included the participant as a random factor. When fitting the models, statistical outliers were excluded when their standardized model residuals were further than three standard deviations away from 0. When applying these models, some variables were log10-transformed to account for heteroscedasticity in the model residuals.

Type-III sum-of-squares p-values were calculated for the main effects using the "car" package, whereas p-values for the post hoc tests were calculated using the "emmeans" package [31]. Additionally, p-values of <0.05 were deemed statistically significant. The R Project for Statistical Computing software version 3.4.3 for Windows (The R Project for Statistical Computing, Auckland City, Auckland, New Zealand) was used for statistical analysis [32].

3. Results

3.1. Baseline Characteristics

A total of 60 out of the 66 participants completed the intervention. At baseline, the intervention group had significantly lower HbA1c and FPG and significantly higher BMI compared with the usual care group (Table 1). Moreover, age tended to be higher in the usual care group ($p = 0.06$). In both groups, the average HbA1c levels were below the target level for people with type 2 diabetes, which is 7% (53 mmol/mol) in The Netherlands [21].

Table 1. Baseline characteristics by treatment group.

Characteristic	Usual Care	Intervention	p-Value
n	60	60	
Men/women (n)	34/26	29/31	NS
Age (years)	65.2 ± 9.7	63.4 ± 7.9	0.06
Body height (m)	1.73 ± 0.10	1.72 ± 0.10	NS
Bodyweight (kg)	90.4 ± 15.1	96.3 ± 16.1	NS
BMI	29.9 ± 5.0	32.6 ± 4.8	0.035
HbA1c (%) HbA1c (mmol/mol)	6.7 ± 3.4 49.7 ± 13.9	6.0 ± 2.8 42.6 ± 7.4	<0.001
FPG (mmol/L)	8.3 ± 4.0	7.0 ± 1.5	0.005
SBP (mmHg)	136 ± 19	137 ± 14	NS
DBP (mmHg)	82 ± 11	83 ± 10	NS
Total cholesterol (mmol/L)	5.9 ± 1.9 †	5.7 ± 1.1	NS
HDL-cholesterol (mmol/L)	1.3 ± 0.5 †	1.3 ± 0.3	NS
Triglycerides (mmol/L)	3.5 ± 5.4 †	2.2 ± 1.0	NS

Data are the mean ± standard deviation, unless otherwise indicated. † $n \approx 20$, not available for all controls and after outlier removal. BMI = body mass index; HbA1c = glycated hemoglobin; FPG = fasting plasma glucose; SBP = systolic blood pressure; DBP = diastolic blood pressure; HDL = high-density lipoprotein; NS = not significant.

3.2. Intervention Effects Compared with Usual Care

After 13 weeks, body weight ($p < 0.001$) and HbA1c ($p < 0.001$) were significantly lower compared with baseline in the intervention group, whilst there were no significant changes in the usual care group (Supplemental Table S2). After one and two years of follow-up, body weight ($p < 0.001$) and HbA1c ($p < 0.001$ at one year and $p < 0.01$ at two years) remained significantly lower compared with baseline in the intervention group. In the usual care group, body weight ($p < 0.01$) was reduced compared with baseline at the two-year follow-up only.

In the intervention group, total cholesterol (−0.47 mmol/L; $p < 0.01$), triglycerides (−0.58 mmol/L; $p < 0.001$), and waist circumference (−11 cm; $p < 0.001$) decreased after the intervention. These data were not available for the usual care group, as these markers are not measured regularly in usual care.

3.3. Diabetes Remission

Table 2 shows the fraction of participants who were classified as "in remission" for the usual care and intervention group. The results are shown as the fraction of participants diagnosed with T2DM at baseline, as our study population also included participants with prediabetes. The intervention group achieved significantly more T2DM remission after 13 weeks compared with the usual care group ($p = 0.0002$). In the intervention group, two participants started using glucose-lowering medication during the follow-up period of the study. For the usual care group, no medication data were available for follow-up, so it was unclear what proportion of participants were still in remission at the one- and two-year follow-ups.

Table 2. Remission data * for the intervention and usual care groups after the intervention (week 13) and at the one- and two-year follow-ups (week 52 and 104), expressed as the number and percentage of participants with T2DM at baseline **.

	Usual Care		Intervention	
	($n = 41$)	(%)	($n = 25$)	(%)
13 weeks	5	22.0	19	75.0
52 weeks	-	-	13	52.4
104 weeks	-	-	7	28.6

* Remission was defined as fasting plasma glucose ≤ 6.9 mmol/L and HbA1c < 6.5% (48 mmol/mol), no use of glucose-lowering medication, and meeting these targets at 12 and 24 months of follow-up; medication data were not available at follow-up for the usual care group. ** In other words, subjects with prediabetes at baseline were excluded from this table, as the remission definition does not apply to people with prediabetes.

For the intervention group, participants that achieved remission after 13 weeks showed significantly more weight loss than participants that did not achieve remission (−10.7 kg resp. −4.6 kg; $p < 0.001$).

Of the participants with prediabetes at baseline, 89% remained prediabetic, whilst 11% progressed to T2DM during the study. Those participants that progressed to T2DM showed significantly less weight loss than participants that remained prediabetic ($p = 0.05$).

3.4. Changes in the Diabetic Phenotype in the Intervention Group

At baseline, 11 participants had hepatic IR (HIR), 7 participants had muscle and hepatic IR (combined IR; CIR), 9 participants had isolated poor BCF (PB), 28 participants had PB-HIR, and 5 participants had PB-CIR. At baseline, there were no participants with a healthy, MIR, or PB-MIR subtype. A substantial redistribution of participants over the subtypes was found after 13 weeks of intervention (Figure 2). The most noticeable trend was seen for the HIR subtype, with 55% of the participants converting into a healthy subtype after the intervention. For the PB-HIR and CIR subtype this was 29%, whereas for the PB and PB-CIR subtypes, it was 22% and 20%, respectively.

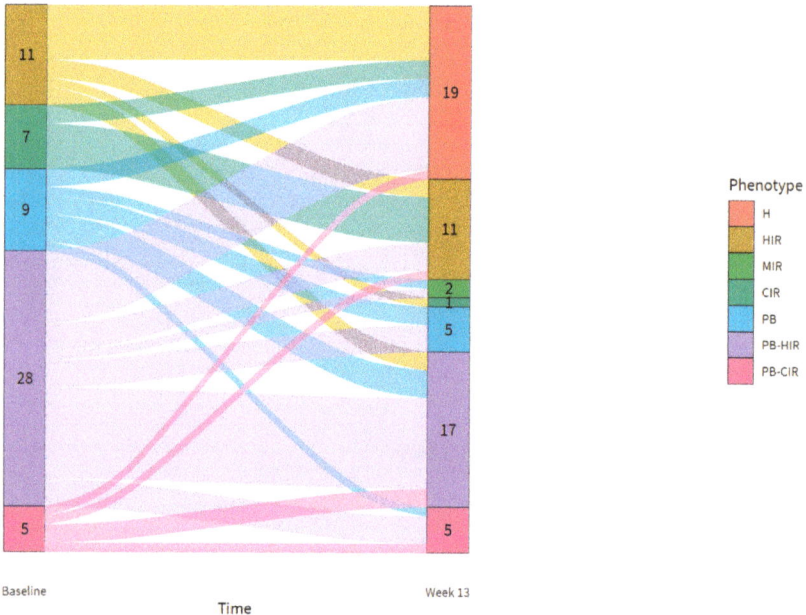

Figure 2. Flow diagram showing the shift in subtypes for participants from baseline to 13 weeks. A shift upwards illustrates a shift toward a less complex phenotype. H = healthy; HIR = moderate BCF and liver IR; MIR = moderate BCF and muscle IR; CIR = moderate BCF and combined IR; PB = low BCF and no IR; PB-HIR = low BCF and liver IR; PB-CIR = low BCF and combined IR.

In total, 32% of the participants ($n = 19$) obtained a healthy subtype (normal BCF without IR) after 13 weeks of intervention, of which 7 participants met the criteria for T2DM remission, 11 had prediabetes at baseline, and one participant reached a HbA1c of 5.4% (36 mmol/mol) and FPG of 7.0 mmol/L at 13 weeks. Including the participant with borderline remission and a healthy subtype, in total, 10 participants could be classified as T2DM after 13 weeks of intervention, of which 6 had the PB-HIR subtype and 3 the PB-CIR subtype.

3.5. Changes in the Glucose Metabolism in the Intervention Group

Liver IR significantly improved (HIRI of -80.2; $p < 0.001$) after 13 weeks. Postprandial glucose (PPG) decreased significantly (-1.34 mmol/L; $p < 0.001$) after 13 weeks. The disposition index and MISI did not change over time ($p = 0.231$, resp. $p = 0.945$).

Furthermore, the 13-week intervention significantly decreased HIRI in all subtypes with liver IR (unknown for subgroup PB-CIR, as no p-value could be calculated due to missing data; Table 3). FPG decreased in two of these subgroups (HIR and PB-HIR).

Table 3. Changes in oral glucose tolerance test response from baseline to 13 weeks (end of intervention) for the main type 2 diabetes subtypes.

Subtype	FPG	PPG	DI	HIRI	MISI
HIR ($n = 11$)	-1.2 **	-1.1	2.19	-1145 **	0.41
CIR ($n = 7$)	-0.3	-3.1 *	1.44	-619 *	-1.71 †
PB ($n = 9$)	0.3	0.2	0.33	138	0.09
PB-HIR ($n = 28$)	-1.2 **	-0.3	0.80 *	-22 **	1.58 **
PB-CIR ($n = 5$)	-0.6	-8.4 †	0.87	2525 †	-2.16 ‡

The data are deltas between baseline and 13 weeks of intervention. FPG = fasting plasma glucose; PPG = postprandial glucose; DI = disposition index; HIRI = hepatic insulin resistance index; MISI = muscle insulin sensitivity index; HIR = moderate BCF and liver IR; CIR = moderate BCF and combined IR; PB = low BCF and no IR; PB-HIR = low BCF and liver IR; PB-CIR = low BCF and combined IR. * $p < 0.01$ and ** $p < 0.001$ compared with baseline; † no p-value available due to missing data; ‡ trend toward a decrease ($p = 0.0590$).

Unexpectedly, MISI increased in the PB-HIR subgroup, indicating a decrease in muscle insulin sensitivity, although the mean MISI was still within the healthy range (-2.87 ± 1.27). Postprandial glucose improved in the CIR subgroup only. The disposition index only improved in the PB-HIR subgroup.

3.6. Long-Term Intervention Effects

All subgroups showed a significant reduction in body weight after the intervention, which was maintained at one and two years of follow-up for all subgroups, except for the group with PB-CIR (+3.3 kg; $p < 0.05$) (Table 4).

Table 4. Changes in body weight, FPG, and HbA1c from baseline (week 0) to the end of the intervention (week 13) and to the one- and two-year follow-ups (weeks 52 and 104) for the type 2 diabetes subtypes.

	HIR ($n = 11$)	CIR ($n = 7$)	PB ($n = 9$)	PB-HIR ($n = 28$)	PB-CIR ($n = 5$)
Bodyweight (kg)					
Weeks 0–13	-10.2 ***	-13.1 ***	-5.6 **	-8.8 ***	-5.7 *
Weeks 0–52	-9.1 ***	-7.3 **	-4.8 ***	-6.0 ***	2.0
Weeks 0–104	-8.4 ***	-7.1 **	-2.3 *	-6.0 ***	3.3 *
Fasting glucose (mmol/L)					
Weeks 0–13	-1.1 ***	-0.3	0.3	-1.1 ***	-0.5
Weeks 0–52	-1.3 ***	-0.2	0.0	-0.7 ***	0.4
Weeks 0–104	-1.0 ***	-0.2	0.4	-0.7 ***	-0.3
HbA1c (mmol/mol)					
Weeks 0–13	-3.4 ***	-3.3 *	0.0	-6.2 ***	-2.2
Weeks 0–52	-4.3 **	-1.3	-1.3	-4.9 ***	-1.5
Weeks 0–104	-2.4 *	-0.4	1.8	-2.5 **	-1.3

The data are deltas comparing baseline to week 13 (end of intervention), week 52 (one year follow-up), and week 104 (two years follow-up). HIR = moderate BCF and liver IR; CIR = moderate BCF and combined IR; PB = low BCF and no IR; PB-HIR = low BCF and liver IR; PB-CIR = low BCF and combined IR. * $p < 0.05$, ** $p < 0.01$, and *** $p < 0.001$ compared with baseline.

In the HIR and PB-HIR subgroups, FPG and HbA1c decreased after the intervention, which was maintained up to two years of follow-up. In the CIR subgroup, HbA1c was significantly reduced after the intervention, but this effect was not maintained at follow-up. For all other subgroups, no significant changes in FPG or HbA1c were found.

4. Discussion

In this study, we showed that diabetes subtyping and subsequent tailored lifestyle interventions in a primary care setting are more effective in improving T2DM-related parameters than usual care. Bodyweight and HbA1c were significantly reduced after 13 weeks of intervention, whilst no changes in these markers were seen with usual care. Additionally, the improvements in health status were maintained up to two years after the intervention. Our results suggest that a (V)LCD may be more effective in improving liver IR, whilst resistance training may be more effective in improving muscle IR.

Unique to our study was the use of an extended OGTT in a primary care setting for identifying the diabetic phenotype and subsequently using this knowledge for a tailored lifestyle treatment. Various clinical studies have shown that persons with T2DM may differ in their metabolic profile, resulting in differential responses to lifestyle interventions [13,15,17,33–36]. However, in these studies, participants were assigned to a dietary pattern at random and subtype effects were identified retrospectively. To the best of our knowledge, this is the first study in which the metabolic profiling of people with T2DM was performed prospectively and used for a phenotype-based sub-diagnosis and adjacent tailored lifestyle treatment in a real-life primary care setting.

Our results suggest that these tailored treatments indeed induce differential effects. The specific improvements in HIRI and FPG for the groups with liver IR, and the improvements in PPG in the groups with combined IR (CIR), suggest that the tailored treatment may have added value over a one-size-fits-all approach. However, as there were no participants with isolated muscle IR (with or without low BCF), future research is needed to investigate the effects of a solely physical activity intervention in people with muscle IR. Previous research has shown that improving MISI is more difficult or may take longer [36,37]. The lack of effect, or even a small negative effect in the PB-HIRI group, on MISI in our study may be a result of weight loss. Weight loss may have included a loss of muscle mass, which may negatively affect MISI. However, in the PROBE trial, the lack of effect on MISI coincided with an improved muscle mass [36].

Average weight loss in our study after one year was 7.1 kg, and this resulted in improvements in T2DM-related health parameters. Caloric restriction has been shown to reduce pancreatic and hepatic fat content and hepatic IR and improve BCF [19,38]. In our study, weight loss was strongly correlated with achieving remission, with an average weight loss of −10.7 kg in the group that achieved remission and −4.7 kg in the group without remission. These results indicate a relationship between T2DM remission achievement and weight loss, as also shown in the DiRECT trial [3]. Modest weight loss of 5–10% has also been previously linked to improvements in cardiovascular risk factors, including HbA1c [39]. Non-responders predominantly had a complex phenotype with combined IR, decreased BCF, or both, indicating that achieving remission is more difficult with a more progressed disease status. Karter et al. observed an association between the rate of remission and years since diagnosis [40], and Taylor et al. linked non-response to a lifestyle intervention to a more advanced, irreversible stage of β-cell dysfunction. In our study, subgroups with combined insulin resistance with or without poor BCF or poor BCF only (CIR, PB, and PB-CIR) showed only short-term or no improvements in FPG or HbA1c [6], whereas subgroups with hepatic insulin resistance with or without decreased BCF (HIR and PB-HIR) had long-term improvements in FPG and HbA1c. Interestingly, persons with combined insulin resistance (CIR) did achieve a sustained bodyweight reduction of 7 kg after two years of follow-up that did not result in reduced hyperglycemia. Therefore, the subgroups with isolated liver IR (HIR and PB-HIR) benefitted most from the lifestyle treatment, as shown by improved bodyweight, HIRI, FPG, and HbA1c after the intervention period, and improved FPG and HbA1c after one and two years of follow-up.

The percentage of participants in remission after the intervention was 75.0%. However, when looking at the diabetic phenotype of the included participants, based on indices for organ-specific insulin sensitivity and β-cell function, only 28% of the participants with T2DM at baseline had a fully remitted and healthy subtype (normal BCF and no IR) after the intervention. T2DM is indeed a multi-factorial disease affecting multiple organs, and normalization of HbA1c and/or FPG levels can still coincide with reduced organ function and β-cell dysfunction [41]. It is therefore recommended for individuals who achieve remission to remain under the supervision of healthcare professionals [42].

Increasing focus on the functioning of organs involved in the pathophysiology of T2DM (liver, adipose tissue, skeletal muscle, and pancreas) may therefore provide more insight into the effects of interventions and disease status, instead of merely focusing on remission numbers. We therefore suggest performing an extended OGTT to assess diabetes pathophysiology so that disease progression or regression before and after an intervention can be more accurately determined over time. Indeed, in a pilot study using the same subtyping methodology in a population with a longer T2DM disease duration, none of the participants were able to achieve a healthy subtype, even though improvements in HbA1c and FPG were observed [37]. Additionally, the diabetes subtyping methodology allows for a more tailored lifestyle intervention, which may improve intervention success. For this, our subtyping method can be used, which uses blood glucose and insulin response to a five-point OGTT as a measure of diabetes pathophysiology [20,43]. Besides our subtyping model, other models exist, using established T2DM genetic loci to identify several diabetic phenotypes [44], using clinical parameters to cluster adult-onset diabetes [45,46], or using patterns of specific glycemic responses called "glucotypes" [47]. The importance of differences in organ function was also suggested in the Diogenes and Maastricht studies, which showed an altered metabolic profile in persons with obesity and liver IR compared with persons with obesity and muscle IR [15,48,49]. However, our subtyping method is, to the best of our knowledge, the first that provides a complete picture of the underlying pathophysiology of T2DM and offers the opportunity for tailored treatment.

A few limitations need to be discussed. An important limitation of this explorative study was that participants in the usual care group were not accurately matched with the intervention group for BMI and age, due to a limited available patient database. Additionally, or maybe consequently, the usual care group had higher baseline FPG and HbA1c values compared with the intervention group. Additionally, as OGTTs are not performed in usual care, no data on type 2 diabetes subtypes and the comparability of the distribution thereof with the intervention group were available. Considering the higher baseline FPG and HbA1c values, the participants in the usual care group, although newly diagnosed, without treatment for type 2 diabetes and with an average HbA1c level below the target, could all have had a poor BCF, which would explain the scarce response in this group. Furthermore, no data on medication were available for the usual care group, except for baseline, where oral medication was used as the exclusion criterium. Possibly, in the usual care group, the use of glucose-lowering medication could have started throughout the trial. These differences between the usual care and intervention groups may have influenced our results. A future efficacy study with a prospective control arm randomized for BMI, age, FPG, HbA1c, and BCF status, as well as careful registration of medicine use is needed to confirm the current results from diabetes subtyping and tailored lifestyle intervention.

In The Netherlands, people are screened for T2DM by determining FPG levels and sometimes HbA1c levels. As 2 h blood glucose is not measured, participants with isolated IGT, which is defined as 2 h glucose levels of 7.8–11.1 mmol [50], are missed. This may have caused the underrepresentation of participants with muscle IR in our study. To improve the early detection of and treatment for participants with isolated IGT, we suggest always performing an OGTT or at least measuring 2 h blood glucose levels.

In the intervention group, the number of participants was relatively small per diabetes subtype, especially for the PB-CIR, CIR, and PB groups. Despite the small diabetes subtype groups, we were still able to reach statistical significance for some of the variables, providing interesting insights into the underlying pathophysiology of type 2 diabetes and how lifestyle interventions can interact with this. For a follow-up study, a larger study population is required to confirm and validate these findings. It will remain difficult, however, to influence equal distribution over the diabetes subtypes, as this follows from the OGTT. Lastly, the frequency of visits to a healthcare professional, including visits to the GP assistant, as well as to dieticians and/or physiotherapists, was probably lower in the control group as compared with the intervention group, which could have resulted in differences in intervention adherence, thereby affecting the study results. However, this more intensive guidance, as well as referral to lifestyle professionals such as dieticians and physiotherapists may be required to help people with newly diagnosed T2DM to initiate behavior change.

5. Conclusions

This was the first study to provide tailored treatment based on the diabetic phenotype of people with T2DM in a primary care setting. The tailored approach resulted in differential effects on T2DM phenotypes, with the largest and most persistent improvement in participants with isolated liver IR (with or without low BCF). Our results suggest that a (V)LCD may be more effective in improving liver IR, whilst resistance training may be more effective in improving muscle IR. Future research, including participants with isolated muscle IR, a prospective control arm matching the intervention arm, and a larger number of study participants to have larger subgroups of diabetes subtypes, should confirm these findings. Even though diabetes remission was achieved by the majority of participants in the intervention group, organ-specific IR and BCF were not fully recovered. This calls for continued monitoring to avoid relapse, and long-term adherence to a tailored-lifestyle treatment may be required for people who achieve T2DM remission. Lastly, this study showed that the tailored approach can be implemented in current primary care and can result in remission or reversal of the disease in the first three months after T2DM diagnosis.

Supplementary Materials: The following are available online at https://www.mdpi.com/article/10.3390/biomedicines10030643/s1: Table S1: Deviating indices and associated treatment plan for all seven type 2 diabetes subtypes and the "healthy" subgroup; Table S2: Means (SDs) and significant changes in the variables after 13 weeks of intervention and one or two years of follow-up for the usual care and intervention groups.

Author Contributions: B.v.O., S.W., W.J.P. and A.B. designed and planned the study. W.J.P., A.B. and I.M.d.H. prepared and conducted the study and collected the data. All authors contributed to writing the manuscript. All authors have read and agreed to the published version of the manuscript.

Funding: This research received no external funding and was funded from internal sources from The Netherlands Organization for Applied Scientific Research (TNO).

Institutional Review Board Statement: This study was conducted according to the guidelines of the Declaration of Helsinki, and approved by the Medical Ethics Committee Brabant (METC Brabant; NL48742.028.14). This study was registered at clinicaltrials.gov (NCT02196350).

Informed Consent Statement: Informed consent was obtained from all subjects involved in the study.

Data Availability Statement: The data presented in this study are available on reasonable request from the corresponding author.

Acknowledgments: General Practitioners Edwin Wallaart, practice Elsbroek, Hillegom, The Netherlands, and Jos Mulders, practice Hillegom Zuid, Hillegom, The Netherlands, are gratefully acknowledged for their effort to conduct the study in their healthcare centers. Ellen Witteman-van Lierop and Marijke van Noort, practice Elsbroek, Hillegom, The Netherlands, Lenneke Elderbroek, dietician Care and Cure, Hillegom, The Netherlands, and Fianne van Veenendaal, physiotherapist, practice van Veenendaal, Hillegom, The Netherlands, are gratefully acknowledged for the coaching of the participants. Hanneke van Engel, AtalMedial, Hillegom, The Netherlands, is gratefully acknowledged for the performance of the tests in the Hillegom care centers. The authors would like to thank Ilse Geerars, TNO, Zeist, The Netherlands, for her role in setting up the study; Adriana Israël, Maarten Costerius, and Martien Caspers, TNO, Zeist, The Netherlands, for their role in data collection; Tim van den Broek, TNO, Zeist, The Netherlands, for his role in data analysis; and Mark Begieneman, TNO, Zeist, The Netherlands, for his help in drafting the manuscript. Last but not least, the authors would like to thank all participants in this study. All authors read and approved the final manuscript.

Conflicts of Interest: The authors declare no conflict of interest.

References

1. Defronzo, R.A. From the triumvirate to the ominous octet: A new paradigm for the treatment of type 2 diabetes mellitus. *Diabetes* 2009, *58*, 773–795. [CrossRef] [PubMed]
2. Buse, J.B.; Caprio, S.; Cefalu, W.T.; Ceriello, A.; Del Prato, S.; Inzucchi, S.E.; McLaughlin, S.; Phillips, G.L.; Robertson, R.P.; Rubino, F.; et al. How Do We Define Cure of Diabetes? *Diabetes Care* 2009, *32*, 2133–2135. [CrossRef] [PubMed]
3. Lean, M.E.; Leslie, W.S.; Barnes, A.C.; Brosnahan, N.; Thom, G.; McCombie, L.; Peters, C.; Zhyzhneuskaya, S.; Al-Mrabeh, A.; Hollingsworth, K.G.; et al. Primary care-led weight management for remission of type 2 diabetes (DiRECT): An open-label, cluster-randomised trial. *Lancet* 2018, *391*, 541–551. [CrossRef]
4. Lean, M.E.J.; Leslie, W.S.; Barnes, A.C.; Brosnahan, N.; Thom, G.; McCombie, L.; Peters, C.; Zhyzhneuskaya, S.; Al-Mrabeh, A.; Hollingsworth, K.G.; et al. Durability of a primary care-led weight-management intervention for remission of type 2 diabetes: 2-year results of the DiRECT open-label, cluster-randomised trial. *Lancet Diabetes Endocrinol.* 2019, *7*, 344–355. [CrossRef]
5. Colberg, S.R. Physical activity: The forgotten tool for type 2 diabetes management. *Front. Endocrinol.* 2012, *3*, 70. [CrossRef]
6. Taylor, R.; Al-Mrabeh, A.; Zhyzhneuskaya, S.; Peters, C.; Barnes, A.C.; Aribisala, B.S.; Hollingsworth, K.G.; Mathers, J.C.; Sattar, N.; Lean, M.E.J. Erratum: Remission of Human Type 2 Diabetes Requires Decrease in Liver and Pancreas Fat Content but Is Dependent upon Capacity for β Cell Recovery. *Cell Metab.* 2018, *28*, 667, Erratum in *Cell Metab.* 2018, *28*, 547–556.e3. [CrossRef]
7. Knowler, W.C.; Barrett-Connor, E.; Fowler, S.E.; Hamman, R.F.; Lachin, J.M.; Walker, E.A.; Nathan, D.M.; Diabetes Prevention Program Research Group. Reduction in the incidence of type 2 diabetes with lifestyle intervention or metformin. *N. Engl. J. Med.* 2002, *346*, 393–403.
8. Steven, S.; Hollingsworth, K.G.; Al-Mrabeh, A.; Avery, L.; Aribisala, B.; Caslake, M.; Taylor, R. Very Low-Calorie Diet and 6 Months of Weight Stability in Type 2 Diabetes: Pathophysiological Changes in Responders and Nonresponders. *Diabetes Care* 2016, *39*, 808–815. [CrossRef]
9. Ried-Larsen, M.; Johansen, M.Y.; MacDonald, C.S.; Hansen, K.B.; Christensen, R.; Wedell-Neergaard, A.; Pilmark, N.S.; Langberg, H.; Vaag, A.A.; Pedersen, B.K.; et al. Type 2 diabetes remission 1 year after an intensive lifestyle intervention: A secondary analysis of a randomized clinical trial. *Diabetes Obes. Metab.* 2019, *21*, 2257–2266. [CrossRef]
10. Kahn, S.E.; Cooper, M.E.; Del Prato, S. Pathophysiology and treatment of type 2 diabetes: Perspectives on the past, present, and future. *Lancet* 2014, *383*, 1068–1083. [CrossRef]
11. Galicia-Garcia, U.; Benito-Vicente, A.; Jebari, S.; Larrea-Sebal, A.; Siddiqi, H.; Uribe, K.B.; Ostolaza, H.; Martín, C. Pathophysiology of Type 2 Diabetes Mellitus. *Int. J. Mol. Sci.* 2020, *21*, 6275. [CrossRef] [PubMed]
12. Meigs, J.B.; Muller, D.C.; Nathan, D.M.; Blake, D.R.; Andres, R.; Baltimore Longitudinal Study of Aging. The natural history of progression from normal glucose tolerance to type 2 diabetes in the Baltimore Longitudinal Study of Aging. *Diabetes* 2003, *52*, 1475–1484. [CrossRef] [PubMed]
13. Pearson, E.R. Type 2 diabetes: A multifaceted disease. *Diabetologia* 2019, *62*, 1107–1112. [CrossRef]
14. Abdul-Ghani, M.A.; Tripathy, D.; DeFronzo, R.A. Contributions of β-cell dysfunction and insulin resistance to the pathogenesis of impaired glucose tolerance and impaired fasting glucose. *Diabetes Care* 2006, *29*, 1130–1139. [CrossRef]
15. Van Der Kolk, B.W.; Kalafati, M.; Adriaens, M.; Van Greevenbroek, M.M.J.; Vogelzangs, N.; Saris, W.H.M.; Astrup, A.; Valsesia, A.; Langin, D.; Van Der Kallen, C.J.H.; et al. Subcutaneous adipose tissue and systemic inflammation are associated with peripheral but not hepatic insulin resistance in humans. *Diabetes* 2019, *68*, 2247–2258. [CrossRef]
16. Hjorth, M.F.; Astrup, A.; Zohar, Y.; Urban, L.E.; Sayer, R.D.; Patterson, B.W.; Herring, S.J.; Klein, S.; Zemel, B.S.; Foster, G.D.; et al. Personalized nutrition: Pretreatment glucose metabolism determines individual long-term weight loss responsiveness in individuals with obesity on low-carbohydrate versus low-fat diet. *Int. J. Obes.* 2019, *43*, 2037–2044. [CrossRef]
17. Blanco-Rojo, R.; Alcala-Diaz, J.F.; Wopereis, S.; Perez-Martinez, P.; Quintana-Navarro, G.M.; Marin, C.; Ordovas, J.M.; van Ommen, B.; Perez-Jimenez, F.; Delgado-Lista, J.; et al. The insulin resistance phenotype (muscle or liver) interacts with the type of diet to determine changes in disposition index after 2 years of intervention: The CORDIOPREV-DIAB randomised clinical trial. *Diabetologia* 2016, *59*, 67–76. [CrossRef]
18. Kirwan, J.P.; Solomon, T.P.J.; Wojta, D.M.; Staten, M.A.; Holloszy, J.O. Effects of 7 days of exercise training on insulin sensitivity and responsiveness in type 2 diabetes mellitus. *Am. J. Physiol. Metab.* 2009, *297*, E151–E156. [CrossRef]
19. Lim, E.L.; Hollingsworth, K.G.; Aribisala, B.S.; Chen, M.J.; Mathers, J.C.; Taylor, R. Reversal of type 2 diabetes: Normalisation of beta cell function in association with decreased pancreas and liver triacylglycerol. *Diabetologia* 2011, *54*, 2506–2514. [CrossRef]

20. Van Ommen, B.; Wopereis, S.; van Empelen, P.; van Keulen, H.M.; Otten, W.; Kasteleyn, M.; Molema, J.J.W.; de Hoogh, I.M.; Chavannes, N.H.; Numans, M.E.; et al. From diabetes care to diabetes cure-the integration of systems biology, ehealth, and behavioral change. *Front. Endocrinol.* **2018**, *8*, 381. [CrossRef]
21. Barents, E.; Bilo, H.; Donk, M.; Hart, H.; Verburg-Oorthuizen, A.; Wiersma, T. NHG-Standaard Diabetes Mellitus Type 2-Pagina 1 NHG-Standaard Diabetes Mellitus Type 2 (M01). 2018. Available online: https://richtlijnen.nhg.org/standaarden/diabetes-mellitus-type-2 (accessed on 19 January 2022).
22. Bergman, R.N.; Phillips, L.S.; Cobelli, C. Physiologic evaluation of factors controlling glucose tolerance in man: Measurement of insulin sensitivity and beta-cell glucose sensitivity from the response to intravenous glucose. *J. Clin. Investig.* **1981**, *68*, 1456–1467. [CrossRef]
23. Kahn, S.E.; Prigeon, R.L.; McCulloch, D.K.; Boyko, E.J.; Bergman, R.N.; Schwartz, M.W.; Neifing, J.L.; Ward, W.K.; Beard, J.C.; Palmer, J.P. Quantification of the relationship between insulin sensitivity and beta-cell function in human subjects. Evidence for a hyperbolic function. *Diabetes* **1993**, *42*, 1663–1672. [CrossRef] [PubMed]
24. Breda, E.; Cavaghan, M.K.; Toffolo, G.; Polonsky, K.S.; Cobelli, C. Oral glucose tolerance test minimal model indexes of beta-cell function and insulin sensitivity. *Diabetes* **2001**, *50*, 150–158. [CrossRef] [PubMed]
25. Matsuda, M.; DeFronzo, R.A. Insulin sensitivity indices obtained from oral glucose tolerance testing: Comparison with the euglycemic insulin clamp. *Diabetes Care* **1999**, *22*, 1462–1470. [CrossRef] [PubMed]
26. Abdul-Ghani, M.A.; Matsuda, M.; Balas, B.; DeFronzo, R.A. Muscle and Liver Insulin Resistance Indexes Derived from the Oral Glucose Tolerance Test. *Diabetes Care* **2007**, *30*, 89–94. [CrossRef]
27. Larsen, T.M.; Dalskov, S.; van Baak, M.; Jebb, S.; Kafatos, A.; Pfeiffer, A.; Martinez, J.A.; Handjieva-Darlenska, T.; Kunešová, M.; Holst, C.; et al. The Diet, Obesity and Genes (Diogenes) Dietary Study in eight European countries—A comprehensive design for long-term intervention. *Obes. Rev.* **2010**, *11*, 76–91. [CrossRef]
28. Delgado-Lista, J.; Perez-Martinez, P.; Garcia-Rios, A.; Alcala-Diaz, J.F.; Perez-Caballero, A.I.; Gomez-Delgado, F.; Fuentes, F.; Quintana-Navarro, G.; Lopez-Segura, F.; Ortiz-Morales, A.M.; et al. CORonary Diet Intervention with Olive oil and cardiovascular PREVention study (the CORDIOPREV study): Rationale, methods, and baseline characteristics. *Am. Heart J.* **2016**, *177*, 42–50. [CrossRef]
29. Wopereis, S.; Stroeve, J.H.M.; Stafleu, A.; Bakker, G.C.M.; Burggraaf, J.; van Erk, M.J.; Pellis, L.; Boessen, R.; Kardinaal, A.A.F.; van Ommen, B. Multi-parameter comparison of a standardized mixed meal tolerance test in healthy and type 2 diabetic subjects: The PhenFlex challenge. *Genes Nutr.* **2017**, *12*, 21. [CrossRef]
30. Bates, D.; Mächler, M.; Bolker, B.; Walker, S. Fitting Linear Mixed-Effects Models Using Lme4. *J. Stat. Softw.* **2015**, *67*, 1–48. [CrossRef]
31. Fox, J.; Weisberg, S. *An R Companion to Applied Regression*, 3rd ed.; SAGE Publications: Thousand Oaks, CA, USA, 2019; ISBN 9781544336473.
32. R Core Team. R: A Language and Environment for Statistical Computing [Internet]. 2019. Available online: http://www.r-project.org/index.html (accessed on 19 January 2022).
33. Yubero-Serrano, E.M.; Delgado-Lista, J.; Tierney, A.C.; Perez-Martinez, P.; Garcia-Rios, A.; Alcala-Diaz, J.F.; Castaño, J.P.; Tinahones, F.J.; Drevon, C.A.; Defoort, C.; et al. Insulin resistance determines a differential response to changes in dietary fat modification on metabolic syndrome risk factors: The LIPGENE study. *Am. J. Clin. Nutr.* **2015**, *102*, 1509–1517. [CrossRef]
34. Blaak, E.E. Current metabolic perspective on malnutrition in obesity: Towards more subgroup-based nutritional approaches? *Proc. Nutr. Soc.* **2020**, *32*, 331–337. [CrossRef] [PubMed]
35. Trouwborst, I.; Bowser, S.M.; Goossens, G.H.; Blaak, E.E. Ectopic Fat Accumulation in Distinct Insulin Resistant Phenotypes; Targets for Personalized Nutritional Interventions. *Front. Nutr.* **2018**, *5*, 77. [CrossRef] [PubMed]
36. Pasman, W.J.; Memelink, R.G.; de Vogel-Van den Bosch, J.; Begieneman, M.P.V.; van den Brink, W.J.; Weijs, P.J.M.; Wopereis, S. Obese Older Type 2 Diabetes Mellitus Patients with Muscle Insulin Resistance Benefit from an Enriched Protein Drink during Combined Lifestyle Intervention: The PROBE Study. *Nutrients* **2020**, *12*, 2979. [CrossRef] [PubMed]
37. de Hoogh, I.M.; Oosterman, J.E.; Otten, W.; Krijger, A.-M.; Berbée-Zadelaar, S.; Pasman, W.J.; van Ommen, B.; Pijl, H.; Wopereis, S. The Effect of a Lifestyle Intervention on Type 2 Diabetes Pathophysiology and Remission: The Stevenshof Pilot Study. *Nutrients* **2021**, *13*, 2193. [CrossRef]
38. Zhyzhneuskaya, S.V.; Al-Mrabeh, A.; Peters, C.; Barnes, A.; Aribisala, B.; Hollingsworth, K.G.; McConnachie, A.; Sattar, N.; Lean, M.E.J.; Taylor, R. Time Course of Normalization of Functional β-Cell Capacity in the Diabetes Remission Clinical Trial After Weight Loss in Type 2 Diabetes. *Diabetes Care* **2020**, *43*, 813–820. [CrossRef]
39. Wing, R.R.; Lang, W.; Wadden, T.A.; Safford, M.; Knowler, W.C.; Bertoni, A.G.; Hill, J.O.; Brancati, F.L.; Peters, A.; Wagenknecht, L. Benefits of modest weight loss in improving cardiovascular risk factors in overweight and obese individuals with type 2 diabetes. *Diabetes Care* **2011**, *34*, 1481–1486. [CrossRef]
40. Karter, A.J.; Nundy, S.; Parker, M.M.; Moffet, H.H.; Huang, E.S. Incidence of remission in adults with type 2 diabetes: The diabetes & aging study. *Diabetes Care* **2014**, *37*, 3188–3195. [CrossRef]
41. Dutia, R.; Brakoniecki, K.; Bunker, P.; Paultre, F.; Homel, P.; Carpentier, A.C.; McGinty, J.; Laferrere, B. Limited Recovery of β-Cell Function after Gastric Bypass Despite Clinical Diabetes Remission. *Diabetes* **2014**, *63*, 1214–1223. [CrossRef]
42. Nagi, D.; Hambling, C.; Taylor, R. Remission of type 2 diabetes: A position statement from the Association of British Clinical Diabetologists (ABCD) and the Primary Care Diabetes Society (PCDS). *Br. J. Diabetes* **2019**, *19*, 73–76. [CrossRef]

43. Yu, E.A.; Le, N.A.; Stein, A.D. Measuring Postprandial Metabolic Flexibility to Assess Metabolic Health and Disease. *J. Nutr.* **2021**, *151*, 3284–3291. [CrossRef]
44. Udler, M.S.; Kim, J.; von Grotthuss, M.; Bonàs-Guarch, S.; Cole, J.B.; Chiou, J.; Boehnke, M.; Laakso, M.; Atzmon, G.; Glaser, B.; et al. Type 2 diabetes genetic loci informed by multi-trait associations point to disease mechanisms and subtypes: A soft clustering analysis. *PLOS Med.* **2018**, *15*, e1002654. [CrossRef] [PubMed]
45. Ahlqvist, E.; Storm, P.; Käräjämäki, A.; Martinell, M.; Dorkhan, M.; Carlsson, A.; Vikman, P.; Prasad, R.B.; Aly, D.M.; Almgren, P.; et al. Novel subgroups of adult-onset diabetes and their association with outcomes: A data-driven cluster analysis of six variables. *Lancet Diabetes Endocrinol.* **2018**, *6*, 361–369. [CrossRef]
46. Ahlqvist, E.; Prasad, R.B.; Groop, L. Subtypes of Type 2 Diabetes Determined From Clinical Parameters. *Diabetes* **2020**, *69*, 2086–2093. [CrossRef] [PubMed]
47. Hall, H.; Perelman, D.; Breschi, A.; Limcaoco, P.; Kellogg, R.; McLaughlin, T.; Snyder, M. Glucotypes reveal new patterns of glucose dysregulation. *PLoS Biol.* **2018**, *16*, e2005143. [CrossRef] [PubMed]
48. Vogelzangs, N.; van der Kallen, C.J.H.; van Greevenbroek, M.M.J.; van der Kolk, B.W.; Jocken, J.W.E.; Goossens, G.H.; Schaper, N.C.; Henry, R.M.A.; Eussen, S.J.P.M.; Valsesia, A.; et al. Metabolic profiling of tissue-specific insulin resistance in human obesity: Results from the Diogenes study and the Maastricht Study. *Int. J. Obes.* **2020**, *44*, 1376–1386. [CrossRef]
49. van der Kolk, B.W.; Vogelzangs, N.; Jocken, J.W.E.; Valsesia, A.; Hankemeier, T.; Astrup, A.; Saris, W.H.M.; Arts, I.C.W.; van Greevenbroek, M.M.J.; Blaak, E.E. Plasma lipid profiling of tissue-specific insulin resistance in human obesity. *Int. J. Obes.* **2019**, *43*, 989–998. [CrossRef]
50. World Health Organization & International Diabetes Federation. *Definition and Diagnosis of Diabetes Mellitus and Intermediate Hyperglycaemia: Report of a WHO/IDF Consultation*; WHO Document Production Services: Geneva, Switzerland, 2006.

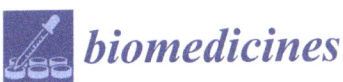

Review

Novel Biomarkers of Inflammation for the Management of Diabetes: Immunoglobulin-Free Light Chains

Akira Matsumori

Clinical Research Center, Kyoto Medical Center, 1-1 Fukakusa Mukaihata-cho, Fushimi-ku, Kyoto 612-8555, Japan; amat@kuhp.kyoto-u.ac.jp

Abstract: Virus infection, inflammation and genetic factors are important factors in the pathogenesis of diabetes mellitus. The nuclear factor-kappa B (NF-κB) is a family of transcription factors that bind the enhancer of the κ light chain gene of B cell immunoglobulin. NF-κB plays an essential role in the activation and development of B cells, and the activation of NF-κB is critical in the inflammation and development of diabetes mellitus. Recently, immunoglobulin-free light chain (FLC) λ was found to be increased in the sera of patients with diabetes mellitus, and the FLC λ and κ/λ ratios are more specific and sensitive markers for the diagnosis of diabetes relative to glycated hemoglobin A1c. Thus, FLCs may be promising biomarkers of inflammation that could relate to the activation of NF-κB. We suggest that NF-κB could be a target for an anti-inflammatory strategy in preventing and treating diabetes when FLCs are modified. FLCs could be a surrogate endpoint in the management of diabetes. In this review, the role of inflammation in the pathogenesis of diabetes, as well as the novel inflammatory biomarkers of FLCs for the management of diabetes, are discussed.

Keywords: anti-inflammation; B cells; biomarker; diabetes; hepatitis C virus; immunoglobulin; inflammation; light chain; nuclear factor-kappa B; virus

1. Introduction

Diabetes mellitus is caused by chronic high glucose levels in the blood as a result of the incapability of β cells in the pancreas to produce adequate insulin or ineffective insulin utilization by cells in the body [1]. There is evidence that virus infection, inflammation and genetic factors play important roles in the pathogenesis of diabetes [2–5]. Experimental and clinical studies suggest the inflammatory hypothesis, and clinical trials are ongoing to confirm the therapeutic effects targeting inflammation to treat or prevent diabetes [6,7].

The nuclear factor-kappa B (NF-κB) was originally identified as a family of transcription factors that binds the immunoglobulin κ light chain gene enhancer, plays an essential role in the activation and development of B cells, and the activation of NF-κB is critical in the inflammation and development of diabetes mellitus [8–10]. Recently, we found that immunoglobulin-free light chains (FLCs) are novel biomarkers of inflammation and found that FLCs are sensitive biomarkers for the diagnosis of inflammatory heart diseases such as heart failure, myocarditis and atrial fibrillation and diabetes [11–13]. In this review, the role of inflammation in the pathogenesis of diabetes, and novel inflammatory biomarkers of FLCs for the management of diabetes, are discussed.

2. Role of Virus in the Pathogenesis of Diabetes Mellitus

Type 1 diabetes mellitus (T1DM) is believed to be caused by genetic and environmental factors, and viruses are the most well-studied environmental triggers. T1DM is an autoimmune disease in which pancreatic β cells, which produce insulin in normal circumstances, are destroyed. Although multiple genes have been identified to play a role in the development of T1DM, environmental factors may be necessary for its progression to clinical disease [14,15]. Enteroviruses, rotavirus, herpesviruses, and other viruses are

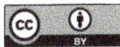

thought to be triggers of T1DM [2,3,16–18]. Molecular mimicry, direct pancreatic infection, infection-induced changes to the gut mucosa, and interactions between the immune system and infection have been proposed as mechanisms of pathogenesis [14,16,17,19]. Enteroviruses are studied most frequently; however, a growing body of research shows the potential influence of rotavirus on T1DM [20]. Hepatitis C virus (HCV), the most common cause of hepatic failure, is frequently associated with the development of diabetes mellitus, especially type 2 (T2DM) [21].

A recent meta-analysis showed that the odds ratio of risk between non-autoimmune diabetes and virus infections was 10.8 for severe acute respiratory syndrome coronavirus 2 (SARS-CoV-2), 3.6 for HCV, 2.7 for human herpesvirus 8, 2.1 for influenza H1N1 virus, 1.6 for hepatitis B virus, 1.5 for herpes simplex virus 1, 3.5 for cytomegalovirus, 2.9 for Torque teno virus, 2. 6 for parvovirus B19, 0.7 for coxsackie B virus, and 0.2 for hepatitis G virus [22].

2.1. SARS-CoV-2

The mechanism of diabetes development in coronavirus disease 2019 (COVID-19) remains to be clarified [23]. COVID-19 affects people with or without diabetes, and hyperglycemia, which is frequently seen in patients with severe COVID-19, is considered as a marker of disease severity [24,25]. A study of COVID-19 patients reported that 22% had a history of diabetes, 21% had newly diagnosed diabetes, and 28% were diagnosed with dysglycemia [25]. A number of studies have reported that new-onset diabetes associated with the presence of COVID-19 was classified as either T1DM or T2DM [23].

Patients with new-onset diabetes have higher levels of inflammatory markers such as C-reactive protein, white blood cell count, and erythrocyte sedimentation rate [25]. A cytokine storm can worsen insulin resistance [26], and neutrophils, d-dimers, and inflammatory biomarkers are higher in individuals with hyperglycemia than in those with normal blood glucose [27]. The proinflammatory cytokines and acute-phase reactants due to COVID-19 may cause inflammation and damage of pancreatic beta cells [28]. A recent study showed that SARS-CoV-2 could infect pancreatic cells, and that the virus entered endocrine islets and exocrine acinar and ductal cells in human pancreatic cultures and postmortem pancreatic tissues from COVID-19 patients [29]. Further studies are needed to investigate the direct effects of SARS-CoV-2 on pancreatic β-cells and other islet cells by experimentation and to assess inflammatory biomarkers in order to understand new-onset COVID-19-related diabetes.

2.2. Hepatitis C Virus

Extrahepatic manifestations are frequently seen in chronic HCV infection. About 70% of patients have one or more extrahepatic manifestations over the course of chronic HCV infection, which are often the first and only clinical signs and symptoms of infection. A causal association between extrahepatic manifestations such as cardiovascular disease, insulin resistance, T2DM, mixed cryoglobulinemia, non-Hodgkin lymphoma, neurological and psychiatric diseases, and rheumatic disease and HCV infection has been supported by experimental and clinical evidence [21,30].

Meta-analyses have shown an approximately 3.5- to 3.6-fold increase in HCV infection risk in individuals with T2D [22,31], and HCV infection seems to be strongly associated with non-autoimmune diabetes. An analysis reported an approximately 1.7-fold increase in T2DM risk in HCV infected individuals compared with non-infected individuals [32,33], and HCV infection is associated with an increased risk of T2DM independent of the severity of the associated liver disease. Patients with chronic HCV have higher insulin resistance compared with body mass index–matched controls, and viral eradication improves global, hepatic, and adipose tissue insulin sensitivity [34], suggesting that HCV infection precedes non-autoimmune diabetes.

HCV replicates in pancreatic cells and affects insulin signaling pathways through its structural and non-structural proteins [35]. The indirect mechanisms of insulin resistance involve HCV-induced oxidative stress, the release of inflammatory cytokines, and the upregulation of gluconeogenic genes such as glucose 6 phosphatase and phosphoenolpyruvate carboxy kinase 2 [36]. Recent studies have shown that clearance of HCV by direct-acting antiviral agents (DAAs) leads to improvement or regression of insulin resistance, improves control of glucose homeostasis in patients both with and without T2DM, and reduces the incidence of T2DM [37,38]. A prospective study of over 2400 HCV patients demonstrated an 81% reduction in the risk of developing T2DM in those who were treated with DAAs compared to those who were untreated [37]. These studies suggest that HCV plays a central role in the increased risk of developing insulin resistance and T2DM, and that eliminating the HCV can reverse insulin resistance and prevent the development of T2DM [39].

2.3. A New Concept of Pathogenesis of HCV-Induced Diseases

HCV infection is frequently associated with heart diseases such as myocarditis, dilated cardiomyopathy, arrhythmogenic right ventricular cardiomyopathy and hypertrophic cardiomyopathy. Various arrhythmias, conduction disturbances and QT prolongation were also associated with HCV infection [21,40–43]. We found that CD68-positive monocytes/macrophages were a primary target of HCV infection [44]. HCV-core antibodies stained mostly mononuclear cells in various body organs such as the liver, heart, kidney and bone marrow, but not hepatocytes or myocytes. Antibodies against the NS4 protein stained the mononuclear cells of peripheral blood and various tissues, confirming that HCV replicates in the mononuclear cells [44].

The presence of multiple extrahepatic organ involvement could be explained by the effect of HCV-infected monocytes/macrophages by immune escape and viral modulation of host immune responses. The virus may also spread through the lymphatic system, where it reaches the peripheral lymph nodes, which may cause immune cell infection prior to recirculation. Thus, HCV may cause diabetes by inflammation in the pancreas induced by monocytes/macrophages infected with HCV.

The major human histocompatibility complex (MHC) is located on the short arm of chromosome 6 and codes for several cell surface proteins involved in immune function, such as complement system components. There are marked differences in the MHC-related disease susceptibility for HCV-associated cardiomyopathies, which suggests that HCV-associated cardiomyopathies are controlled by different pathogenic mechanisms [45,46]. Therefore, HCV-induced diabetes might associate with different MHCs [3].

3. Role of Inflammation in the Pathogenesis of Diabetes Mellitus

Diet influences inflammation. Orally absorbed advanced glycation and lipoxidation end-products that are formed during the processing of foods are linked to overnutrition and hence obesity and inflammation. Furthermore, high-glycemic-load foods, such as isolated sugars and refined grains can cause increased oxidative stress that activates inflammatory genes [47]. Physical inactivity can increase the risk for diabetes because it is linked to obesity, and excessive visceral adipose tissue is a significant trigger of inflammation [47].

3.1. Inflammatory Cytokines

Circulating levels of acute-phase proteins are elevated in diabetes, such as serum amyloid A, C-reactive protein (CRP), fibrinogen, haptoglobin, plasminogen activator inhibitor, sialic acid, interleukin (IL)-1β, IL-1 receptor antagonist (IL-1Ra), IL-6 and tumor necrosis factor (TNF)-α [48–51]. Elevated circulating CRP, IL-1β, IL-1Ra and IL-6 are predictive markers for the development of T2DM [49,52–55]. The production of TNF-α is increased by adipose tissues during obesity, and insulin sensitivity is improved by a TNF-α antagonist [56]. Macrophages and other immune cells exist in adipose tissues and may release TNF-α, IL-1β, IL-6 and IL-33 [57–59]. It is now well-established that tissue inflammation plays a critical role in insulin resistance [6,7].

Inflammation may play an important role in defective insulin action and insulin secretion. Increased cytokine expressions and immune cell infiltration of pro-inflammatory macrophages are seen in pancreatic islets of patients with T2DM [60,61]. This chronic inflammatory process is associated with fibrosis and amyloid deposits, which are observed in the islets of most patients with T2DM [7].

3.2. Nuclear Factor-Kappa B (NF-κB)

Nuclear factor-kappa B (NF-κB) is a key molecule in the pathogenesis of diabetes. The NF-κB pathway is activated by genotoxic, oxidative and inflammatory stress, and regulates the expression of cytokines, growth factors and genes that regulate apoptosis, cell-cycle progression and inflammation [8]. Pharmacologic and genetic suppression implicated that NF-κB activation causes insulin resistance and glucose metabolism [9]. Upregulation of NF-κB signaling in hepatocytes results in a T2DM [10], and innate immune activation and inflammatory response that may underlie T2DM [62]. Therefore, NF-κB activation in numerous tissues, including adipose tissue, pancreas and liver, contributes to the pathogenesis of T2DM.

4. Novel Biomarkers of Inflammation: Immunoglobulin-Free Light Chains (FLCs)

4.1. FLCs as Novel Biomarkers of Chronic Inflammation

NF-κB was originally identified as a family of transcription factors that binds the immunoglobulin κ light chain gene enhancer. FLCs are synthesized de novo and secreted into circulation by B cells. FLCs emerge as an excess byproduct of antibody synthesis by B cells; elevated FLCs have been proposed to be a biomarker of B cell activity in many inflammatory and autoimmune conditions [63]. Polyclonal FLCs are a predictor of mortality in the general population, measured by the sum of κ and λ concentrations [64]. Increased FLCκ, and the higher κ/λ ratio, occurred more in rheumatic disease than in healthy blood donors [65]. FLCs in inflammatory and autoimmune diseases correlate with disease activity, suggesting their role as potential therapeutic targets in such conditions.

As discussed above, HCV infection can induce insulin resistance and cause diabetes [20–38]. High concentrations of FLC κ have been observed in HCV-positive patients, and an alteration in the κ/λ ratio is positively correlated with an increasing HCV-related lymphoproliferative disorder severity [66]. Furthermore, it has been suggested that the κ/λ ratio may be useful in the evaluation of therapeutic efficacy [67].

4.2. FLCs as Markers of Heart Failure and Myocarditis

We found that FLCs were increased in a mouse model of heart failure due to viral myocarditis [68]. Recently, we conducted additional research with patients in heart failure, and we observed that circulating FLC λ were increased while the κ/λ ratio was decreased in sera from patients with heart failure resulting from myocarditis, as compared to a group of healthy controls. These findings demonstrated that the FLC λ and κ/λ ratio together showed good diagnostic potential for the identification of myocarditis. In addition, the FLC κ/λ ratio could also be used as an independent prognostic factor for overall patient survival [11].

As shown in our previous studies, HCV infection has often been associated with myocarditis [21,40–45]. In our study on FLCs using sera from the U.S. Multicenter Myocarditis Treatment Trial, myocardial injury was more severe in patients with HCV infection than in non-infected patients. The level of FLC κ was lower, FLC λ was higher, and the κ/λ ratio decreased in patients with myocarditis, both with and without biopsy-confirmation according to the Dallas criteria, as compared to normal volunteers. These changes were more prominent in patients with HCV infection, as compared to those without infection. HCV infection may enhance the production of FLC λ while decreasing FLC κ [69,70]. Although the mechanisms of these changes require clarification, the detection of FLCs might be helpful for the diagnosis of myocarditis with heart failure and also be useful in differentiating patients with HCV infection from those without infection [69,70]. In heart failure patients, LV end-diastolic and end-systolic diameters, pulmonary arterial pressure, and N-terminal pro-brain natriuretic peptide correlated positively with FLC λ and negatively with the κ/λ ratio. Left ventricular ejection fraction was also negatively correlated with the κ/λ ratio [70].

4.3. FLCs and COVID-19 and Heart Diseases

The recent review of 316 cases of postmortem examination of COVID-19 patients demonstrated that cardiac abnormalities, either on gross pathology or histology, were identified in almost all cases. Most autopsies demonstrated chronic cardiac pathologies such as hypertrophy (27%), fibrosis (23%), amyloidosis (4%), cardiac dilatation (20%), acute ischemia (8%), intracardiac thrombi (2.5%), pericardial effusion (2.5%), and myocarditis (1.5%). SARS-CoV-2 was detected within the myocardium of 47% of studied hearts [71]. However, the Dallas criteria was satisfied in only five of these cases. In an additional 35 cases, minimal lymphocytic or mononuclear infiltration was reported, and they did not satisfy the Dallas criteria for myocarditis. Lymphocytic infiltration was scarce but could be detected in the pericardium, myocardium, epicardium, or endothelium. Therefore, cellular infiltration may be rare in COVID-19 myocarditis and, therefore, the Dallas criteria may not be accurate in the diagnosis of COVID-19 myocarditis, as it is the same in the case of HCV myocarditis [21,69].

An increase in blood troponin levels in COVID-19 is an indicator of myocardial damage. Several studies have documented a strong association between COVID-19 progression and elevated blood troponin. Reports from China found that elevated circulating cardiac troponin was present in 7–28% of COVID-19 patients, suggesting the existence of myocardial injury or myocarditis [72,73]. In hospitalized patients with COVID-19, mortality in the elevated-blood-troponin group was 51.2–59.6%, a range markedly higher than in the 4.5–8.9% in the normal-blood-troponin group [74].

We have studied how frequently myocardial injury or myocarditis occurs in COVID-19 patients [75]. Troponin T was positive in 63% of patients, NT-proBNP was elevated in 68% of patients, and elevated creatine kinase was noted in 43% of patients at admission. NT-proBNP showed a significant correlation with the length of hospital management and the severity of pulmonary CT findings. In addition, the existence of enhanced inflammatory biomarkers such as CRP and ferritin suggested that myocardial injury may be caused by inflammatory myocardial processes. D-dimer was also elevated frequently, suggesting that coagulation abnormality occurs frequently in COVID-19 patients [75]. Thus, COVID-19 has been frequently associated with myocardial injury, suggesting that SARS-CoV-2 causes myocarditis.

We also measured FLCs and IL-6 in COVID-19 patients. FLC κ and λ was elevated in 73% and 80% of patients, respectively, and the frequency of the elevated levels was higher than those of troponin T, NT-proBNP, creatine kinase, and IL-6. IL-6 has been frequently measured in COVID 19 patients, but elevated levels of IL-6 were less frequent, as compared to other parameters [69,75].

4.4. FLCs as Markers of Atrial Fibrillation

Atrial fibrillation is the most common arrhythmia, which is an important cause of stroke. Diabetes is a risk factor for the development of atrial fibrillation. Diabetes in patients with atrial fibrillation is associated with increased cardiovascular and cerebrovascular mortality [76]. The pathogenesis of diabetes-related atrial fibrillation remains to be clarified, but may be related to structural, electrical, electromechanical, and autonomic remodeling.

Abnormal atrial histology compatible with a diagnosis of myocarditis was uniformly found in patients with lone atrial fibrillation. Patients with atrial fibrillation exhibited a higher concentration of cytokines, higher NF-κB activity and more severe lymphocyte infiltration than those in sinus rhythm. These observations imply local inflammatory responses in the atria in atrial fibrillation [12]. The concentrations of circulating FLC κ and λ in patients with lone atrial fibrillation were significantly different from the healthy group. The mechanism by which FLCs cause atrial fibrillation remains to be clarified. However, the inflammation associated with FLCs directly induces atrial fibrillation. Moreover, FLCs might cause a change in membrane fluidity, which, in turn, could alter ion channel function [12].

4.5. FLCs as Biomarkers of Diabetes

Since we found that FLCs could be biomarkers of NF-κB, immune responses and inflammation, FLCs were measured in the patients with T2DM. Circulating levels of FLC λ were higher, and the κ/λ ratio was lower in patients with T2DM than in controls (Figure 1) [13].

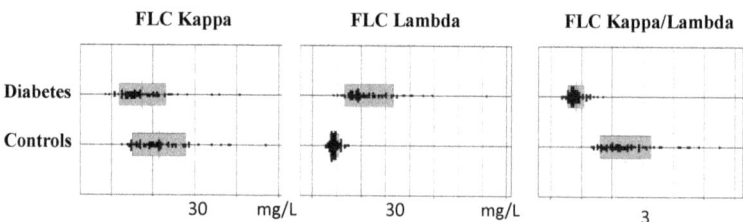

Figure 1. Immunoglobulin-free light chains (FLCs) in patients with type 2 diabetes and healthy controls (Adapted from [13]).

A statistical analysis showed that the area under the receiver operating curve (ROC-AUC) of the FLC λ and κ/λ ratio was significantly larger than glycated hemoglobin (HbA1c) [13]. The diagnostic ability for distinguishing between T2DM and controls had a sensitivity of 0.96, a specificity of 1, a positive predictive value of 1 and a negative predictive value of 0.96, with an optimal cutoff value of 1.3 for the FLC κ/λ ratio,. The odds ratio was 0.000018. The ROC-AUC, sensitivity, and specificity for HbA1c were 0.95, 0.86 and 0.94, respectively, on the cutoff value of 6.2% (Figures 2 and 3).

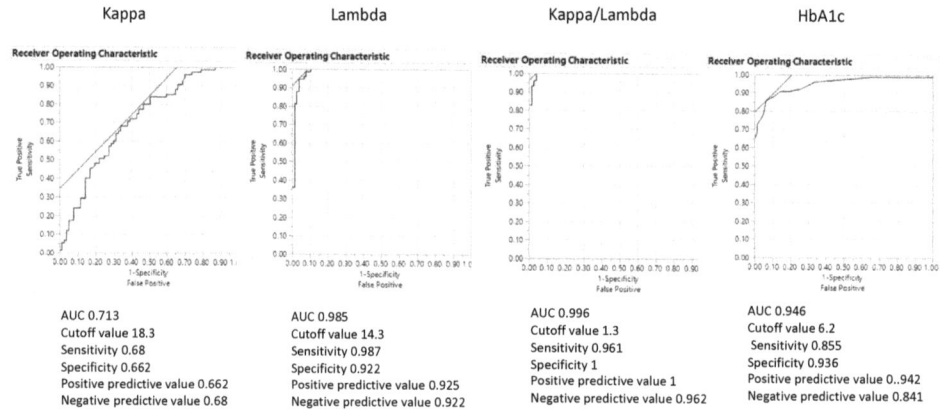

Figure 2. The area under the receiver operating curve (ROC-AUC) of the FLC κ, λ and κ/λ ratio and glycated hemoglobin (HbA1c). ROC-AUC of the FLC κ/λ ratio showed the largest compared with other FLC variables (Adapted from [13]).

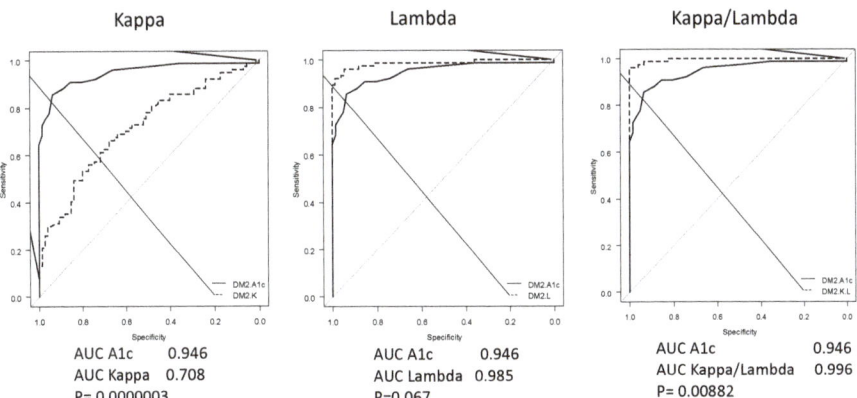

Figure 3. Comparisons of ROC-AUC between FLC variables and HbA1c. The ROC-AUC of the FLC κ/λ ratio was larger than that of HbA1c (Adapted from [13]).

In our preliminary study, urine FLC λ and the κ/λ ratio were well correlated with sera, suggesting that urine FLCs could be a suitable and non-invasive biomarker of diabetes (unpublished observation). Since HbA$_{1c}$ cannot be measured in urine, FLCs would be more beneficial biomarkers of diabetes than HbA1c. Since FLCs are a marker of inflammation/immune activation, their presence in diabetes confirms the inflammatory /immune character of the disease.

Since NF-κB activation is a critical mechanism of the inflammatory cascade in developing T2DM as discussed above [8–10], it is interesting that FLC λ and κ/λ ratio are more specific and sensitive markers for the diagnosis for T2DM than HbA1c. Therefore, FLCs represent promising potential biomarkers of inflammation that may reflect the activation of NF-κB.

Recently, we also found that FLC λ was higher, and the κ/λ ratio was lower in patients with T1DM, as seen in those with T2DM (unpublished observation). The reason why the specific activation of FLC λ occurred is unknown. B lymphocytes and plasma cells, which produce FLC λ, may be specifically activated in diabetes [13]. Another possibility is that FLC κ and λ are differently regulated because NF-κB may not exercise control of the production of FLC κ and λ in the same manner [13]. NF-κB could be a target for new types of anti-inflammatory therapy for diabetes when FLCs are changed and could be a surrogate endpoint in the management of diabetes.

5. Targeting Inflammation for the Management of Diabetes

Several therapeutic approaches or pharmacologic agents used for diabetes are reported to have anti-inflammatory properties in addition to their major mechanisms of action. Conversely, some anti-inflammatory approaches may affect glucose metabolism and cardiovascular health. It is suggested that targeting the inflammation may differentially affect hyperglycemia and atherothrombosis. Clarifying the underlying pathogenetic mechanisms may contribute to the development of effective new therapies for the optimal management of both metabolic and atherothrombotic disease states [6,7].

5.1. Metformin

Cytokines and chemokines play important roles in inflammation, and some of them are therapeutic targets for attenuating chronic inflammatory diseases [77,78]. In a large-scale treatment trial of newly diagnosed diabetic patients, metformin decreased the neutrophil-to-lymphocyte ratio, a marker of systemic inflammation. Metformin also inhibited circulating cytokines and chemokines in a non-diabetic heart failure trial. These findings show that metformin has anti-inflammatory effects in both diabetic and non-diabetic patients [79].

Metformin attenuates the production of IL-6 and TNF-α induced by lipopolysaccharide (LPS) and reduces the activation of NF-κB induced by TNF-α. NF-κB inhibition by metformin also reduces IL-1β production [80]. Metformin was shown to inhibit LPS-stimulated chemokine expression by activating AMP-activated protein kinase (AMPK), and to inhibit the phosphorylation of I-κBα and p65 in a macrophage cell line [78]. Metformin also attenuated LPS-stimulated acute lung injury by activating AMPK; reducing inflammatory cytokine, neutrophil, and macrophage infiltration; and reducing myeloperoxidase activity [81]. Metformin therapy reduced acute phase serum amyloid A, a pro-inflammatory adipokine that is upregulated in patients with obesity and insulin resistance [82]. The anti-inflammatory actions of metformin seem to be independent of glycemia and are most prominent in immune cells and vascular tissues [6].

5.2. Dipeptidyl Peptidase-4 Inhibitors

Dipeptidyl peptidase-4 (DPP-4) is a transmembrane glycoprotein known as CD26, expressed on T lymphocytes, macrophages and endothelial cells, and regulates the actions of chemokines and cytokines involved in T cell activation. DPP-4 inhibitors suppress the actions of NLRP3 inflammasomes, TLR4 and IL-1β in macrophages [83]. Sitagliptin and other DPP-4 inhibitors reduce the expression or activity of TNF-α, jun amino terminal kinase (JNK)1, Toll-like receptor (TLR) 2, TLR4, β subunit of IκB kinase and the chemokine receptor CCR2 [84].

5.3. The Glucagon-Like Peptide 1 Receptor Agonists

The glucagon-like peptide 1 (GLP-1) receptor agonists reduce circulating inflammatory biomarkers even in the absence of substantial weight loss. Markers of inflammation, are reduced including reactive oxygen species, NF-κB activity, the expression of mRNAs of IL-1β, TNF-α, JNK1, TLR2, TLR4 and SOCS-3 in mononuclear cells, and circulating concentrations of IL-6, monocyte chemoattractant protein-1, matrix metalloproteinase-9, and serum amyloid A [85,86].

5.4. SGLT2 Inhibitors

SGLT2 inhibitors improve cardiovascular and renal outcomes in large cardiovascular outcome trials in patients with diabetes. SGLT2 inhibitors reduce adipose tissue-mediated inflammation and pro-inflammatory cytokine production [87,88]. An SGLT2 inhibitor, canagliflozin, was reported to decrease circulating levels of IL-6, TNF receptor 1, fibronectin 1 and matrix metalloproteinase 7, and contributes to improving molecular processes related to inflammation, extracellular matrix turnover and fibrosis [89]. Empagliflozin may contribute to cardiovascular benefits in heart failure by repleting AMP kinase activation-mediated energy and reducing inflammation [90].

5.5. Anti-IL-1 Agents

Anakinra (recombinant human IL-1 receptor antagonist) improved glycemia, reduced CRP levels and improved β-cell secretory function [91]. The CANTOS study demonstrated that anti–IL-1β antibody (canakinumab) treatment lowered cardiovascular events over placebo [92]. IL-1β antagonism significantly decreased HBA1c in a subanalysis on metabolic endpoints [93]. A T2DM meta-analysis, following the CANTOS study, demonstrated a substantial reduction in HbA1c [94].

Therapeutic approaches to reduce inflammation may include weight-reducing diets and lifestyles, pharmacologic or surgical approaches to weight management, statin therapy and antidiabetic drugs. Serial measurements of FLCs in these interventions may be helpful in the evaluation of their therapeutic efficacy as anti-inflammatory interventions. The determination of FLCs seems suitable as an initial health screening in the general population. When the abnormalities of FLCs are found, secondary tests such as HbA1c would be performed and followed up for diabetes.

Figure 4 summarizes the risk factors, inflammation, FLCs and anti-inflammatory therapy for diabetes.

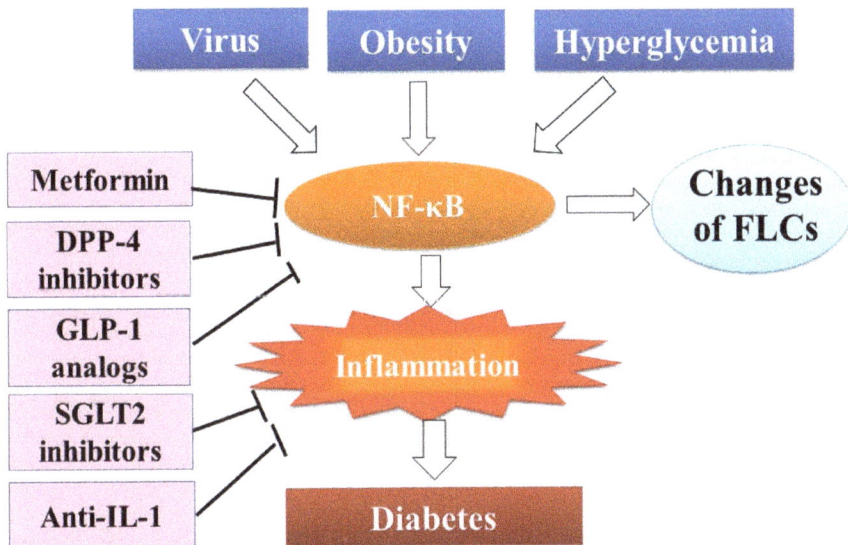

Figure 4. FLCs as inflammatory biomarkers of diabetes. Risk factors of diabetes such as viral infection, hyperglycemia and obesity activate nuclear factor kappa B (NF-κB), which regulates transcription of immunoglobulin-free light chains in the immunoglobulin-producing B cells and plasma cells and production of many inflammatory molecules, leading to inflammation. Thus, FLCs were proposed to be biomarkers of NF-κB activation and inflammation. Metformin, DPP-4 inhibitors and GLP-1 receptor agonists inhibit NF-κB activation and inflammation, and SGLT2 inhibitors and anti-IL-1 therapy inhibit inflammation.

6. Conclusions

Virus infection and inflammation are important factors in the pathogenesis of diabetes mellitus. Enteroviruses are studied most frequently; however, a growing body of research shows the potential influence of HCV and SARS-CoV-2 infections in the pathogenesis of T1DM and T2DM. Circulating FLCs are specific and sensitive diagnostic markers for diabetes mellitus. They may represent promising potential biomarkers of inflammation, which may reflect activation of NF-κB. NF-κB could be a target for new types of anti-inflammatory prevention and treatment for diabetes when FLCs are changed. FLCs could be a surrogate endpoint in the management of diabetes. Anti-inflammatory approaches may be promising for the prevention and treatment of diabetes mellitus. Clarifying the underlying pathogenetic mechanisms may contribute to the development of effective new therapies for optimal management of both metabolic and cardiovascular diseases.

Funding: This research received no external funding.

Institutional Review Board Statement: Not applicable.

Informed Consent Statement: Not applicable.

Data Availability Statement: Not applicable.

Conflicts of Interest: The authors declare no conflict of interest.

References

1. Alberti, K.G.; Zimmet, P.Z. Definition, diagnosis and classification of diabetes mellitus and its complications. Part 1: Diagnosis and classification of diabetes mellitus provisional report of a WHO consultation. *Diabet. Med.* **1998**, *15*, 539–553. [CrossRef]
2. Yoon, J.W.; Austin, M.; Onodera, T.; Notkins, A.L. Isolation of a virus from the pancreas of a child with diabetic ketoacidosis. *N. Engl. J. Med.* **1979**, *300*, 1173–1179. [CrossRef] [PubMed]
3. Sakurami, T.; Nabeya, N.; Nagaoka, K.; Matsumori, A.; Kuno, S.; Honda, A. Antibodies to Coxsackie B viruses and HLA in Japanese with juvenile-onset Type 1 (insulin-dependent) diabetes mellitus. *Diabetologia* **1982**, *22*, 375–377. [CrossRef] [PubMed]
4. Tracy, S.; Drescher, K.M.; Jackson, J.D.; Kim, K.; Kono, K. Enteroviruses, type 1 diabetes and hygiene: A complex relationship. *Rev. Med Virol.* **2010**, *20*, 106–116. [CrossRef]
5. Oever, I.A.M.V.D.; Raterman, H.G.; Nurmohamed, M.T.; Simsek, S. Endothelial dysfunction, inflammation, and apoptosis in diabetes mellitus. *Mediat. Inflamm.* **2010**, *2010*, 792393. [CrossRef]
6. Goldfine, A.B.; Shoelson, S.E. Therapeutic approaches targeting inflammation for diabetes and associated cardiovascular risk. *J. Clin. Investig.* **2017**, *127*, 83–93. [CrossRef] [PubMed]
7. Donath, M.Y.; Meier, D.T.; Boni-Schnethler, M. Inflammation in the pathophysiology and therapy of cardiometabolic disease. *Endocr. Rev.* **2019**, *40*, 1080–1091. [CrossRef] [PubMed]
8. Sultuybek, G.K.; Soydas, T.; Yenmis, G. NF-κB as the mediator of metformin's effect on ageing and ageing-related diseases. *Clin. Exp. Pharmacol. Physiol.* **2019**, *46*, 413–422. [CrossRef]
9. Yuan, M.; Konstantopoulos, N.; Lee, J.; Hansen, L.; Li, Z.W.; Karin, M.; Shoelson, S.E. Reversal of obesity- and diet-induced insulin resistance with salicylates or targeted disruption of Ikk beta. *Science* **2001**, *293*, 1673–1677. [CrossRef] [PubMed]
10. Cai, D.; Yuan, M.; Frantz, D.F.; Melendez, P.A.; Hansen, L.; Lee, J.; Shoelson, S.E. Local and systemic insulin resistance resulting from hepatic activation of IKK-beta and NF-kappaB. *Nat. Med.* **2005**, *11*, 183–190. [CrossRef]
11. Matsumori, A.; Shimada, T.; Nakatani, E.; Shimada, M.; Tracy, S.; Chapman, N.M.; Drayson, M.T.; Hartz, V.L.; Mason, J.W. Immunoglobulin free light chains as an inflammatory biomarker of heart failure with myocarditis. *Clin. Immunol.* **2020**, *217*, 108455. [CrossRef]
12. Matsumori, A.; Shimada, T.; Shimada, M.; Otani, H.; Drayson, M.T.; Mason, J.W. Immunoglobulin free light chains as inflammatory biomarkers of atrial fibrillation. *Circ. Arrhythmia Electrophysiol.* **2020**, *13*, e009017. [CrossRef] [PubMed]
13. Matsumori, A.; Shimada, T.; Shimada, M.; Drayson, M.T. Immunoglobulin free light chains: An inflammatory biomarker of diabetes. *Inflamm. Res.* **2020**, *69*, 715–718, Correction in *Inflamm. Res.* **2020**, *69*, 719. [CrossRef] [PubMed]
14. Katsarou, A.; Gudbjörnsdottir, S.; Rawshani, A.; Dabelea, D.; Bonifacio, E.; Anderson, B.J.; Jacobsen, L.M.; Schatz, D.A.; Lernmark, Å. Type 1 *Diabetes mellitus*. *Nat. Rev. Dis. Primers* **2017**, *3*, 17016. [CrossRef] [PubMed]
15. Rogers, M.A.M.; Kim, C.; Banerjee, T.; Lee, J.M. Fluctuations in the incidence of type 1 diabetes in the United States from 2001 to 2015: A longitudinal study. *BMC Med.* **2017**, *15*, 199. [CrossRef] [PubMed]
16. Rewers, M.; Ludvigsson, J. Environmental risk factors for type 1 diabetes. *Lancet* **2016**, *387*, 2340–2348. [CrossRef]
17. Filippi, C.M.; von Herrath, M.G. Viral trigger for type 1 diabetes: Pros and cons. *Diabetes* **2008**, *57*, 2863–2871. [CrossRef] [PubMed]
18. Rodriguez-Calvo, T.; Sabouri, S.; Anquetil, F.; von Herrath, M.G. The viral paradigm in type 1 diabetes: Who are the main suspects? *Autoimmun. Rev.* **2016**, *15*, 964–969. [CrossRef]
19. Smatti, M.K.; Cyprian, F.S.; Nasrallah, G.K.; Al Thani, A.A.; Almishal, R.O.; Yassine, H.M. Viruses and Autoimmunity: A review on the potential interaction and molecular mechanisms. *Viruses* **2019**, *11*, 762. [CrossRef]
20. Burke, R.M.; Tate, J.E.; Jiang, B.; Parashar, U.D. Rotavirus and type 1 diabetes—Is there a connection? A synthesis of the evidence. *J. Infect. Dis.* **2020**, *222*, 1076–1083. [CrossRef] [PubMed]
21. Haykal, M.; Matsumori, A.; Saleh, A.; Fayez, M.; Negm, H.; Shalaby, M.; Bassuony, S. Diagnosis and treatment of HCV heart diseases. *Expert Rev. Cardiovasc. Ther.* **2021**, *19*, 493–499. [CrossRef] [PubMed]
22. Lontchi-Yimagou, E.; Feutseu, C.; Kenmoe, S.; Zune, A.L.D.; Ekali, S.F.K.; Nguewa, J.L.; Choukem, S.P.; Mbanya, J.C.; Gautier, J.F.; Sobngwi, E. Non-autoimmune diabetes mellitus and the risk of virus infections: A systematic review and meta-analysis of case-control and cohort studies. *Sci. Rep.* **2021**, *11*, 8968. [CrossRef] [PubMed]
23. Khunti, K.; Prato, D.P.; Mathieu, C.; Kahn, S.E.; Gabbay, R.A.; Buse, J.B. COVID-19, hyperglycemia, and new-onset diabetes. *Diabetes Care* **2021**, *44*, 2645–2655. [CrossRef] [PubMed]
24. Bode, B.; Garrett, V.; Messler, J.; McFarland, R.; Crowe, J.; Booth, R.; Klonoff, D.C. Glycemic characteristics and clinical out-comes of COVID-19 patients hospitalized in the United States. *J. Diabetes Sci. Technol.* **2020**, *14*, 813–821. [CrossRef] [PubMed]
25. Li, H.; Tian, S.; Chen, T.; Cui, Z.; Shi, N.; Zhong, X.; Qiu, K.; Zhang, J.; Zeng, T.; Chen, L.; et al. Newly diagnosed diabetes is associated with a higher risk of mortality than known diabetes in hospitalized patients with COVID-19. *Diabetes Obes. Metab.* **2020**, *22*, 1897–1906. [CrossRef]
26. Accili, D. Can COVID-19 cause diabetes? *Nat. Metab.* **2021**, *3*, 123–125. [CrossRef]
27. Coppelli, A.; Giannarelli, R.; Aragona, M.; Penno, G.; Falcone, M.; Tiseo, G.; Ghiadoni, L.; Barbieri, G.; Monzani, F.; Virdis, A.; et al. Hyperglycemia at hospital admission is associated with severity of the prognosis in patients hospitalized for COVID-19: The Pisa COVID-19 study. *Diabetes Care* **2020**, *43*, 2345–2348. [CrossRef] [PubMed]
28. Ahlqvist, E.; Storm, P.; Käräjämäki, A.; Martinell, M.; Dorkhan, M.; Carlsson, A.; Vikman, P.; Prasad, R.B.; Aly, D.M.; Almgren, P.; et al. Novel subgroups of adult-onset diabetes and their association with outcomes: A data-driven cluster analysis of six variables. *Lancet Diabetes Endocrinol.* **2018**, *6*, 361–369. [CrossRef]

29. Shaharuddin, S.H.; Wang, V.; Santos, R.S.; Gross, A.; Wang, Y.; Jawanda, H.; Zhang, Y.; Hasan, W.; Garcia, G.J.; Arumugaswami, V.; et al. Deleterious effects of SARS-CoV-2 infection on human pancreatic cells. *Front. Cell. Infect. Microbiol.* **2021**, *11*, 678482. [CrossRef]
30. Mazzaro, C.; Quartuccio, L.; Adinolfi, L.E.; Roccatello, D.; Pozzato, G.; Nevola, R.; Tonizzo, M.; Gitto, S.; Andreone, P.; Gattei, V. A review on extrahepatic manifestations of chronic hepatitis C virus infection and the impact of direct-acting antiviral therapy. *Viruses* **2021**, *13*, 2249. [CrossRef] [PubMed]
31. Guo, X.; Jin, M.; Yang, M.; Liu, K.; Li, J.-W. Type 2 diabetes mellitus and the risk of hepatitis C virus infection: A systematic review. *Sci. Rep.* **2013**, *3*, srep02981. [CrossRef] [PubMed]
32. White, D.; Ratziu, V.; El-Serag, H.B. Hepatitis C infection and risk of diabetes: A systematic review and meta-analysis. *J. Hepatol.* **2008**, *49*, 831–844. [CrossRef] [PubMed]
33. Naing, C.; Mak, J.W.; Ahmed, S.I.; Maung, M. Relationship between hepatitis C virus infection and type 2 diabetes mellitus: Meta-analysis. *World J. Gastroenterol.* **2012**, *18*, 1642–1651. [CrossRef]
34. Lim, T.R.; Hazlehurst, J.M.; Oprescu, A.I.; Armstrong, M.J.; Abdullah, S.F.; Davies, N.; Flintham, R.; Balfe, P.; Mutimer, D.J.; McKeating, J.A.; et al. Hepatitis C virus infection is associated with hepatic and adipose tissue insulin resistance that improves after viral cure. *Clin. Endocrinol.* **2018**, *90*, 440–448. [CrossRef] [PubMed]
35. Nevola, R.; Acierno, C.; Pafundi, P.C.; Adinolfi, L.E. Chronic hepatitis C infection induces cardiovascular disease and type 2 diabetes: Mechanisms and management. *Minerva Med.* **2020**, *112*, 118–200. [CrossRef] [PubMed]
36. Adinolfi, L.E.; Restivo, L.; Guerrera, B.; Sellitto, A.; Ciervo, A.; Iuliano, N.; Rinaldi, L.; Santoro, A.; Vigni, G.L.; Marrone, A. Chronic HCV infection is a risk factor of ischemic stroke. *Atherosclerosis* **2013**, *231*, 22–26. [CrossRef]
37. Adinolfi, L.E.; Petta, S.; Fracanzani, A.L.; Coppola, C.; Narciso, V.; Nevola, R.; Rinaldi, L.; Calvaruso, V.; Staiano, L.; Di Marco, V.; et al. Impact of hepatitis C virus clearance by direct-acting antiviral treatment on the incidence of major cardiovascular events: A prospective multicentre study. *Atherosclerosis* **2020**, *296*, 40–47. [CrossRef]
38. Adinolfi, L.E.; Nevola, R.; Guerrera, B.; D'Alterio, G.; Marrone, A.; Giordano, M.; Rinaldi, L. Hepatitis C virus clearance by direct-acting antiviral treatments and impact on insulin resistance in chronic hepatitis C patients. *J. Gastroenterol. Hepatol.* **2018**, *33*, 1379–1382. [CrossRef] [PubMed]
39. Butt, A.A.; Yan, P.; Aslam, S.; Shaikh, O.S.; Abou-Samra, A.B. Hepatitis C virus (HCV) treatment with directly acting agents reduces the risk of incident diabetes: Results from electronically retrieved cohort of HCV infected veterans (ERCHIVES). *Clin. Infect. Dis.* **2020**, *70*, 1153–1160. [CrossRef]
40. Matsumori, A.; Matoba, Y.; Sasayama, S. Dilated cardiomyopathy associated with hepatitis C virus infection. *Circulation* **1995**, *92*, 2519–2525. [CrossRef]
41. Matsumori, A.; Yutani, C.; Ikeda, Y.; Kawai, S.; Sasayama, S. Hepatitis C virus from the hearts of patients with myocarditis and cardiomyopathy. *Lab. Investig.* **2000**, *80*, 1137–1142. [CrossRef] [PubMed]
42. Matsumori, A. Hepatitis C virus and cardiomyopathy. *Circ. Res.* **2005**, *9*, 144–147. [CrossRef] [PubMed]
43. Matsumori, A.; Shimada, T.; Chapman, N.M.; Tracy, S.M.; Mason, J.W. Myocarditis and heart Failure associated with hepatitis C virus infection. *J. Card. Fail.* **2006**, *12*, 293–298. [CrossRef] [PubMed]
44. Matsumori, A.; Shimada, M.; Obata, T. Leukocytes are the major target of hepatitis C virus infection: Possible mechanism of multiorgan involvement including the heart. *Glob. Heartl* **2010**, *5*, 51–58. [CrossRef]
45. Shichi, D.; Kikkawa, E.F.; Ota, M.; Katsuyama, Y.; Kimura, A.; Matsumori, A.; Kulski, J.K.; Naruse, T.K.; Inoko, H. The hap-lotype block, NFKBIL1-ATP6V1G2-BAT1-MICB-MICA, within the class III-class I boundary region of the human major his-tocompatibility complex may control susceptibility to hepatitis C virus-associated dilated cardiomyopathy. *Tissue Antigens* **2005**, *66*, 200–208. [CrossRef] [PubMed]
46. Shichi, D.; Matsumori, A.; Naruse, T.K.; Inoko, H.; Kimura, A. HLA-DPbeta chain may confer the susceptibility to hepatitis C virus-associated hypertrophic cardiomyopathy. *Int. J. Immunogenet.* **2008**, *35*, 37–43. [PubMed]
47. Furman, D.; Campisi, J.; Verdin, E.; Carrera-Bastos, P.; Targ, S.; Franceschi, C.; Ferrucci, L.; Gilroy, D.W.; Fasano, A.; Miller, G.W.; et al. Chronic inflammation in the etiology of disease across the life span. *Nat. Med.* **2019**, *25*, 1822–1832. [CrossRef]
48. Pickup, J.C.; Mattock, M.B.; Chusney, G.D.; Burt, D. NIDDM as a disease of the innate immune system: Association of acute-phase reactants and interleukin-6 with metabolic syndrome X. *Diabetologia* **1997**, *40*, 1286–1292. [CrossRef] [PubMed]
49. Spranger, J.; Kroke, A.; Mohlig, M.; Hoffmann, K.; Bergmann, M.M.; Ristow, M.; Boeing, H.; Pfeiffer, A.F. Inflammatory cyto-kines and the risk to develop type 2 diabetes: Results of the prospective population-based European Prospective Investigation into Cancer and Nutrition (EPIC)-Potsdam Study. *Diabetes* **2003**, *52*, 812–817. [CrossRef]
50. Herder, C.; Illig, T.; Rathmann, W.; Martin, S.; Haastert, B.; Müller-Scholze, S.; Holle, R.; Thorand, B.; Koenig, W.; Wichmann, H.E.; et al. Inflammation and type 2 diabetes: Results from KORA Augsburg. *Das Gesundheitswesen* **2005**, *67*, 115–121. [CrossRef]
51. Herder, C.; Brunner, E.J.; Rathmann, W.; Strassburger, K.; Tabak, A.G.; Schloot, N.C.; Witte, D.R. Elevated levels of the anti-inflammatory interleukin-1 receptor antagonist precede the onset of type 2 diabetes: The Whitehall II study. *Diabetes Care* **2009**, *32*, 421–423. [CrossRef] [PubMed]
52. Fröhlich, M.; Imhof, A.; Berg, G.; Hutchinson, W.L.; Pepys, M.B.; Boeing, H.; Muche, R.; Brenner, H.; Koenig, W. Association between C-reactive protein and features of the metabolic syndrome: A population-based study. *Diabetes Care* **2000**, *23*, 1835–1839. [CrossRef]

53. Meier, C.A.; Bobbioni, E.; Gabay, C.; Assimacopoulos-Jeannet, F.; Golay, A.; Dayer, J.M. IL-1 receptor antagonist serum levels are increased in human obesity: A possible link to the resistance to leptin? *J. Clin. Endocrinol. Metab.* **2002**, *87*, 1184–1188. [CrossRef]
54. Carstensen, M.; Herder, C.; Kivimaki, M.; Jokela, M.; Roden, M.; Shipley, M.J.; Witte, D.R.; Brunner, E.J.; Tabak, A.G. Accel-erated increase in serum interleukin-1 receptor antagonist starts 6 years before diagnosis of type 2 diabetes: Whitehall II pro-spective cohort study. *Diabetes* **2010**, *59*, 1222–1227. [CrossRef] [PubMed]
55. Marculescu, R.; Endler, G.; Schillinger, M.; Iordanova, N.; Exner, M.; Hayden, E.; Huber, K.; Wagner, O.; Mannhalter, C. In-terleukin-1 receptor antagonist genotype is associated with coronary atherosclerosis in patients with type 2 diabetes. *Diabetes* **2002**, *51*, 3582–3585. [CrossRef] [PubMed]
56. Hotamisligil, G.S.; Shargill, N.S.; Spiegelman, B.M. Adipose expression of tumor necrosis factor-alpha: Direct role in obesi-ty-linked insulin resistance. *Science* **1993**, *259*, 87–91. [CrossRef] [PubMed]
57. Weisberg, S.P.; McCann, D.; Desai, M.; Rosenbaum, M.; Leibel, R.L.; Ferrante, A.W., Jr. Obesity is associated with macrophage accumulation in adipose tissue. *J. Clin. Investig.* **2003**, *112*, 1796–1808. [CrossRef] [PubMed]
58. Xu, H.; Barnes, G.T.; Yang, Q.; Tan, G.; Yang, D.; Chou, C.J.; Sole, J.; Nichols, A.; Ross, J.S.; Tartaglia, L.A.; et al. Chronic inflammation in fat plays a crucial role in the development of obesity-related insulin resistance. *J. Clin. Investig.* **2003**, *112*, 1821–1830. [CrossRef]
59. Mathis, D. Immunological Goings-on in Visceral Adipose Tissue. *Cell Metab.* **2013**, *17*, 851–859. [CrossRef]
60. Hotamisligil, G.S. Inflammation, metaflammation and immunometabolic disorders. *Nature* **2017**, *542*, 177–185. [CrossRef] [PubMed]
61. Maedler, K.; Sergeev, P.; Ris, F.; Oberholzer, J.; Joller-Jemelka, H.I.; Spinas, G.A.; Kaiser, N.; Halban, P.A.; Donath, M.Y. Glucose-induced beta cell production of IL-1beta contributes to glucotoxicity in human pancreatic islets. *J. Clin. Investig.* **2002**, *110*, 851–860. [CrossRef]
62. Nosadini, R.; Avogaro, A.; Trevisan, A.; Valerio, A.; Tessari, P.; Duner, E.; Tiengo, A.; Velussi, M.M.; Prato, S.D.; Kreutzenberg, S.D.; et al. Effect of metformin on insulin-stimulated glucose turnover and insulin binding to receptors in type II diabetes. *Diabetes Care* **1987**, *10*, 62–67. [CrossRef] [PubMed]
63. Hampson, J.; Turner, A.; Stockley, R. Polyclonal free light chains: Promising new biomarkers in inflammatory disease. *Curr. Biomark. Find.* **2014**, *4*, 139. [CrossRef]
64. Dispenzieri, A.; Katzmann, J.A.; Kyle, R.A.; Larson, D.R.; Therneau, T.M.; Colby, C.L.; Clark, R.J.; Mead, G.P.; Kumar, S.; Melton, L.J., 3rd; et al. Use of nonclonal serum immunoglobulin free light chains to predict overall survival in the general population. *Mayo Clin. Proc.* **2012**, *87*, 517–523. [CrossRef] [PubMed]
65. Gulli, F.; Napodano, C.; Marino, M.; Ciasca, G.; Pocino, K.; Basile, V.; Visentini, M.; Stefanile, A.; Todi, L.; De Spirito, M.; et al. Serum immunoglobulin free light chain levels in systemic autoimmune rheumatic diseases. *Clin. Exp. Immunol.* **2019**, *199*, 163–171. [CrossRef] [PubMed]
66. Terrier, B.; Sène, D.; Saadoun, D.; Ghillani-Dalbin, P.; Thibault, V.; Delluc, A.; Piette, J.-C.; Cacoub, P. Serum-free light chain assessment in hepatitis C virus-related lymphoproliferative disorders. *Ann. Rheum. Dis.* **2009**, *68*, 89–93. [CrossRef] [PubMed]
67. Basile, U.; Gragnani, L.; Piluso, A.; Gulli, F.; Urraro, T.; Dell'Abate, M.T.; Torti, E.; Stasi, C.; Monti, M.; Rapaccini, G.L.; et al. Assessment of free light chains in HCV-positive patients with mixed cryoglobulinaemia vasculitis undergoing rituximab treatment. *Liver Int.* **2015**, *35*, 2100–2107. [CrossRef]
68. Matsumori, A.; Shimada, M.; Jie, X.; Higuchi, H.; Kormelink, T.G.; Redegeld, F.A. Effects of Free Immunoglobulin Light Chains on Viral Myocarditis. *Circ. Res.* **2010**, *106*, 1533–1540. [CrossRef]
69. Matsumori, A. Viral myocarditis from animal models to human diseases. In *Advances in Medicine and Biology*; Berhardt, L.V., Ed.; Nova Medicine & Health: New York, NY, USA, 2022; pp. 40–74.
70. Matsumori, A. Novel biomarkers for diagnosis and management of myocarditis and heart Failure: Immunoglobulin free light chains. *21st Century Cardiol.* **2022**, *2*, 114.
71. Roshdy, A.; Zaher, S.; Fayed, H.; Coghlan, J.G. COVID-19 and the Heart: A systematic review of cardiac autopsies. *Front. Cardiovasc. Med.* **2020**, *7*, 626975. [CrossRef] [PubMed]
72. Chung, M.K.; Zidar, D.A.; Bristow, M.R.; Cameron, S.J.; Chan, T.; Harding, C.V., III; Kwon, D.H.; Singh, T.; Tilton, J.C.; Tsai, E.J.; et al. COVID-19 and cardiovascular disease. From bench to bedside. *Circ. Res.* **2021**, *128*, 1214–1236. [CrossRef] [PubMed]
73. Matsumori, A.; Mason, J.W. The new FLC biomarker for a novel treatment of myocarditis, COVID-19 disease and other in-flammatory disorders. *Intern. Cardiovasc. Forum J.* **2022**, in press.
74. Komiyama, M.; Hasegawa, K.; Matsumori, A. Dilated cardiomyopathy risk in patients with coronavirus disease 2019: How to identify and characterise it early? *Eur. Cardiol. Rev.* **2020**, *15*, e49. [CrossRef] [PubMed]
75. Saleh, A.; Matsumori, A.; Abdelrazek, S.; Eltaweel, S.; Salous, A.; Neumann, F.-J.; Antz, M. Myocardial involvement in coronavirus disease. *Herz* **2020**, *45*, 719–725. [CrossRef] [PubMed]
76. Wang, A.; Green, J.B.; Halperin, J.L.; Piccini, J.P. Atrial fibrillation and diabetes mellitus. *J. Am. Coll. Cardiol.* **2019**, *74*, 1107–1115. [CrossRef]
77. Feng, X.; Chen, W.; Ni, X.; Little, P.J.; Xu, S.; Tang, L.; Weng, J. Metformin, macrophage dysfunction and atherosclerosis. *Front. Immunol.* **2021**, *12*, 682853. [CrossRef] [PubMed]

78. Ye, J.; Zhu, N.; Sun, R.; Liao, W.; Fan, S.; Shi, F.; Lin, H.; Jiang, S.; Ying, Y. Metformin inhibits chemokine expression through the AMPK/NF-Kappab signaling pathway. *J. Interferon Cytokine Res.* **2018**, *38*, 63–369. [CrossRef]
79. Cameron, A.R.; Morrison, V.L.; Levin, D.; Mohan, M.; Forteath, C.; Beall, C.; McNeilly, A.D.; Balfour, D.J.K.; Savinko, T.; Wong, A.K.F.; et al. Anti-Inflammatory effects of metformin irrespective of diabetes status. *Circ. Res.* **2016**, *119*, 652–665. [CrossRef] [PubMed]
80. Kelly, B.; Tannahill, G.M.; Murphy, M.P.; O'Neill, L.A. Metformin inhibits the production of reactive oxygen species from NADH: Ubiquinone oxidoreductase to limit induction of interleukin-1β (IL-1β) and boosts interleukin-10 (IL-10) in lipopoly-saccharide (LPS)-activated macrophages. *J. Biol. Chem.* **2015**, *290*, 20348–20359. [CrossRef] [PubMed]
81. Zhang, X.; Shang, F.; Hui, L.; Zang, K.; Sun, G. The alleviative effects of metformin for lipopolysaccharide-induced acute lung injury rat model and its underlying mechanism. *Saudi Pharm. J.* **2017**, *25*, 666–670. [CrossRef] [PubMed]
82. Tan, B.K.; Adya, R.; Shan, X.; Aghilla, M.; Lehnert, H.; Keay, S.D.; Randeva, H.S. The Anti-atherogenic aspect of metformin treatment in insulin resistant women with the polycystic ovary syndrome: Role of the newly established pro-inflammatory adipokine acute-phase serum amyloid A; Evidence of an adipose tissue-monocyte axis. *Atherosclerosis* **2011**, *216*, 402–408. [CrossRef]
83. Dai, Y.; Dai, D.; Wang, X.; Ding, Z.; Mehta, J.L. DPP-4 inhibitors repress NLRP3 inflammasome and interleukin-1 beta via GLP-1 receptor in macrophages through protein kinase C pathway. *Cardiovasc. Drugs Ther.* **2014**, *28*, 425–432. [CrossRef] [PubMed]
84. Ussher, J.R.; Drucker, D.J. Cardiovascular biology of the incretin system. *Endocr. Rev.* **2012**, *33*, 187–215. [CrossRef] [PubMed]
85. Chaudhuri, A.; Ghanim, H.; Vora, M.; Sia, C.L.; Korzeniewski, K.; Dhindsa, S.; Makdissi, A.; Dandona, P. Exenatide exerts a potent antiinflammatory effect. *J. Clin. Endocrinol. Metab.* **2012**, *97*, 198–207. [CrossRef] [PubMed]
86. Yang, F.; Zeng, F.; Luo, X.; Lei, Y.; Li, J.; Lu, S.; Huang, X.; Lan, Y.; Liu, R. GLP-1 Receptor: A New Target for Sepsis. *Front. Pharmacol.* **2021**, *12*, 706908. [CrossRef]
87. Cowie, M.R.; Fisher, M. SGLT2 inhibitors: Mechanisms of cardiovascular benefit beyond glycaemic control. *Nat. Rev. Cardiol.* **2020**, *17*, 761–772. [CrossRef] [PubMed]
88. Lopaschuk, G.D.; Verma, S. Mechanisms of cardiovascular benefits of sodium glucose co-transporter 2 (SGLT2) Inhibitors: A state-of-the-art review. *JACC Basic Transl. Sci.* **2020**, *5*, 632–644. [CrossRef] [PubMed]
89. Heerspink, H.J.L.; Perco, P.; Mulder, S.; Leierer, J.; Hansen, M.K.; Heinzel, A.; Mayer, G. Canagliflozin reduces inflammation and fibrosis biomarkers: A potential mechanism of action for beneficial effects of SGLT2 inhibitors in diabetic kidney disease. *Diabetologia* **2019**, *62*, 1154–1166. [CrossRef] [PubMed]
90. Koyani, C.N.; Plastira, I.; Sourij, H.; Hallström, S.; Schmidt, A.; Rainer, P.P.; Bugger, H.; Frank, S.; Malle, E.; von Lewinski, D. Empagliflozin protects heart from inflammation and energy depletion via AMPK activation. *Pharmacol. Res.* **2020**, *158*, 104870. [CrossRef] [PubMed]
91. Larsen, C.M.; Faulenbach, M.; Vaag, A.; Vølund, A.; Ehses, J.A.; Seifert, B.; Mandrup-Poulsen, T.; Donath, M.Y. Interleu-kin-1-receptor antagonist in type 2 diabetes mellitus. *N. Engl. J. Med.* **2007**, *356*, 1517–1526. [CrossRef] [PubMed]
92. Ridker, P.M.; Everett, B.M.; Thuren, T.; MacFadyen, J.G.; Chang, W.H.; Ballantyne, C.; Fonseca, F.; Nicolau, J.; Koenig, W.; Anker, S.D.; et al. CANTOS Trial Group. Antiinflammatory therapy with canakinumab for athrosclerotic disease. *N. Engl. J. Med.* **2017**, *377*, 1119–1131. [CrossRef] [PubMed]
93. Everett, B.M.; Donath, M.Y.; Pradhan, A.D.; Thuren, T.; Pais, P.; Nicolau, J.C.; Glynn, R.J.; Libby, P.; Ridker, P.M. Anti-inflammatory therapy with canakinumab for the prevention and management of diabetes. *J. Am. Coll. Cardiol.* **2018**, *71*, 2392–2401. [CrossRef] [PubMed]
94. Kataria, Y.; Ellervik, C.; Mandrup-Poulsen, T. Treatment of type 2 diabetes by targeting interleukin-1: A meta-analysis of 2921 patients. *Semin. Immunopathol.* **2019**, *41*, 413–425. [CrossRef] [PubMed]

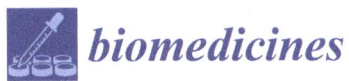 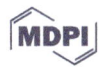

Review

Dysregulation of β-Cell Proliferation in Diabetes: Possibilities of Combination Therapy in the Development of a Comprehensive Treatment

Natsuki Eguchi, Arvin John Toribio, Michael Alexander, Ivana Xu, David Lee Whaley, Luis F. Hernandez, Donald Dafoe and Hirohito Ichii *

Department of Surgery, University of California, Irvine, CA 92697, USA; neguchi@hs.uci.edu (N.E.); atoribi1@uci.edu (A.J.T.); michaela@hs.uci.edu (M.A.); ivanax@uci.edu (I.X.); whaleyd@uci.edu (D.L.W.); luisfh2@uci.edu (L.F.H.); ddafoe@hs.uci.edu (D.D.)
* Correspondence: hichii@hs.uci.edu

Abstract: Diabetes mellitus (DM) is a metabolic disorder characterized by chronic hyperglycemia as a result of insufficient insulin levels and/or impaired function as a result of autoimmune destruction or insulin resistance. While Type 1 DM (T1DM) and Type 2 DM (T2DM) occur through different pathological processes, both result in β-cell destruction and/or dysfunction, which ultimately lead to insufficient β-cell mass to maintain normoglycemia. Therefore, therapeutic agents capable of inducing β-cell proliferation is crucial in treating and reversing diabetes; unfortunately, adult human β-cell proliferation has been shown to be very limited (~0.2% of β-cells/24 h) and poorly responsive to many mitogens. Furthermore, diabetogenic insults result in damage to β cells, making it ever more difficult to induce proliferation. In this review, we discuss β-cell mass/proliferation pathways dysregulated in diabetes and current therapeutic agents studied to induce β-cell proliferation. Furthermore, we discuss possible combination therapies of proliferation agents with immunosuppressants and antioxidative therapy to improve overall long-term outcomes of diabetes.

Keywords: pancreatic β-cells; proliferation; antioxidative therapy; immunosuppression; diabetes

1. Introduction

Diabetes Mellitus (DM) is a metabolic disorder characterized by chronic hyperglycemia that affects an estimated 34.2 million people in the United States [1]. Diabetes is commonly associated with a plethora of complications, including diabetic nephropathy, retinopathy, and cardiovascular disease, and thus, early diagnosis and management is crucial to improve outcomes. T1DM and T2DM are distinguished by different pathological processes that ultimately lead to insufficient insulin levels to maintain normoglycemia. While T1DM results from autoimmune destruction of pancreatic β cells, T2DM is found in patients with insulin resistance, which initially results in β-cell overdrive and increased insulin secretion, which eventually drives β-cell exhaustion. Current treatments for both T1DM and T2DM focus on increasing insulin levels by improving β-cell function and/or by administering exogenous insulin. However, exogenous insulin is not sufficient to prevent the progression of DM and only works to delay the onset of comorbidities associated with long-term DM. Therefore, current research focuses on identifying islet cell regeneration methods by inducing β-cell proliferation and/or transdifferentiation. Unfortunately, this approach has been met with several obstacles, primarily that adult human β-cell proliferation has been shown to be very limited (~0.2% of β cells/24 h) and poorly responsive to many mitogens [2]. Furthermore, diabetogenic insults result in the dysregulation of pathways modulating β-cell masses, making it ever more difficult to induce proliferation. This review first briefly discusses alterations in β-cell function and mass in DM, followed by β-cell mass/proliferation pathways dysregulated in DM and current therapeutic agents studied

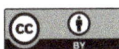

to induce β-cell proliferation. Lastly, we discuss possible combination therapies with proliferation agents to improve overall long-term outcomes of DM.

2. Diminished β-Cell Function and Mass in DM

Pancreatic β-cells are endocrine cells that modulate blood sugar levels mainly through secreting insulin under basal conditions in a pulsatile manner and when stimulated by high glucose exposure after a meal. In this section, we discuss the impact of diabetogenic insult on β-cell function and health.

2.1. Pancreatic β-Cell Function in T2DM

Oral glucose tolerance test (OGTT) is commonly used to measure β-cell function by measuring blood glucose pattern following glucose administration. T2DM and healthy patients display distinctive glucose curve patterns during OGTT; patients with T2DM commonly (67.8%) show a monophasic blood glucose curve, even under treatment with metformin, to a prevalence of 80.9% in pre-diabetic patients with impaired glucose tolerance, while normal glucose tolerant patients exhibit biphasic curves [3,4]. Insulin sensitivity (homeostasis model of insulin sensitivity, HOMA2-S) for T2DM patients are similar regardless of the shape of their OGTT curve and is lower than would be seen in a normal population [3,5]. However, β-cell function adjusted for insulin resistance was significantly to be lower in patients with a monophasic curve, compared with patients with normal biphasic response, suggesting that the altered OGTT curve seen in T2DM is primarily a result of impaired β-cell function [4].

One theory of how β-cell function becomes impaired in T2DM is as insulin sensitivity decreases; β-cell increases their insulin production to compensate [6]. In turn, hyperinsulinemia leads to endoplasmic reticulum stress response, oxidative stress, and accumulation of reactive oxygen species leading to β-cell death [7–9]. As glycemia increases, insulin secretion rates from the β-cells become less responsive to changes in the glucose level, especially compared with non-diabetic subjects [10]. It is still unknown whether this dysfunction is caused by a reduction in β-cell mass or by a decrease in glucose sensitivity [11]. The alternative theory is that β-cell impairment on the first phase of insulin secretion leads toward T2DM [12]. Pancreatic β-cells release insulin in a pulsatile manner [13]. Normally, autocrine action of insulin in β-cell increases the packing of mature insulin into granules for exocytosis (first-phase insulin response), followed by negative feedback that prevents continuous insulin secretion [14,15]. In β-cells treated with fatty acids to imitate T2DM, insulin granules with synaptotagmin-9 were lost [14]. This dysfunction impairs the β-cell resting period in DM, characterized by increased levels of pro-insulin, as there is less time for intracellular insulin processing to proceed normally [16]. The impairment of β-cell insulin pulsatility has a potential genetic background, where the offspring and relatives of T2DM patients exhibit impaired insulin pulsatility [17,18]. A plethora of genes have been associated with an increased risk of β-cell dysfunction, including TCF7L2, CDKAL1, HHEX, CDKNA/2B, IGF2BP2, SLC30A8, and JAZF1 (accurately reviewed in [19–21]).

2.2. Pancreatic β-Cell Damage and Death in DM

Diminishing β-cell mass in diabetes occurs primarily through three pathways: apoptosis, necrosis, autophagy, and potentially ferroptosis [22]. In T1D, macrophage-derived IL-1 cytokine was found to be a strong intermediary that increases inducible nitric oxide synthase (iNOS) and nitric oxide production in β-cell, leading to β-cell death [22]. In contrast, in T2D patients, first, increased apoptosis was found, accompanied by reduced β-cell replication [23]. Additionally, autophagy pathway is normally responsible for maintaining normal islet homeostasis, especially in response to a high fat diet [24]. However, in T2D, gene expression of the normal autophagy pathway was altered, leading to accumulation of cytoplasmic vacuoles and increased β-cell death. This damage was found to be reversible by metformin treatment [25]. Therefore, while loss of β-cell mass in T1DM results from autoimmune destruction, diabetogenic insults result in β-cell dysfunction and death in

T2DM. In the following section, we discuss β-cell mass regulating pathways that have been found to be dysregulated in T2DM.

3. Dysregulation of Pathways Regulating β-Cell Mass in DM

Loss of β-cell mass in T1DM and T2DM occurs through distinctive methods. While T1DM results in β-cell mass loss through destruction by autoreactive immune cells, in T2DM, diabetogenic insults, most commonly hyperglycemia and hyperlipidemia, result in β-cell apoptosis, proliferation pathway dysregulation, and dedifferentiation. Stewart AF et al. have published a comprehensive review of proliferation pathways regulating human β-cell mass [26]. In this section, we focus on pathways regulating β-cell mass that have been shown to be dysregulated in T2DM conditions: PI3K-AKT/PKB pathway, Ras/Raf/Extracellular signal-regulated kinase (ERK) pathway, and cell cycle regulation (Figure 1).

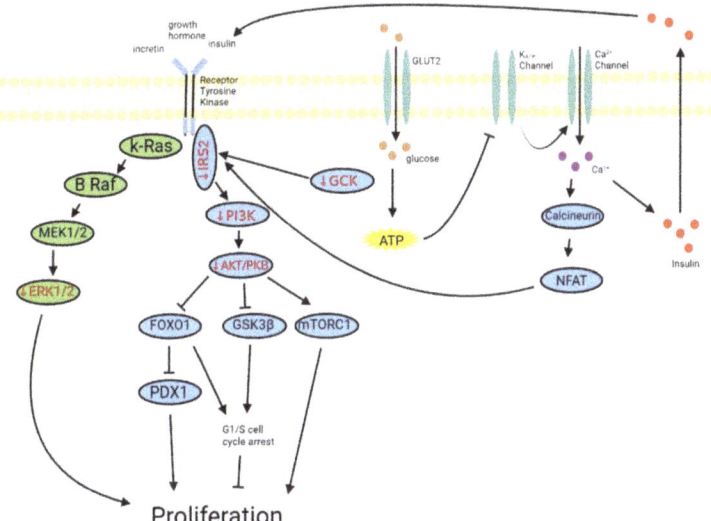

Figure 1. Pathways dysregulated in human T2DM islets and their potential downstream consequences (based on rodent and human studies). Downregulated genes found in T2DM human islets are indicated by the red color and arrow. T2DM β-cells exhibit alteration in gene expression of key upstream components of major pathways regulating β-cell mass, which may contribute to the reduced β-cell mass evident in T2DM patients.

3.1. PI3K-AKT/PKB Pathway

The PI3K-AKT/PKB pathway plays a crucial role in the regulation of β-cell function and proliferation through modulating insulin secretion and key proliferation genes including Forkhead box protein O1 (FOXO1), glycogen synthase kinase—3 (GSK3), and mammalian target rapamycin (mTOR) [27–29]. Importantly, islet cells of T2DM patients exhibit a significant reduction in AKT2 and a downward trend of PI3K expression [30]. Under physiological conditions, the AKT/PKB pathway is stimulated by insulin, growth factors, incretins, and glucose [31]. Both insulin and growth factors act through the stimulation of Insulin receptor substrate 2 (IRS2) receptors, which has been shown to play a central role in maintaining β-cell mass. IRS2-deficient β-cells in mice exhibit reduced proliferation and an inability to respond to external insulin stimulation, while overexpression of IRS2 receptors in β-cells induces proliferation in rats and decreases apoptosis in humans β-cells under hyperglycemic treatment in vitro [32,33]. Importantly, it has been demonstrated that islet cells of T2DM patients exhibit significantly lower the levels of IRS2 receptors compared with normal glucose tolerant patients [30,34]. Glucose metabolism also stimulates the AKT/PKB pathway through the IRS2 receptors. In addition to activating IRS2 receptors through stimulating insulin secretion, glucose metabolism also directly increases IRS2 receptor expression through glucokinase (GCK) activity and calcineurin/NFAT pathway [35–37]. GCK may be an important point of intervention as T2DM patients exhibit downregulation of GCK expression and a patient with a GCK mutation that resulted in 8.5 times higher affinity for glucose demonstrated significantly higher β-cell proliferation rates compared to control patients [30,38,39].

The inhibition of FOXO1 and GSK3β, and the activation of mTORC1 are important downstream targets of the AKT/PKB pathway. FOXO1 has been described as a double-edged sword as it has both protective and harmful effects. Under oxidative stress conditions, FOXO1 activates expression of Neuro D and MAF BZIP transcription factor A(MafA), two insulin 2 gene transcription factors important for β-cell identity and function [40]. On the other hand, the constitutive nuclear expression of FOXO1 prevents pancreatic and duodenal homeobox 1 (PDX-1) induced β-cell proliferation by downregulating expression of PDX-1 [41]. Furthermore, mice with IRSKO exhibit nuclear restriction of FOXO1 in β-cells, significantly reduced β-cell mass, and suffers from β-cell failure; however, the ablation of one allele of FOXO1 is sufficient to restore β-cell proliferation, indicating that FOXO1 is an important target of IRS2 for regulation of proliferation [41,42]. mTORC1 is another downstream target of the PI3K-AKT/PKB pathway that has been shown to be important in inducing β-cell proliferation. Counterintuitively however, it has been shown that islets of T2DM patients exhibit elevated mTORC1 levels [43]. In mice, forcing mTORC1 expression in islet cells significantly increases islet cell mass consistent with the consensus on the importance of mTORC1 on β-cell proliferation, but the islets demonstrated transcription pattern consistent with neonatal immature islets [44]. Supporting this study, Jia YF et al. showed that the treatment of T2DM patient islets with diabetogenic insults results in reduced β-cell proliferation secondary to upregulation of TBK1 and subsequent downregulation of mTORC1. Interestingly, the upregulation of mTORC1 through the inhibition of TBK1 in INS-1 832/13 β-cells augments β-cell proliferation while compromising the expression of function maintaining genes under basal conditions [45]. These results are in line with previous studies that showed an inverse relation between proliferative capacity and β-cell maturity [46]. Lastly, the inhibition of GSK3β through phosphorylation by AKT also plays an important role in maintaining β-cell mass. Active GSK3β phosphorylates Cyclin D2 and Cyclin D3 and causes G1/S cell cycle arrest, which is further discussed below [29]. Furthermore, activated GSK3β phosphorylates PDX-1, promoting its degradation by proteasomes [47]. Importantly, hyperglycemic treatment of human islets in vitro caused hyperactivation of GSK3β and subsequent increased phosphorylation and degradation of PDX-1 [47]. In addition to decreasing proliferation, the suppression of PDX-1 resulted in the downregulation of glucose transporter 2 (GLUT2); since this would result in decreased glucose metabolism, this may aggravate the reduced activation of PI3K-AKT/PKB pathway in DM [47]. Studies evaluating the expression levels of Glut2 in T2DM islets have yielded conflicted results; while some reported downregulation, others reported no change [30,38].

3.2. ERK1/2 Pathway

ERKs are one of the classical mitogen activated protein kinase (MAPK) signaling that has been extensively studied for their role in regulation of cell proliferation in pancreatic β-cells [26]. ERKs are commonly activated by growth factors, and its activation is mediated by MAPK3s (Raf isoforms) and MAP2Ks (MEK1/2 isoforms) [48]. The importance of ERK1/2 for β-cell proliferation has been demonstrated primarily in rodent models. Mek1- and Mek2-deficient mice with abrogation of ERK signaling in β-cells exhibit insufficient insulin production with lower β-cell proliferation and reduced β-cell mass [49]. Pharmacological agents such as Trefoil factor 2, genistein, and Epoxypukalide induced mice β-cell proliferation in vitro and in vivo through ERK1/2 activation, an effect abrogated with ERK1/2 inhibition [50–52]. Although fewer studies have been conducted in human islets, it has been shown that genistein also induces human β-cell proliferation through activation of ERK 1/2 pathway in vitro, and ERK 1/2 inhibition results in abrogation of this effect [51]. Furthermore, the inhibition of men1, inhibitor of k-Ras and downstream ERK1/2, stimulates human β-cell proliferation in vitro [53]. Importantly, pancreatic islets of T2DM patients exhibit significantly lower levels of phosphorylated ERK 1/2 [49]. Supporting this finding, human islets from type 2 DM donors were reported to be 80% deficient in the p21 (Cdc42/Rac)-activated kinase, PAK1, which has been shown to be important for activation of ERK1/2 amongst other things in both rodent and human [54]. Furthermore, HNFα-deficient mice islets exhibit impaired ERK 1/2 phosphorylation in response to EGF treatment, suggesting that HNFα is required for ERK1/2 activation; interestingly, T2DM islets also exhibit downregulation of HNF-α as well [30,55].

3.3. Altered Cell Cycle Dynamics

In addition to disruption of the PI3K-AKT/PKB and ERK1/2 pathways, alterations in cell cycle regulators may also play a part in reduced β-cell mass in T2DM. The difficulty of inducing human β-cell proliferation even under physiological conditions is well known, and this has been suggested to be partly due to the majority of G1/S proteins involved in cell cycle progression being expressed cytoplasmically rather than in the nucleus [56]. Compounding these issues, islets from T2DM patients exhibit elevated proliferating cell nuclear antigen (PCNA) expression with concomitant downregulation of cyclin dependent kinase 2 (CDK2) and p27-kip1, suggesting that diabetic islets from T2DM patients are able to enter the cell cycle but are unable to proliferate due to G1/S phase arrest [57]. p27-kip1 has dual effect in regulating cell cycle progression: (1) inhibition through inhibiting cyclin A/cyclin E/cdk1/cdk2) and (2) promotion through stimulating the nuclear translocation of CDK2/4 and Cyclin D [58]. However, it has not been evaluated whether Cyclin D and CDK2/4 nuclear expression is downregulated in T2DM islets, and thus, whether the downregulation of p27-kip1 has beneficial or harmful effects is unclear. On the other hand, the downregulation of CDK2 has clear consequences; pancreatic CDK2-deficient mice exhibit β-cell dysfunction and defects in β-cell proliferation [59]. Furthermore, in human islets, it has been shown that CDK2 binds to and phosphorylates FOXO1 in a glucose dependent manner, causing nuclear exclusion; thus, the downregulation of CDK2 would result in constitutive expression of FOXO1 in the nucleus and subsequent β-cell dysfunction [59]. Moreover, FOXO1 has been shown to downregulate cyclin D2, which plays an important role in G1 phase progression, feeding into a vicious cycle [60]. A possible explanation of the downregulation of CDK2 in T2DM is the downregulation of IRS receptors in T2DM patients. IR-deficient β-cells in mice exhibited high levels of nuclear FOXO1 with concomitant downregulation of CDK2; CDK4; and cyclin D2, D3, and E expression (CKD2: virtually absent, CDK4: ~85% reduction, cyclin D2 and D3: >80% reduction, cyclin E: 42% reduction in IR-deficient β-cell compared with the control) [57]. The expression of human insulin receptor B isoform in IR-deficient β cells in mice restored FOXO1 cytoplasmic expression and phosphorylation, and CDK2, CDK4, and cyclin E protein expression, further highlighting the importance of proper IRS expression and function in restoring β-cell masses [57]. Lastly, the overexpression of CDK6 and Cyclin D2 in human β-cells increased proliferation to 13% of β-cells from negligible levels in vitro [61–63]. Additionally, in vivo, transplanting 1500 islet equivalent (IEQ) of CDK6 and cyclinD2 overexpressing human islets into non-obese diabetic (NOD)-SCID mice yielded similar blood glucose and intraperitoneal glucose tolerance test (IPGTT) results to those transplanted with 4000 IEQ of untreated human islets, suggesting increased proliferation and function in vivo [61]. Thus, all in all, T2DM patients exhibit dysregulation of cell cycle regulators, and further studies must be conducted to evaluate the efficacy and safety of therapeutic agents targeted at stimulating cell cycle regulators.

4. Current Therapeutic Agents

Both T1DM and T2DM pathogeneses involve the loss of β-cell mass, and the identification of mitogenic factors that may stimulate β-cell proliferation is crucial in developing a therapeutic regimen to improve prognosis of DM. Unfortunately, adult human β-cell proliferation has been shown to be very limited (~0.2% of β-cells/24 h) and poorly responsive to many mitogens that have been shown to induce expansion in rodent models, including glucagon-like peptide 1 (GLP-1) analogs, IGF-1, and hepatocyte growth factors, to name a few [2]. Furthermore, recent studies have identified age-dependent factors in humans that influences the ability of β-cells to respond to specific mitogens; thus, juvenile and adult pancreatic β-cells require different mitogens for expansion. This section discusses therapeutic agents that have been shown to induce proliferation in juvenile and adult human pancreatic β-cells.

4.1. Therapeutic Agents for Juvenile Human Pancreatic β-Cells

4.1.1. GLP-1 Analogs

GLP-1 analogs are a class of anti-diabetic medication currently approved for the treatment of T2DM. It has been shown to be effective in improving Hemoglobin A1C (HbA1C) by 0.6–1.5% over a three year period predominately through augmentation of glucose-stimulated insulin secretion [64]. While GLP-1 analogs have been shown to promote β-cell expansion in rodent models, prior studies investigating the effect of GLP-1 analogs on human β-cell proliferation have yielded conflicting results [65,66]. Although liraglutide, a GLP-1 agonist, indeed induced the proliferation of β-cells (0.042% vs. 0.082% control vs. liraglutide, $p < 0.05$) in an in vitro study, this increase would not be sufficient to serve as a treatment for DM [67]. This discrepancy may partly be a result of the age of donors. Dai C et al. recently demonstrated that exendin-4, a GLP1 analog, induced proliferation in juveniles (ages 0.5–9 years) through the activation of the calcineurin/nuclear factor of activated T cells (NFAT) pathway but not in adult human β-cells (ages 20 and up) [68]. The basal juvenile β-cell proliferation rate decreased with age and the increase in proliferation rate in response to exendin-4 treatment was inversely correlated with age.

4.1.2. Prolactin

Prolactin is a hormone produced by the anterior pituitary gland. While it is most well-known for its function in lactation and homeostatic control, it has also been shown to play a crucial role in β-cell adaptation during pregnancy [69,70]. During pregnancy, β-cell mass is increased two- to threefold in rodent models and 40% in humans [71,72]. Furthermore, low prolactin levels in non-pregnant human models show a higher prevalence of DM and impaired glucose regulation [73]. Importantly however, the frequency of β-cell proliferation was not increased in pregnancy, as evidenced by the non-significant change in Ki67% insulin+ cells [72]. Instead of proliferation, it has been suggested that islet cell neogenesis may be responsible for the increased β-cell mass evident during pregnancy [72]. Supporting this finding, a study demonstrated that, while human recombinant prolactin treatment of human pancreatic β-cells increased in vitro survival by 37%, there was no apparent increase in proliferation [74]. Furthermore, while the unresponsiveness of β-cells to prolactin has partly been attributed to the fact that adult human β-cells express little to no prolactin receptors (PRLR), restoration of human PRLR on human β-cells rescued the JAK/STAT5 signaling pathway but failed to activate proliferation [71]. On the other hand, fetal pancreatic islets during late gestation express high levels of PRLR [75]. Currently, no studies have assessed the effect of prolactin on juvenile β-cell proliferation, and therefore, further studies in this field will be crucial to determine if prolactin could be used as therapy for early T1DM.

4.1.3. PDGF

Platelet-derived growth factor (PDGF) is a serum growth factor that has been shown to be involved in β-cell proliferation. In a rodent model, a decrease in PDGF-AA serum produced by osteoblast cells in bones decreased β-cell proliferation in vitro [76]. The proliferative capacity of PDGF appears to be age dependent, however, as PDGF treatment increased β-cell proliferation in juvenile mice but not in adult mice. Similar effects were seen in human β-cells; PDGF treatment increased β-cell proliferation in juveniles through activation of ERK1/2 pathway but not in adults [77]. This is likely due to PDGF receptors not being expressed in adults as overexpression of human PDGFR-a in β-cells of adult transgenic mice increased β-cell proliferation [78]. Thus, PDGF may be a promising therapy to enhance β-cell proliferation in children with early onset T1DM.

4.1.4. WISP1

Wnt-induced signaling protein 1 (WISP1) is a circulating factor involved in a wide range of tissue specific biological functions including cell growth, tumorigenesis, as well as β-cell proliferation in both rodents and humans. WISP1-deficient mice lead to reduced β-cell proliferation during the early postnatal period; in addition, injecting recombinant mouse Wisp1 in WISP 1-deficient mice showed a 1.7- to 2-fold increase in β-cell proliferation compared with saline treatment in both juvenile and adult mice [79]. Similarly, treatment of human islets (average age of 54.1 years) with recombinant human WISP1 increased β-cell proliferation up to 2% through the activation of the AKT/PKB pathway, evidenced by the abrogation of proliferative effects of WISP1 when rodent and human β-cells were co-treated with WISP1 and an AKT inhibitor. Importantly, children aged 2–5 years have been shown to have significantly higher circulating WISP1 levels compared with adults aged 28–45 years; thus, usage of young blood factors is a potential way to increase β-cell proliferation in adult humans [79]. However, further studies must be conducted to confirm safety of WISP1 treatment as it has a plethora of target sites throughout the body that may lead to pathological conditions including cancer.

4.2. Therapeutic Agents for Adult Human Pancreatic β-Cells

4.2.1. Gastrin

The ability of gastrin to improve glycemic control in T2DM has been indirectly demonstrated by clinical trials that demonstrated improved HbA1C in patients receiving proton pump inhibitors (PPIs), which indirectly elevates serum gastrin levels [80–82]. Whether this is through improving β-cell function or altering β-cell mass is not known. Gastrin has been shown to be a potent inducer of rodent β-cell proliferation; however, studies evaluating the effect of gastrin on human β-cell proliferation have yielded conflicting results [83,84]. Consistent with the experimental data in rodents, gastrin treatment increased proliferation of human 1.1B4 β-cells in vitro [85]. Supporting this, Meier et al. reported high rates of β-cell proliferation adjacent to gastrinomas, gastrin producing tumors, in the adult human pancreas [86]. In contrast with this report, Bruer et al. reported that there was no difference in β-cell area and replication between DM patients receiving PPI treatment and those without [87]. Furthermore, in an in vitro study, while gastrin alone was able to increase survival of insulin + cells when human islets from healthy donors were incubated with gastrin, gastrin alone failed to increase the number of insulin+ cells [88]. However, interestingly, treatment of pancreatic cells in gastrin or gastrin + epidermal growth factor (EGF) increased the expression of β-cell transcription factors PDX-1 and Insulin in CD19+ pancreatic duct cells. Thus, it is possible that gastrin may induce β-cell neogenesis through transdifferentiation of pancreatic duct cells, an effect augmented to significant levels with cotreatment with EGF [88]. However, further studies must be conducted to elucidate this effect.

Gastrin may also contribute to β-cell mass through maintaining β-cell identity under diabetic conditions. For example, gastrin treatment of islets from DM patients resulted in increased expression of insulin (INS), PDX-1, MAFA, NKX homeobox 1 (NKX6.1), NK2 homeobox 2 (NKX2.2), monitor neuron and pancreas homeobox 1 (MNX1), and common β-cell markers [89]. Islets from patients with higher HbA1C, signifying higher average blood glucose level in the prior 3 months, experienced a more profound increase in these β-cell transcription factors compared with those with lower HbA1C [89]. This is possibly due to the increased gastrin receptor expression, cholecystokinin B receptor (CCKBR), in insulin positive cells from donors with higher HbA1C [89]. Interestingly, while PPI treatment of patients with HbA1C ≤ 7% only resulted in an average of 0.05% decrease in HbA1C, patients with HbA1C > 7% and HbA1C > 9% showed 0.5% and 1.2% reduction in HbA1C, respectively [82,90]. Thus, further studies elucidating the mechanism in which PPI and gastrin improve glycemic control may help in directing this treatment approach to the appropriate patient population. Lastly, while PPI benefited T2DM patients, a clinical trial that studied the efficacy of combination therapy with sitagliptin and lansoprazole(PPI) in patients with recent onset T1DM demonstrated no changes in C peptide levels and HbA1C levels between patients receiving PPI and those without [91]. Thus, while combination therapies with drugs that increase gastrin levels are promising avenues to improve glycemic control in T2DM, possibly through increasing β-cell mass, further studies must be conducted to discover novel combination therapies with gastrin to treat T1DM.

4.2.2. DYRK1A Inhibitors

Small molecule inhibitors of dual specificity tyrosine phosphorylation regulated kinase 1A (DYRK1A) have gained widespread interest due to its potent ability to induce human β-cell proliferation. Among the known DYRK1A inhibitors that have been shown to induce human β-cell proliferation including aminopyrazines, thiadiazine, and 5-IT, harmine has been the most studied [92–94]. Harmine treatment in vitro of human pancreatic β-cells increased proliferation to approximately 1.3% from negligible levels through activation of DYRK1A -NFAT pathway, which has been shown to upregulate transcription of proliferation related genes including cell cycle regulators and IRS-2 receptors [37,95]. Similarly, when human islets were transplanted into the renal capsule of NOD-SCID mice, harmine treatment in vivo increased BrdU and Ki67 labeling in β-cells by 2 to 3 folds compared with saline treatment, and improved blood glucose levels and intraperitoneal glucose tolerance test [96]. Several combinations have been explored to improve the potency of harmine. First, harmine and TGFβ inhibitor combination resulted in increased Ki67 positive β-cells to 5–8% compared with the 1–3% in harmine alone in vitro [97]. Secondly, harmine and GLP1 combination treatment of human islets resulted in an average proliferation rate of 5%, similar to the combination with TGFβ. Importantly, blood glucose levels after transplantation of 1500 IEQ or 500 IEQ with harmine and exendin-4 treatment in streptozotocin (STZ) diabetic NOD scid gamma mouse (NSG) mice showed no significant difference, a result that was accompanied by a 3-fold increase in proliferation in the harmine + exendin-4 treatment arm compared with the saline group [66]. Furthermore, while the concern of increased proliferation in β-cell is the worry of naive phenotype, both harmine + TGFβ and harmine + GLP-1 analog treatment of normal and T2DM human islets resulted in an increased expression of key β-cell markers including PDX1, NKX6.1, MAFA, and MAFB [66,97]. With its potent ability to induce β-cell proliferation, DYRK1A inhibitors appear to be a promising regeneration treatment for both T1DM and T2DM; however, clinical utility is hampered by central nervous system off target effects. To curtail these effects, several derivatives of current inhibitors have been evaluated for increased kinase selectivity, and decreased off-target effects and cytotoxicity [93,98–101].

4.2.3. GABA

The neurotransmitter γ-aminobutyric acid (GABA) is a signaling molecule secreted from β-cells. It has been reported to be important in insulin exocytosis and glucose stimulated insulin secretion in human β-cells, and GABA signaling has been shown to be dysregulated in β cells from T2DM patients [102]. In addition to its role in insulin regulation, GABA has also been shown to stimulate β-cell proliferation in both rodent and human β cells [103,104]. In a rodent model, GABA treatment prevented the development of DM and reversed DM through preservation and restoration of β-cell mass in STZ-induced NOD Mice [103]. The in vivo GABA treatment of NOD-Scid mice or STZ-induced C57BL/6J mice transplanted with human islets increased Ki67+ insulin+ islet cells and decreased apoptotic islet cells [104,105]. Purwana I et al. demonstrated that, in human β-cells, GABA evokes Ca^{2+} influx, which subsequently results in AKT and cAMP response element binding protein (CREB) phosphorylation, suggesting that GABA signals through the PI3K/AKT pathway. Furthermore, GABA treatment increased IRS-2 mRNA expression [105]. The therapeutic effects of GABA have been thought to be due to its ability to induce β-cell proliferation and to augment insulin secretion but also its anti-inflammatory and immunosuppressive properties. In rodent models, GABA treatment reduced circulating inflammatory cytokines including IL-1β, TNF-α, IFN-γ, and IL-12 in STZ-induced mice, and in vitro, GABA reduced CD4+ and CD8+ T cells and increased regulatory T cells [103]. Furthermore, the activation of GABA(A) receptor has been shown to inhibit proliferation in T cells isolated from human peripheral blood mononuclear cells in vitro [106]. Based on these compelling data, clinical trials with GABA have been initiated for prevention and treatment for new onset T1DM; however, its safety and efficacy has not been reported thus far [107]. Lastly, GABA has been shown to improve insulin resistance through increasing peripheral expression of Glut4, reducing inflammation, and decreasing blood glucose levels [108]. Oral treatment with GABA inhibited the high-fat-diet-induced glucose intolerance, insulin resistance, and obesity through its anti-inflammatory effects in C57BL/6J mice [109]. Thus, GABA is a promising treatment for both T1DM and T2DM, and further studies evaluating its efficacy and safety is warranted.

Several other agents such as GSK3β inhibitors, transforming growth factor β (TGFβ) inhibitors, IKKε and EBP1, and Serpin B1 have been evaluated for their ability to induce β-cell proliferation in human islets [110,111]. GSK 3β inhibitors, LiCl and 1-Akp, in combination with glucose, stimulated mTOR-dependent DNA synthesis, cell cycle progression, and proliferation of human β-cells [112]. Additionally, pharmacological agents with dual GSK3β and DYRK1A inhibition have been shown to increase β-cell proliferation to 3–6% from negligible levels in human islets [92,100]. However, whether the proliferated β-cells exhibit mature phenotype has not been evaluated yet. TGFβ inhibitors have also been shown to induce proliferation. Combination treatment in vitro with small molecule menin-MLL inhibitors and TGFβ inhibitors synergistically increased human β-cell proliferation through the downregulation of cell cycle inhibitors without affecting insulin production, suggesting sustained mature phenotype. Furthermore, in vivo, TGF-β inhibitors also successfully increased Ki67+ β-cells from approximately 0.1% to 0.5% in human islets transplanted in NSG mice [113]. TGF-β has also been tested in combination with DYRK1a as discussed earlier [114]. While promising, clinical utility of TG-β has been questioned due to its potential harmful effects to other organs at evaluated doses.

5. New Therapeutic Approach

In both T1DM and T2DM, β-cells face multi-prong challenges that limit their function, survival, and proliferative capacity. Therapeutic approaches solely focused on increasing β-cell proliferation are not sufficient in improving the long-term outcomes of DM. Combination therapy focused on protecting β-cells from apoptosis/dedifferentiation from diabetogenic insults in the case of T2DM or protecting islets from activated autoreactive immune cells for T1DM is crucial to developing a comprehensive approach. Here, in this section, we discuss potential combination therapy with nuclear factor erythroid factor 2 related factor 2 (Nrf2) activators and immunosuppressive medication to magnify the beneficial effects of β-cell proliferation agents in the treatment of T1DM and T2DM.

5.1. T2DM

T2DM is caused by a combination of two factors: (1) impaired insulin secretion and death of pancreatic β-cells and (2) insulin resistance. Thus, while β-cell proliferation is an attractive therapeutic approach in improving prognosis of T2DM, without targeting insulin resistance, β-cell proliferation may serve only as a temporary bandage. Unfortunately, current treatment options for insulin resistance are very limited and are primarily focused on weight management [115]. Worse yet, the chronic hyperglycemia resulting from insulin resistance results in β-cell dysfunction and death, promoting a vicious cycle. The effects of hyperglycemia on β-cells have been extensively studied, and more recently, oxidative stress has been highlighted as one of the major downstream consequences that has detrimental impact on β-cell function and survival possibly due to the limited antioxidative capacity of β-cells [116]. Compared with α-cells, β-cells have a significantly lower expression of catalase and glutathione peroxidase, and exposure to oxidative stress conditions results in significantly lower survival and viability of β-cells, reducing the β/α cell ratio [117]. Thus, combination therapy with therapeutic agents targeted at alleviating oxidative stress may improve outcomes through providing protection of newly proliferated β-cells.

Nrf2 activators hold tremendous potential to fulfill this role. The Nrf2 pathway is an important regulator of cellular defense against oxidants and in human pancreatic islets, controls the expression of key antioxidants including NAD(P)H: Quinone oxidoreductase, Heme oxygenase 1 (HO-1), glucose 6 phosphate dehydrogenase (G6Pd), sulfiredoxin-1, and thioredoxin reductase1 (TXNRD1) [118]. Pharmacological activation of Nrf2 pathway by dimethyl fumarate (DMF), oltipraz, dh404, curcumin, sulforaphane, vitexin in human and/or rodent β-cells have been shown to protect β-cells under different stressors, including glucolipotoxicity and oxidative stress, by preserving β-cell function and mass [118–122]. Furthermore, Nrf2 activation has been shown to be sufficient to drive human β-cell proliferation in vitro, supporting the beneficial effect of Nrf2 activation on proliferation [123,124]. Lastly, a cross sectional study that evaluated TNF-α, HO-1, and Nrf2 levels in β-cells of normal glucose tolerant, prediabetic and T2DM patients found that while TNF-α levels increased with progressing DM, HO-1 and Nrf2 levels decreased, indicating an impaired antioxidative system in DM conditions [34]. In addition to offering protection from diabetogenic insults, more recent studies have also elucidated the potential beneficial effect of Nrf2 activators on insulin resistance. Thus, in T2DM, elevating Nrf2 levels to improve β-cell function and survival while increasing β-cell mass through proliferation agents may be a novel holistic approach to improve long-term outcomes of T2DM.

5.2. T1DM

Several immunosuppressive regimen have been tested for the treatment of T1DM. Immunotherapy against new-onset T1DM is largely grouped into three categories: therapies targeting T cells, targeting B cells, and anti-inflammatories and cytokines. Of the therapies targeting T cells including cyclosporine and anti-thymocyte globulin, anti-CD3 monoclonal antibody(teplizumab) showed the most promising results, delaying the diagnosis by at least 2 years versus the placebo. However, 20 to 55% of teplizumab-treated participants developed antidrug antibodies, and thus, the long-term efficacy has not been established yet [125]. For B cell therapy, while rituximab improved HbA1C in T1DM patients, its effects were only seen temporarily as immune tolerance was not induced [126,127]. Anti-inflammatory therapy, IL-6Ra blockade recently showed no clinical efficacy while TNF-α blockade successfully delayed C-peptide loss in new-onset T1DM. However, whether TNF-α can prevent or delay T1DM onset has not been evaluated [126]. Thus, evaluation of new immunosuppressant with long-term efficacy and without β-cell toxicity combined with β-cell proliferation agent is fundamental to improving the overall outcomes of T1DM.

DMF is an immunosuppressant with anti-inflammatory and antioxidative properties that has also been shown to have protective effects on pancreatic β-cells [120,128]. DMF has been successfully used to treat multiple sclerosis (MS) and psoriasis. In the MS clinical trial, DMF treatment significantly decreased both T and B cell counts in MS patients [129]. Importantly, the effect of DMF differs based on the T cell subpopulation, and it has been shown that DMF increased CD4/CD8 and naive/memory T cells while reducing the frequency of T helper 1 (Th1) and Th17 inflammatory cells in DMF-treated MS patients [130]. Furthermore, DMF has also been shown to decrease follicular helper T cell, a subset of T cells critical for B cell activation to increase proliferation and antibody production [131]. In addition to altering T and B cell population, DMF has also been shown to alter activity of macrophages. Although yet to be studied in humans, animal models have demonstrated that DMF decreased M1(pro-inflammatory)/M2(anti-inflammatory) macrophage polarization and absolute number. DMF treatment of a mouse model of immune thrombocytopenia, an autoimmune disease characterized by immune mediated platelet destruction, demonstrated reduced number of CD68+ macrophages in the spleen, and in an in vitro study, DMF induced apoptosis of macrophages dose dependently. Lastly, in support of these findings, we previously reported that DMF significantly delayed the onset of T1DM in non-obese diabetic mice and reduced the onset of autoimmune DM. The insulitis score was significantly lower, and these results were accompanied by a significant reduction in serum level of proinflammatory cytokines and chemokines [132]. Thus, combination therapy with DMF is a novel approach that may augment the efficacy of proliferation agents by providing protection from autoreactive immune cell destruction.

6. Conclusions

In conclusion, in both T1DM and T2DM, pancreatic β-cells face several obstacles hampering their ability to regulate blood glucose levels. In contrast, in T1DM, β-cell destruction by autoreactive immune cells causes reduced β-cell mass; in T2DM, diabetogenic insults result in major changes in pathways (PI3K-AKT/PKB, Ras/Raf/ERK, cell cycle regulators) that impair the ability of β-cells to proliferate. Thus, there has been a focus on identifying therapeutic agents capable of inducing β-cell proliferation in human islets, most importantly, gastrin, DYRK1A, and GABA, as discussed earlier. While promising, further studies on combination therapy with proliferation agents must be conducted to develop a comprehensive treatment regimen for both T1DM and T2DM. Nrf2 activators for T2DM and DMF for T1DM have tremendous potential in fulfilling these roles to provide protection of newly proliferated β-cells. Evaluating other therapeutic agents that could be used in the combination therapy is an exciting avenue to explore.

Author Contributions: N.E. and H.I. conceived and designed the review; N.E., A.J.T. and M.A. drafted the manuscript; N.E., A.J.T., M.A., I.X., D.L.W., L.F.H., D.D. and H.I. edited and revised the manuscript. All authors have read and agreed to the published version of the manuscript.

Funding: This research received no external funding.

Institutional Review Board Statement: Not applicable.

Informed Consent Statement: Not applicable.

Data Availability Statement: The data are contained within the article.

Conflicts of Interest: The authors declare no conflict of interest.

Abbreviations

T1DM	Type 1 Diabetes
T2DM	Type 2 Diabetes
OGTT	Oral Glucose Tolerance Test
HOMA2	Homeostasis Model Assessment
iNOS	Nitric Oxide Synthase
PI3K—AKT/PKB	Phosphoinositide 3 Kinases-AKT/Protein Kinase B
FOXO1	Forkhead Box Protein O1
GSK3	Glycogen Synthase Kinase-3
mTOR	Mammalian Target Rapamycin
IRS2	Insulin Receptor Substrate 2
GCK	Glucokinase
ERK	Extracellular Signal-Regulated Kinase
MAPK	Mitogen-Activated Protein Kinase
MafA	MAF BZIP Transcription Factor A
PDX-1	Pancreatic and Duodenal Homeobox 1

GLUT2	Glucose Transporter 2
PCNA	Proliferating Cell Nuclear Antigen
CDK2	Cyclin-Dependent Kinase 2
NOD mouse	Non-Obese Diabetic Mouse
IPGTT	Intraperitoneal Glucose Tolerance Test
GLP1	Glucagon-Like Peptide 1
HbA1C	Hemoglobin A1C
NFAT	Nuclear Factor of Activated T-Cells
PRLR	Prolactin Receptor
PDGF	Platelet-Derived Growth Factor
WISP1	Wnt-Induced Signaling Protein 1
PPI	Proton Pump Inhibitors
EGF	Epidermal Growth Factor
INS	nsulin
NKX1.6	NKX Homeobox 1
NKX2.2	NK2 Homeobox 2
MNX1	Motor Neuron and Pancreas Homeobox 1
CCKBR	Dholecystokinin B Receptor
DYRK1A	Dual Specificity Tyrosine Phosphorylation Regulated Kinase 1A
IEQ	Islet Equivalent
GABA	γ-Aminobutyric Acid
CREB	cAMP Response Element Binding Protein
TGF β	Transforming Growth Factor β
STZ	Streptozotocin
NSG mouse	NOD Scid Gamma Mouse
Nrf2	Nuclear Factor Erythroid Factor 2-Related Factor 2
HO-1	Heme Oxygenase 1
G6PD	Glucose 6 Phosphate Dehydrogenase
TXNRD1	Thioredoxin Reductase 1
DMF	Dimethyl Fumarate
MS	Multiple Sclerosis
Th1	T-Helper 1

References

1. *Disease, National Institute of Diabetes and Digestive and Kidney*; National Institute of Health: Bethesda, MD, USA, 2020.
2. Kulkarni, R.N.; Mizrachi, E.B.; Ocana, A.G.; Stewart, A.F. Human Beta-Cell Proliferation and Intracellular Signaling: Driving in the Dark without a Road Map. *Diabetes* **2012**, *61*, 2205–2213. [CrossRef]
3. Utzschneider, K.M.; Younes, N.; Rasouli, N.; Barzilay, J.I.; Banerji, M.A.; Cohen, R.M.; Gonzalez, E.V.; Ismail-Beigi, F.; Mather, K.J.; Raskin, P.; et al. Shape of the Ogtt Glucose Response Curve: Relationship with Beta-Cell Function and Differences by Sex, Race, and Bmi in Adults with Early Type 2 Diabetes Treated with Metformin. *BMJ Open Diabet. Res. Care* **2021**, *9*, e002264. [CrossRef]
4. Kanauchi, M.; Kimura, K.; Saito, Y. Beta-cell function and insulin sensitivity contribute to the shape of plasma glucose curve during an oral glucose tolerance test in non-diabetic individuals. *Int. J. Clin. Pract.* **2005**, *59*, 427–432. [CrossRef]
5. Wallace, T.M.; Levy, J.C.; Matthews, D.R. Use and Abuse of HOMA Modeling. *Diabet. Care* **2004**, *27*, 1487–1495. [CrossRef]
6. Schofield, C.J.; Sutherland, C. Disordered insulin secretion in the development of insulin resistance and Type 2 diabetes. *Diabet. Med.* **2012**, *29*, 972–979. [CrossRef]
7. Marchetti, P.; Bugliani, M.; De Tata, V.; Suleiman, M.; Marselli, L. Pancreatic Beta Cell Identity in Humans and the Role of Type 2 Diabetes. *Front. Cell Dev. Biol.* **2017**, *5*, 55. [CrossRef]
8. Supale, S.; Li, N.; Brun, T.; Maechler, P. Mitochondrial Dysfunction in Pancreatic Beta Cells. *Trends Endocrinol. Metab.* **2012**, *23*, 477–487. [CrossRef] [PubMed]
9. Gerber, P.A.; Rutter, G.A. The Role of Oxidative Stress and Hypoxia in Pancreatic Beta-Cell Dysfunction in Diabetes Mellitus. *Antioxid. Redox Signal.* **2017**, *26*, 501–518. [CrossRef] [PubMed]
10. Ferrannini, E.; Gastaldelli, A.; Miyazaki, Y.; Matsuda, M.; Mari, A.; DeFronzo, R.A. Beta-Cell Function in Subjects Spanning the Range from Normal Glucose Tolerance to Overt Diabetes: A New Analysis. *J. Clin. Endocrinol. Metab.* **2005**, *90*, 493–500. [CrossRef] [PubMed]
11. Ferrannini, E. The Stunned Beta Cell: A Brief History. *Cell Metab.* **2010**, *11*, 349–352. [CrossRef] [PubMed]

12. Kanauchi, M.; Nakajima, M.; Saito, Y.; Kanauchi, K. Pancreatic beta-cell function and insulin sensitivity in japanese subjects with impaired glucose tolerance and newly diagnosed type 2 diabetes mellitus. *Metabolism* **2003**, *52*, 476–481. [CrossRef] [PubMed]
13. Laurenti, M.; Matveyenko, A.; Vella, A. Measurement of Pulsatile Insulin Secretion: Rationale and Methodology. *Metabolites* **2021**, *11*, 409. [CrossRef] [PubMed]
14. Kreutzberger, A.J.B.; Kiessling, V.; Doyle, C.A.; Schenk, N.; Upchurch, C.M.; Elmer-Dixon, M.; Ward, A.E.; Preobraschenski, J.; Hussein, S.S.; Tomaka, W.; et al. Distinct insulin granule subpopulations implicated in the secretory pathology of diabetes types 1 and 2. *eLife* **2020**, *9*, e62506. [CrossRef] [PubMed]
15. Goginashvili, A.; Zhang, Z.; Erbs, E.; Spiegelhalter, C.; Kessler, P.; Mihlan, M.; Pasquier, A.; Krupina, K.; Schieber, N.; Cinque, L.; et al. Insulin Granules. Insulin Secretory Granules Control Autophagy in Pancreatic Beta Cells. *Science* **2015**, *347*, 878–882. [CrossRef]
16. Laedtke, T.; Kjems, L.; Pørksen, N.; Schmitz, O.; Veldhuis, J.; Kao, P.C.; Butler, P. Overnight inhibition of insulin secretion restores pulsatility and proinsulin/insulin ratio in type 2 diabetes. *Am. J. Physiol. Metab.* **2000**, *279*, E520–E528. [CrossRef]
17. Stadler, M.; Pacini, G.; Petrie, J.; Luger, A.; Anderwald, C.; on behalf of the RISC Investigators. Beta cell (dys)function in non-diabetic offspring of diabetic patients. *Diabetologia* **2009**, *52*, 2435–2444. [CrossRef]
18. O'Rahilly, S.; Turner, R.C.; Matthews, D.R. Impaired Pulsatile Secretion of Insulin in Relatives of Patients with Non-Insulin-Dependent Diabetes. *N. Engl. J. Med.* **1988**, *318*, 1225–1230. [CrossRef]
19. Petrie, J.R.; Pearson, E.; Sutherland, C. Implications of genome wide association studies for the understanding of type 2 diabetes pathophysiology. *Biochem. Pharmacol.* **2011**, *81*, 471–477. [CrossRef]
20. Thomsen, S.K.; Gloyn, A.L. The Pancreatic Beta Cell: Recent Insights from Human Genetics. *Trends Endocrinol. Metab.* **2014**, *25*, 425–434. [CrossRef]
21. Kettunen, J.; Tuomi, T.; Jarno, L.K. Human Physiology of Genetic Defects Causing Beta-cell Dysfunction. *J. Mol. Biol.* **2020**, *432*, 1579–1598. [CrossRef]
22. Cerf, M.E. Beta Cell Dysfunction and Insulin Resistance. *Front. Endocrinol.* **2013**, *4*, 37. [CrossRef]
23. Karaca, M.; Magnan, C.; Kargar, C. Functional pancreatic beta-cell mass: Involvement in type 2 diabetes and therapeutic intervention. *Diabetes Metab.* **2009**, *35*, 77–84. [CrossRef]
24. Ebato, C.; Uchida, T.; Arakawa, M.; Komatsu, M.; Ueno, T.; Komiya, K.; Azuma, K.; Hirose, T.; Tanaka, K.; Kominami, E.; et al. Autophagy Is Important in Islet Homeostasis and Compensatory Increase of Beta Cell Mass in Response to High-Fat Diet. *Cell Metab.* **2008**, *8*, 325–332. [CrossRef]
25. Marchetti, P.; Masini, M. Autophagy and the pancreatic beta-cell in human type 2 diabetes. *Autophagy* **2009**, *5*, 1055–1056. [CrossRef]
26. Stewart, A.F.; Hussain, M.A.; Garcia-Ocana, A.; Vasavada, R.C.; Bhushan, A.; Bernal-Mizrachi, E.; Kulkarni, R.N. Human Beta-Cell Proliferation and Intracellular Signaling: Part 3. *Diabetes* **2015**, *64*, 1872–1885. [CrossRef]
27. Kaneko, K.; Ueki, K.; Takahashi, N.; Hashimoto, S.; Okamoto, M.; Awazawa, M.; Okazaki, Y.; Ohsugi, M.; Inabe, K.; Umehara, T.; et al. Class Ia Phosphatidylinositol 3-Kinase in Pancreatic Beta Cells Controls Insulin Secretion by Multiple Mechanisms. *Cell Metab.* **2010**, *12*, 619–632. [CrossRef]
28. Jiang, W.J.; Peng, Y.C.; Yang, K.M. Cellular Signaling Pathways Regulating Beta-Cell Proliferation as a Promising Therapeutic Target in the Treatment of Diabetes. *Exp. Ther. Med.* **2018**, *16*, 3275–3285.
29. Balcazar Morales, N.; de Plata, C.A. Role of Akt/Mtorc1 Pathway in Pancreatic Beta-Cell Proliferation. *Colomb. Med.* **2012**, *43*, 235–243. [CrossRef]
30. Gunton, J.E.; Kulkarni, R.N.; Yim, S.; Okada, T.; Hawthorne, W.J.; Tseng, Y.H.; Roberson, R.S.; Ricordi, C.; O'Connell, P.J.; Gonzalez, F.J.; et al. Loss of Arnt/Hif1beta Mediates Altered Gene Expression and Pancreatic-Islet Dysfunction in Human Type 2 Diabetes. *Cell* **2005**, *122*, 337–349. [CrossRef]
31. Elghazi, L.; Bernal-Mizrachi, E. Akt and Pten: Beta-Cell Mass and Pancreas Plasticity. *Trends Endocrinol. Metab.* **2009**, *20*, 243–251. [CrossRef]
32. Assmann, A.; Ueki, K.; Winnay, J.N.; Kadowaki, T.; Kulkarni, R.N. Glucose Effects on Beta-Cell Growth and Survival Require Activation of Insulin Receptors and Insulin Receptor Substrate 2. *Mol. Cell. Biol.* **2009**, *29*, 3219–3228. [CrossRef]
33. Mohanty, S.; Spinas, G.A.; Maedler, K.; Zuellig, R.A.; Lehmann, R.; Donath, M.Y.; Trub, T.; Niessen, M. Overexpression of Irs2 in Isolated Pancreatic Islets Causes Proliferation and Protects Human Beta-Cells from Hyperglycemia-Induced Apoptosis. *Exp. Cell Res.* **2005**, *303*, 68–78. [CrossRef]
34. Liu, Y.; Zeng, Y.; Miao, Y.; Cheng, X.; Deng, S.; Hao, X.; Jiang, Y.; Wan, Q. Relationships among Pancreatic Beta Cell Function, the Nrf2 Pathway, and Irs2: A Cross-Sectional Study. *Postgrad. Med.* **2020**, *132*, 720–726. [CrossRef]
35. Terauchi, Y.; Takamoto, I.; Kubota, N.; Matsui, J.; Suzuki, R.; Komeda, K.; Hara, A.; Toyoda, Y.; Miwa, I.; Aizawa, S.; et al. Glucokinase and Irs-2 Are Required for Compensatory Beta Cell Hyperplasia in Response to High-Fat Diet-Induced Insulin Resistance. *J. Clin. Investig.* **2007**, *117*, 246–257. [CrossRef]
36. Nakamura, A.; Terauchi, Y.; Ohyama, S.; Kubota, J.; Shimazaki, H.; Nambu, T.; Takamoto, I.; Kubota, N.; Eiki, J.; Yoshioka, N.; et al. Impact of Small-Molecule Glucokinase Activator on Glucose Metabolism and Beta-Cell Mass. *Endocrinology* **2009**, *150*, 1147–1154. [CrossRef]

37. Demozay, D.; Tsunekawa, S.; Briaud, I.; Shah, R.; Rhodes, C.J. Specific Glucose-Induced Control of Insulin Receptor Substrate-2 Expression Is Mediated Via Ca2+-Dependent Calcineurin/Nfat Signaling in Primary Pancreatic Islet Beta-Cells. *Diabetes* **2011**, *60*, 2892–2902. [CrossRef]
38. Del Guerra, S.; Lupi, R.; Marselli, L.; Masini, M.; Bugliani, M.; Sbrana, S.; Torri, S.; Pollera, M.; Boggi, U.; Mosca, F.; et al. Functional and Molecular Defects of Pancreatic Islets in Human Type 2 Diabetes. *Diabetes* **2005**, *54*, 727–735. [CrossRef]
39. Kassem, S.; Bhandari, S.; Rodriguez-Bada, P.; Motaghedi, R.; Heyman, M.; Garcia-Gimeno, M.A.; Cobo-Vuilleumier, N.; Sanz, P.; Maclaren, N.K.; Rahier, J.; et al. Large Islets, Beta-Cell Proliferation, and a Glucokinase Mutation. *N. Engl. J. Med.* **2010**, *362*, 1348–1350. [CrossRef]
40. Kitamura, Y.I.; Kitamura, T.; Kruse, J.P.; Raum, J.C.; Stein, R.; Gu, W.; Accili, D. Foxo1 Protects against Pancreatic Beta Cell Failure through Neurod and Mafa Induction. *Cell Metab.* **2005**, *2*, 153–163. [CrossRef]
41. Kitamura, T.; Nakae, J.; Kitamura, Y.; Kido, Y.; Biggs, W.H., 3rd; Wright, C.V.; White, M.F.; Arden, K.C.; Accili, D. The Forkhead Transcription Factor Foxo1 Links Insulin Signaling to Pdx1 Regulation of Pancreatic Beta Cell Growth. *J. Clin. Investig.* **2002**, *110*, 1839–1847. [CrossRef]
42. Ueberberg, S.; Tannapfel, A.; Schenker, P.; Viebahn, R.; Uhl, W.; Schneider, S.; Meier, J.J. Differential expression of cell-cycle regulators in human beta-cells derived from insulinoma tissue. *Metabolism* **2016**, *65*, 736–746. [CrossRef]
43. Yuan, T.; Rafizadeh, S.; Gorrepati, K.D.D.; Lupse, B.; Oberholzer, J.; Maedler, K.; Ardestani, A. Reciprocal regulation of mTOR complexes in pancreatic islets from humans with type 2 diabetes. *Diabetologia* **2016**, *60*, 668–678. [CrossRef]
44. Jaafar, R.; Tran, S.; Shah, A.N.; Sun, G.; Valdearcos, M.; Marchetti, P.; Masini, M.; Swisa, A.; Giacometti, S.; Bernal-Mizrachi, E.; et al. Mtorc1 to Ampk Switching Underlies Beta-Cell Metabolic Plasticity During Maturation and Diabetes. *J. Clin. Investig.* **2019**, *129*, 4124–4137. [CrossRef]
45. Jia, Y.F.; Jeeva, S.; Xu, J.; Heppelmann, C.J.; Jang, J.S.; Slama, M.Q.; Tapadar, S.; Oyelere, A.K.; Kang, S.M.; Matveyenko, A.V.; et al. Tbk1 Regulates Regeneration of Pancreatic Beta-Cells. *Sci. Rep.* **2020**, *10*, 19374. [CrossRef]
46. Puri, S.; Roy, N.; Russ, H.A.; Leonhardt, L.; French, E.K.; Roy, R.; Bengtsson, H.; Scott, D.K.; Stewart, A.F.; Hebrok, M. Replication Confers Beta Cell Immaturity. *Nat. Commun.* **2018**, *9*, 485. [CrossRef]
47. Sacco, F.; Seelig, A.; Humphrey, S.; Krahmer, N.; Volta, F.; Reggio, A.; Marchetti, P.; Gerdes, J.; Mann, M. Phosphoproteomics Reveals the GSK3-PDX1 Axis as a Key Pathogenic Signaling Node in Diabetic Islets. *Cell Metab.* **2019**, *29*, 1422–1432.e3. [CrossRef]
48. Sidarala, V.; Kowluru, A. The Regulatory Roles of Mitogen-Activated Protein Kinase (Mapk) Pathways in Health and Diabetes: Lessons Learned from the Pancreatic Beta-Cell. *Recent Pat. Endocr. Metab. Immune Drug Discov.* **2017**, *10*, 76–84. [CrossRef]
49. Ikushima, Y.M.; Awazawa, M.; Kobayashi, N.; Osonoi, S.; Takemiya, S.; Kobayashi, H.; Suwanai, H.; Morimoto, Y.; Soeda, K.; Adachi, J.; et al. Mek/Erk Signaling in Beta-Cells Bifunctionally Regulates Beta-Cell Mass and Glucose-Stimulated Insulin Secretion Response to Maintain Glucose Homeostasis. *Diabetes* **2021**, *70*, 1519–1535. [CrossRef]
50. Orime, K.; Shirakawa, J.; Togashi, Y.; Tajima, K.; Inoue, H.; Ito, Y.; Sato, K.; Nakamura, A.; Aoki, K.; Goshima, Y.; et al. Trefoil Factor 2 Promotes Cell Proliferation in Pancreatic Beta-Cells through Cxcr-4-Mediated Erk1/2 Phosphorylation. *Endocrinology* **2013**, *154*, 54–64. [CrossRef]
51. Fu, Z.; Zhang, W.; Zhen, W.; Lum, H.; Nadler, J.; Bassaganya-Riera, J.; Jia, Z.; Wang, Y.; Misra, H.; Liu, D. Genistein Induces Pancreatic Beta-Cell Proliferation through Activation of Multiple Signaling Pathways and Prevents Insulin-Deficient Diabetes in Mice. *Endocrinology* **2010**, *151*, 3026–3037. [CrossRef]
52. Lopez-Acosta, J.F.; Moreno-Amador, J.L.; Jimenez-Palomares, M.; Diaz-Marrero, A.R.; Cueto, M.; Perdomo, G.; Cozar-Castellano, I. Epoxypukalide Induces Proliferation and Protects against Cytokine-Mediated Apoptosis in Primary Cultures of Pancreatic Beta-Cells. *PLoS ONE* **2013**, *8*, e52862.
53. Chamberlain, C.E.; Scheel, D.W.; McGlynn, K.; Kim, H.; Miyatsuka, T.; Wang, J.; Nguyen, V.; Zhao, S.; Mavropoulos, A.; Abraham, A.G.; et al. Menin Determines K-Ras Proliferative Outputs in Endocrine Cells. *J. Clin. Investig.* **2014**, *124*, 4093–4101. [CrossRef]
54. Wang, Z.; Oh, E.; Clapp, D.W.; Chernoff, J.; Thurmond, D.C. Inhibition or Ablation of p21-activated Kinase (PAK1) Disrupts Glucose Homeostatic Mechanisms in Vivo. *J. Biol. Chem.* **2011**, *286*, 41359–41367. [CrossRef]
55. Gupta, R.K.; Gao, N.; Gorski, R.K.; White, P.; Hardy, O.T.; Rafiq, K.; Brestelli, J.E.; Chen, G.; Stoeckert, C.J., Jr.; Kaestner, K.H. Expansion of Adult Beta-Cell Mass in Response to Increased Metabolic Demand Is Dependent on Hnf-4alpha. *Genes Dev.* **2007**, *21*, 756–769. [CrossRef]
56. Fiaschi-Taesch, N.M.; Kleinberger, J.W.; Salim, F.G.; Troxell, R.; Wills, R.; Tanwir, M.; Casinelli, G.; Cox, A.E.; Takane, K.K.; Scott, D.K.; et al. Human Pancreatic Beta-Cell G1/S Molecule Cell Cycle Atlas. *Diabetes* **2013**, *62*, 2450–2459. [CrossRef]
57. Folli, F.; Okada, T.; Perego, C.; Gunton, J.; Liew, C.W.; Akiyama, M.; D'Amico, A.; la Rosa, S.; Placidi, C.; Lupi, R.; et al. Altered Insulin Receptor Signalling and Beta-Cell Cycle Dynamics in Type 2 Diabetes Mellitus. *PLoS ONE* **2011**, *6*, e28050. [CrossRef]
58. Fiaschi-Taesch, N.M.; Kleinberger, J.W.; Salim, F.G.; Troxell, R.; Wills, R.; Tanwir, M.; Casinelli, G.; Cox, A.E.; Takane, K.K.; Srinivas, H.; et al. Cytoplasmic-Nuclear Trafficking of G1/S Cell Cycle Molecules and Adult Human Beta-Cell Replication: A Revised Model of Human Beta-Cell G1/S Control. *Diabetes* **2013**, *62*, 2460–2470. [CrossRef]
59. Kim, S.Y.; Lee, J.H.; Merrins, M.J.; Gavrilova, O.; Bisteau, X.; Kaldis, P.; Satin, L.S.; Rane, S.G. Loss of Cyclin-Dependent Kinase 2 in the Pancreas Links Primary Beta-Cell Dysfunction to Progressive Depletion of Beta-Cell Mass and Diabetes. *J. Biol. Chem.* **2017**, *292*, 3841–3853. [CrossRef]

60. Glauser, D.A.; Schlegel, W. The Emerging Role of Foxo Transcription Factors in Pancreatic Beta Cells. *J. Endocrinol.* **2007**, *193*, 195–207. [CrossRef]
61. Fiaschi-Taesch, N.; Bigatel, T.A.; Sicari, B.; Takane, K.K.; Salim, F.; Velazquez-Garcia, S.; Harb, G.; Selk, K.; Cozar-Castellano, I.; Stewart, A.F. Survey of the Human Pancreatic Beta-Cell G1/S Proteome Reveals a Potential Therapeutic Role for Cdk-6 and Cyclin D1 in Enhancing Human Beta-Cell Replication and Function in Vivo. *Diabetes* **2009**, *58*, 882–893. [CrossRef]
62. Takane, K.K.; Kleinberger, J.W.; Salim, F.G.; Fiaschi-Taesch, N.M.; Stewart, A.F. Regulated and Reversible Induction of Adult Human Beta-Cell Replication. *Diabetes* **2012**, *61*, 418–424. [CrossRef]
63. Fiaschi-Taesch, N.M.; Salim, F.; Kleinberger, J.; Troxell, R.; Cozar-Castellano, I.; Selk, K.; Cherok, E.; Takane, K.K.; Scott, D.K.; Stewart, A.F. Induction of Human Beta-Cell Proliferation and Engraftment Using a Single G1/S Regulatory Molecule, Cdk6. *Diabetes* **2010**, *59*, 1926–1936. [CrossRef]
64. Gupta, V. Glucagon-Like Peptide-1 Analogues: An Overview. *Indian J. Endocrinol. Metab.* **2013**, *17*, 413–421. [CrossRef]
65. Parnaud, G.; Bosco, D.; Berney, T.; Pattou, F.; Kerr-Conte, J.; Donath, M.Y.; Bruun, C.; Mandrup-Poulsen, T.; Billestrup, N.; Halban, P.A. Proliferation of Sorted Human and Rat Beta Cells. *Diabetologia* **2008**, *51*, 91–100. [CrossRef]
66. Ackeifi, C.; Wang, P.; Karakose, E.; Fox, J.E.M.; Gonzalez, B.J.; Liu, H.; Wilson, J.; Swartz, E.; Berrouet, C.; Li, Y.; et al. Glp-1 Receptor Agonists Synergize with Dyrk1a Inhibitors to Potentiate Functional Human Beta Cell Regeneration. *Sci. Transl. Med.* **2020**, *12*, eaaw9996. [CrossRef]
67. Rutti, S.; Sauter, N.S.; Bouzakri, K.; Prazak, R.; Halban, P.A.; Donath, M.Y. In Vitro Proliferation of Adult Human Beta-Cells. *PLoS ONE* **2012**, *7*, e35801. [CrossRef]
68. Dai, C.; Hang, Y.; Shostak, A.; Poffenberger, G.; Hart, N.; Prasad, N.; Phillips, N.; Levy, S.E.; Greiner, D.L.; Shultz, L.D.; et al. Age-Dependent Human Beta Cell Proliferation Induced by Glucagon-Like Peptide 1 and Calcineurin Signaling. *J. Clin. Investig.* **2017**, *127*, 3835–3844. [CrossRef]
69. Bole-Feysot, C.; Goffin, V.; Edery, M.; Binart, N.; Kelly, P.A. Prolactin (Prl) and Its Receptor: Actions, Signal Transduction Pathways and Phenotypes Observed in Prl Receptor Knockout Mice. *Endocr. Rev.* **1998**, *19*, 225–268. [CrossRef]
70. Shengold, L. An Attempt at Soul Murder. Rudyard Kipling's Early Life and Work. *Psychoanal. Study Child* **1975**, *30*, 683–724. [CrossRef]
71. Chen, H.; Kleinberger, J.W.; Takane, K.K.; Salim, F.; Fiaschi-Taesch, N.; Pappas, K.; Parsons, R.; Jiang, J.; Zhang, Y.; Liu, H.; et al. Augmented Stat5 Signaling Bypasses Multiple Impediments to Lactogen-Mediated Proliferation in Human Beta-Cells. *Diabetes* **2015**, *64*, 3784–3797. [CrossRef]
72. Butler, A.E.; Cao-Minh, L.; Galasso, R.; Rizza, R.A.; Corradin, A.; Cobelli, C.; Butler, P.C. Adaptive Changes in Pancreatic Beta Cell Fractional Area and Beta Cell Turnover in Human Pregnancy. *Diabetologia* **2010**, *53*, 2167–2176. [CrossRef]
73. Wang, T.; Lu, J.; Xu, Y.; Li, M.; Sun, J.; Zhang, J.; Xu, B.; Xu, M.; Chen, Y.; Bi, Y.; et al. Circulating Prolactin Associates with Diabetes and Impaired Glucose Regulation: A Population-Based Study. *Diabetes Care* **2013**, *36*, 1974–1980. [CrossRef]
74. Yamamoto, T.; Mita, A.; Ricordi, C.; Messinger, S.; Miki, A.; Sakuma, Y.; Timoneri, F.; Barker, S.; Fornoni, A.; Molano, R.D.; et al. Prolactin Supplementation to Culture Medium Improves Beta-Cell Survival. *Transplantation* **2010**, *89*, 1328–1335. [CrossRef]
75. Freemark, M.; Driscoll, P.; Maaskant, R.; Petryk, A.; Kelly, P.A. Ontogenesis of Prolactin Receptors in the Human Fetus in Early Gestation Implications for Tissue Differentiation and Development. *J. Clin. Investig.* **1997**, *99*, 1107–1117. [CrossRef]
76. Liu, X.; Zhang, F.; Chai, Y.; Wang, L.; Yu, B. The Role of Bone-Derived Pdgf-Aa in Age-Related Pancreatic Beta Cell Proliferation and Function. *Biochem. Biophys. Res. Commun.* **2020**, *524*, 22–27. [CrossRef]
77. Welsh, M.; Claesson-Welsh, L.; Hallberg, A.; Welsh, N.; Betsholtz, C.; Arkhammar, P.; Nilsson, T.; Heldin, C.H.; Berggren, P.O. Coexpression of the platelet-derived growth factor (PDGF) B chain and the PDGF beta receptor in isolated pancreatic islet cells stimulates DNA synthesis. *Proc. Natl. Acad. Sci. USA* **1990**, *87*, 5807–5811. [CrossRef]
78. Chen, H.; Gu, X.; Liu, Y.; Wang, J.; Wirt, S.E.; Bottino, R.; Schorle, H.; Sage, J.; Kim, S.K. Pdgf Signalling Controls Age-Dependent Proliferation in Pancreatic Beta-Cells. *Nature* **2011**, *478*, 349–355. [CrossRef]
79. Fernandez-Ruiz, R.; García-Alamán, A.; Esteban, Y.; Mir-Coll, J.; Serra-Navarro, B.; Fontcuberta-PiSunyer, M.; Broca, C.; Armanet, M.; Wojtusciszyn, A.; Kram, V.; et al. Wisp1 is a circulating factor that stimulates proliferation of adult mouse and human beta cells. *Nat. Commun.* **2020**, *11*, 5982. [CrossRef]
80. Takebayashi, K.; Inukai, T. Effect of proton pump inhibitors on glycemic control in patients with diabetes. *World J. Diabetes* **2015**, *6*, 1122–1131. [CrossRef]
81. Boj-Carceller, D.; Bocos-Terraz, P.; Moreno-Vernis, M.; Sanz-Paris, A.; Trincado-Aznar, P.; Albero-Gamboa, R. Are Proton Pump Inhibitors a New Antidiabetic Drug? A Cross Sectional Study. *World J. Diabet.* **2011**, *2*, 217–220. [CrossRef]
82. Peng, C.C.; Tu, Y.K.; Lee, G.Y.; Chang, R.H.; Huang, Y.; Bukhari, K.; Tsai, Y.C.; Fu, Y.; Huang, H.K.; Munir, K.M. Effects of Proton Pump Inhibitors on Glycemic Control and Incident Diabetes: A Systematic Review and Meta-Analysis. *J. Clin. Endocrinol. Metab.* **2021**, *106*, 3354–3366. [CrossRef]
83. Rooman, I.; Lardon, J.; Bouwens, L. Gastrin Stimulates Beta-Cell Neogenesis and Increases Islet Mass from Transdifferentiated but Not from Normal Exocrine Pancreas Tissue. *Diabetes* **2002**, *51*, 686–690. [CrossRef]
84. Wang, M.; Racine, J.J.; Song, X.; Li, X.; Nair, I.; Liu, H.; Avakian-Mansoorian, A.; Johnston, H.F.; Liu, C.; Shen, C.; et al. Mixed Chimerism and Growth Factors Augment Beta Cell Regeneration and Reverse Late-Stage Type 1 Diabetes. *Sci. Transl. Med.* **2012**, *4*, 133ra59. [CrossRef]

85. Khan, D.; Vasu, S.; Moffett, R.C.; Irwin, N.; Flatt, P.R. Expression of Gastrin Family Peptides in Pancreatic Islets and Their Role in Beta-Cell Function and Survival. *Pancreas* **2018**, *47*, 190–199. [CrossRef]
86. Meier, J.J.; Butler, A.E.; Galasso, R.; Rizza, R.A.; Butler, P.C. Increased Islet Beta Cell Replication Adjacent to Intrapancreatic Gastrinomas in Humans. *Diabetologia* **2006**, *49*, 2689–2696. [CrossRef]
87. Breuer, T.G.K.; Borker, L.; Quast, D.R.; Tannapfel, A.; Schmidt, W.E.; Uhl, W.; Meier, J.J. Impact of proton pump inhibitor treatment on pancreatic beta-cell area and beta-cell proliferation in humans. *Eur. J. Endocrinol.* **2016**, *175*, 467–476. [CrossRef]
88. Suarez-Pinzon, W.L.; Lakey, J.R.; Brand, S.J.; Rabinovitch, A. Combination Therapy with Epidermal Growth Factor and Gastrin Induces Neogenesis of Human Islet {Beta}-Cells from Pancreatic Duct Cells and an Increase in Functional {Beta}-Cell Mass. *J. Clin. Endocrinol. Metab.* **2005**, *90*, 3401–3409. [CrossRef]
89. Lenz, A.; Lenz, G.; Ku, H.; Ferreri, K.; Kandeel, F. Islets from human donors with higher but not lower hemoglobin A1c levels respond to gastrin treatment in vitro. *PLoS ONE* **2019**, *14*, e0221456. [CrossRef]
90. Hove, K.D.; Færch, K.; Bödvarsdóttir, T.B.; Karlsen, A.E.; Petersen, J.S.; Vaag, A.A. Treatment with a proton pump inhibitor improves glycaemic control in type 2 diabetic patients—A retrospective analysis. *Diabet. Res. Clin. Pract.* **2010**, *90*, e72–e74. [CrossRef]
91. Griffin, K.J.; Thompson, P.A.; Gottschalk, M.; Kyllo, J.H.; Rabinovitch, A. Combination Therapy with Sitagliptin and Lansoprazole in Patients with Recent-Onset Type 1 Diabetes (Repair-T1d): 12-Month Results of a Multicentre, Randomised, Placebo-Controlled, Phase 2 Trial. *Lancet Diabet. Endocrinol.* **2014**, *2*, 710–718. [CrossRef]
92. Shen, W.; Taylor, B.; Jin, Q.; Nguyen-Tran, V.; Meeusen, S.; Zhang, Y.Q.; Kamireddy, A.; Swafford, A.; Powers, A.F.; Walker, J.; et al. Inhibition of Dyrk1a and Gsk3b Induces Human Beta-Cell Proliferation. *Nat. Commun.* **2015**, *6*, 8372. [CrossRef]
93. Kumar, K.; Ung, P.M.; Wang, P.; Wang, H.; Li, H.; Andrews, M.K.; Stewart, A.F.; Schlessinger, A.; DeVita, R.J. Novel Selective Thiadiazine Dyrk1a Inhibitor Lead Scaffold with Human Pancreatic Beta-Cell Proliferation Activity. *Eur. J. Med. Chem.* **2018**, *157*, 1005–1016. [CrossRef]
94. Dirice, E.; Walpita, D.; Vetere, A.; Meier, B.C.; Kahraman, S.; Hu, J.; Dancik, V.; Burns, S.M.; Gilbert, T.J.; Olson, D.E.; et al. Inhibition of Dyrk1a Stimulates Human Beta-Cell Proliferation. *Diabetes* **2016**, *65*, 1660–1671. [CrossRef]
95. Heit, J.J.; Apelqvist, A.A.; Gu, X.; Winslow, M.M.; Neilson, J.R.; Crabtree, G.R.; Kim, S.K. Calcineurin/Nfat Signalling Regulates Pancreatic Beta-Cell Growth and Function. *Nature* **2006**, *443*, 345–349. [CrossRef]
96. Wang, P.; Alvarez-Perez, J.C.; Felsenfeld, D.P.; Liu, H.; Sivendran, S.; Bender, A.; Kumar, A.; Sanchez, R.; Scott, D.K.; Garcia-Ocana, A.; et al. A High-Throughput Chemical Screen Reveals That Harmine-Mediated Inhibition of Dyrk1a Increases Human Pancreatic Beta Cell Replication. *Nat. Med.* **2015**, *21*, 383–388. [CrossRef]
97. Wang, P.; Karakose, E.; Liu, H.; Swartz, E.; Ackeifi, C.; Zlatanic, V.; Wilson, J.; González, B.J.; Bender, A.; Takane, K.K.; et al. Combined Inhibition of DYRK1A, SMAD, and Trithorax Pathways Synergizes to Induce Robust Replication in Adult Human Beta Cells. *Cell Metab.* **2018**, *29*, 638–652.e5. [CrossRef]
98. Allegretti, P.A.; Horton, T.M.; Abdolazimi, Y.; Moeller, H.P.; Yeh, B.; Caffet, M.; Michel, G.; Smith, M.; Annes, J.P. Generation of Highly Potent Dyrk1a-Dependent Inducers of Human Beta-Cell Replication Via Multi-Dimensional Compound Optimization. *Bioorg. Med. Chem.* **2020**, *28*, 115193. [CrossRef]
99. Kumar, K.; Wang, P.; Wilson, J.; Zlatanic, V.; Berrouet, C.; Khamrui, S.; Secor, C.; Swartz, E.A.; Lazarus, M.; Sanchez, R.; et al. Synthesis and Biological Validation of a Harmine-Based, Central Nervous System (Cns)-Avoidant, Selective, Human Beta-Cell Regenerative Dual-Specificity Tyrosine Phosphorylation-Regulated Kinase a (Dyrk1a) Inhibitor. *J. Med. Chem.* **2020**, *63*, 2986–3003. [CrossRef]
100. Liu, Y.A.; Jin, Q.; Zou, Y.; Ding, Q.; Yan, S.; Wang, Z.; Hao, X.; Nguyen, B.; Zhang, X.; Pan, J.; et al. Selective Dyrk1a Inhibitor for the Treatment of Type 1 Diabetes: Discovery of 6-Azaindole Derivative Gnf2133. *J. Med. Chem.* **2020**, *63*, 2958–2973. [CrossRef]
101. Kumar, K.; Wang, P.; Sanchez, R.; Swartz, E.A.; Stewart, A.F.; DeVita, R.J. Development of Kinase-Selective, Harmine-Based Dyrk1a Inhibitors That Induce Pancreatic Human Beta-Cell Proliferation. *J. Med. Chem.* **2018**, *61*, 7687–7699. [CrossRef]
102. Korol, S.V.; Jin, Z.; Jin, Y.; Bhandage, A.K.; Tengholm, A.; Gandasi, N.R.; Barg, S.; Espes, D.; Carlsson, P.O.; Laver, D.; et al. Functional Characterization of Native, High-Affinity Gabaa Receptors in Human Pancreatic Beta Cells. *EBioMedicine* **2018**, *30*, 273–282. [CrossRef]
103. Soltani, N.; Qiu, H.; Aleksic, M.; Glinka, Y.; Zhao, F.; Liu, R.; Li, Y.; Zhang, N.; Chakrabarti, R.; Ng, T.; et al. Gaba Exerts Protective and Regenerative Effects on Islet Beta Cells and Reverses Diabetes. *Proc. Natl. Acad. Sci. USA* **2011**, *108*, 11692–11697. [CrossRef]
104. Tian, J.; Dang, H.; Chen, Z.; Guan, A.; Jin, Y.; Atkinson, M.A.; Kaufman, D.L. Gamma-Aminobutyric Acid Regulates Both the Survival and Replication of Human Beta-Cells. *Diabetes* **2013**, *62*, 3760–3765. [CrossRef]
105. Purwana, I.; Zheng, J.; Li, X.; Deurloo, M.; Son, D.O.; Zhang, Z.; Liang, C.; Shen, E.; Tadkase, A.; Feng, Z.P.; et al. Gaba Promotes Human Beta-Cell Proliferation and Modulates Glucose Homeostasis. *Diabetes* **2014**, *63*, 4197–4205. [CrossRef]
106. Sparrow, E.L.; James, S.; Hussain, K.; Beers, S.A.; Cragg, M.S.; Bogdanov, Y.D. Activation of Gaba(a) Receptors Inhibits T Cell Proliferation. *PLoS ONE* **2021**, *16*, e0251632. [CrossRef]
107. Choat, H.M.; Martin, A.; Mick, G.J.; Heath, K.E.; Tse, H.M.; McGwin, G., Jr.; McCormick, K.L. Effect of Gamma Aminobutyric Acid (Gaba) or Gaba with Glutamic Acid Decarboxylase (Gad) on the Progression of Type 1 Diabetes Mellitus in Children: Trial Design and Methodology. *Contemp. Clin. Trials* **2019**, *82*, 93–100. [CrossRef]
108. Soltani, N.; Rezazadeh, H.; Sharifi, M.R. Insulin resistance and the role of gamma-aminobutyric acid. *J. Res. Med. Sci.* **2021**, *26*, 39. [CrossRef]

109. Tian, J.; Dang, H.N.; Yong, J.; Chui, W.S.; Dizon, M.P.; Yaw, C.K.; Kaufman, D.L. Oral Treatment with Gamma-Aminobutyric Acid Improves Glucose Tolerance and Insulin Sensitivity by Inhibiting Inflammation in High Fat Diet-Fed Mice. *PLoS ONE* **2011**, *6*, e25338. [CrossRef]
110. El Ouaamari, A.; Dirice, E.; Gedeon, N.; Hu, J.; Zhou, J.Y.; Shirakawa, J.; Hou, L.; Goodman, J.; Karampelias, C.; Qiang, G.; et al. Serpinb1 Promotes Pancreatic Beta Cell Proliferation. *Cell Metab.* **2016**, *23*, 194–205. [CrossRef]
111. Shen, W.; Tremblay, M.S.; Deshmukh, V.A.; Wang, W.; Filippi, C.M.; Harb, G.; Zhang, Y.Q.; Kamireddy, A.; Baaten, J.E.; Jin, Q.; et al. Small-Molecule Inducer of Beta Cell Proliferation Identified by High-Throughput Screening. *J. Am. Chem. Soc.* **2013**, *135*, 1669–1672. [CrossRef]
112. Liu, H.; Remedi, M.S.; Pappan, K.L.; Kwon, G.; Rohatgi, N.; Marshall, C.A.; McDaniel, M.L. Glycogen Synthase Kinase-3 and Mammalian Target of Rapamycin Pathways Contribute to DNA Synthesis, Cell Cycle Progression, and Proliferation in Human Islets. *Diabetes* **2009**, *58*, 663–672. [CrossRef] [PubMed]
113. Pahlavanneshan, S.; Behmanesh, M.; Oropeza, D.; Furuyama, K.; Tahamtani, Y.; Basiri, M.; Herrera, P.L.; Baharvand, H. Combined inhibition of menin-MLL interaction and TGF-β signaling induces replication of human pancreatic beta cells. *Eur. J. Cell Biol.* **2020**, *99*, 151094. [CrossRef]
114. Dhawan, S.; Dirice, E.; Kulkarni, R.N.; Bhushan, A. Inhibition of Tgf-Beta Signaling Promotes Human Pancreatic Beta-Cell Replication. *Diabetes* **2016**, *65*, 1208–1218. [CrossRef]
115. Freeman, A.M.; Pennings, N. *Insulin Resistance*; Statpearls: Treasure Island, FL, USA, 2021.
116. Eguchi, N.; Vaziri, N.D.; Dafoe, D.C.; Ichii, H. The Role of Oxidative Stress in Pancreatic Beta Cell Dysfunction in Diabetes. *Int. J. Mol. Sci.* **2021**, *22*, 1509. [CrossRef] [PubMed]
117. Miki, A.; Ricordi, C.; Sakuma, Y.; Yamamoto, T.; Misawa, R.; Mita, A.; Molano, R.D.; Vaziri, N.D.; Pileggi, A.; Ichii, H. Divergent Antioxidant Capacity of Human Islet Cell Subsets: A Potential Cause of Beta-Cell Vulnerability in Diabetes and Islet Transplantation. *PLoS ONE* **2018**, *13*, e0196570. [CrossRef] [PubMed]
118. Masuda, Y.; Vaziri, N.D.; Li, S.; Le, A.; Hajighasemi-Ossareh, M.; Robles, L.; Foster, C.E.; Stamos, M.J.; Al-Abodullah, I.; Ricordi, C.; et al. The Effect of Nrf2 Pathway Activation on Human Pancreatic Islet Cells. *PLoS ONE* **2015**, *10*, e0131012. [CrossRef] [PubMed]
119. Den Hartogh, D.J.; Gabriel, A.; Tsiani, E. Antidiabetic Properties of Curcumin I: Evidence from In Vitro Studies. *Nutrients* **2020**, *12*, 118. [CrossRef]
120. Schultheis, J.; Beckmann, D.; Mulac, D.; Müller, L.; Esselen, M.; Düfer, M. Nrf2 Activation Protects Mouse Beta Cells from Glucolipotoxicity by Restoring Mitochondrial Function and Physiological Redox Balance. *Oxidative Med. Cell. Longev.* **2019**, *2019*, 7518510. [CrossRef]
121. Song, M.Y.; Kim, E.K.; Moon, W.S.; Park, J.W.; Kim, H.J.; So, H.S.; Park, R.; Kwon, K.B.; Park, B.H. Sulforaphane Protects against Cytokine- and Streptozotocin-Induced Beta-Cell Damage by Suppressing the Nf-Kappab Pathway. *Toxicol. Appl. Pharmacol.* **2009**, *235*, 57–67. [CrossRef]
122. Ganesan, K.; Ramkumar, K.M.; Xu, B. Vitexin Restores Pancreatic Beta-Cell Function and Insulin Signaling through Nrf2 and Nf-Kappab Signaling Pathways. *Eur. J. Pharmacol.* **2020**, *888*, 173606. [CrossRef]
123. Kumar, A.; Katz, L.S.; Schulz, A.M.; Kim, M.; Honig, L.B.; Li, L.; Davenport, B.; Homann, D.; Garcia-Ocana, A.; Herman, M.A.; et al. Activation of Nrf2 Is Required for Normal and Chrebpalpha-Augmented Glucose-Stimulated Beta-Cell Proliferation. *Diabetes* **2018**, *67*, 1561–1575. [CrossRef] [PubMed]
124. Baumel-Alterzon, S.; Katz, L.S.; Brill, G.; Garcia-Ocaña, A.; Scott, D.K. Nrf2: The Master and Captain of Beta Cell Fate. *Trends Endocrinol. Metab.* **2020**, *32*, 7–19. [CrossRef] [PubMed]
125. Herold, K.C.; Bundy, B.N.; Long, S.A.; Bluestone, J.A.; DiMeglio, L.A.; Dufort, M.J.; Gitelman, S.E.; Gottlieb, P.A.; Krischer, J.P.; Linsley, P.S.; et al. An Anti-Cd3 Antibody, Teplizumab, in Relatives at Risk for Type 1 Diabetes. *N. Engl. J. Med.* **2019**, *381*, 603–613. [CrossRef] [PubMed]
126. Bluestone, J.A.; Buckner, J.H.; Herold, K.C. Immunotherapy: Building a Bridge to a Cure for Type 1 Diabetes. *Science* **2021**, *373*, 510–516. [CrossRef] [PubMed]
127. Chatenoud, L.; Warncke, K.; Ziegler, A.-G. Clinical Immunologic Interventions for the Treatment of Type 1 Diabetes. *Cold Spring Harb. Perspect. Med.* **2012**, *2*, a007716. [CrossRef]
128. Fu, J.; Zheng, H.; Wang, H.; Yang, B.; Zhao, R.; Lu, C.; Liu, Z.; Hou, Y.; Xu, Y.; Zhang, Q.; et al. Protective Role of Nuclear Factor E2-Related Factor 2 against Acute Oxidative Stress-Induced Pancreatic Beta -Cell Damage. *Oxid. Med. Cell. Longev.* **2015**, *2015*, 639191. [CrossRef]
129. Marastoni, D.; Buriani, A.; Pisani, A.I.; Crescenzo, F.; Zuco, C.; Fortinguerra, S.; Sorrenti, V.; Marenda, B.; Romualdi, C.; Magliozzi, R.; et al. Increased Nk Cell Count in Multiple Sclerosis Patients Treated with Dimethyl Fumarate: A 2-Year Longitudinal Study. *Front. Immunol.* **2019**, *10*, 1666. [CrossRef]
130. Hosseini, A.; Masjedi, A.; Baradaran, B.; Hojjat-Farsangi, M.; Ghalamfarsa, G.; Anvari, E.; Jadidi-Niaragh, F. Dimethyl fumarate: Regulatory effects on the immune system in the treatment of multiple sclerosis. *J. Cell. Physiol.* **2018**, *234*, 9943–9955. [CrossRef]
131. Holm Hansen, R.; Hojsgaard Chow, H.; Sellebjerg, F.; Rode von Essen, M. Dimethyl fumarate therapy suppresses B cell responses and follicular helper T cells in relapsing-remitting multiple sclerosis. *Mult. Scler. J.* **2019**, *25*, 1289–1297. [CrossRef]
132. Li, S.; Vaziri, N.; Swentek, L.; Takasu, C.; Vo, K.; Stamos, M.; Ricordi, C.; Ichii, H. Prevention of Autoimmune Diabetes in NOD Mice by Dimethyl Fumarate. *Antioxidants* **2021**, *10*, 193. [CrossRef]

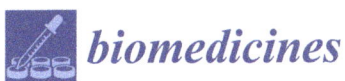

Article

MORG1—A Negative Modulator of Renal Lipid Metabolism in Murine Diabetes

Eric Jankowski, Sophie Wulf, Nadja Ziller, Gunter Wolf [†] and Ivonne Loeffler [*,†]

Department of Internal Medicine III, Jena University Hospital, Am Klinikum 1, D-07747 Jena, Germany; Eric.Jankowski@med.uni-jena.de (E.J.); Sophie.Wulf@med.uni-jena.de (S.W.); Nadja.ziller@med.uni-jena.de (N.Z.); gunter.wolf@med.uni-jena.de (G.W.)
* Correspondence: ivonne.loeffler@med.uni-jena.de; Tel.: +49-3641-9324630
† These authors contributed equally to this work.

Abstract: Renal fatty acid (FA) metabolism is severely altered in type 1 and 2 diabetes mellitus (T1DM and T2DM). Increasing evidence suggests that altered lipid metabolism is linked to tubulointerstitial fibrosis (TIF). Our previous work has demonstrated that mice with reduced MORG1 expression, a scaffold protein in HIF and ERK signaling, are protected against TIF in the db/db mouse model. Renal TGF-ß1 expression and EMT-like changes were reduced in mice with single-allele deficiency of MORG1. Given the well-known role of HIF and ERK signaling in metabolic regulation, here we examined whether protection was also associated with a restoration of lipid metabolism. Despite similar features of TIF in T1DM and T2DM, diabetes-associated changes in renal lipid metabolism differ between both diseases. We found that de novo synthesis of FA/cholesterol and β-oxidation were more strongly disrupted in T1DM, whereas pathological fat uptake into tubular cells mediates lipotoxicity in T2DM. Thus, diminished MORG1 expression exerts renoprotection in the diabetic nephropathy by modulating important factors of TIF and lipid dysregulation to a variable extent in T1DM and T2DM. Prospectively, targeting MORG1 appears to be a promising strategy to reduce lipid metabolic alterations in diabetic nephropathy.

Keywords: type 1 diabetes mellitus; T1DM; type 2 diabetes mellitus; T2DM; diabetic nephropathy; kidney; lipid metabolism; fatty acid metabolism; MORG1; mitogen-activated protein kinase organizer 1; WDR83

Citation: Jankowski, E.; Wulf, S.; Ziller, N.; Wolf, G.; Loeffler, I. MORG1—A Negative Modulator of Renal Lipid Metabolism in Murine Diabetes. *Biomedicines* **2022**, *10*, 30. https://doi.org/10.3390/biomedicines10010030

Academic Editor: Maria Grau

Received: 1 December 2021
Accepted: 21 December 2021
Published: 23 December 2021

Publisher's Note: MDPI stays neutral with regard to jurisdictional claims in published maps and institutional affiliations.

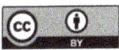

Copyright: © 2021 by the authors. Licensee MDPI, Basel, Switzerland. This article is an open access article distributed under the terms and conditions of the Creative Commons Attribution (CC BY) license (https://creativecommons.org/licenses/by/4.0/).

1. Introduction

One of the most important complications of type 1 (T1DM) and type 2 diabetes mellitus (T2DM) is diabetic nephropathy (DN) [1,2]. Early in DN, the interstitium becomes dilated, leading to tubulointerstitial fibrosis (TIF) and tubular atrophy [3,4]. In TIF, myofibroblast accumulation is observed, accompanied by excessive extracellular matrix (ECM) deposition and, in later stages, destruction of renal tubules [5,6]. Fibrosis-promoting cytokines (e.g., transforming growth factor beta 1 (TGF-β1), connective tissue growth factor (CTGF)) are produced in fibrogenic signaling phase of TIF [7]. In contemporary understanding of renal fibrosis, multiple cell types and different mechanisms appear to be responsible for ECM accumulation and remodeling [8–15]. Recently, it has been demonstrated that the downregulation of key enzymes and regulators of fatty acid oxidation (FAO), as well as increased lipid accumulation in proximal tubular epithelial cells, is directly linked to TIF [16]. Under physiological conditions, tubular cells rely on fatty acids (FAs) as their main energy source. Therefore, uptake of FAs, FA oxidation and FA synthesis are tightly balanced in these cells [16–19]. Conversely, injured tubular cells display dramatic metabolic rearrangements, including profound suppression of FAO [17]. This altered renal lipid metabolism has been described in DN, where sustained hyperglycemia promotes FA synthesis and triglyceride accumulation [20]. The elevated serum triglycerides, together with free FAs and modified cholesterol, can cause lipid accumulation in non-adipose tissues, a process termed lipotoxicity [20].

Various pathological stimuli in the diabetic milieu, such as TGF-β1 and hypoxia, are known to induce an imbalance in lipid metabolism [21–23]. Tissue hypoxia in patients with chronic kidney disease results from an altered renal oxygen supply, thus leading to the stabilization of the hypoxia-dependent transcription factors HIF1/2 (hypoxia-inducible factor 1/2) in the kidneys [24]. HIF1α and HIF2α function mainly as transcriptional activators, regulating several biological processes, such as metabolism of glucose, cholesterol and FAs [25–27]. In contrast to the apparent role of HIF in carbohydrate metabolism, its effects on lipid metabolism have recently been investigated [21]. In addition to the HIF pathway, the MEK/ERK pathway also appears to be involved in lipid metabolism, as extracellular signal-regulated kinases 1/2 (ERK1/2) can influence several master regulators of cellular lipid metabolism [28–31].

MORG1 (mitogen-activated protein kinase organizer 1, also known as WDR83) is identified as a scaffold protein in both ERK1/2 and HIF pathways. It is a member of the WD-40 domain protein family with a molecular mass of 34.5 kDa and is ubiquitously expressed in different organs, including the heart, brain and kidney [32]. MORG1 was first isolated as a binding partner of the ERK pathway scaffold protein MP1 (MEK partner 1) in 2004 [32]. It also specifically associates with multiple-components of the mitogen-activated protein kinase (MAPK) cascade and stabilizes their assembly into an oligomeric complex [32]. Furthermore, MORG1 biphasically modulates the activation of the ERK cascade: at low concentrations, MORG1 enhances ERK activation, whereas high concentrations lead rather to the inhibition of ERK activation [32]. In addition to its central role in the MAPK pathway, MORG1 also functions as a scaffold protein in HIF signaling. Our group has identified MORG1 as a scaffold protein of PHD3 (prolyl hydroxylase domain protein 3) that regulates the degradation of HIF-1α and HIF-2α under normoxic conditions [24,33]. MORG1 was found to interact with PHD3, leading to the stabilization of PHD3. In this way, MORG1 works together with PHD3 in the regulation and degradation of HIF-α protein [33–35]. By suppression of MORG1 the basal HIF-α protein stability is increased and (as a result) there is reduction in HIF-α degradation [33,36–38]. Several lines of evidence support the notion that MORG1 is involved in the pathophysiology of various diseases. Due to embryonic lethality of homozygous MORG1 knockout mice, studies have been conducted in heterozygous mice that exhibit a normal phenotype. We described that heterozygous MORG1 knockout mice are protected from experimentally induced focal cerebral ischemia [39], from acute renal ischemia-reperfusion injury [40] and from acute kidney damage due to systemic hypoxia [37]. Recent data indicate that they are also protected from kidney damage as a late consequence of T2DM [41]. In the db/db mouse model for type 2 DN, the DN was ameliorated when MORG1 expression was suppressed [41]. We hypothesize that the attenuated TIF is, at least partly, a consequence of reduced EMT (epithelial-to-mesenchymal transition)-like changes in tubular cells [41].

In this study, we aimed to investigate whether a reduction of MORG1 in kidneys of diabetic mice leads to a restoration of a potentially disrupted lipid metabolism. Here, we compare two different diabetes models: insulin-dependent (STZ-induced T1DM-like phenotype) and insulin-independent diabetes mellitus (db/db mouse model for T2DM).

2. Materials and Methods

2.1. Animals

All animal experiments were approved by the Local Ethics Committee of Thüringer-Landesamt für Verbraucherschutz (approval numbers UKJ-17-024 and 02-039/15) and were performed in accordance with the German Animal Protection Law. The animals were housed in a pathogen-free facility with a 12-h light–dark cycle and raised on standard chow and water ad libitum. MORG1 knockout mice were derived from the C57BL6/J strain and generated by homologous recombination, using standard techniques [42]. A cassette containing various selection markers and the gene for green fluorescence protein was placed in the exons 1–5 of the MORG1 gene to disrupt the MORG1 coding sequence and to detect the expression. Individuals involved in this study were backcrossed to the C57BLKS background for at least 10 generations. MORG1$^{+/-}$ (heterozygous) mice exhibited a normal phenotype; however, MORG1$^{-/-}$ (homozygous) animals exhibited embryonal lethality between embryonic days 8.5 and 10.5, probably due to diffuse vascularization of the embryo and malformations in the neural tube (unpublished observations).

Mouse model for T1DM-like phenotype: Mild insulin-dependent diabetes mellitus was induced in wild-type ($n = 7$) and MORG1 heterozygous mice ($n = 7$) at 12–15 weeks of age by intraperitoneal administration of 50 mg/kg streptozotocin (STZ; Sigma-Aldrich, St. Louis, MO, USA; in sterile 10 mM sodium citrate, pH 5.5) for 4 consecutive days. Due to their genetic background, which contains proportions of DBA/2, the animals used were very good STZ responders [43]. Therefore, the used STZ protocol was sufficient to keep fasting blood glucose stable above 15 mmol/L (on average) and to avoid ketonuria. Non-diabetic control animals received daily intraperitoneal injections of placebo (10 mM sodium citrate, pH 5.5) for 4 days. After 3 months of inducing diabetes, the mice were euthanized and their kidneys were removed. One half of the kidney was fixed in 4% phosphate buffered formalin and for histological studies embedded in paraffin. Remaining tissue was snap-frozen for mRNA analysis.

T2DM mouse model: The mouse line used for our T2DM model was generated by crossing mice from the db/db strain (BKS.Cg-Dock7m+/+Leprdb/J; C57BLKS/J background; obtained from Charles River Laboratory (Brussels, Belgium)) with mice from the MORG1 strain. Based on their genotype, the animals were divided into four groups: MORG1 wild-type non-diabetic control (db/m; MORG1$^{+/+}$) ($n = 10$), MORG1 wild-type diabetic T2DM (db/db; MORG1$^{+/+}$) ($n = 8$), MORG1 heterozygous non-diabetic control (db/m; MORG1$^{+/-}$) ($n = 5$) and MORG1 heterozygous diabetic T2DM (db/db; MORG1$^{+/-}$) ($n = 6$). At the age of 25–28 weeks, mice were euthanized, and their kidneys were removed. One half of a kidney was fixed in 4% phosphate buffered formalin and for histological studies embedded in paraffin. Remaining tissue was snap-frozen for mRNA analysis and Oil Red O staining.

2.2. Immunohistochemistry and Oil Red O Staining

In preparation for immunohistochemical staining, the 3 μm paraffin sections were dewaxed/deparaffinized and rehydrated. A heat-mediated antigen retrieval procedure in citrate buffer (pH 6.0) was performed. Blocking of endogenous peroxidase was achieved by incubation with 3% H2O2 (Roth, Karlsruhe, Germany) for 10 min at room temperature. Following the blocking with Roti-Block, the sections were incubated with primary antibodies overnight at 4 °C. The following primary antibodies were used: rabbit polyclonal anti-fatty acid synthase (FAS) antibody (Abcam, Camebridge, UK), mouse monoclonal anti-MTCO1 antibody (Abcam, Camebridge, UK) and rabbit polyclonal anti-PPARα antibody (Abcam, Cambridge, UK). After incubation with peroxidase-labeled goat anti-rabbit IgG antibody (KPL, Gaithersburg, MD, USA) or anti-mouse IgG antibody (SeraCare, Milford, MA, USA), di-aminobenzidine (DAB) (DAB-peroxidase substrate kit; Vector Laboratories, Burlingame, CA, USA) was used as a chromogen.

For Oil Red O staining, snap-frozen renal sections (thickness 10 μm) were stained by using Oil Red O solution 0.5% in iso-propanol (Sigma-Aldrich, Merck, Darmstadt, Germany).

2.3. Immunofluorescence

Protein expression via immunofluorescence was analyzed on paraffin-embedded kidney sections (thickness 3 μm). After deparaffination, hydration and heat-mediated antigen retrieval in citrate buffer (pH 6.0), blocking with 5% BSA (bovine serum albumin, Roth, Karlsruhe, Germany) was performed for one hour at room temperature. The kidney sections were incubated with recombinant anti-CD36 antibody (Abcam, Camebridge, UK) at 4 °C overnight. As secondary antibody anti-rabbit IgG DY-light 594 (Vector Laboratories, Burlingame, CA, USA) was used. Nuclei were counterstained with 4′,6-diamidino-2-phenylindole (DAPI, Sigma-Aldrich, Merck, Darmstadt, Germany).

2.4. Quantification

For quantification, at least 10 non-overlapping high-power fields (magnification ×200) for each kidney sample were examined by AxioVision 4.8 software monochrome modus of the AxioCamHRc camera (both Zeiss, Jena, Germany) and analyzed by using an ImageJ Macro. ZeissVisionImage (.zvi) format was exported to TIFF format. Gained data were analyzed by using the thresholding function of ImageJ. For each staining, an individual threshold was customized and applied to all images of that staining. Staining was segmented into relevant and irrelevant. As an example, the used MACRO for FAS staining can be found in the Supplementary Materials and Section 2.

Obtained data of relevantly stained area per image were averaged for each mouse. To compare individuals of different groups, all mice were normalized to the mean value of samples from the MORG1 wild-type non-diabetic control group (db/m; MORG1$^{+/+}$).

2.5. cDNA Synthesis and Semi-Quantitative Real-Time PCR

For isolation of total RNA from kidney cortex, the NucleoSpin 8 RNA Kit (Macherey-Nagel, Düren, Germany) was used. Elimination of possible DNA contamination was performed with the RNase-Free DNase Set (Qiagen, Hilden, Germany), and 1 µg total RNA was reverse-transcripted into cDNA with the Reverse-Transcription System Promega (Promega, Madison, WI, USA). Determination of gene-expression levels was performed by semi-quantitative real-time PCR by use of the LightCycler-FastStart DNA Master SYBR Green 1 (Roche Diagnostics, Mannheim, Germany) and a thermocycler (qTower, Analytik Jena, Jena, Germany). PCRs were carried out with sense and antisense primers at a concentration of 0.25 µM each (purchased from TIB Molbiol, Berlin, Germany). Temperatures and sequences of all primer pairs are shown in Table 1. Hypoxanthine phosphoribosyltransferase 1 (HPRT1) was used as the housekeeping gene. Relative expression ratio was quantified by the ΔΔCT method, and transcript levels were normalized to the mean value of the MORG1 wild-type non-diabetic control group.

Table 1. List of primer pairs and annealing temperatures.

Gene	Sense and Antisense Primers	T$_{ann.}$
ACOX1	5'-GCCCAACTGTGACTTCCATC-3' 5'-GCCAGGACTATCGCATGATT-3'	60 °C [44]
CPT1	5'-TCCATGCATACCAAAGTGGA-3' 5'-TGGTAGGAGAGCAGCACCTT-3'	60 °C [45]
CTGF	5'-TGCTGTGCAGGTGATAAAGC-3' 5'-AAGGCCATTTGTTCACCAAC-3'	58 °C [46]
FAS	5'-CCTGGATAGCATTCCGAACCT-3' 5'-ACACATCTCGAAGGCTACACA-3'	61 °C [47]
HMG-CoA-Red	5'-AGCCGAAGCAGCACATGAT-3' 5'-CTTGTGGAATGCCTTGTGATTG-3'	57 °C [48]
HPRT1	5'-TGGATACAGGCCAGACTTTGTT-3' 5'-CAGATTCAACTTGCGCTCATC-3'	59 °C [49]
KIM1	5'-ATGAATCAGATTCAAGTCTTC-3' 5'-TCTGGTTTGTGAGTCCATGTG-3'	58 °C [50]
SREBP2	5'-CAAGTCTGGCGTTCTGAGGAA-3' 5'-ATGTTCTCCTGGCGAAGCT-3'	61 °C [51]

ACOX1 = Acyl-CoA Oxidase 1, CPT1 = carnitine palmitoyltransferase 1, CTGF = connective tissue growth factor, FAS = fatty acid synthase, HMG-CoA-Red = 3-hydroxy-3-methylglutaryl-Coenzyme A reductase, HPRT1 = hypoxanthine phosphoribosyl transferase 1, KIM1 = kidney injury molecule-1, SREBP2 = sterol regulatory element-binding protein 2, T$_{ann.}$ = annealing temperature.

2.6. Statistics

The data from the four experimental groups are shown as box/whisker-dot plots, drawn using SPSS statistics (IBM company, Armonk, NY, USA). The boxes' boundaries mark the 25th percentile in the bottom and the 75th percentile on the top. The line in the center of the box indicates the median of values and the whiskers, drawn below and above the box, span from the 10th to the 90th percentile. Values with a distance of ≥1.5*IQR (interquartile range) to the first and third quartile are defined as outliers. Outliers (presented as single dots outside the whiskers) were excluded from statistical analysis. Effects (main effects and interactions) were assessed by using two-way analysis of variance (ANOVA) with phenotype (non-diabetic control or diabetic (STZ-T1DM/T2DM)) and genotype (wild-type or heterozygous) as the two factors. Interaction determines whether the one main effect depends on the level of the other main effect. For intergroup comparison, Mann–Whitney U test was used to test the statistically significance between two independent groups (MORG1 wild-type control vs. MORG1 wild-type STZ-T1DM/T2DM; MORG1 wild-type control vs. MORG1 heterozygous control; MORG1 heterozygous control vs. MORG1 heterozygous STZ-T1DM/T2DM; MORG1 wild-type STZ-T1DM/T2DM vs. MORG1 heterozygous STZ-T1DM/T2DM).

To analyze the correlation between tested lipid metabolism markers and CTGF, KIM1 or lipid accumulation, all groups were included, and the Pearson correlation coefficient (ρ) was calculated by using SPSS statistics. To analyze the correlation between PPARα and FAS or CD36 expression, only non-diabetic mice were included, and the Pearson correlation coefficient (ρ) was calculated. We classified Pearson's correlations as reasonable according to medical standards, with ρ of 0.3 to 0.5 as fair, 0.6 to 0.7 as moderate and >0.7 as very strong [52].

A p-value of ≤0.05 was considered statistically significant. The p-values from ≥0.05 to ≤0.1 were considered biologically relevant.

3. Results and Discussion

3.1. Different Role of MORG1 in Renal Fatty Acid and Cholesterol Synthesis in STZ-T1DM and T2DM

A tubule epithelial lipid accumulation was found in patients with manifested DN. Lipid droplets are round membrane-coated organelles, which contain potentially toxic triglycerides and cholesterol esters [20]. It is believed that genes involved in triglyceride, as well as cholesterol, metabolism are dysregulated in DN. In diabetic kidneys, increased uptake of FAs, de novo synthesis of FAs and triglycerides and decreased expression of master regulators of FAO may contribute to lipid storage, thus contributing to the altered expression of receptors or transporters regulating the influx/efflux of cholesterol [16,17,19,20].

Firstly, we investigated the expression of markers for FA and cholesterol synthesis in our models. Sterol regulatory element binding proteins (SREBPs) serve as the master regulators of cellular FA and cholesterol synthesis, whereas SREBP-2 regulates cholesterol synthesis. FA synthesis is regulated by SREBP-1 and catalyzed through FA synthase (FAS) and acetyl-CoA carboxylase (ACC) [20,21]. Our analysis revealed differences not only between the types of diabetes, but also regarding the MORG1 genotype in this condition (Figures 1 and 2). In mice with T1DM-like phenotype, FAS protein, as well as HMG-CoA-Red and SREBP2 mRNA, was upregulated (Figures 1A and 2A,C), and this correlates with previous data [20]. Whereas the single-allele deficiency of MORG1 resulted in the restoration of diabetes-induced FAS dysregulation (Figure 1A), the upregulation of cholesterol synthesis was independent of MORG1 genotype (Figure 2C). Analysis of variance (represented in tables below the graphs) confirms a significant diabetes effect on FA and cholesterol synthesis (Figures 1A and 2A,C) and a profound interaction between diabetes phenotype and MORG1 genotype on protein expression of FAS (Figure 1A).

The similar analysis of kidneys from T2DM mice (Figures 1B and 2B,D) did not yield significant results, except that the non-diabetic control animals with MORG1 heterozygous genotype showed significantly higher FAS expression compared to the wild-type control (Figure 1B). This could also be observed in the non-diabetic animals of the STZ-T1DM model (Figure 1A). A possible explanation is the HIF1/2 stabilization in MORG1 heterozygous mice, which was shown in previous work [37,41]. An HIF1-dependent activation of SREBP1 and, thus, increased expression of FAS have been described [21].

Studies of a possible diabetes effects on renal MORG1 expression revealed that neither T2DM nor STZ-induced diabetes affected tubular MORG1 protein expression in our models. Thus, renal MORG1 levels are similar in non-diabetic and diabetic kidneys, with an overall reduction of MORG1 of approximately 20–25% in heterozygous mice (Supplementary Materials Figure S1 and Reference [41]).

In summary, we demonstrated that there is a significant interaction between MORG1 expression and STZ-T1DM in the synthesis of FA. The results further suggest that, in our T2DM model, increased FA or cholesterol synthesis does not play a role in lipid accumulation. On the contrary and consistent with the trend observed in wild-type animals with T2DM (Figure 2D), gene expression analyses in kidney biopsies of patients with DN (with T2DM) showed decreased FAS, as well as SREBP2 [20].

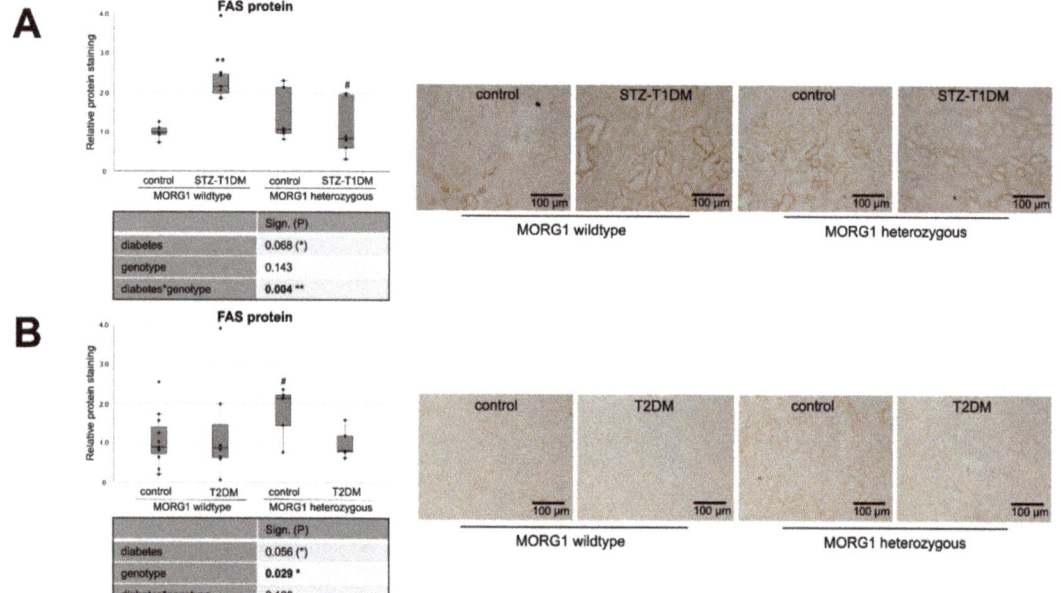

Figure 1. Role of MORG1 in de novo synthesis of fatty acids in tubular cells. (**A**,**B**) Immunohistochemistry of FAS (fatty acid synthase) in STZ-T1DM and T2DM and semi-quantitative analysis of the staining. Representative images are shown next to the graphs (magnification ×200). The significances shown in the tables were assessed by two-way ANOVA with diabetes (control or STZ-T1DM/T2DM) and genotype (MORG1 wild-type or MORG1 heterozygous) as the two factors. Diabetes, genotype: main effect of diabetes/genotype, respectively. Diabetes*genotype: interaction. Bold: statistically significant. (*) Biologically relevant. Significances shown next to each bar were assessed by using Mann–Whitney U test; ** $p \leq 0.01$ in between same genotype; # $p \leq 0.05$ in between different genotypes.

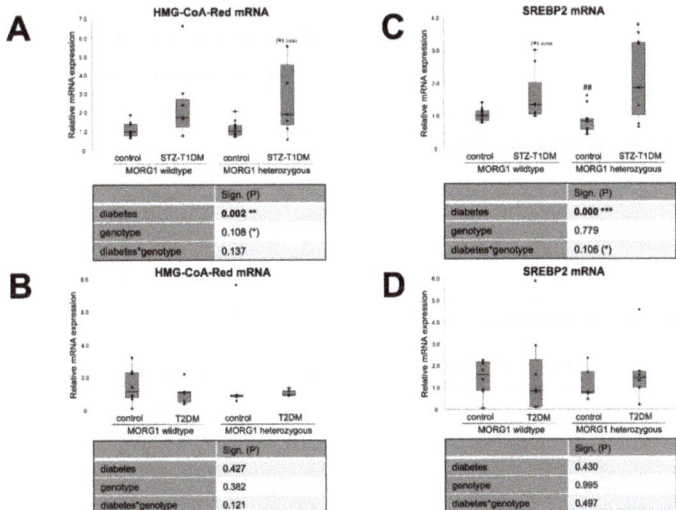

Figure 2. Effect of MORG1 and diabetes on renal expression of key enzymes of cholesterol synthesis. (**A,B**) Real-time analysis of HMG-CoA-Red (3-hydroxy-3-methylglutaryl-CoA-reductase) mRNA expression in STZ-T1DM and T2DM. (**C,D**) Real-time mRNA analysis of SREBP2 (sterol regulatory element-binding protein 2) in STZ-T1DM and T2DM. (**A–D**) The significances shown in the tables were assessed by two-way ANOVA with diabetes (control or STZ-T1DM/T2DM) and genotype (MORG1 wild-type or MORG1 heterozygous) as the two factors. Diabetes, genotype: main effect of diabetes/genotype, respectively. Diabetes*genotype: interaction. Bold: statistically significant. (*) Biologically relevant. Significances shown next to each bar were assessed by using Mann–Whitney U test; * $p \leq 0.05$ in between same genotype; ## $p \leq 0.01$ in between different genotypes; (*) biological relevant in between same genotypes.

3.2. Expression of Fat Transporters in Tubular Cells Depends on Type of Diabetes and MORG1 Level

Intracellular lipid accumulation can result from de novo synthesis of FAs and cholesterol or from exogenous FAs uptake and cholesterol influx. CD36 (cluster of differentiation 36) is a scavenger receptor class B that mediates binding and uptake of long-chain FAs, oxidized lipids and phospholipids, advanced oxidation protein products, advanced glycation end-products (AGEs) and thrombospondin [53]. In the kidney, CD36 is mainly expressed in tubular epithelial cells, podocytes and mesangial cells, and multiple ligands regulate its expression and intracellular location [53]. Moreover, we have demonstrated for the first time that the scavenger receptor class B type I, a specific receptor for HDL is mainly expressed in proximal tubular cells and is downregulated by angiotensin II (ANG II) [54]. Since local ANG II concentrations are high in DN [2], this mechanism may contribute to severe lipid abnormalities in DN.

Experimental induction of a T1DM-like phenotype significantly reduces tubular CD36 protein in our model, which is further decreased by reduction of MORG1 (Figure 3A). Variance analysis reveals significant diabetes–MORG1 interaction. The data suggest that, in this diabetes model, increased de novo synthesis, but not increased uptake, contributes to impaired lipid metabolism.

However, a somewhat different situation emerges in the T2DM model (Figure 3B). Although not statistically significant across all animals tested in the intergroup comparison, we found accelerated CD36 expression in the kidneys of some mice with T2DM (Figure 3B). This is consistent with the finding that patients with diagnosed type 2 DN showed increased fat uptake receptor expression in kidneys (e.g., CD36) [20].

HK-2 tubular cells line cultured with high glucose (HG) showed exacerbated lipid deposition. The effect was partly due to increased CD36 expression via the AKT-PPARγ signaling pathway. This underlines/emphasizes the relevance of FA or cholesterol uptake in intracellular lipid accumulation [55,56]. Furthermore, CD36 is involved in HG-induced EMT in renal tubular epithelial cells [57]. This is of great interest because we also observed EMT-like changes in the kidneys in our db/db mouse model; for example, the expression of the transcription factor Snail1 was increased and the tubular epithelial marker E-cadherin was reduced [41]. Although hyperglycemia is a clinical hallmark in T1DM and EMT-like changes could already be detected in the STZ model [58], but in our mice with a T1DM-like phenotype, both the HG-CD36 and the CD36-EMT axis do not play a major role.

In the T2DM model, however, a reduction of MORG1 expression inhibits both TGF-β1 and EMT-like changes [41], conforming the CD36 expression pattern shown here in heterozygous MORG1 mice (Figure 3B).

In line with the increased FAS in non-diabetic MORG1 knockout mice, the CD36 protein is also highly expressed when MORG1 is reduced (Figure 3A,B). This is intriguing, as the uptake of extracellular FA and triacylglycerol synthesis are promoted by transcription factor PPARγ, which is directly activated by HIF1 [21].

Consistent with CD36 expression in the STZ-induced T1DM model, there is also a significant diabetes*MORG1 genotype interaction in T2DM, but this results from different and partially opposing effects. However, in mice with the single-allele deficiency of MORG1, there is significantly lower renal CD36 expression compared to non-diabetic kidneys, independent of diabetes type.

It is believed that lipotoxicity in patients with DN can mechanistically results from cell-specific stress (e.g., CD36-mediated cellular stress in tubular cells), as well as from generic cellular stress (e.g., altered mitochondrial energy production) [59]. Mitochondrial dysfunction is a well-recognized pathologic feature which triggers fibrosis [60]. Mitochondrially encoded cytochrome c oxidase subunit 1 (MTCO1) is one of the core subunits of complex IV (the final enzyme of electron transport chain of mitochondrial oxidative phosphorylation) and can be used as a mitochondrial marker. Recently, Haraguchi et al. showed an accumulation of oxidative modified mitochondria in the damaged diabetic proximal renal tubules after 10 weeks of STZ-induced T1DM in C57BL/6J mice [61]. We also selected MTCO1 as a mitochondrial target, but could not confirm diabetes-induced accumulation of mitochondria in STZ-T1DM (Figure 3C). In contrast to the model of Haraguchi et al., our mice have a different genetic background (namely, C57BLKS and not C57BL/6J) and administered with a lower dose of STZ (50 mg/kg body weight for 4 consecutive days vs. 70 mg/kg body weight for 5 consecutive days) [61].

Similarly, in our T2DM model, we did not detect any diabetic effect on MTCO1 levels (Figure 3D). Interestingly, kidneys with reduced MORG1 expression (MORG1 heterozygous) showed significantly intense MTCO1 staining (Figure 3D). We interpret higher levels of MTCO1 with increased mitochondrial fission. Mitochondrial fission generates new organelles, facilitates quality control and is a mechanism for preconditioning to be prepared for metabolic stress [62]. Various studies have demonstrated that hypoxia-preconditioning, pharmacologic and/or genetic activation of HIF protects from kidney injury [37,40,41,63–65]. Considering the fact that mitochondrial fission is regulated via ERK1/2 signaling [66], and, at low concentrations, MORG1 also enhances ERK activation [32]; this novel finding confirms that the MORG1 heterozygous mice are protected because of preconditioning. Supporting our hypothesis, it has been shown that increased expression of the key transcriptional regulator of mitochondrial biogenesis, PGC-1α, in renal tubule cells protects against chronic kidney disease [67].

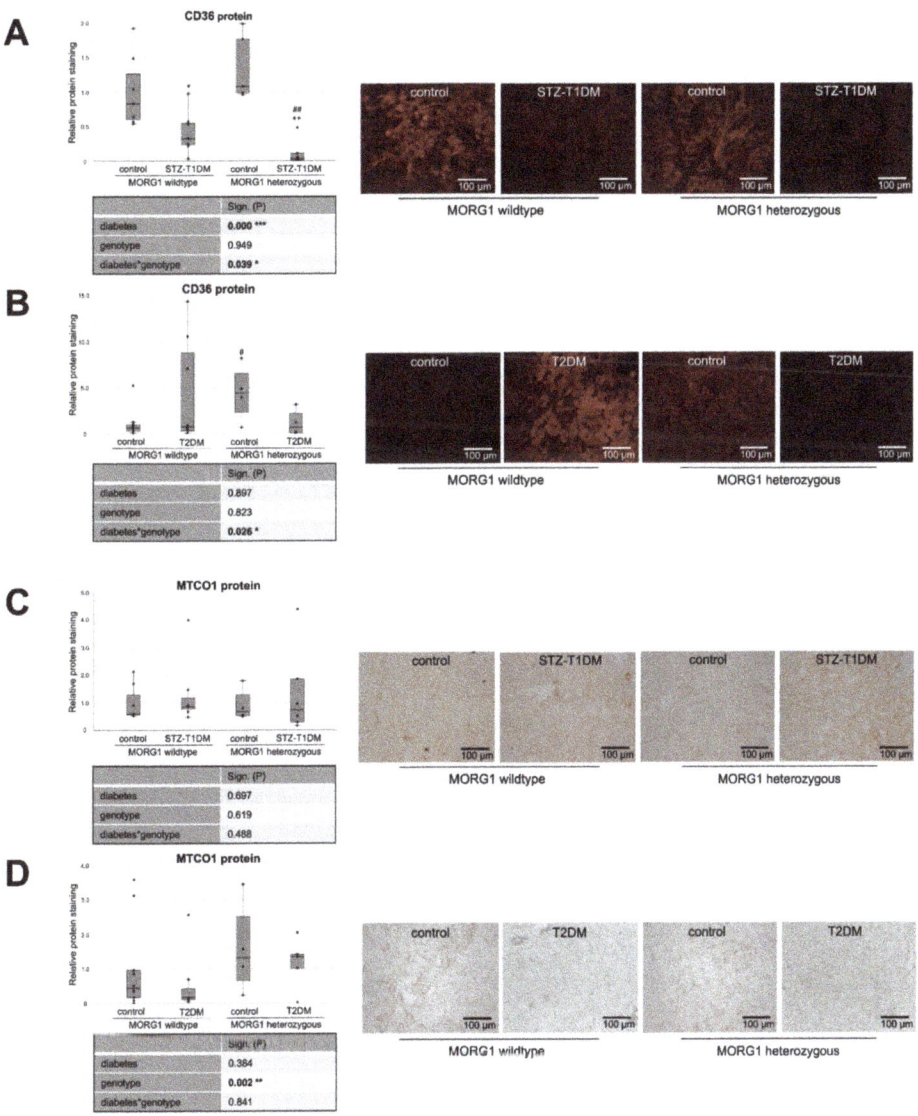

Figure 3. Analysis of fat uptake and metabolic stress in kidneys of diabetic animals. (**A,B**) Immunofluorescence staining of CD36 (cluster of differentiation 36) and semi-quantitative analysis of the staining in STZ-T1DM and T2DM. (**C,D**) Immunohistochemistry of MTCO1 (mitochondrially encoded cytochrome C oxidase 1) in STZ-T1DM and T2DM and semi-quantitative analysis of the staining. (**A–D**) Representative images are shown next to the graph (magnification ×200). The significances shown in the tables were assessed by two-way ANOVA with diabetes (control or STZ-T1DM/T2DM) and genotype (MORG1 wild-type or MORG1 heterozygous) as the two factors. Diabetes, genotype: main effect of diabetes/genotype, respectively. Diabetes*genotype: interaction. Bold: statistically significant. Significances shown next to each bar were assessed by using Mann–Whitney U test; * $p \leq 0.05$ in between same genotype; ** $p \leq 0.01$ in between same genotype; # $p \leq 0.05$ in between different genotypes; ## $p \leq 0.01$ in between different genotypes.

3.3. Single-Allele Deficiency of MORG1 Restores Pathological Changes in Renal FAO

Tubular cells have a high basal level of energy demand, which is mostly produced by the β-oxidation of FA, due to greater ATP yield compared to oxidation of only glucose [16,18,68]. Decreased FAO in these renal epithelial cells has been reported to play a particular role in kidney fibrosis: on the one hand, the inhibition of FAO leads to a fibrotic phenotype, and, on the other hand, restoring FA metabolism protected mice from TIF [16].

Therefore, we investigated the expression of key enzymes of FAO pathways: peroxisome proliferator activated receptor alpha (PPARα), carnitine palmitoyltransferase 1 (CPT1) and acyl-CoA oxidase (ACOX1) (Figures 4 and 5). PPARα is the key transcriptional factor that directly controls genes involved in β-oxidation, FA uptake and triglyceride catabolism [68]. FAs undergo transport into mitochondria, where FAO takes place, by CPT1 and degradation (β-oxidation) by ACOX1 [20,21].

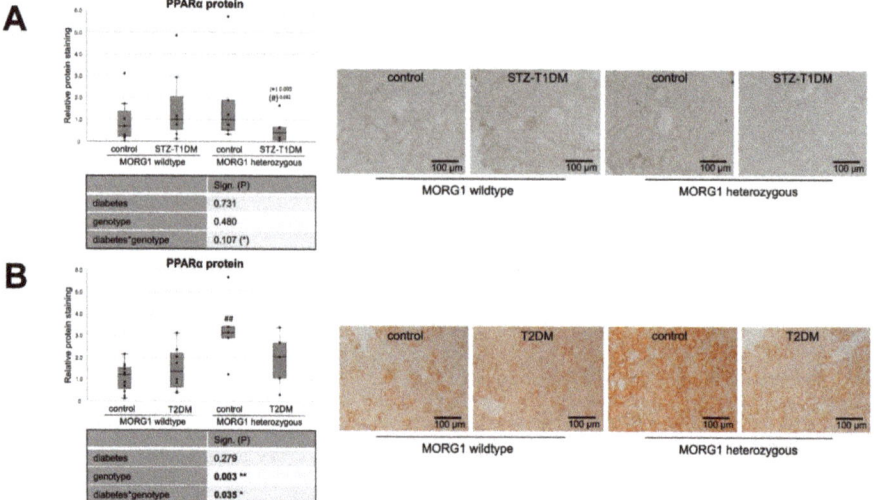

Figure 4. Role of MORG1 in renal expression of transcriptional factor of β-oxidation. (**A,B**) Immunohistochemistry of PPARα (peroxisome proliferator activated receptor alpha) protein in STZ-T1DM and T2DM with 10 non-overlapping images per animal and semi-quantitative analysis of the staining. Representative images are shown next to the graphs (magnification ×200). The significances shown in the tables were assessed by two-way ANOVA with diabetes (control or STZ-T1DM/T2DM) and genotype (MORG1 wild-type or MORG1 heterozygous) as the two factors. Diabetes, genotype: main effect of diabetes/genotype, respectively. Diabetes*genotype: interaction. Bold: statistically significant. (*) Biologically relevant. Significances shown next to each bar was assessed by using Mann–Whitney U test; * $p \leq 0.05$ in between same genotype; ## $p \leq 0.01$ in between different genotypes; (*) biological relevant in between same genotype; (#) biological relevant in between different genotypes.

Whereas our wild-type animals, in contrast to the literature, showed no changes in tubular PPARα protein expression in either STZ-T1DM or T2DM (Figure 4), there is the expected diabetic effect (in this study: significant in STZ-T1DM and tangential in T2DM) in the expression of CPT1 and ACOX1 (Figure 5). The diabetes-induced decrease in both FAO markers is abolished in mice with single-allele deficiency of MORG1, which translates into a significant diabetes*genotype interaction in STZ-T1DM (for CPT1 and ACOX1) and T2DM (for ACOX1). One possible explanation as to why there is no detectable change in expression of PPARα while its target genes CPT1 and ACOX1 are reduced is that TGF-β1 influences FAO. TGF-β1, which is upregulated in both T1DM and T2DM, can decrease FAO by classical signaling (via Smad3 and ERK1/2 pathway) by reducing PPARα and its target genes CPT1 and ACOX1; additionally, it can also inhibit PGC-1α and PPAR at epigenetic levels [16,67].

Interestingly, in non-diabetic animals with reduced MORG1 expression PPARα is increased. Because this is consistent with the expression patterns for FAS and CD36 (compare Figure 4B with Figures 1B and 3B and Figure 4A with Figures 1A and 3A), we assume a feedback mechanism here to maintain physiological lipid metabolism. Correlation analysis of non-diabetic control animals revealed a strong positive correlation (ρ 0.74**) between PPARα and FAS in the T2DM model (compare Figure 4B with Figure 1B).

In the presence of diabetes and lower MORG1 expression, PPARα values return to basal levels. There is a biological relevance in STZ diabetes (Figure 4A) and even a significant interaction between diabetes and MORG1 genotype in T2DM (Figure 4B). This may be related to increased HIF2α expression/stabilization in these animals, as it was shown in the fatty liver that HIF2α-mediated activation of ERK decreases PPARα activity [69]. Previous studies in the db/db model showed that diabetic animals with single-allele deficiency of MORG1 had significantly higher HIF2α levels [41], which was also confirmed in the STZ-T1DM model (data not shown).

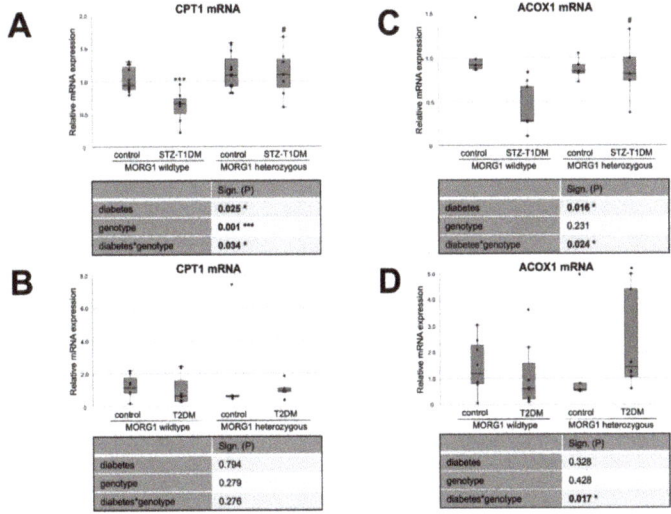

Figure 5. MORG1 effect on expression of key enzymes of FAO (fatty acid oxidation) in diabetic kidneys. (**A,B**) Real-time analysis of CPT1 (carnitine palmitoyl transferase 1) mRNA expression in STZ-T1DM and T2DM. (**C,D**) Real-time analysis of ACOX1 (Acyl-CoA Oxidase 1) mRNA expression in STZ-T1DM and T2DM. (**A–D**) The significances shown in the tables were assessed by two-way ANOVA with diabetes (control or STZ-T1DM/T2DM) and genotype (MORG1 wild-type or MORG1 heterozygous) as the two factors. Diabetes, genotype: main effect of diabetes/genotype, respectively. Diabetes*genotype: interaction. Bold: statistically significant. Significances shown next to each bar was assessed by using Mann–Whitney U test; * $p \leq 0.05$ in between same genotype; *** $p \leq 0.001$ in between same genotype; # $p \leq 0.05$ in between different genotypes.

3.4. Reduction of MORG1 Ameliorates Renal Fibrosis and Lipid Accumulation

It has been reported that altered lipid metabolism, especially defective FAO, can promote TIF [16]. In addition, gene-expression analyses of a large number of human renal tubule samples showed that genes with metabolic functions represent the largest group of dysregulated genes in renal fibrosis [67]. Therefore, we investigated the expression of fibrosis-promoting factors CTGF and kidney injury molecule 1 (KIM1) (Figure 6). For KIM1, a type I membrane protein, a high induction of expression after acute injury and in fibrotic kidneys has been shown [70,71]. KIM1 is an early biomarker of AKI and has furthermore a potential role in predicting the long-term renal outcome [71]. It has also been shown that KIM1 expression correlates with proinflammatory chemokine MCP1 expression [70].

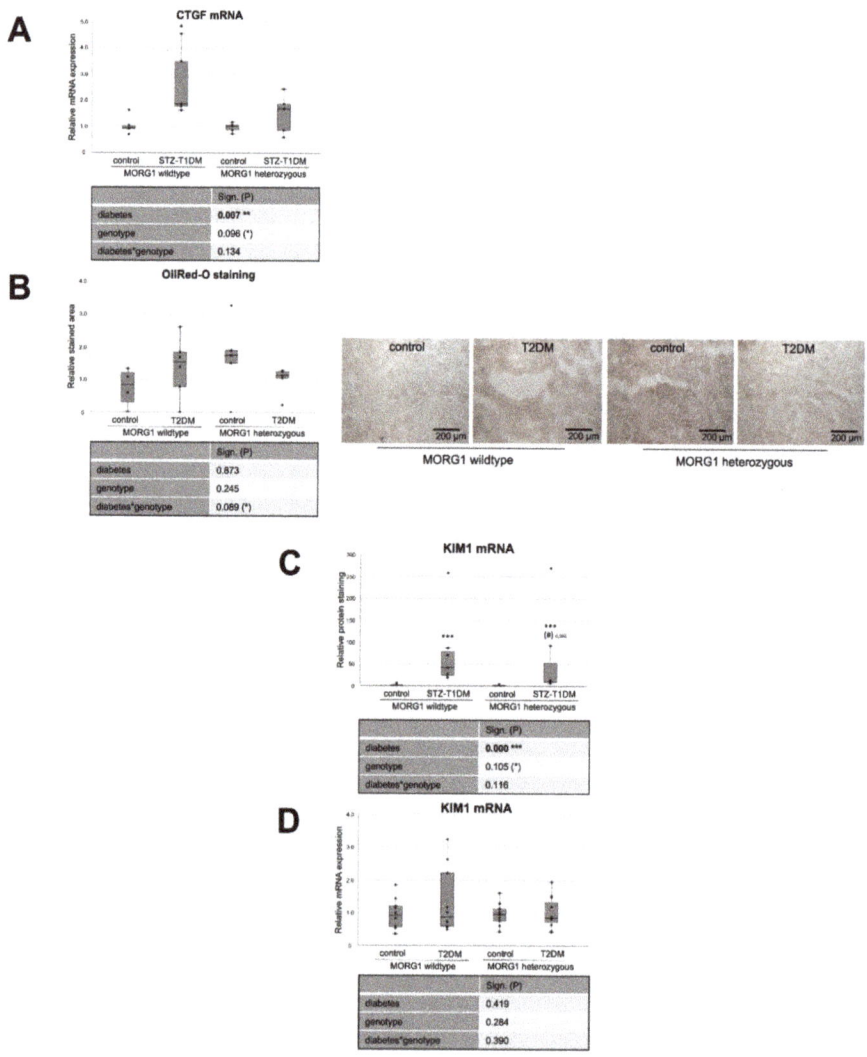

Figure 6. Effect of diabetes and MORG1 on TIF and lipid accumulation. (**A**) Real-time analysis of CTGF (connective tissue growth factor) mRNA expression in STZ-T1DM. (**B**) Quantitative analysis of OilRedO staining of kidney sections from T2DM animals (graph) and representative images next to the graph (magnification ×100). (**C,D**) Real-time analysis of KIM1 (kidney injury molecule-1) mRNA expression in STZ-T1DM and T2DM (**A**–**D**) The significances shown in the tables were assessed by two-way ANOVA with diabetes (control or STZ-T1DM/T2DM) and genotype (MORG1 wild-type or MORG1 heterozygous) as the two factors. Diabetes, genotype: main effect of diabetes/genotype, respectively. Diabetes*genotype: interaction. Bold: statistically significant. (*) Biologically relevant. Significances shown next to each bar were assessed by using Mann–Whitney U test; * $p \leq 0.05$ in between same genotype; *** $p \leq 0.001$ in between same genotype; (#) biological relevant in between different genotypes.

In the STZ-T1DM model, a clear and significant diabetes effect was detected on both CTGF and KIM1 mRNA expression (Figure 6A,C). However, diabetic conditions do not have such a strong effect on fibrosis marker expression when MORG1 is reduced. There is no statistical significance in heterozygous genotype between diabetic and non-diabetic animals (in the case of CTGF; Figure 6A). However, a direct group comparison of diabetic heterozygous animals with those of the MORG1 wild type shows a decrease with biological relevance (in case of KIM1; Figure 6C). Correlation analyses showed moderately significant inverse correlations between renal fibrosis and FAO (CTGF mRNA vs. CPT1 mRNA ρ—0.6**; CTGF mRNA vs. ACOX1 mRNA ρ—0.7***). In addition, a fair to moderately significant inverse correlation between damaged tubules and FAO (KIM1 mRNA vs. CPT1 mRNA ρ—0.4**; KIM1 mRNA vs. ACOX1 mRNA ρ—0.7***) was demonstrated.

We have already examined TIF in the T2DM animals with different MORG1 genotypes in our previous study [41]. The results obtained in a previous study correlate with the current findings for STZ-T1DM. Diabetes-induced CTGF mRNA and protein expression, as well as collagen I and fibronectin accumulation in the tubulointerstitium of the *db/db* mice, were less pronounced when a heterozygous MORG1 knockout genotype was present in addition to diabetes [41]. KIM1 expression analysis in the T2DM model showed no significance among the mice studied here, but a trend showing the same pattern as the other fibrosis markers from the previous study (Figure 6D and Reference [41]).

Our analyses of the expression of key proteins and enzymes of lipid metabolism in the kidneys of mice with T1DM-like phenotype and T2DM show clear evidence of alterations that may be causative for accumulation of fat in kidney tissue. To investigate the extent to which visible lipid droplets are already present, we applied Oil Red O staining. While no renal intracellular fat was detectable in the STZ mice (data not shown), lipid droplets could be visualized in type 2 diabetic kidneys (Figure 6C). This is consistent with the findings in kidney biopsies of patients with diagnosed type 2 DN [20]. In the background of the MORG1 heterozygous knockout, less lipid deposition was detectable in diabetic kidneys than in non-diabetic ones. However, a significance analysis across all groups indicates a statistical interaction between the T2DM and the MORG1 genotype that we consider to be biologically relevant, with $p = 0.089$ (Figure 6B). The results shown so far suggest that the accumulation of lipid droplets in db/db mice is not due to the increased synthesis of FA, and it is also less because of downregulated FAO. Rather, in this model, there is an oversupply of circulating lipids due to obesity per se that may be transported via CD36 into the kidney cells. Hence, the correlation analysis reveals a moderate positive correlation between tubular lipid accumulation and lipid uptake (OilRedO vs. CD36 protein ρ 0.6**).

As discussed above, we hypothesize a feedback mechanism in response to increased FA levels as an explanation for the elevated PPARα expression in non-diabetic heterozygous animals (see Figure 4). Oil Red O staining confirms increased lipid accumulation in these animals, to which the cells apparently respond by increasing PPARα. The efficacy of thereby decreasing renal lipid accumulation was demonstrated by pharmacological activation of PPARα by, for example, fenofibrate [72].

Evidence suggests that renal lipid accumulation may be the consequence, as well as the cause, of diabetic kidney injury [73]. In kidneys that show increased intracellular lipid droplets, β-oxidation pathways were downregulated [20]. Although we found a marked downregulation of the CPT1 and ACOX1 genes in STZ-T1DM, no lipid accumulation could be visualized. However, because the expression of fibrosis markers was already upregulated, it can be assumed that, in the STZ-T1DM model, changes in lipid metabolism are the consequence rather than the cause of early damage. In obesity-associated T2DM, it seems to be the other way around: lipid droplets are clearly visible, whereas fibrotic changes are still comparatively minor.

Of great interest in this context is a very recent study with the finding that overexpression of CPT1 in renal tubule cells protects against renal injury and fibrosis by restoring metabolic gain of function in FAO and mitochondrial homeostasis [74]. This is a promising finding, especially because overexpression of CPT1 attenuated the fibrotic phenotype even after FA-induced injury [74]. One negative aspect of this study, according to Reidy and Ross [75], is that all three employed murine models of renal fibrosis have well-known limitations regarding their relevance to human chronic kidney disease.

4. Conclusions

In this animal-based study, key markers of de novo FA/cholesterol synthesis, lipid uptake and FAO were examined in parallel for both major diabetes types and related to TIF and lipid accumulation. Alterations in lipid metabolism are present in both STZ-T1DM and T2DM, but therapeutic targets on lipid metabolism, such as PPAR agonists or CD36 antagonists, to prevent diabetes-induced TIF should be adapted to the diabetes type. Another and possibly better target is MORG1, which appears to play different roles in lipid metabolism, depending on the underlying diabetes type. Although our current study has not yet fully established a causal link between MORG1 expression and the observed changes in gene expression levels, the results, in agreement with several previous observations, support a potential implication of MORG1 in pathogenesis of lipid-associated kidney fibrosis. In other words, reducing MORG1 levels restores physiological lipid metabolism and is renoprotective, regardless of the diabetes type.

Supplementary Materials: The following are available online at https://www.mdpi.com/article/10.3390/biomedicines10010030/s1. Method S1: MACRO used for FAS-staining, exemplary for all IHC evaluations. Figure S1: MORG1 protein expression in STZ-T1DM model.

Author Contributions: Conceptualization, I.L. and G.W.; validation, I.L.; data curation, E.J. and I.L.; formal analysis, E.J. and I.L.; investigation, E.J., S.W., N.Z. and I.L.; writing—original draft preparation, I.L. and E.J.; writing—review and editing, E.J., S.W., N.Z., G.W. and I.L.; supervision, I.L.; project administration, I.L. All authors have read and agreed to the published version of the manuscript.

Funding: This research received no external funding.

Institutional Review Board Statement: All animal experiments were conducted in accordance with the German Animal Protection Law and were approved by the Local Ethics Committee of ThüringerLandesamt für Verbraucherschutz (STZ experiments: approval number 02-039/15, date of approval 14 March 2017; db/db experiments: approval number UKJ-17-024, date of approval 6 December 2017).

Informed Consent Statement: Not applicable.

Data Availability Statement: The data presented in this study are available on request from the corresponding author.

Acknowledgments: We would like to acknowledge Simone Schönfelder and Simone Goebel for the technical support. We further thank Tzvetanka Bondeva and Marita Liebisch for the help with STZ animal experiments. Many thanks to Seerat Bajwa for editing of English language and style throughout the manuscript.

Conflicts of Interest: The authors declare no conflict of interest.

Abbreviations

ACC, acetyl-CoA carboxylase; ACOX1, acyl-CoA oxidase; AGE, advanced glycation end-products; ANG II, angiotensin II; BSA, bovine serum albumin; CD36, cluster of differentiation 36; CPT1, carnitine palmitoyltransferase 1; CTGF, connective tissue growth factor; DAB, diabminobenzidine; DAPI, 4′,6-diamidino-2-phenylindole; DN, diabetic nephropathy; ECM, extracellular matrix; EMT, epithelial-to-mesenchymal transition; EPO, erythropoietin; ERK1/2, extracellular signal-regulated kinase; ESRD, end-stage renal disease; FA, fatty acid; FAO, fatty acid oxidation; FAS, fatty acid synthase; HDL, high density lipoprotein; HIF1/2, hypoxia-inducible factor; HMG-CoA-Red, 3-hydroxy-3-methylglutaryl-Coenzyme A reductase; HPRT1, hypoxanthine phospho-ribosyltransferase 1; KIM1, kidney injury molecule-1; MAPK, mitogen-activated protein kinase; MCP1, monocyte chemoattractantprotein-1; MORG1, mitogen-activated protein kinase organizer 1; MP1, MEK partner

1; MTCO1,mitochondrially encoded cytochrome C oxidase I; PGC-1α, peroxisome proliferator-activated receptor gamma coactivator 1-alpha; PHD3, prolyl hydroxylase domain protein 3; PPARα, peroxisome proliferator activated receptor alpha; SCD1, stearoyl-CoA desaturase 1; RAF, rapidly accelerated fibrosarcoma; SREBP2, sterol regulatory element binding proteins; STZ, streptozotocin; T1DM, type 1 diabetes mellitus; T2DM, type 2 diabetes mellitus; TGF-β1, transforming growth factor β1; TIF, tubulointerstitial fibrosis.

References

1. Martinez-Castelao, A.; Navarro-Gonzalez, J.F.; Gorriz, J.L.; de Alvaro, F. The Concept and the Epidemiology of Diabetic Nephropathy Have Changed in Recent Years. *J. Clin. Med.* **2015**, *4*, 1207–1216. [CrossRef] [PubMed]
2. Wolf, G. New insights into the pathophysiology of diabetic nephropathy: From haemodynamics to molecular pathology. *Eur. J. Clin. Investig.* **2004**, *34*, 785–796. [CrossRef]
3. Ina, K.; Kitamura, H.; Tatsukawa, S.; Takayama, T.; Fujikura, Y.; Shimada, T. Transformation of interstitial fibroblasts and tubulointerstitial fibrosis in diabetic nephropathy. *Med. Electron. Microsc.* **2002**, *35*, 87–95. [CrossRef]
4. Kolset, S.O.; Reinholt, F.P.; Jenssen, T. Diabetic nephropathy and extracellular matrix. *J. Histochem. Cytochem.* **2012**, *60*, 976–986. [CrossRef]
5. Iwano, M.; Neilson, E.G. Mechanisms of tubulointerstitial fibrosis. *Curr. Opin. Nephrol. Hypertens.* **2004**, *13*, 279–284. [CrossRef]
6. Li, R.; Chung, A.C.; Dong, Y.; Yang, W.; Zhong, X.; Lan, H.Y. The microRNA miR-433 promotes renal fibrosis by amplifying the TGF-beta/Smad3-Azin1 pathway. *Kidney Int.* **2013**, *84*, 1129–1144. [CrossRef] [PubMed]
7. Eddy, A.A. Molecular basis of renal fibrosis. *Pediatr. Nephrol.* **2000**, *15*, 290–301. [CrossRef] [PubMed]
8. Loeffler, I.; Wolf, G. Epithelial-to-Mesenchymal Transition in Diabetic Nephropathy: Fact or Fiction? *Cells* **2015**, *4*, 631–652. [CrossRef] [PubMed]
9. Kriz, W.; Kaissling, B.; Le Hir, M. Epithelial-mesenchymal transition (EMT) in kidney fibrosis: Fact or fantasy? *J. Clin. Investig.* **2011**, *121*, 468–474. [CrossRef]
10. Zeisberg, M.; Duffield, J.S. Resolved: EMT produces fibroblasts in the kidney. *J. Am. Soc. Nephrol.* **2010**, *21*, 1247–1253. [CrossRef]
11. Liu, Y. New insights into epithelial-mesenchymal transition in kidney fibrosis. *J. Am. Soc. Nephrol.* **2010**, *21*, 212–222. [CrossRef] [PubMed]
12. Grgic, I.; Duffield, J.S.; Humphreys, B.D. The origin of interstitial myofibroblasts in chronic kidney disease. *Pediatr. Nephrol.* **2012**, *27*, 183–193. [CrossRef]
13. Quaggin, S.E.; Kapus, A. Scar wars: Mapping the fate of epithelial-mesenchymal-myofibroblast transition. *Kidney Int.* **2011**, *80*, 41–50. [CrossRef]
14. Simonson, M.S. Phenotypic transitions and fibrosis in diabetic nephropathy. *Kidney Int.* **2007**, *71*, 846–854. [CrossRef]
15. Loeffler, I.; Wolf, G. Transforming growth factor-beta and the progression of renal disease. *Nephrol. Dial. Transplant.* **2014**, *29* (Suppl. S1), i37–i45. [CrossRef]
16. Kang, H.M.; Ahn, S.H.; Choi, P.; Ko, Y.A.; Han, S.H.; Chinga, F.; Park, A.S.; Tao, J.; Sharma, K.; Pullman, J.; et al. Defective fatty acid oxidation in renal tubular epithelial cells has a key role in kidney fibrosis development. *Nat. Med.* **2015**, *21*, 37–46. [CrossRef] [PubMed]
17. Lovisa, S.; Zeisberg, M.; Kalluri, R. Partial Epithelial-to-Mesenchymal Transition and Other New Mechanisms of Kidney Fibrosis. *Trends Endocrinol. Metab.* **2016**, *27*, 681–695. [CrossRef] [PubMed]
18. Simon, N.; Hertig, A. Alteration of Fatty Acid Oxidation in Tubular Epithelial Cells: From Acute Kidney Injury to Renal Fibrogenesis. *Front. Med.* **2015**, *2*, 52. [CrossRef]
19. Stadler, K.; Goldberg, I.J.; Susztak, K. The evolving understanding of the contribution of lipid metabolism to diabetic kidney disease. *Curr. Diabetes Rep.* **2015**, *15*, 40. [CrossRef] [PubMed]
20. Herman-Edelstein, M.; Scherzer, P.; Tobar, A.; Levi, M.; Gafter, U. Altered renal lipid metabolism and renal lipid accumu-lation in human diabetic nephropathy. *J. Lipid. Res.* **2014**, *55*, 561–572. [CrossRef] [PubMed]
21. Mylonis, I.; Simos, G.; Paraskeva, E. Hypoxia-Inducible Factors and the Regulation of Lipid Metabolism. *Cells* **2019**, *8*, 214. [CrossRef]
22. Wang, Z.; Jiang, T.; Li, J.; Proctor, G.; McManaman, J.L.; Lucia, S.; Chua, S.; Levi, M. Regulation of renal lipid metabolism, lipid accumulation, and glomerulosclerosis in FVBdb/db mice with type 2 diabetes. *Diabetes* **2005**, *54*, 2328–2335. [CrossRef]
23. Yuan, Y.; Sun, H.; Sun, Z. Advanced glycation end products (AGEs) increase renal lipid accumulation: A pathogenic factor of diabetic nephropathy (DN). *Lipids Health Dis.* **2017**, *16*, 126. [CrossRef] [PubMed]
24. Loeffler, I.; Wolf, G. The role of hypoxia and Morg1 in renal injury. *Eur. J. Clin. Investig.* **2015**, *45*, 294–302. [CrossRef]
25. Gaspar, J.M.; Velloso, L.A. Hypoxia Inducible Factor as a Central Regulator of Metabolism—Implications for the Development of Obesity. *Front. Neurosci.* **2018**, *12*, 813. [CrossRef] [PubMed]
26. Greer, S.N.; Metcalf, J.L.; Wang, Y.; Ohh, M. The updated biology of hypoxia-inducible factor. *EMBO J.* **2012**, *31*, 2448–2460. [CrossRef] [PubMed]

27. Semenza, G.L. Oxygen sensing, hypoxia-inducible factors, and disease pathophysiology. *Annu. Rev. Pathol.* **2014**, *9*, 47–71. [CrossRef] [PubMed]
28. Collier, J.B.; Whitaker, R.M.; Eblen, S.T.; Schnellmann, R.G. Rapid Renal Regulation of Peroxisome Proliferator-activated Receptor gamma Coactivator-1alpha by Extracellular Signal-Regulated Kinase 1/2 in Physiological and Pathological Condi-tions. *J. Biol. Chem.* **2016**, *291*, 26850–26859. [CrossRef] [PubMed]
29. Kotzka, J.; Muller-Wieland, D.; Roth, G.; Kremer, L.; Munck, M.; Schurmann, S.; Knebel, B.; Krone, W. Sterol regulatory element binding proteins (SREBP)-1a and SREBP-2 are linked to the MAP-kinase cascade. *J. Lipid. Res.* **2000**, *41*, 99–108. [CrossRef]
30. Roth, G.; Kotzka, J.; Kremer, L.; Lehr, S.; Lohaus, C.; Meyer, H.E.; Krone, W.; Muller-Wieland, D. MAP kinases Erk1/2 phosphorylate sterol regulatory element-binding protein (SREBP)-1a at serine 117 in vitro. *J. Biol. Chem.* **2000**, *275*, 33302–33307. [CrossRef]
31. Wang, L.; Xie, W.; Zhang, L.; Li, D.; Yu, H.; Xiong, J.; Peng, J.; Qiu, J.; Sheng, H.; He, X.; et al. CVB3 Nonstructural 2A Protein Modulates SREBP1a Signaling via the MEK/ERK Pathway. *J. Virol.* **2018**, *92*, e01060-18. [CrossRef] [PubMed]
32. Vomastek, T.; Schaeffer, H.J.; Tarcsafalvi, A.; Smolkin, M.E.; Bissonette, E.A.; Weber, M.J. Modular construction of a sig-naling scaffold: MORG1 interacts with components of the ERK cascade and links ERK signaling to specific agonists. *Proc. Natl. Acad. Sci. USA* **2004**, *101*, 6981–6986. [CrossRef] [PubMed]
33. Hopfer, U.; Hopfer, H.; Jablonski, K.; Stahl, R.A.; Wolf, G. The novel WD-repeat protein Morg1 acts as a molecular scaffold for hypoxia-inducible factor prolyl hydroxylase 3 (PHD3). *J. Biol. Chem.* **2006**, *281*, 8645–8655. [CrossRef] [PubMed]
34. Meister, M.; Tomasovic, A.; Banning, A.; Tikkanen, R. Mitogen-Activated Protein (MAP) Kinase Scaffolding Proteins: A Recount. *Int. J. Mol. Sci.* **2013**, *14*, 4854–4884. [CrossRef]
35. Loeffler, I.; Wolf, G. Mechanisms of Interstitial Fibrosis in Diabetic Nephropathy. In *Diabetic Nephropathy: Pathophysiology and Clinical Aspects*; Roelofs, J.J., Vogt, L., Eds.; Springer International Publishing: Cham, Switzerland, 2019; pp. 227–251. [CrossRef]
36. Bondeva, T.; Heinzig, J.; Ruhe, C.; Wolf, G. Advanced glycated end-products affect HIF-transcriptional activity in renal cells. *Mol. Endocrinol.* **2013**, *27*, 1918–1933. [CrossRef]
37. Loeffler, I.; Wolf, G. Morg1 heterozygous deficiency ameliorates hypoxia-induced acute renal injury. *Am. J. Physiol. Renal Physiol.* **2015**, *308*, F511–F521. [CrossRef] [PubMed]
38. Loeffler, I.; Wolf, G. MORG1 (Mitogen-Activated Protein Kinase Organizer 1). In *Encyclopedia of Signaling Molecules*; Choi, S., Ed.; Springer International Publishing: Cham, Switzerland, 2018; p. 6060.
39. Stahr, A.; Frahm, C.; Kretz, A.; Bondeva, T.; Witte, O.W.; Wolf, G. Morg1(+/−) heterozygous mice are protected from ex-perimentally induced focal cerebral ischemia. *Brain Res.* **2012**, *1482*, 22–31. [CrossRef]
40. Hammerschmidt, E.; Loeffler, I.; Wolf, G. Morg1 heterozygous mice are protected from acute renal ischemia-reperfusion injury. *Am. J. Physiol. Renal. Physiol.* **2009**, *297*, F1273–F1287. [CrossRef] [PubMed]
41. Loeffler, I.; Liebisch, M.; Daniel, C.; Amann, K.; Wolf, G. Heterozygosity of mitogen-activated protein kinase organizer 1 ameliorates diabetic nephropathy and suppresses epithelial-to-mesenchymal transition-like changes in db/db mice. *Nephrol. Dial. Transplant.* **2017**, *32*, 2017–2034. [CrossRef]
42. Capecchi, M.R. Altering the genome by homologous recombination. *Science* **1989**, *244*, 1288–1292. [CrossRef]
43. Deeds, M.C.; Anderson, J.M.; Armstrong, A.S.; Gastineau, D.A.; Hiddinga, H.J.; Jahangir, A.; Eberhardt, N.L.; Kudva, Y.C. Single dose streptozotocin-induced diabetes: Considerations for study design in islet transplantation models. *Lab. Anim.* **2011**, *45*, 131–140. [CrossRef]
44. Ozawa, T.; Maehara, N.; Kai, T.; Arai, S.; Miyazaki, T. Dietary fructose-induced hepatocellular carcinoma development manifested in mice lacking apoptosis inhibitor of macrophage (AIM). *Genes Cells* **2016**, *21*, 1320–1332. [CrossRef] [PubMed]
45. Helsley, R.N.; Varadharajan, V.; Brown, A.L.; Gromovsky, A.D.; Schugar, R.C.; Ramachandiran, I.; Fung, K.; Kabbany, M.N.; Banerjee, R.; Neumann, C.K.; et al. Obesity-linked suppression of membrane-bound O-acyltransferase 7 (MBOAT7) drives non-alcoholic fatty liver disease. *eLife* **2019**, *8*, e49882. [CrossRef]
46. Simon-Tillaux, N.; Hertig, A. Snail and kidney fibrosis. *Nephrol. Dial. Transplant.* **2017**, *32*, 224–233. [CrossRef]
47. Ni, X.; Wang, H. Silymarin attenuated hepatic steatosis through regulation of lipid metabolism and oxidative stress in a mouse model of nonalcoholic fatty liver disease (NAFLD). *Am. J. Transl. Res.* **2016**, *8*, 1073–1081. [PubMed]
48. Munkacsi, A.B.; Hammond, N.; Schneider, R.T.; Senanayake, D.S.; Higaki, K.; Lagutin, K.; Bloor, S.J.; Ory, D.S.; Maue, R.A.; Chen, F.W.; et al. Normalization of Hepatic Homeostasis in the Npc1(nmf164) Mouse Model of Niemann-Pick Type C Dis-ease Treated with the Histone Deacetylase Inhibitor Vorinostat. *J. Biol. Chem.* **2017**, *292*, 4395–4410. [CrossRef] [PubMed]
49. Saito, M.; Kaneda, A.; Shigeto, H.; Hanata, N.; Otokuni, K.; Matsuoka, H. Development of an optimized 5-stage protocol for the in vitro preparation of insulin-secreting cells from mouse ES cells. *Cytotechnology* **2016**, *68*, 987–998. [CrossRef]
50. Bai, X.; Geng, J.; Zhou, Z.; Tian, J.; Li, X. MicroRNA-130b improves renal tubulointerstitial fibrosis via repression of Snail-induced epithelial-mesenchymal transition in diabetic nephropathy. *Sci. Rep.* **2016**, *6*, 20475. [CrossRef]
51. Knight, B.L.; Patel, D.D.; Humphreys, S.M.; Wiggins, D.; Gibbons, G.F. Inhibition of cholesterol absorption associated with a PPAR alpha-dependent increase in ABC binding cassette transporter A1 in mice. *J. Lipid. Res.* **2003**, *44*, 2049–2058. [CrossRef]
52. Chan, Y.H. Biostatistics 104: Correlational analysis. *Singap. Med. J.* **2003**, *44*, 614–619.
53. Yang, X.; Okamura, D.M.; Lu, X.; Chen, Y.; Moorhead, J.; Varghese, Z.; Ruan, X.Z. CD36 in chronic kidney disease: Novel insights and therapeutic opportunities. *Nat. Rev. Nephrol.* **2017**, *13*, 769–781. [CrossRef] [PubMed]

54. Wolf, G.; Wenzel, U.; Jablonski, K.; Brundert, M.; Rinninger, F. Angiotensin II down-regulates the SR-BI HDL receptor in proximal tubular cells. *Nephrol. Dial. Transplant.* **2005**, *20*, 1222–1227. [CrossRef] [PubMed]
55. Feng, L.; Gu, C.; Li, Y.; Huang, J. High Glucose Promotes CD36 Expression by Upregulating Peroxisome Prolifera-tor-Activated Receptor γ Levels to Exacerbate Lipid Deposition in Renal Tubular Cells. *BioMed Res. Int.* **2017**, *2017*, 1414070. [CrossRef] [PubMed]
56. Susztak, K.; Ciccone, E.; McCue, P.; Sharma, K.; Bottinger, E.P. Multiple metabolic hits converge on CD36 as novel mediator of tubular epithelial apoptosis in diabetic nephropathy. *PLoS Med.* **2005**, *2*, e45. [CrossRef] [PubMed]
57. Hou, Y.; Wu, M.; Wei, J.; Ren, Y.; Du, C.; Wu, H.; Li, Y.; Shi, Y. CD36 is involved in high glucose-induced epithelial to mesenchymal transition in renal tubular epithelial cells. *Biochem. Biophys. Res. Commun.* **2015**, *468*, 281–286. [CrossRef]
58. Loeffler, I.; Liebisch, M.; Wolf, G. Collagen VIII influences epithelial phenotypic changes in experimental diabetic nephropathy. *Am. J. Physiol. Renal. Physiol.* **2012**, *303*, F733–F745. [CrossRef]
59. Murea, M.; Freedman, B.I.; Parks, J.S.; Antinozzi, P.A.; Elbein, S.C.; Ma, L. Lipotoxicity in diabetic nephropathy: The po-tential role of fatty acid oxidation. *Clin. J. Am. Soc. Nephrol.* **2010**, *5*, 2373–2379. [CrossRef] [PubMed]
60. Ishii, K.; Kobayashi, H.; Taguchi, K.; Guan, N.; Li, A.; Tong, Z.; Davidoff, O.; Tran, P.V.; Sharma, M.; Chandel, N.S.; et al. Kidney epithelial targeted mitochondrial transcription factor A deficiency results in progressive mitochondrial depletion associated with severe cystic disease. *Kidney Int.* **2021**, *99*, 657–670. [CrossRef] [PubMed]
61. Haraguchi, R.; Kohara, Y.; Matsubayashi, K.; Kitazawa, R.; Kitazawa, S. New Insights into the Pathogenesis of Diabetic Nephropathy: Proximal Renal Tubules Are Primary Target of Oxidative Stress in Diabetic Kidney. *Acta Histochem. Cytochem.* **2020**, *53*, 21–31. [CrossRef] [PubMed]
62. Youle, R.J.; van der Bliek, A.M. Mitochondrial fission, fusion, and stress. *Science* **2012**, *337*, 1062–1065. [CrossRef]
63. Zhang, W.; Liu, L.; Huo, Y.; Yang, Y.; Wang, Y. Hypoxia-pretreated human MSCs attenuate acute kidney injury through enhanced angiogenic and antioxidative capacities. *BioMed Res. Int.* **2014**, *2014*, 462472. [CrossRef] [PubMed]
64. Yu, X.; Fang, Y.; Liu, H.; Zhu, J.; Zou, J.; Xu, X.; Jiang, S.; Ding, X. The balance of beneficial and deleterious effects of hy-poxia-inducible factor activation by prolyl hydroxylase inhibitor in rat remnant kidney depends on the timing of admin-istration. *Nephrol. Dial. Transplant.* **2012**, *27*, 3110–3119. [CrossRef] [PubMed]
65. Kapitsinou, P.P.; Sano, H.; Michael, M.; Kobayashi, H.; Davidoff, O.; Bian, A.; Yao, B.; Zhang, M.Z.; Harris, R.C.; Duffy, K.J.; et al. Endothelial HIF-2 mediates protection and recovery from ischemic kidney injury. *J. Clin. Investig.* **2014**, *124*, 2396–2409. [CrossRef] [PubMed]
66. Cook, S.J.; Stuart, K.; Gilley, R.; Sale, M.J. Control of cell death and mitochondrial fission by ERK1/2 MAP kinase signalling. *FEBS J.* **2017**, *284*, 4177–4195. [CrossRef] [PubMed]
67. Li, S.Y.; Susztak, K. The Role of Peroxisome Proliferator-Activated Receptor gamma Coactivator 1alpha (PGC-1alpha) in Kidney Disease. *Semin. Nephrol.* **2018**, *38*, 121–126. [CrossRef] [PubMed]
68. Chung, K.W.; Lee, E.K.; Lee, M.K.; Oh, G.T.; Yu, B.P.; Chung, H.Y. Impairment of PPARalpha and the Fatty Acid Oxidation Pathway Aggravates Renal Fibrosis during Aging. *J. Am. Soc. Nephrol.* **2018**, *29*, 1223–1237. [CrossRef]
69. Mooli, R.G.R.; Rodriguez, J.; Takahashi, S.; Solanki, S.; Gonzalez, F.J.; Ramakrishnan, S.K.; Shah, Y.M. Hypoxia via ERK Signaling Inhibits Hepatic PPARα to Promote Fatty Liver. *Cell. Mol. Gastroenterol. Hepatol.* **2021**, *12*, 585–597. [CrossRef]
70. Humphreys, B.D.; Xu, F.; Sabbisetti, V.; Grgic, I.; Movahedi Naini, S.; Wang, N.; Chen, G.; Xiao, S.; Patel, D.; Henderson, J.M.; et al. Chronic epithelial kidney injury molecule-1 expression causes murine kidney fibrosis. *J. Clin. Investig.* **2013**, *123*, 4023–4035. [CrossRef] [PubMed]
71. Song, J.; Yu, J.; Prayogo, G.W.; Cao, W.; Wu, Y.; Jia, Z.; Zhang, A. Understanding kidney injury molecule 1: A novel immune factor in kidney pathophysiology. *Am. J. Transl. Res.* **2019**, *11*, 1219–1229.
72. Balakumar, P.; Kadian, S.; Mahadevan, N. Are PPAR alpha agonists a rational therapeutic strategy for preventing abnor-malities of the diabetic kidney? *Pharmacol. Res.* **2012**, *65*, 430–436. [CrossRef]
73. Bobulescu, I.A. Renal lipid metabolism and lipotoxicity. *Curr. Opin. Nephrol. Hypertens.* **2010**, *19*, 393–402. [CrossRef] [PubMed]
74. Miguel, V.; Tituana, J.; Herrero, J.I.; Herrero, L.; Serra, D.; Cuevas, P.; Barbas, C.; Puyol, D.R.; Marquez-Exposito, L.; Ruiz-Ortega, M.; et al. Renal tubule Cpt1a overexpression protects from kidney fibrosis by restoring mitochondrial homeo-stasis. *J. Clin. Investig.* **2021**, *131*, e140695. [CrossRef]
75. Reidy, K.J.; Ross, M.J. Re-energizing the kidney: Targeting fatty acid metabolism protects against kidney fibrosis. *Kidney Int.* **2021**, *100*, 742–744. [CrossRef] [PubMed]

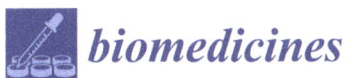

Article

Impact of Plasma Xanthine Oxidoreductase Activity on the Mechanisms of Distal Symmetric Polyneuropathy Development in Patients with Type 2 Diabetes

Midori Fujishiro [1,2,*], Hisamitsu Ishihara [1], Katsuhiko Ogawa [2,3], Takayo Murase [4], Takashi Nakamura [5], Kentaro Watanabe [1], Hideyuki Sakoda [6], Hiraku Ono [7], Takeshi Yamamotoya [8], Yusuke Nakatsu [8], Tomoichiro Asano [8] and Akifumi Kushiyama [9]

[1] Division of Diabetes and Metabolic Diseases, Department of Internal Medicine, Nihon University School of Medicine, 30-1 Oyaguchi Kami-cho, Itabashi-ku, Tokyo 173-8610, Japan; ishihara.hisamitsu@nihon-u.ac.jp (H.I.); watanabe.kentaro@nihon-u.ac.jp (K.W.)
[2] Department of Internal Medicine, Nihon University Hospital, 1-6 Kanda-Surugadai, Chiyoda-ku, Tokyo 101-8309, Japan; ogawa.katsuhiko@nihon-u.ac.jp
[3] Division of Neurology, Department of Internal Medicine, Nihon University School of Medicine, 30-1 Oyaguchi Kami-cho, Itabashi-ku, Tokyo 173-8610, Japan
[4] Radioisotope and Chemical Analysis Center, Pharmaceuticals Research Laboratories, Sanwa Kagaku Kenkyusho Co., Ltd., 363 Shiosaki, Hokusei-cho, Inabe-shi 511-0406, Mie, Japan; ta_murase@skk-net.com
[5] Medical Affairs Department, Sanwa Kagaku Kenkyusho Co., Ltd., 35 Higashisotobori-cho, Higashi-ku, Nagoya 461-8631, Aichi, Japan; ta_nakamura@mb4.skk-net.com
[6] Division of Neurology, Respirology, Endocrinology and Metabolism, Department of Internal Medicine, Faculty of Medicine, University of Miyazaki, 5200 Kihara, Kiyotake 889-1692, Miyazaki, Japan; hideyuki_sakoda@med.miyazaki-u.ac.jp
[7] Department of Clinical Cell Biology, Graduate School of Medicine, Chiba University, 1-8-1 Inohana, Chuo-ku, Chiba 260-8670, Chiba, Japan; hono@chiba-u.jp
[8] Department of Medical Science, Graduate School of Medicine, Hiroshima University, 1-2-3 Kasumi, Minami-ku, Hiroshima 734-8551, Hiroshima, Japan; ymmty@hiroshima-u.ac.jp (T.Y.); nakatsu@hiroshima-u.ac.jp (Y.N.); tasano@hiroshima-u.ac.jp (T.A.)
[9] Department of Pharmacotherapy, Meiji Pharmaceutical University, 2-522-1 Noshio, Kiyose 204-8588, Tokyo, Japan; kushiyama@my-pharm.ac.jp
* Correspondence: fujishiro.midori@nihon-u.ac.jp; Tel.: +81-3-3972-8111

Citation: Fujishiro, M.; Ishihara, H.; Ogawa, K.; Murase, T.; Nakamura, T.; Watanabe, K.; Sakoda, H.; Ono, H.; Yamamotoya, T.; Nakatsu, Y.; et al. Impact of Plasma Xanthine Oxidoreductase Activity on the Mechanisms of Distal Symmetric Polyneuropathy Development in Patients with Type 2 Diabetes. *Biomedicines* 2021, 9, 1052. https://doi.org/10.3390/biomedicines9081052

Academic Editor: Yih-Hsin Chang

Received: 30 June 2021
Accepted: 16 August 2021
Published: 19 August 2021

Publisher's Note: MDPI stays neutral with regard to jurisdictional claims in published maps and institutional affiliations.

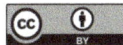

Copyright: © 2021 by the authors. Licensee MDPI, Basel, Switzerland. This article is an open access article distributed under the terms and conditions of the Creative Commons Attribution (CC BY) license (https://creativecommons.org/licenses/by/4.0/).

Abstract: To unravel associations between plasma xanthine oxidoreductase (XOR) and diabetic vascular complications, especially distal symmetric polyneuropathy (DSP), we investigated plasma XOR activities using a novel assay. Patients with type 2 diabetes mellitus (T2DM) with available nerve conduction study (NCS) data were analyzed. None were currently taking XOR inhibitors. XOR activity of fasting blood samples was assayed using a stable isotope-labeled substrate and LC-TQMS. JMP Clinical version 5.0. was used for analysis. We analyzed 54 patients. Mean age was 64.7 years, mean body mass index was 26.0 kg/m^2, and mean glycated hemoglobin was 9.4%. The logarithmically transformed plasma XOR activity (ln-XOR) correlated positively with hypoxanthine, xanthine, visceral fatty area, and liver dysfunction but negatively with HDL cholesterol. ln-XOR correlated negatively with diabetes duration and maximum intima-media thickness. Stepwise multiple regression analysis revealed ln-XOR to be among selected explanatory factors for various NCS parameters. Receiver operating characteristic curves showed the discriminatory power of ln-XOR. Principal component analysis revealed a negative relationship of ln-XOR with F-waves as well as positive relationships of ln-XOR with hepatic steatosis and obesity-related disorders. Taken together, our results show plasma XOR activity to be among potential disease status predictors in T2DM patients. Plasma XOR activity measurements might reliably detect pre-symptomatic DSP.

Keywords: type 2 diabetes; xanthine oxidoreductase; distal symmetric polyneuropathy

1. Introduction

Type 2 diabetes mellitus (T2DM) is a metabolic disease that leads to various vascular complications involving multiple organs, ultimately reducing the lifespans of affected patients [1]. Diabetes prevalence rose in the second decade of the 21st century and continues to increase. In 2019, diabetes prevalence worldwide was estimated to be 463 million people [2], and 4.2 million people were estimated to have died from diabetes and its complications [3]. Prevention or early detection of T2DM and its complications is hugely important but occult and asymptomatic complications are difficult to detect. Distal symmetric polyneuropathy (DSP) especially often precedes other complications and can progress to become a life-threatening disorder [4]. However, the progression of DSP is very difficult to evaluate and employs routine outpatient examinations. Consensus definitions consistently recommend a combination of neuropathic symptoms and signs in addition to specific nerve conduction study (NCS) abnormalities as criteria for diagnosing DSP and it is essential to confirm that the diagnosis of this condition is accurate [5].

Though the mechanisms by which diabetic vascular complications develop remain to be elucidated, oxidative stress and chronic inflammation, as well as longstanding hyperglycemia, associated metabolic derangements including increased polyol flux, accumulation of advanced glycation end products, and lipid alterations among other metabolic abnormalities, are thought to be among the key factors contributing to the development of DSP [6,7]. Obesity, especially when accompanied by visceral fat accumulation, hypertension, hyperglycemia, hyperinsulinemia, and fatty change in the liver are considered to be parameters predicting upregulation of oxidative stress and/or chronic inflammation as risk factors for diabetic complications [8]. The serum uric acid (UA) level is also associated with obesity and insulin resistance [9,10], and a high serum UA level has been proposed to be an independent risk factor for various diabetic complications such as diabetic nephropathy [11,12], as well as diabetic retinopathy (DR) [13] and neuropathy [14]. Xanthine oxidoreductase (XOR), the rate-limiting enzyme of UA production, was recently reported to be upregulated in fat, liver, kidneys, and the vasculature of patients with T2DM and other metabolic diseases [15,16]. XOR produces UA by catalyzing the oxidation of purines such as hypoxanthine to xanthine and xanthine to UA. Excessive purine derivatives derived from biological activities such as ATP depletion due to exercise, intake of fructose or alcohol, intake of a purine-rich diet or a pathological event such as ischemia, or degradation of RNA and DNA induced by cell turnover, are broken down by the purine metabolism system, in which XOR plays an essential role [17]. On the other hand, xanthine dehydrogenase (XDH) is converted to xanthine oxidase (XO) in response to tissue injury [18]. XO can reduce molecular oxygen to superoxide and hydrogen peroxide and is thought to be one of the key enzymes producing reactive oxygen species (ROS) [19] which serve as important messengers inducing inflammation [20,21].

However, XOR activity measurement has not been sufficiently established because the level of plasma XOR activity is quite low in humans as compared with that in rodents [17]. Recently, a novel human plasma XOR activity assay using a combination of liquid chromatography (LC) and triple quadrupole mass spectrometry (TQMS) to detect [13C2,15N2]-UA using [13C2,15N2]-xanthine as a substrate was developed [22]. At present, plasma XOR activity levels during the clinical courses of T2DM patients remain unclear. Thus, to unravel the associations of early vascular complications such as DSP with XOR activity, we investigated the relationships between clinical features of T2DM and plasma XOR levels measured employing this novel assay.

2. Materials and Methods

2.1. Study Subjects

We enrolled 127 patients with T2DM who visited the department of diabetes and metabolic diseases in our hospital during the period from August 2017 to October 2020. Of these patients, we analyzed those who had complete NCS data. The key inclusion criteria were as follows: (1) confirmed diagnosis of T2DM, (2) 18 years or older, and (3) no liver dysfunction. The exclusion criteria were: (4) pregnant, breastfeeding, or not using contraception for women of childbearing age, (5) currently taking XOR inhibitors, and/or (6) judged by their primary doctors to be inappropriate for trial enrollment due to safety concerns or for any other reasons. This investigation conformed with the principles outlined in the Declaration of Helsinki. The study protocol was approved by the Institutional Ethics Committee of Nihon University Hospital (approval number 20170701) and was registered at UMIN Clinical Trials Registry with the ID number UMIN000029257. All patients provided written informed consent for study participation.

2.2. Clinical Parameters and Procedures

Patient profiles, including diabetic microangiopathy, were collected from medical records. The intra-abdominal visceral fat area (VFA) was evaluated from computed tomography cross-sectional scans at the level of the umbilicus, as previously reported [23]. Diabetic nephropathy was clinically diagnosed by attending physicians based on microalbuminuria or overt proteinuria with no evidence of other kidney or urological diseases [24] and was classified into four stages (patients receiving dialysis therapy were excluded) according to the classification of diabetic nephropathy promulgated in 2014 by a joint committee on diabetic nephropathy in Japan [25]. DR includes non-proliferative DR diagnosed by the presence of microaneurysms and retinal hemorrhages [26], and all DR cases were confirmed by ophthalmologists. DR was subdivided as follows: no apparent diabetic retinopathy (NDR), simple diabetic retinopathy (SDR), and proliferative diabetic retinopathy (PDR). For the estimation of diabetic autonomic neuropathy, the coefficient of variation of the R-R intervals at rest and in deep breathing was measured with CardiMax FCP-8800® (Fukuda Denshi Corporation, Tokyo, Japan) as previously described [27]. To estimate DSP, the vibratory sensation was tested by measuring the perception time for a fork vibration using a 128 Hz tuning fork at the lateral malleoli. We measured the sensory nerve conduction velocity of the sural nerve as well as motor nerve conduction velocity and F-wave parameters of the peroneal nerve and tibial nerves using NeuropackX1® (Nihon Kohden Corporation, Tokyo, Japan) as previously described [27]. For estimation of macrovascular complications, we measured the cardio-ankle vascular index as well as the ankle-brachial index (ABI) using the VaSera VS-3000TN® (Fukuda Denshi Corporation, Tokyo, Japan). We measured carotid ultrasonographic variables such as the intima-media thickness (IMT) and the plaque score of the common carotid artery as previously reported [28] using the Aplio 500® (Toshiba Medical Systems Corporation, Tokyo, Japan). We usually performed the examinations, other than NCS, employed in this protocol as part of a comprehensive annual check-up aimed at detecting complications in patients with T2DM followed at our hospital.

To measure XOR activity, fasted blood samples were centrifuged at 3000 g for 15 min at 4 °C when collected in the early morning and the obtained plasma was stored at −80 °C until analysis. The XOR activity assay was performed using a stable isotope-labeled substrate and LC-TQMS together with the measurement of metabolites as previously reported [22,29]. In brief, 100 µL plasma samples pooled at −80 °C (purified by Sephadex G25 column) were mixed with Tris buffer (pH 8.5) containing [13C2,15N2]-xanthine as a substrate, NAD+, and [13C3,15N3]-UA as the internal standard. The mixtures were incubated at 37 °C for 90 min. Subsequently, the mixtures were combined with 500 µL of methanol and centrifuged at 2000× g for 15 min at 4 °C. The supernatants were transferred to new tubes and dried with a centrifugal evaporator. The residues were reconstituted with 150 µL of distilled water, filtered through an ultrafiltration membrane, and measured using LC/TQMS. We used LC/TQMS consisting of a Nano Space SI-2 LC system (Shiseido, Ltd., Tokyo, Japan) and a TSQ-TQMS (Thermo Fisher Scientific, Bremen, Germany) equipped with an ESI interface. Calibration standard samples of [13C2,15N2]-UA were also measured, and the amounts of [13C2,15N2]-UA production were quantitated from the calibration curve. XOR activities were expressed as [13C2,15N2]-UA in pmol/mL/h.

2.3. Statistical Analysis

JMP Clinical version 5.0 (SAS Institute, Cary, NC, USA) was used for all statistical analyses. Data are presented as the mean ± standard deviation, or as a number with the percentage. F-wave latency was corrected by height as previously described, that is, it was multiplied by 160 then divided by height (cm) [30]. We used Student's *t*-test for continuous variables. Percentage data were examined using the Chi-square test or Fisher's exact test as appropriate. Stepwise multiple regression analysis was performed using various NCV parameters stratified by the thresholds identified for prediction of incident DSP as described in a previous report [31] as the objective variable, as well as variables including XOR activity which had been natural logarithm-transformed to normalize the skewed distribution, sex, age, height, duration of diabetes, body mass index (BMI), waist circumference, fasting blood glucose (FBG), and maximum IMT as explanatory variables. To reveal the relationships between plasma XOR, DSP parameters, and other parameters in detail, we performed principal component analysis (PCA). When NCS values were undetectable, the longest F-wave latency in the dataset from another subject as well as a value of "0" for amplitude or conduction velocity was used as a substitute value for the purposes of the regression analysis as previously reported [32,33]. All *p*-values are two-sided, and $p < 0.05$ was considered to indicate a statistically significant difference.

3. Results

3.1. Characteristics of the Enrolled Patients

The characteristics and principal parameters of enrolled patients are listed in Table 1. We enrolled 54 patients with T2DM (37 males and 17 females, mean age 64.7 ± 12.2 years). Mean diabetes duration was 146 ± 130 months, glycated hemoglobin 9.4 ± 1.9%, BMI 26.0 ± 5.9 kg/m^2, and waist circumference 94.1 ± 14.8 cm. As for antidiabetic drugs, 13 patients (24%) were prescribed various forms of insulin, 9 (17%) sulfonylureas or glinides, 27 (50%) dipeptidyl peptidase-4 inhibitors or GLP-1 agonists, 12 (22%) sodium-glucose cotransporter 2 inhibitors, 15 (28%) biguanides, 2 (4%) thiazolidinediones, 5 (9%) α-glucosidase inhibitors, and 1 (2%) epalrestat, as indicated in Table 1. As for antihypertensive agents, 17 patients (31%) were taking angiotensin-converting enzyme inhibitors/angiotensin receptor blockers, 15 (28%) calcium channel blockers, 3 (6%) diuretics, and 6 (11%) β-blockers.

Table 1. Baseline characteristics of study participants.

Variable (n = 54) *	n or Mean ± SD	(Median)
Sex (male/female)	37/17	
Age (years)	64.7 ± 12.2	(66.5)
Height (cm)	162.5 ± 9.6	(163.3)
BMI (kg/m^2)	26.0 ± 5.9	(24.0)
Waist circumference (cm)	94.1 ± 14.8	(93.5)
VFA (cm^2)	180.8 ± 78.3	(171.4)
SBP (mmHg)	131 ± 19	(130)
DBP (mmHg)	79 ± 13	(78)
Pulse Rate (bpm)	76 ± 12	(77)
Duration of diabetes (M)	146 ± 130	(108)
Brinkman index	443 ± 677	(0)
Vibration (sec)	7.3 ± 3.5	(7.0)
CVRR (%)	148 ± 130	(106)
Minimum ABI	1.07 ± 0.13	(1.11)
Maximum IMT (mm)	2.3 ± 1.2	(2.2)
Laboratory measurements		
XOR activity (pmol/h/mL)	216 ± 441	(78.3)
Hypoxanthine (μM)	1.7 ± 0.8	(1.5)
Xanthine (μM)	0.63 ± 0.30	(0.49)
UA by LC/TQMS (mg/dL)	5.0 ± 1.4	(4.8)
FBG (mg/dL)	168 ± 46	(161)
HbA1c (%)	9.4 ± 1.9	(9.2)

Table 1. Cont.

Variable (n = 54) *	n or Mean ± SD	(Median)
Cre (mg/dL)	0.9 ± 0.4	(0.8)
eGFR (mL/min/1.73 m²)	72.9 ± 24.1	(71.1)
ACR (mg/g)	127 ± 288	(30.3)
Plt (×10⁹/L)	223 ± 63	(215)
AST (IU/L)	30 ± 24	(23)
ALT (IU/L)	33 ± 34	(24)
γGTP (IU/L)	54 ± 78	(34)
AAR	1.11 ± 0.61	(1.00)
APRI	0.40 ± 0.37	(0.29)
FIB-4 index	1.92 ± 1.99	(1.50)
Albumin (g/dL)	4.2 ± 0.4	(4.2)
HDL-Chol (mg/dL)	52 ± 15	(49)
LDL-Chol (mg/dL)	122 ± 40	(120)
TG (mg/dL)	136 ± 51	(133)
EPA/AA	0.34 ± 0.31	(0.21)
CRP (mg/dL)	0.3 ± 0.9	(0.1)
BNP (pg/mL)	48.5 ± 28.3	(14.3)

NCS Parameters	Median (Q1, Q3)
Sural Amp (μV)	ND (ND, 3.3)
Sural CV (m/s)	ND (ND, 43.3)
Peroneal Amp (mV)	4.6 (1.4, 6.7)
Peroneal CV (m/s)	43.8 (37.7, 47.0)
Peroneal F-wave (ms)	49.2 (45.8, 52.6)
Tibial Amp (mV)	10.6 (6.4, 17.1)
Tibial CV (m/s)	41.4 (37.7, 45.0)
Tibial F-wave (ms)	51.6 (47.3, 55.4)

Incidence of Diabetic Microangiopathy	n
Nephropathy	27
Stage 1	21
Stage 2	4
Stage 3	2
Stage 4	
Retinopathy	
NDR	32
SDR	8
PDR	14

Use of Antidiabetic Drugs or Other Medications	n (%)
Insulins	13 (24)
SU/Glinides	9 (17)
GLP1RAs/DPP4is	27 (50)
SGLT2is	12 (22)
Biguanides	15 (28)
TZDs	2 (4)
αGIs	5 (9)
Epalrestat	1 (2)
Statins	22 (41)
EPAs	6 (11)
ACEI/ARBs	17 (31)
CCBs	15 (28)
Diuretics	3 (6)
β-blockers	6 (11)

SBP, systolic blood pressure; DBP, diastolic blood pressure; Cre, serum creatinine; eGFR, estimated glomerular filtration rate; ACR, albumin to creatinine ratio; Plt, platelet count; FIB-4 index, fibrosis-4 index; EPA/AA, eicosapentaenoic acid to arachidonic acid ratio; CRP, C-reactive protein; BNP, B-type natriuretic peptide; Amp, amplitude potential; ND, not determined; CV, conduction velocity; F wave, F wave latency Vibration: perception time for a fork vibration. F-wave latency was corrected by height as previously described as described in the "**Patients and Methods**" section. All data are presented as n or means ± standard deviation and medians with or without the first (Q1) and the third (Q3) quartiles. * Visceral fat area from two patients and vibration data from one patient were missing. The coefficient of variation of RR intervals (CVRR) from eight patients with arrhythmias were omitted. SUs, sulfonylureas; GLP-1RAs/DPP4is, GLP-1 agonists/dipeptidyl peptidase-4 inhibitors; SGLT2: sodium-glucose cotransporter 2 inhibitors; αGIs: α-glucosidase inhibitors; TZDs: thiazolidinediones; EPAs, eicosapentaenoic acids; ACEIs: angiotensin-converting enzyme inhibitors; ARBs: angiotensin receptor blockers; CCBs: calcium channel blockers.

3.2. Relationships of Plasma XOR Activity with Individual Parameters

Plasma XOR activity was logarithmically transformed to normalize the skewed distribution to determine correlations between variables using analysis of variance (Figure 1). Correlations of individual parameters with logarithmically transformed plasma XOR activity (ln-XOR) are shown in Figure 2. As shown in panel (A), ln-XOR was significantly and positively correlated with the plasma hypoxanthine level ($r2 = 0.086$, $p = 0.032$) and the plasma level of xanthine ($r2 = 0.439$, $p < 0.0001$), but not with the plasma UA level ($r2 = 0.123$, $p = 0.011$). Ln-XOR showed a significant positive correlation with VFA ($r2 = 0.022$, $p = 0.284$) but with neither BMI ($r2 = 0.024$, $p = 0.265$) nor waist circumference ($r2 = 0.024$, $p = 0.265$). We found that ln-XOR showed a significant negative correlation with the duration of diabetes ($r2 = 0.078$, $p = 0.041$), the Brinkman index (number of cigarettes smoked per day) x (number of years smoked) ($r2 = 0.131$, $p = 0.007$), and maximum IMT ($r2 = 0.176$, $p = 0.002$) but not with sex ($r2 = 0.027$, $p = 0.233$), age ($r2 = 0.014$, $p = 0.400$), height ($r2 = 0.012$, $p = 0.423$), vibration ($r2 = 0.012$, $p = 0.443$), or minimum ABI ($r2 = 0.023$, $p = 0.269$). In addition, ln-XOR showed significant positive correlations with aspartate aminotransferase (AST) ($r2 = 0.568$, $p < 0.0001$), alanine aminotransferase (ALT) ($r2 = 0.619$, $p < 0.0001$), gamma-glutamyl transferase (γ-GTP) ($r2 = 0.188$, $p < 0.0001$), the AST to platelet ratio index (APRI) ($r2 = 0.310$, $p < 0.0001$), and albumin ($r2 = 0.093$, $p = 0.025$), while showing negative correlations with the AST to ALT ratio (AAR) ($r2 = 0.159$, $p = 0.003$) and high density lipoprotein (HDL)-cholesterol ($r2 = 0.129$, $p = 0.008$). The ln-XOR showed no significant correlations with FBG ($r2 = 0.153$, $p = 0.372$), HbA1c ($r2 = 0.0001$, $p = 0.930$), estimated glomerular filtration rate (eGFR) ($r2 = 0.010$, $p = 0.469$), low density lipoprotein (LDL)-cholesterol ($r2 = 0.026$, $p = 0.249$), triglyceride (TG) ($r2 = 0.030$, $p = 0.209$), the eicosapentaenoic acid to arachidonic acid ratio (EPA/AA) ($r2 = 0.0008$, $p = 0.843$), C-reactive protein (CRP) ($r2 = 0.006$, $p = 0.571$), or B-type natriuretic peptide (BNP) ($r2 = 0.066$, $p = 0.061$). We examined relationships of XOR with anti-diabetic drugs, antihyperlipidemic agents, and antihypertensive agents and found that ln-XOR showed a significant negative correlation with GLP-1 agonists/dipeptidyl peptidase-4 inhibitors (GLP-1RAs/DPP4is) ($r2 = 0.162$, $p = 0.003$).

As shown in panel (B), we investigated the correlations between ln-XOR and NCS parameters. For the correlation analysis, we excluded the parameters related to the sural nerve because in half of the analyzed participants (27/54) these parameters were not detectable (Table 1). There were no significant correlations of ln-XOR with peroneal amp ($r2 = 0.013$, $p = 0.434$), tibial amp ($r2 = 0.059$, $p = 0.076$), or tibial F-wave ($r2 = 0.044$, $p = 0.136$). However, we did demonstrate significant positive correlations of ln-XOR with both peroneal conduction velocity ($r2 = 0.135$, $p = 0.008$) and tibial conduction velocity ($r2 = 0.097$, $p = 0.023$), together with a significant negative correlation of ln-XOR with the peroneal F-wave ($r2 = 0.107$, $p = 0.028$).

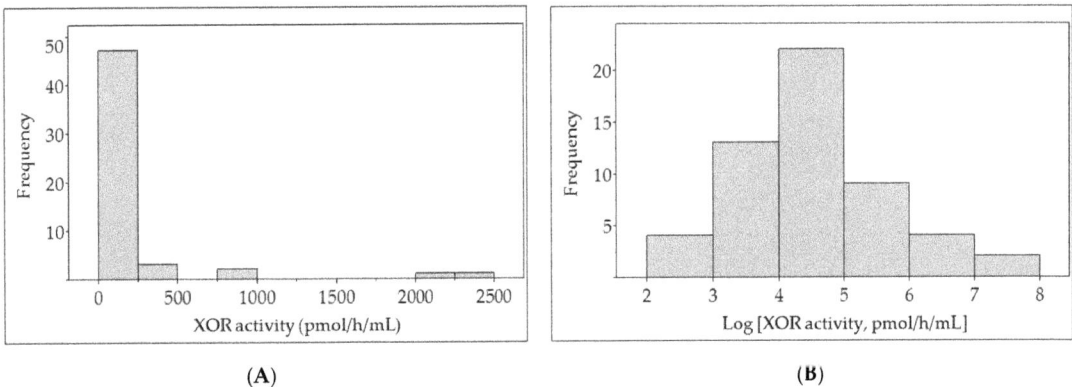

Figure 1. Distribution of plasma XOR activity (**A**) with logarithmically transformed data (**B**) displayed as a histogram.

(**A**)

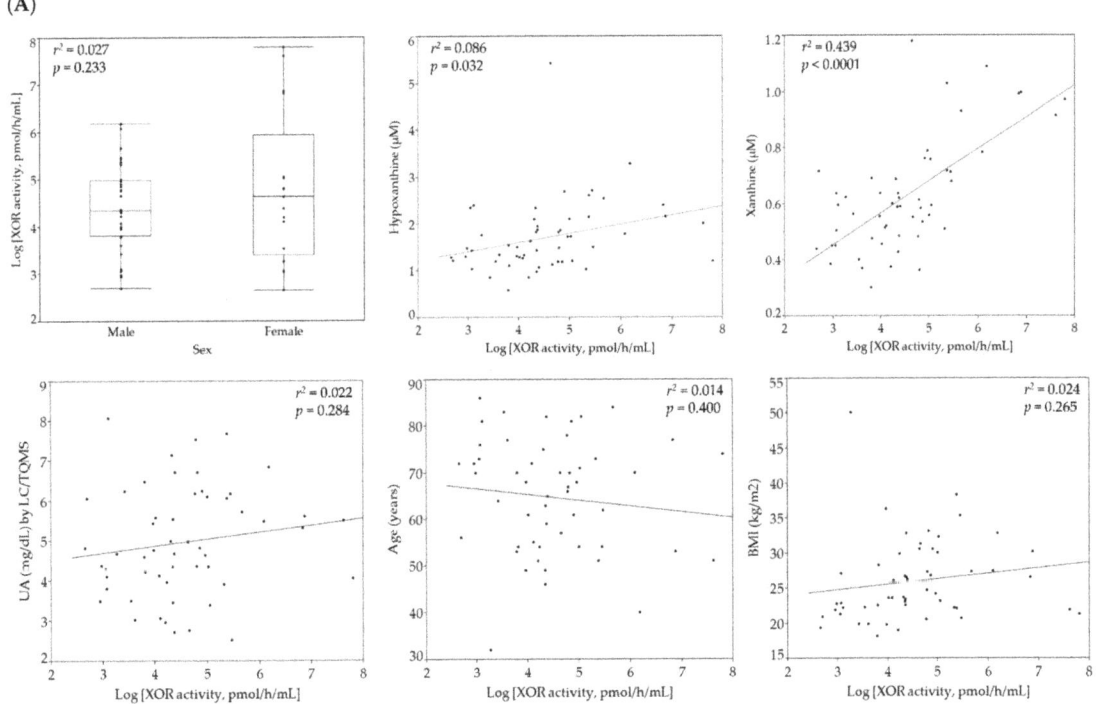

Figure 2. *Cont.*

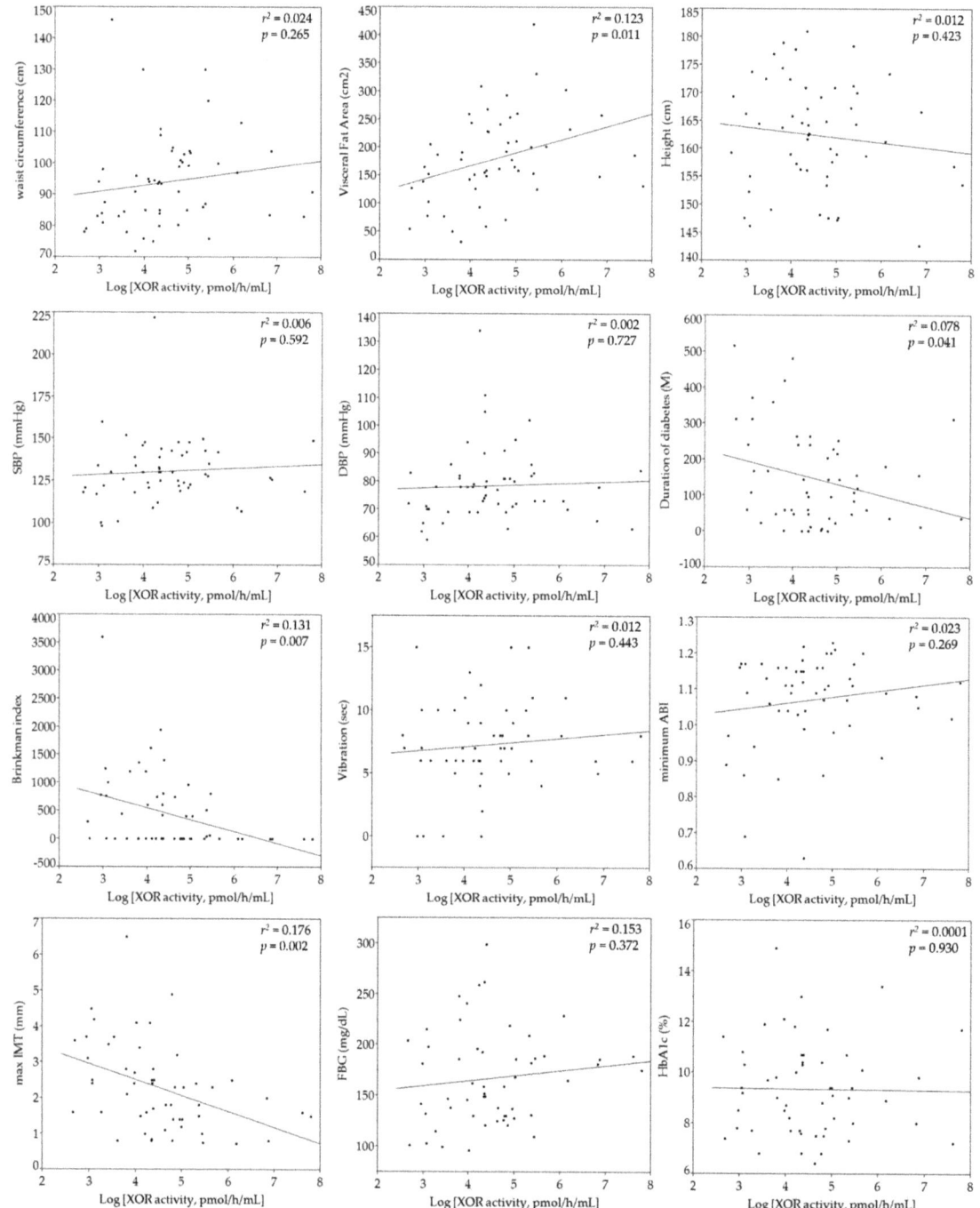

Figure 2. *Cont.*

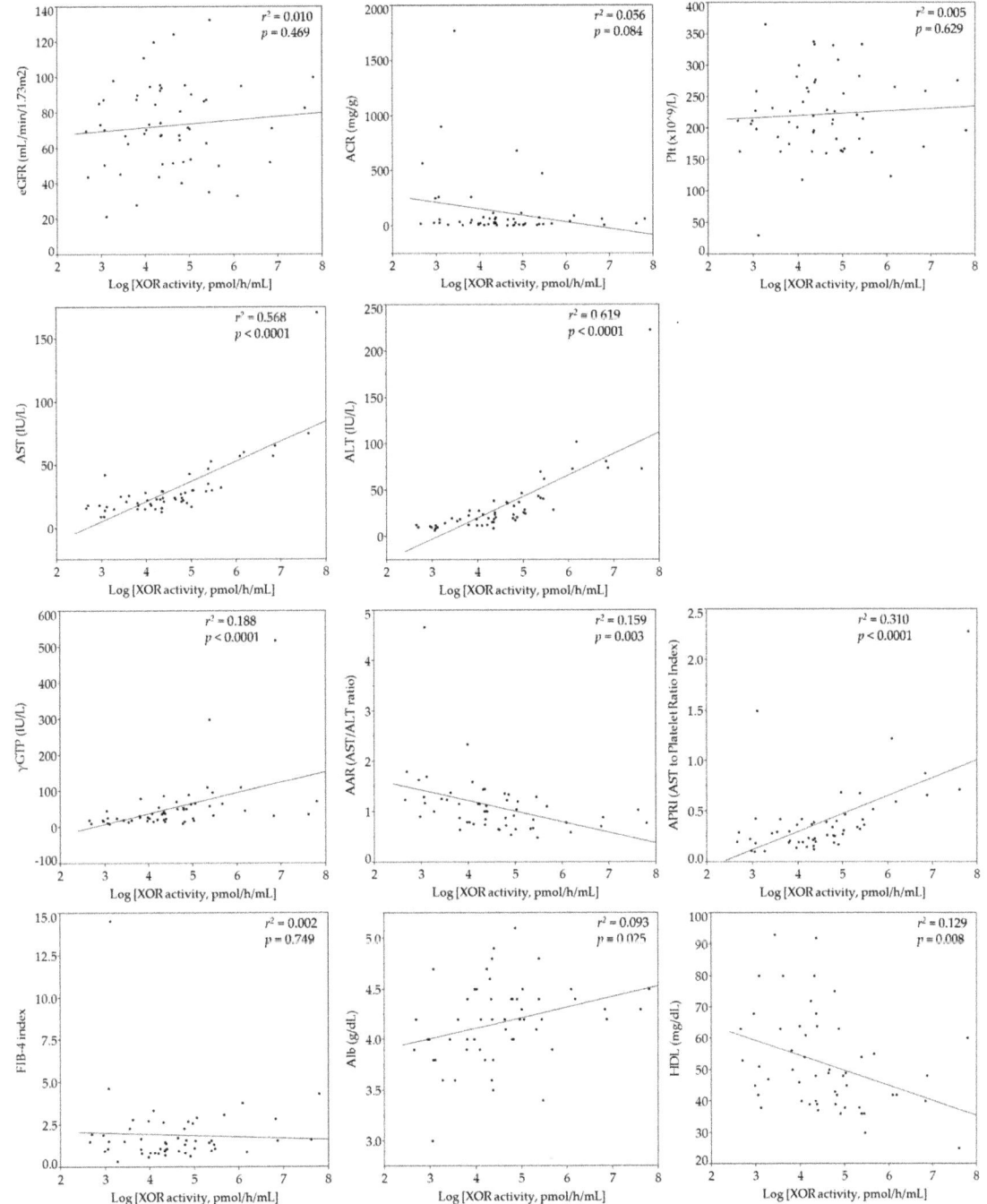

Figure 2. Cont.

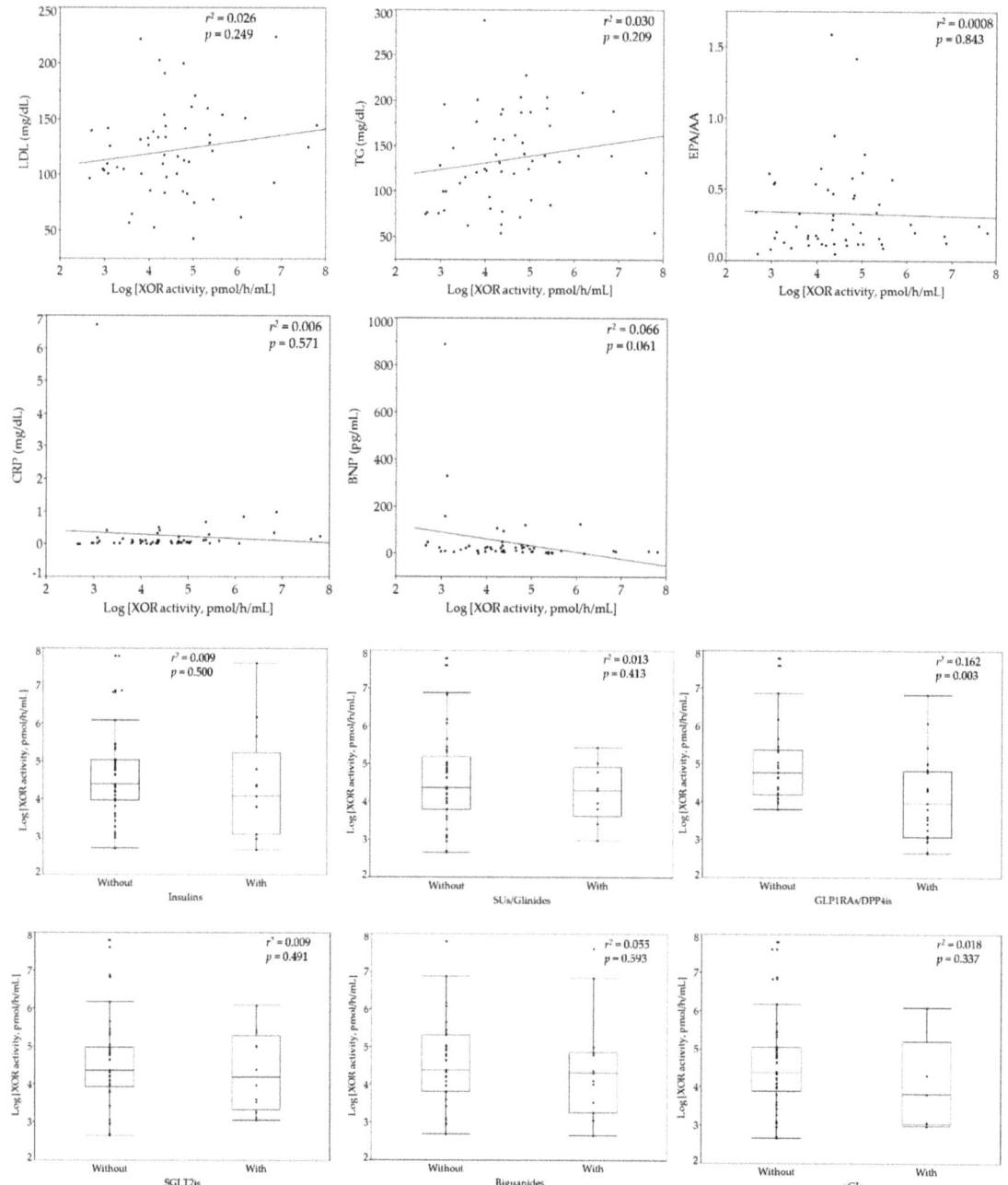

Figure 2. *Cont.*

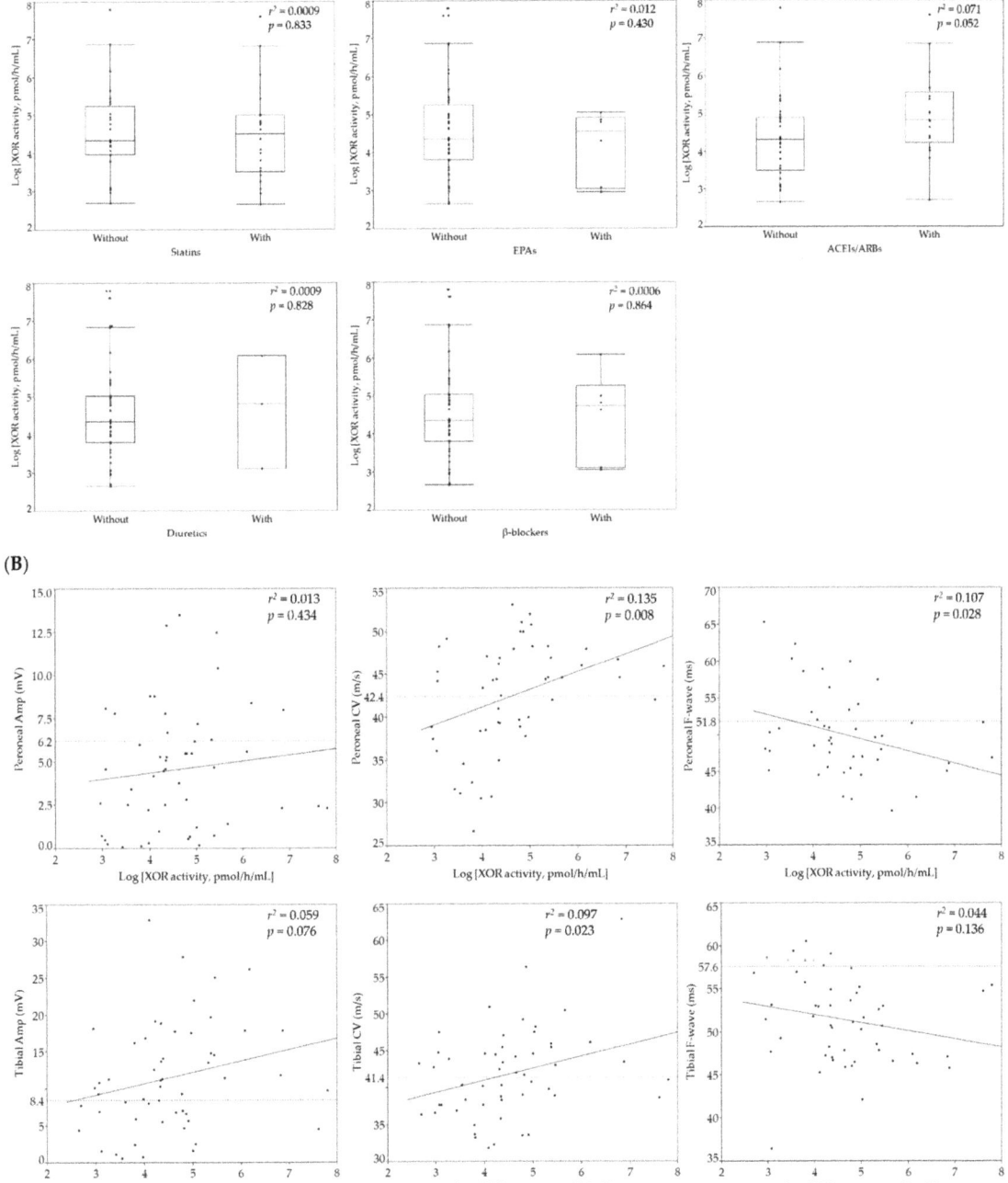

Figure 2. Correlations of individual parameters with logarithmically transformed plasma XOR activity. Results of sex, hypoxanthine, xanthine, UA, age, BMI, waist circumference, VFA, height, SBP, DBP, duration of diabetes, Brinkman index, vibration, minimum ABI, maximum IMT, FBG, HbA1c, Cre, eGFR, ACR, Plt, AST, ALT, γGTP, AAR, APRI, FIB-4 index, Alb, HDL cholesterol, LDL cholesterol, TG, EPA/AA, CRP, BNP, anti-diabetic drugs, antihyperlipidemic agents, and antihypertensive agents are shown in (**A**), those of various NCS parameters in (**B**). Solid lines indicate regression lines, while each dotted line shows the threshold level of each of the NCS parameters in panel (**B**). The thresholds for peroneal/tibial amplitude potential, peroneal/tibial conduction velocity, and peroneal/tibial F-wave for prediction of incident DSP were 6.2/8.4 mV, 42.4/41.4 m/s, and 51.8/57.6 ms, respectively. SBP, systolic blood pressure; DBP, diastolic blood pressure; Cre, serum creatinine; eGFR, estimated glomerular filtration rate; ACR, albumin to creatinine ratio; Plt, platelet count; FIB-4 index, fibrosis-4 index; EPA/AA, eicosapentaenoic acid to arachidonic acid ratio; BNP, B-type natriuretic peptide; CRP, C-reactive protein; αGIs, α-glucosidase inhibitors; GLP-1RAs/DPP4is, GLP-1 agonists/dipeptidyl peptidase-4 inhibitors; SGLT2, sodium-glucose co-transporter 2 inhibitors; ACEIs, angiotensin-converting enzyme inhibitors; ARBs, angiotensin receptor blockers; CCBs, calcium channel blockers; Amp, amplitude potential; CV, conduction velocity; F-wave, F-wave latency. r2: coefficient of determination, vibration: perception time for a fork vibration.

3.3. Relationships of Plasma XOR Activity with NCS Parameters

As for DSP, stepwise multiple regression analysis using various NCS parameters as the objective variable, as well as variables including ln-XOR, sex, age, duration of diabetes, BMI, waist circumference, FBG, minimum ABI, and maximum IMT as explanatory variables, revealed significant correlations of peroneal conduction velocity with ln-XOR, age and waist circumference, peroneal F-wave latency with ln-XOR and BMI, and tibial F-wave latency with ln-XOR when stratified by the thresholds identified for prediction of incident DSP (Table 2). Receiver operating characteristic curves (Figure 3) showed the discriminatory power of the ln-XOR for various NCS parameters, such as peroneal conduction velocity, peroneal F-wave, and tibial F-wave, stratified by the thresholds identified for prediction of incident DSP [31]. Their area under the curve values were 0.83, 0.80, and 0.83, respectively.

Table 2. Univariate and multivariate regression analysis of NCS parameters.

Univariate Analysis				
Objective Variable	Explanatory Variable	OR	<95% CI>	*p*-value
Peroneal Amp (<6.2 mV)	Ln-XOR	0.78	<0.46–1.31>	0.349
Peroneal CV (<42.4 m/s)		0.48	<0.24–0.83>	0.007
Peroneal F-wave (>51.8 ms)		0.39	<0.18–0.73>	0.002
Tibial Amp (<8.4 mV)		0.63	<0.34–1.07>	0.087
Tibial CV (<41.4 m/s)		0.84	<0.51–1.34>	0.454
Tibial F-wave (>57.6 ms)		0.23	<0.07–0.58>	0.001
Multivariate Analysis				
Objective Variable	Explanatory Variable	OR	<95% CI>	*p*-value
Peroneal CV (<42.4 m/s)	Ln-XOR	0.47	<0.22–0.86>	0.013
	Age	0.93	<0.87–0.99>	0.027
	Waist circumference	0.92	<0.86–0.96>	0.0004
Peroneal F-wave (>51.8 ms)	Ln-XOR	0.48	<0.21–0.89>	0.017
	BMI	0.83	<0.69–0.96>	0.007
Tibial F-wave (>57.6 ms)	Ln-XOR	0.23	<0.07–0.58>	0.001

OR, odds ratio; CI, confidence interval; Amp, amplitude potential; CV, conduction velocity; F-wave, F-wave latency. NCV parameters were stratified by the thresholds identified for prediction of incident DSP according to a previous report as described in the "**Patients and Methods**" section, that is, the thresholds for peroneal/tibial amplitude potential, peroneal/tibial conduction velocity, and peroneal/tibial F-wave were 6.2/8.4 mV, 42.4/41.4 m/s, and 51.8/57.6 ms, respectively.

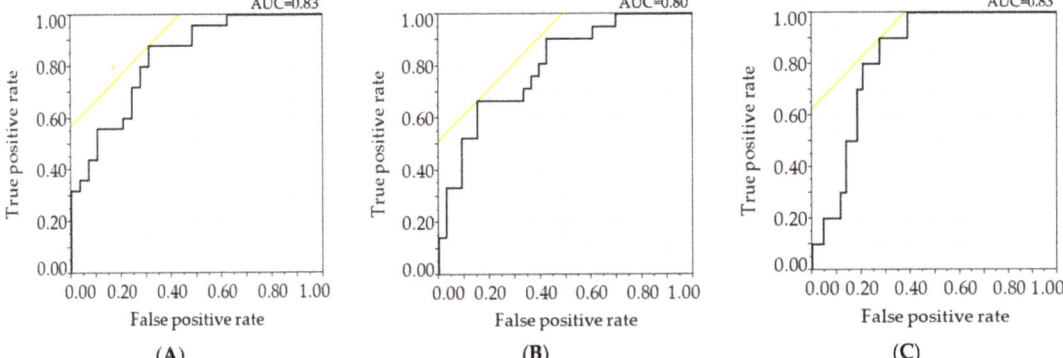

Figure 3. ROC curves for various NCS parameters stratified by the thresholds identified for prediction of incident DSP. (**A**) Peroneal CV, (**B**) peroneal F-wave, (**C**) tibial F-wave. ROC, receiver operating characteristic; AUC, area under the curve; F-wave, F-wave latency. NCV parameters were stratified by the thresholds identified for the prediction of incident DSP according to a previous report as described in the "**Patients and Methods**" section, that is, the thresholds for peroneal conduction velocity, peroneal F-wave, and tibial F-wave were 42.4 m/s, 51.8 ms, and 57.6 ms, respectively.

The PCA biplot (Figure 4) showed distributions of parameters from the axes of three primary components (PC). Along the axis of PC1, ln-XOR correlated strongly with hypoxanthine, xanthine, impaired liver functions (ALT, AST, γGTP, and/or APRI abnormalities, with hepatic steatosis), obesity-related parameters (BMI, VFA, waist circumference, and triglyceride), and various NCS parameters. Ln-XOR also correlated positively with amplitude potentials and conduction velocities and negatively with F-waves for both peroneal and tibial nerves. Factor loadings (Table 3) for PC1 to PC11 showed ln-XOR to have significant loadings in PC1 and PC2. PC1 showed a positive correlation of ln-XOR with impaired liver functions (ALT, AST, γGTP, and/or APRI abnormalities, with hepatic steatosis), xanthine, hypoxanthine, conduction velocity of the peroneal nerve, amplitude potentials (both peroneal and tibial), and obesity-related parameters (BMI, VFA, waist circumference, and triglyceride), as well as negative correlations of ln-XOR with F-waves (both peroneal and tibial), maximum IMT, duration of diabetes, HDL-cholesterol, AAR, GLP1RAs/DPP4is use, retinopathy, ACR, age, and the Brinkman index. PC2 showed positive correlations of ln-XOR with liver dysfunction (APRI, AST, and ALT) and age, while showing inverse relationships of ln-XOR with obesity-related parameters (BMI, waist circumference, and triglyceride), renal function (eGFR and without nephropathy), and peroneal nerve amplitude potential. PC3 showed positive correlations of ln-XOR with F-waves (both peroneal and tibial), height, female gender, FBG, Alb, and minimum AMI, while correlations with age, the AST to ALT ratio, BNP, and CRP together with tibial nerve conduction velocity were negative.

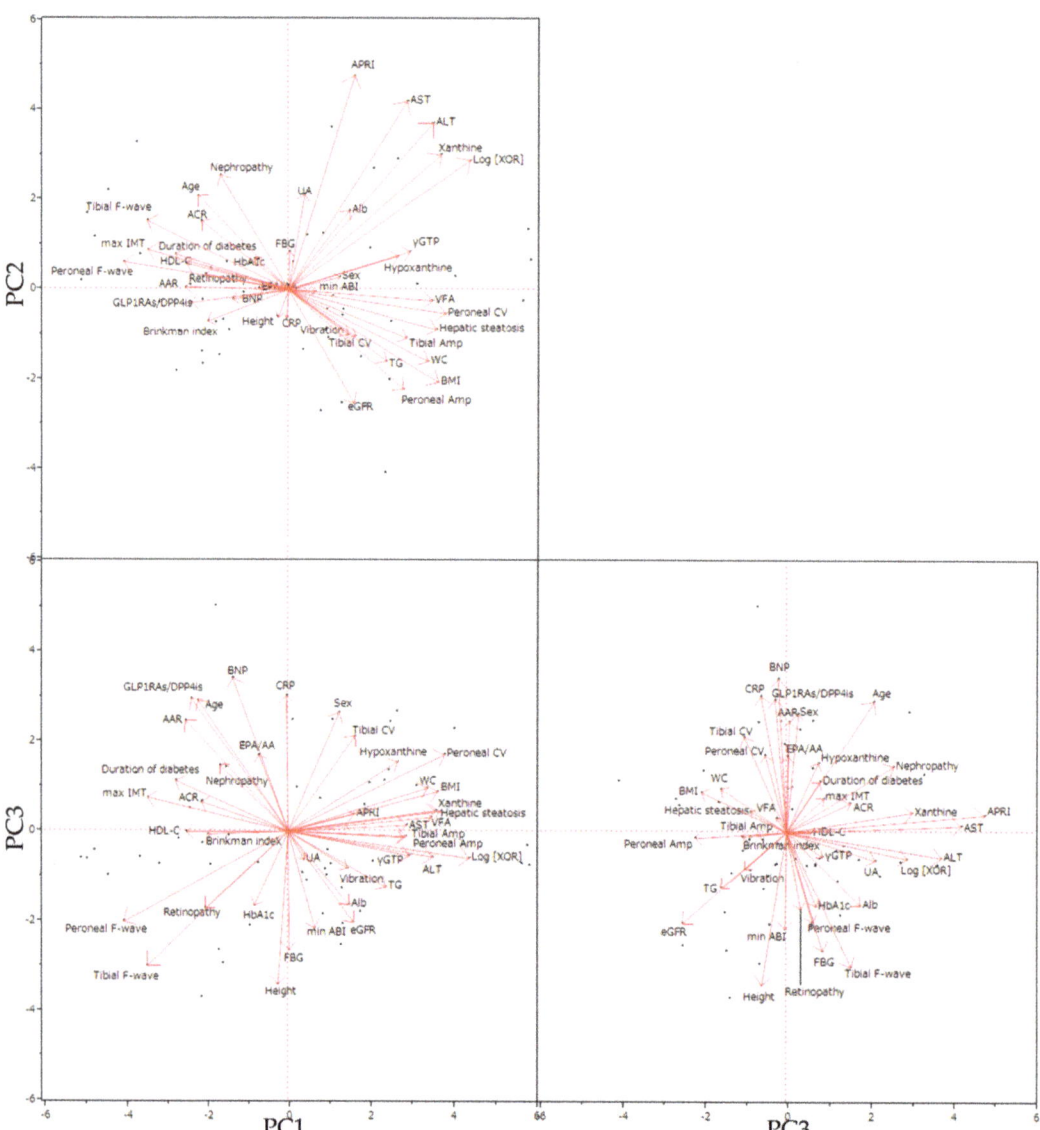

Figure 4. Visualization of correlations between variabilities in PCA biplots. PC, principal component; Amp, amplitude; CV, conduction velocity; WC, waist circumference.

Table 3. Principal component analysis (PCA).

Variables	PC1	PC2	PC3	PC4	PC5	PC6	PC7	PC8	PC9	PC10	PC11
Log [XOR activity, pmol/h/mL]	0.75	0.49									
Peroneal F-wave (ms)	−0.69		−0.34								
Peroneal CV (m/s)	0.65										−0.3
Xanthine (μM)	0.63	0.51									
BMI (kg/m^2)	0.62	−0.35		0.48							
Hepatic steatosis (Without0/Wth1)	0.61										0.35
ALT (IU/L)	0.6	0.64									
Tibial F-wave (ms)	−0.6		−0.51								
Visceral Fat Area (cm^2)	0.6				0.52						
max IMT (mm)	−0.6				0.32						
Waist circumference (cm)	0.58				0.52						
γGTP (IU/L)	0.51										
AST (IU/L)	0.49	0.72									
Tibial Amp (mV)	0.49			−0.34					0.38	−0.43	
Peroneal Amp (mV)	0.48	−0.38						0.46			
Duration of diabetes (M)	−0.48					−0.48					0.35
Hypoxanthine (μM)	0.46			0.31				−0.36		−0.35	
AAR (AST/ALT ratio)	−0.43		0.42			−0.39					
HDL-Chol (mg/dL)	−0.43				0.44						
GLP1RAs/DPP4is (Without0/Wth1)	−0.41		0.51						−0.34		
TG (mg/dL)	0.41			0.56							
Age (years)	−0.38	0.36	0.5					0.36			
ACR (mg/g)	−0.37				0.37			−0.41			
Retinopathy (Without0/Wth1)	−0.35			0.46	−0.33	−0.32					
Brinkman index	−0.34					0.43					0.37
APRI (AST to Platelet Ratio Index)		0.82									
Nephropathy (Without0/Wth1)		0.44						0.32			
eGFR (mL/min/1.73 m^2)		−0.43	−0.35	−0.38	−0.34					0.34	
UA (mg/dL) by LC/TQMS		0.36		0.67				−0.32			
Alb (g/dL)		0.3			0.52		0.35				
BNP (pg/mL)			0.58			0.58					
Height (cm)			−0.58					−0.31			
CRP (mg/dL)			0.52		−0.34	0.64					
Sex (Male0/Female1)			0.45		−0.48			−0.32			
FBG (mg/dL)			−0.45					0.65			
min ABI			−0.37	−0.45	0.49						
Tibial CV (m/s)			0.36					−0.42			
EPA/AA					0.51		0.41			0.41	
HbA1c (%)					−0.51		0.39	0.36			
Vibration (sec)							−0.33		0.5	0.31	

	Eigenvalues of PCs		
	Eigenvalues	Proportion of Variance	Cumulative Proportion
PC1	7.63	0.191	0.191
PC2	3.69	0.092	0.283
PC3	3.61	0.09	0.373
PC4	3.22	0.081	0.454
PC5	2.67	0.067	0.521
PC6	2.21	0.055	0.576
PC7	1.81	0.045	0.621
PC8	1.71	0.043	0.664
PC9	1.33	0.033	0.697
PC10	1.26	0.031	0.729
PC11	1.13	0.028	0.757

PC, principal component. Hepatic steatosis was diagnosed by ultrasonography. We omitted factor loadings with an absolute value less than 0.3 (indicated as blanks).

4. Discussion

We investigated the associations of plasma XOR activity in T2DM patients with individual parameters and diabetic vascular complications. To our knowledge, this study is the first to demonstrate low levels of plasma XOR activity to be associated with an elongation in the F-wave latencies of both tibial and peroneal nerves, which are known to be the most sensitive parameters of DSP [34]. Stepwise analysis using clinical thresholds for prediction of incident DSP applied for various NCS parameters showed significant and independent sensitivity of XOR activity measurement for the detection of DSP. In contrast, we found that high plasma XOR activity levels were associated with a short duration of diabetes and metabolic disorders often found in young diabetic patients such as central obesity and liver dysfunction.

Recently, relationships between various clinical features and the level of plasma XOR activity measured by the procedure used in our present study have been reported. For example, plasma XOR activity is related to obesity and habitual smoking in the general population [35], vascular endothelial dysfunction assessed by flow-mediated dilation in patients with type 1 diabetes [36], liver dysfunction in T2DM patients [37], the prevalence rate of coronary artery spasm [38], and adverse clinical outcomes in patients with heart failure but with a preserved ejection fraction [39], as well as the requirement for cardiovascular intensive care [40]. Previous studies demonstrated that XOR activity is upregulated in patients with diabetic vascular complications [41–44]. Furthermore, XOR was suggested to mediate axonal and myelin loss in a murine model of neural diseases [45]. XOR-derived ROS involvement in the pathogenesis of tissue lesions induced by reperfusion after ischemia is thought to be related to vascular injury resulting from diabetic vascular complications [46]. Taken together, these observations suggest that plasma XOR activity is upregulated in the early period of diabetes and then becomes exhausted with the development of diabetic vascular complications, as suggested in a recent report [47].

Moreover, PCA analysis revealed two patterns of relationships between XOR activity and F-wave latency. One pattern is low XOR activity associated with elongation in the F-wave latency, consistent with our main findings, while the other is an inverse weakly positive relationship, possibly reflecting neuronal injury due to altered XOR activity, as shown in previous studies [41–44]. Importantly, the thresholds for F-wave latency that we used in this study were effective for discriminating DSP due to decreased XOR activity. Interestingly, this study also revealed increases in both incretin and its mimetics, due to the use of GLP1RAs or DPP4is, to be related to low XOR activity, an observation consistent with accumulating evidence that incretins induce anti-inflammatory effects by downregulating ROS production and NF-κB activation in vascular cells [48,49].

Since assessing NCS requires expensive equipment and specialized personnel, in addition to being relatively invasive and time-consuming to perform, the recent position statement from the American Diabetes Association has stressed that diabetic polyneuropathy (DPN) can be clinically diagnosed without assessing NCS results and that NCS is only required in patients with special situations [50]. Diabetologists have been making efforts to establish simpler methods of detecting DPN, but none have been sufficiently reliable to gain worldwide acceptance for diagnosing DPN [51–53]. As noted above, the plasma XOR level may serve as a marker for evaluating the development of DPN. Applying this technique to measure plasma XOR levels is rather complicated, based on utilizing a combination of [13C2,15N2]-xanthine and measurement using LC/TQMS. Improvements of this technique are thus needed before a routine clinical application can be achieved.

This study has limitations. First, the collection of blood samples and various physiological examinations were not consistently performed on the same day which might have resulted in bias. Second, there might have been selection bias as our participants were a group of patients willing to be examined for diabetic complications. Furthermore, in order to study patients who had complete NCS data, we analyzed only a portion of the participants in our database because our physiological laboratory incorporated F-wave parameters into the NCS dataset after December 2018. The final study size was thus determined by referring to previous reports, one with 26 [29] and the other with 71 [36] subjects. In our view, reasonable confidence is achieved above a certain standard when a statistically meaningful difference is demonstrated. Third, this study was cross-sectional and observational such that the relationship between diabetic DSP and plasma XOR activity cannot be assumed to be causal. An interventional study with a much larger sample size is needed to further elucidate the association between DSP and plasma XOR activity.

5. Conclusions

In this cross-sectional analysis, we showed that plasma XOR activity is a potential predictor of diabetes disease status. XOR activity is upregulated in the early period of diabetes and then appears to become exhausted with the development and progression of diabetic vascular complications. As early DSP usually lacks typical symptoms and is very difficult to detect when employing routine outpatient examinations, measurement of plasma XOR activity might serve as a reliable evaluation tool for DSP prior to the development of symptoms.

Author Contributions: Conceptualization, M.F. and A.K.; methodology, M.F. and A.K.; software, M.F.; validation, M.F. and A.K.; formal analysis, A.K.; investigation, T.M. and T.N.; resources, M.F.; data curation, M.F. and A.K.; writing—original draft preparation, M.F.; writing—review and editing, K.O., K.W., H.S., H.O., T.Y., Y.N., T.A., and H.I.; visualization, M.F.; supervision, K.O., K.W., H.S., H.O., T.Y., Y.N., T.A., and H.I.; project administration, H.I.; funding acquisition, none of the authors sought funding. All authors have read and agreed to the published version of the manuscript.

Funding: This research received no external funding.

Institutional Review Board Statement: The study was conducted according to the guidelines of the Declaration of Helsinki, and approved by the Institutional Ethics Committee of Nihon University Hospital (approval number 20170701).

Informed Consent Statement: Informed consent was obtained from all subjects involved in the study.

Acknowledgments: The authors are deeply indebted to the subjects who agreed to participate in the present study.

Conflicts of Interest: H.I. has served on the advisory board of Astellas Pharma, has received lecture fees from Astellas Pharma, MSD, Mitsubishi Tanabe Pharma, Nippon Boehringer Ingelheim, and Novartis Pharma, and has received grants from Ono Pharmaceutical, Nippon Boehringer Ingelheim, Sanofi, Mitsubishi Tanabe Pharma, Eli Lilly, Daiichi-Sankyo, Novo Nordisk Pharma and MSD. M.F., K.O., T.M., T.N., K.W., H.S., H.O., T.Y., Y.N., T.A., and A.K. have no conflict of interest regarding the contents of this article to declare.

Abbreviations

ABI	Ankle-Brachial Index
AST	Aspartate Aminotransferase
ALT	Alanine Aminotransferase
AAR	AST to ALT Ratio
APRI	AST to Platelet Ratio Index
BNP	B-Type Natriuretic Peptide
BMI	Body Mass Index
CRP	C-Reactive Protein
CVRR	Coefficient of Variation of RR Intervals
DR	Diabetic Retinopathy
DPN	Diabetic Polyneuropathy
DSP	Distal Symmetric Polyneuropathy
EPA/AA	Eicosapentaenoic Acid to Arachidonic Acid Ratio
eGFR	Estimated Glomerular Filtration Rate
FBG	Fasting Blood Glucose
γ-GTP	Gamma-Glutamyl Transferase
HDL-Cholesterol	High Density Lipoprotein-Cholesterol
IMT	Intima-Media Thickness
LC	Liquid Chromatography
ln-XOR	Logarithmically Transformed Plasma XOR Activity
LDL-Cholesterol	Low Density Lipoprotein-Cholesterol

NCS	Nerve Conduction Study
NDR	No Apparent Diabetic Retinopathy
PCA	Principal Component Analysis
PDR	Proliferative Diabetic Retinopathy
SDR	Simple Diabetic Retinopathy
TQMS	Triple Quadrupole Mass Spectrometry
T2DM	Type 2 Diabetes Mellitus
TG	Triglyceride
UA	Uric Acid
VFA	Visceral Fat Area
XOR	Xanthine Oxidoreductase

References

1. Rao Kondapally Seshasai, S.; Kaptoge, S.; Thompson, A.; Di Angelantonio, E.; Gao, P.; Sarwar, N.; Whincup, P.H.; Mukamal, K.J.; Gillum, R.F.; Holme, I.; et al. Diabetes mellitus, fasting glucose, and risk of cause-specific death. *N. Engl. J. Med.* **2011**, *364*, 829–841. [CrossRef]
2. Saeedi, P.; Petersohn, I.; Salpea, P.; Malanda, B.; Karuranga, S.; Unwin, N.; Colagiuri, S.; Guariguata, L.; Motala, A.A.; Ogurtsova, K.; et al. Global and regional diabetes prevalence estimates for 2019 and projections for 2030 and 2045: Results from the International Diabetes Federation Diabetes Atlas, 9(th) edition. *Diabetes Res. Clin. Pract.* **2019**, *157*, 107843. [CrossRef]
3. Saeedi, P.; Salpea, P.; Karuranga, S.; Petersohn, I.; Malanda, B.; Gregg, E.W.; Unwin, N.; Wild, S.H.; Williams, R. Mortality attributable to diabetes in 20–79 years old adults, 2019 estimates: Results from the International Diabetes Federation Diabetes Atlas, 9th ed. *Diabetes Res. Clin. Pract.* **2020**, *162*, 108086. [CrossRef] [PubMed]
4. Callaghan, B.C.; Cheng, H.T.; Stables, C.L.; Smith, A.L.; Feldman, E.L. Diabetic neuropathy: Clinical manifestations and current treatments. *Lancet Neurol.* **2012**, *11*, 521–534. [CrossRef]
5. Tesfaye, S.; Boulton, A.J.; Dyck, P.J.; Freeman, R.; Horowitz, M.; Kempler, P.; Lauria, G.; Malik, R.A.; Spallone, V.; Vinik, A.; et al. Diabetic neuropathies: Update on definitions, diagnostic criteria, estimation of severity, and treatments. *Diabetes Care* **2010**, *33*, 2285–2293. [CrossRef] [PubMed]
6. Furman, D.; Campisi, J.; Verdin, E.; Carrera-Bastos, P.; Targ, S.; Franceschi, C.; Ferrucci, L.; Gilroy, D.W.; Fasano, A.; Miller, G.W.; et al. Chronic inflammation in the etiology of disease across the life span. *Nat. Med.* **2019**, *25*, 1822–1832. [CrossRef] [PubMed]
7. Tesfaye, S.; Chaturvedi, N.; Eaton, S.E.; Ward, J.D.; Manes, C.; Ionescu-Tirgoviste, C.; Witte, D.R.; Fuller, J.H. Vascular risk factors and diabetic neuropathy. *N. Engl. J. Med.* **2005**, *352*, 341–350. [CrossRef] [PubMed]
8. Deng, Y.; Scherer, P.E. Adipokines as novel biomarkers and regulators of the metabolic syndrome. *Ann. NY Acad. Sci.* **2010**, *1212*, E1–E19. [CrossRef] [PubMed]
9. Facchini, F.; Chen, Y.D.; Hollenbeck, C.B.; Reaven, G.M. Relationship between resistance to insulin-mediated glucose uptake, urinary uric acid clearance, and plasma uric acid concentration. *JAMA* **1991**, *266*, 3008–3011. [CrossRef] [PubMed]
10. Lin, J.D.; Chiou, W.K.; Chang, H.Y.; Liu, F.H.; Weng, H.F. Serum uric acid and leptin levels in metabolic syndrome: A quandary over the role of uric acid. *Metabolism* **2007**, *56*, 751–756. [CrossRef]
11. Bjornstad, P.; Laffel, L.; Lynch, J.; El Ghormli, L.; Weinstock, R.S.; Tollefsen, S.E.; Nadeau, K.J. Elevated Serum Uric Acid is Associated with Greater Risk for Hypertension and Diabetic Kidney Diseases in Obese Adolescents with Type 2 Diabetes: An Observational Analysis From the Treatment Options for Type 2 Diabetes in Adolescents and Youth (TODAY) Study. *Diabetes Care* **2019**, *42*, 1120–1128. [CrossRef]
12. Spatola, L.; Ferraro, P.M.; Gambaro, G.; Badalamenti, S.; Dauriz, M. Metabolic syndrome and uric acid nephrolithiasis: Insulin resistance in focus. *Metabolism* **2018**, *83*, 225–233. [CrossRef] [PubMed]
13. Zhu, D.D.; Wang, Y.Z.; Zou, C.; She, X.P.; Zheng, Z. The role of uric acid in the pathogenesis of diabetic retinopathy based on Notch pathway. *Biochem. Biophys. Res. Commun.* **2018**, *503*, 921–929. [CrossRef]
14. Yu, S.; Chen, Y.; Hou, X.; Xu, D.; Che, K.; Li, C.; Yan, S.; Wang, Y.; Wang, B. Serum Uric Acid Levels and Diabetic Peripheral Neuropathy in Type 2 Diabetes: A Systematic Review and Meta-analysis. *Mol. Neurobiol.* **2016**, *53*, 1045–1051. [CrossRef]
15. Zhang, J.; Xu, C.; Zhao, Y.; Chen, Y. The significance of serum xanthine oxidoreductase in patients with nonalcoholic fatty liver disease. *Clin. Lab.* **2014**, *60*, 1301–1307. [CrossRef]
16. Kuppusamy, U.R.; Indran, M.; Rokiah, P. Glycaemic control in relation to xanthine oxidase and antioxidant indices in Malaysian Type 2 diabetes patients. *Diabet Med.* **2005**, *22*, 1343–1346. [CrossRef] [PubMed]
17. Parks, D.A.; Granger, D.N. Xanthine oxidase: Biochemistry, distribution and physiology. *Acta Physiol Scand. Suppl.* **1986**, *548*, 87–99. [PubMed]
18. Nishino, T.; Okamoto, K.; Eger, B.T.; Pai, E.F.; Nishino, T. Mammalian xanthine oxidoreductase—Mechanism of transition from xanthine dehydrogenase to xanthine oxidase. *FEBS J.* **2008**, *275*, 3278–3289. [CrossRef] [PubMed]

19. Nishino, T.; Okamoto, K.; Kawaguchi, Y.; Hori, H.; Matsumura, T.; Eger, B.T.; Pai, E.F.; Nishino, T. Mechanism of the conversion of xanthine dehydrogenase to xanthine oxidase: Identification of the two cysteine disulfide bonds and crystal structure of a non-convertible rat liver xanthine dehydrogenase mutant. *J. Biol. Chem.* **2005**, *280*, 24888–24894. [CrossRef]
20. Gibbings, S.; Elkins, N.D.; Fitzgerald, H.; Tiao, J.; Weyman, M.E.; Shibao, G.; Fini, M.A.; Wright, R.M. Xanthine oxidoreductase promotes the inflammatory state of mononuclear phagocytes through effects on chemokine expression, peroxisome proliferator-activated receptor-{gamma} sumoylation, and HIF-1{alpha}. *J. Biol. Chem.* **2011**, *286*, 961–975. [CrossRef]
21. Kushiyama, A.; Nakatsu, Y.; Matsunaga, Y.; Yamamotoya, T.; Mori, K.; Ueda, K.; Inoue, Y.; Sakoda, H.; Fujishiro, M.; Ono, H.; et al. Role of Uric Acid Metabolism-Related Inflammation in the Pathogenesis of Metabolic Syndrome Components Such as Atherosclerosis and Nonalcoholic Steatohepatitis. *Mediat. Inflamm.* **2016**, *2016*, 8603164. [CrossRef] [PubMed]
22. Murase, T.; Nampei, M.; Oka, M.; Miyachi, A.; Nakamura, T. A highly sensitive assay of human plasma xanthine oxidoreductase activity using stable isotope-labeled xanthine and LC/TQMS. *J. Chromatogr. B Analyt. Technol. Biomed. Life Sci.* **2016**, *1039*, 51–58. [CrossRef]
23. Yoshizumi, T.; Nakamura, T.; Yamane, M.; Islam, A.H.; Menju, M.; Yamasaki, K.; Arai, T.; Kotani, K.; Funahashi, T.; Yamashita, S.; et al. Abdominal fat: Standardized technique for measurement at CT. *Radiology* **1999**, *211*, 283–286. [CrossRef]
24. Tanaka, K.; Hara, S.; Hattori, M.; Sakai, K.; Onishi, Y.; Yoshida, T.; Kawazu, S.; Kushiyama, A. Role of elevated serum uric acid levels at the onset of overt nephropathy in the risk for renal function decline in patients with type 2 diabetes. *J. Diabetes Investig.* **2015**, *6*, 98–104. [CrossRef] [PubMed]
25. Haneda, M.; Utsunomiya, K.; Koya, D.; Babazono, T.; Moriya, T.; Makino, H.; Kimura, K.; Suzuki, Y.; Wada, T.; Ogawa, S.; et al. A new classification of Diabetic Nephropathy 2014: A report from Joint Committee on Diabetic Nephropathy. *Clin. Exp. Nephrol.* **2015**, *19*, 1–5. [CrossRef] [PubMed]
26. Mohamed, Q.; Gillies, M.C.; Wong, T.Y. Management of diabetic retinopathy: A systematic review. *JAMA* **2007**, *298*, 902–916. [CrossRef] [PubMed]
27. Ando, A.; Miyamoto, M.; Kotani, K.; Okada, K.; Nagasaka, S.; Ishibashi, S. Cardio-Ankle Vascular Index and Indices of Diabetic Polyneuropathy in Patients with Type 2 Diabetes. *J. Diabetes Res.* **2017**, *2017*, 2810914. [CrossRef] [PubMed]
28. O'Leary, D.H.; Polak, J.F.; Wolfson, S.K., Jr.; Bond, M.G.; Bommer, W.; Sheth, S.; Psaty, B.M.; Sharrett, A.R.; Manolio, T.A. Use of sonography to evaluate carotid atherosclerosis in the elderly. The Cardiovascular Health Study. CHS Collaborative Research Group. *Stroke* **1991**, *22*, 1155–1163. [CrossRef]
29. Washio, K.W.; Kusunoki, Y.; Murase, T.; Nakamura, T.; Osugi, K.; Ohigashi, M.; Sukenaga, T.; Ochi, F.; Matsuo, T.; Katsuno, T.; et al. Xanthine oxidoreductase activity is correlated with insulin resistance and subclinical inflammation in young humans. *Metabolism* **2017**, *70*, 51–56. [CrossRef]
30. Yanagida, H.A.A.; Kenta, O.; Nagasaka, S.; Ishibashi, S.; Kotani, K.; Hasegawa, O.; Taniguchi, N. Determination of reference ranges for nerve conduction studies: Influence of age, height and gender. *Jichi Med. Univ. J.* **2015**, *38*, 27–39.
31. Weisman, A.; Bril, V.; Ngo, M.; Lovblom, L.E.; Halpern, E.M.; Orszag, A.; Perkins, B.A. Identification and prediction of diabetic sensorimotor polyneuropathy using individual and simple combinations of nerve conduction study parameters. *PLoS ONE* **2013**, *8*, e58783. [CrossRef] [PubMed]
32. Armstrong, T.N.; Dale, A.M.; Al-Lozi, M.T.; Franzblau, A.; Evanoff, B.A. Median and ulnar nerve conduction studies at the wrist: Criterion validity of the NC-stat automated device. *J. Occup. Environ. Med.* **2008**, *50*, 758–764. [CrossRef]
33. Lee, H.J.; Kwon, H.K.; Kim, D.H.; Pyun, S.B. Nerve conduction studies of median motor nerve and median sensory branches according to the severity of carpal tunnel syndrome. *Ann. Rehabil. Med.* **2013**, *37*, 254–262. [CrossRef]
34. Andersen, H.; Stålberg, E.; Falck, B. F-wave latency, the most sensitive nerve conduction parameter in patients with diabetes mellitus. *Muscle Nerve* **1997**, *20*, 1296–1302. [CrossRef]
35. Furuhashi, M.; Koyama, M.; Higashiura, Y.; Murase, T.; Nakamura, T.; Matsumoto, M.; Sakai, A.; Ohnishi, H.; Tanaka, M.; Saitoh, S.; et al. Differential regulation of hypoxanthine and xanthine by obesity in a general population. *J. Diabetes Investig.* **2020**, *11*, 878–887. [CrossRef]
36. Washio, K.; Kusunoki, Y.; Tsunoda, T.; Osugi, K.; Ohigashi, M.; Murase, T.; Nakamura, T.; Matsuo, T.; Konishi, K.; Katsuno, T.; et al. Xanthine oxidoreductase activity correlates with vascular endothelial dysfunction in patients with type 1 diabetes. *Acta Diabetol.* **2020**, *57*, 31–39. [CrossRef]
37. Kawachi, Y.; Fujishima, Y.; Nishizawa, H.; Nagao, H.; Nakamura, T.; Akari, S.; Murase, T.; Taya, N.; Omori, K.; Miyake, A.; et al. Plasma xanthine oxidoreductase activity in Japanese patients with type 2 diabetes across hospitalized treatment. *J. Diabetes Investig.* **2020**, *12*, 1512–1520. [CrossRef]
38. Watanabe, K.; Shishido, T.; Otaki, Y.; Watanabe, T.; Sugai, T.; Toshima, T.; Takahashi, T.; Yokoyama, M.; Kinoshita, D.; Murase, T.; et al. Increased plasma xanthine oxidoreductase activity deteriorates coronary artery spasm. *Heart Vessels* **2019**, *34*, 1–8. [CrossRef]
39. Watanabe, K.; Watanabe, T.; Otaki, Y.; Shishido, T.; Murase, T.; Nakamura, T.; Kato, S.; Tamura, H.; Nishiyama, S.; Takahashi, H.; et al. Impact of plasma xanthine oxidoreductase activity in patients with heart failure with preserved ejection fraction. *ESC Heart Fail.* **2020**, *7*, 1735–1743. [CrossRef] [PubMed]
40. Shibata, Y.; Shirakabe, A.; Okazaki, H.; Matsushita, M.; Goda, H.; Shigihara, S.; Asano, K.; Kiuchi, K.; Tani, K.; Murase, T.; et al. Plasma xanthine oxidoreductase (XOR) activity in patients who require cardiovascular intensive care. *Heart Ves-*

sels **2020**, *35*, 1390–1400. [CrossRef] [PubMed]
41. Miric, D.J.; Kisic, B.M.; Filipovic-Danic, S.; Grbic, R.; Dragojevic, I.; Miric, M.B.; Puhalo-Sladoje, D. Xanthine Oxidase Activity in Type 2 Diabetes Mellitus Patients with and without Diabetic Peripheral Neuropathy. *J. Diabetes Res.* **2016**, *2016*, 4370490. [CrossRef]
42. Liu, J.; Wang, C.; Liu, F.; Lu, Y.; Cheng, J. Metabonomics revealed xanthine oxidase-induced oxidative stress and inflammation in the pathogenesis of diabetic nephropathy. *Anal. Bioanal. Chem.* **2015**, *407*, 2569–2579. [CrossRef] [PubMed]
43. Xia, J.; Wang, Z.; Zhang, F. Association between Related Purine Metabolites and Diabetic Retinopathy in Type 2 Diabetic Patients. *Int. J. Endocrinol.* **2014**, *2014*, 651050. [CrossRef] [PubMed]
44. Feoli, A.M.; Macagnan, F.E.; Piovesan, C.H.; Bodanese, L.C.; Siqueira, I.R. Xanthine oxidase activity is associated with risk factors for cardiovascular disease and inflammatory and oxidative status markers in metabolic syndrome: Effects of a single exercise session. *Oxid. Med. Cell Longev.* **2014**, *2014*, 587083. [CrossRef] [PubMed]
45. Honorat, J.A.; Kinoshita, M.; Okuno, T.; Takata, K.; Koda, T.; Tada, S.; Shirakura, T.; Fujimura, H.; Mochizuki, H.; Sakoda, S.; et al. Xanthine oxidase mediates axonal and myelin loss in a murine model of multiple sclerosis. *PLoS ONE* **2013**, *8*, e71329. [CrossRef]
46. Battelli, M.G.; Bolognesi, A.; Polito, L. Pathophysiology of circulating xanthine oxidoreductase: New emerging roles for a multi-tasking enzyme. *Biochim. Biophys. Acta* **2014**, *1842*, 1502–1517. [CrossRef]
47. Okuyama, T.; Shirakawa, J.; Nakamura, T.; Murase, T.; Miyashita, D.; Inoue, R.; Kyohara, M.; Togashi, Y.; Terauchi, Y. Association of the plasma xanthine oxidoreductase activity with the metabolic parameters and vascular complications in patients with type 2 diabetes. *Sci. Rep.* **2021**, *11*, 3768. [CrossRef] [PubMed]
48. Wang, D.; Luo, P.; Wang, Y.; Li, W.; Wang, C.; Sun, D.; Zhang, R.; Su, T.; Ma, X.; Zeng, C.; et al. Glucagon-like peptide-1 protects against cardiac microvascular injury in diabetes via a cAMP/PKA/Rho-dependent mechanism. *Diabetes* **2013**, *62*, 1697–1708. [CrossRef]
49. Lee, Y.S.; Park, M.S.; Choung, J.S.; Kim, S.S.; Oh, H.H.; Choi, C.S.; Ha, S.Y.; Kang, Y.; Kim, Y.; Jun, H.S. Glucagon-like peptide-1 inhibits adipose tissue macrophage infiltration and inflammation in an obese mouse model of diabetes. *Diabetologia* **2012**, *55*, 2456–2468. [CrossRef]
50. Pop-Busui, R.; Boulton, A.J.; Feldman, E.L.; Bril, V.; Freeman, R.; Malik, R.A.; Sosenko, J.M.; Ziegler, D. Diabetic Neuropathy: A Position Statement by the American Diabetes Association. *Diabetes Care* **2017**, *40*, 136–154. [CrossRef]
51. Binns-Hall, O.; Selvarajah, D.; Sanger, D.; Walker, J.; Scott, A.; Tesfaye, S. One-stop microvascular screening service: An effective model for the early detection of diabetic peripheral neuropathy and the high-risk foot. *Diabet. Med.* **2018**, *35*, 887–894. [CrossRef]
52. Alam, U.; Jeziorska, M.; Petropoulos, I.N.; Asghar, O.; Fadavi, H.; Ponirakis, G.; Marshall, A.; Tavakoli, M.; Boulton, A.J.M.; Efron, N.; et al. Diagnostic utility of corneal confocal microscopy and intra-epidermal nerve fibre density in diabetic neuropathy. *PLoS ONE* **2017**, *12*, e0180175. [CrossRef] [PubMed]
53. Selvarajah, D.; Cash, T.; Davies, J.; Sankar, A.; Rao, G.; Grieg, M.; Pallai, S.; Gandhi, R.; Wilkinson, I.D.; Tesfaye, S. SUDOSCAN: A Simple, Rapid, and Objective Method with Potential for Screening for Diabetic Peripheral Neuropathy. *PLoS ONE* **2015**, *10*, e0138224. [CrossRef] [PubMed]

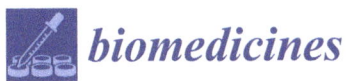

Systematic Review

Optical Coherence Tomography Angiography in Diabetic Patients: A Systematic Review

Ana Boned-Murillo [1,†], Henar Albertos-Arranz [2,†], María Dolores Diaz-Barreda [1], Elvira Orduna-Hospital [3,4], Ana Sánchez-Cano [3,4], Antonio Ferreras [3,5], Nicolás Cuenca [2] and Isabel Pinilla [1,3,6,*]

1. Department of Ophthalmology, Lozano Blesa University Hospital, 50009 Zaragoza, Spain; abonedm@salud.aragon.es (A.B.-M.); mddiaz@salud.aragon.es (M.D.D.-B.)
2. Department of Physiology, Genetics and Microbiology, University of Alicante, 03690 Alicante, Spain; henar.albertos@ua.es (H.A.-A.); cuenca@ua.es (N.C.)
3. Aragón Health Research Institute (IIS Aragón), 50009 Zaragoza, Spain; eordunahospital@unizar.es (E.O.-H.); anaisa@unizar.es (A.S.-C.); aferreras@unizar.es (A.F.)
4. Department of Applied Physics, University of Zaragoza, 50009 Zaragoza, Spain
5. Department of Ophthalmology, Miguel Servet University Hospital, 50009 Zaragoza, Spain
6. Department of Surgery, University of Zaragoza, 50009 Zaragoza, Spain
* Correspondence: ipinilla@unizar.es; Tel.: +34-696-808-295
† These authors contributed equally to this work.

Abstract: Background: Diabetic retinopathy (DR) is the leading cause of legal blindness in the working population in developed countries. Optical coherence tomography (OCT) angiography (OCTA) has risen as an essential tool in the diagnosis and control of diabetic patients, with and without DR, allowing visualisation of the retinal and choroidal microvasculature, their qualitative and quantitative changes, the progression of vascular disease, quantification of ischaemic areas, and the detection of preclinical changes. The aim of this article is to analyse the current applications of OCTA and provide an updated overview of them in the evaluation of DR. Methods: A systematic literature search was performed in PubMed and Embase, including the keywords "OCTA" OR "OCT angiography" OR "optical coherence tomography angiography" AND "diabetes" OR "diabetes mellitus" OR "diabetic retinopathy" OR "diabetic maculopathy" OR "diabetic macular oedema" OR "diabetic macular ischaemia". Of the 1456 studies initially identified, 107 studies were screened after duplication, and those articles that did not meet the selection criteria were removed. Finally, after looking for missing data, we included 135 studies in this review. Results: We present the common and distinctive findings in the analysed papers after the literature search including the diagnostic use of OCTA in diabetes mellitus (DM) patients. We describe previous findings in retinal vascularization, including microaneurysms, foveal avascular zone (FAZ) changes in both size and morphology, changes in vascular perfusion, the appearance of retinal microvascular abnormalities or new vessels, and diabetic macular oedema (DME) and the use of deep learning technology applied to this disease. Conclusion: OCTA findings enable the diagnosis and follow-up of DM patients, including those with no detectable lesions with other devices. The evaluation of retinal and choroidal plexuses using OCTA is a fundamental tool for the diagnosis and prognosis of DR.

Keywords: diabetes mellitus; diabetic retinopathy; foveal avascular zone; FAZ; optical coherence tomography angiography; OCTA; diabetic macular oedema

Citation: Boned-Murillo, A.; Albertos-Arranz, H.; Diaz-Barreda, M.D.; Orduna-Hospital, E.; Sánchez-Cano, A.; Ferreras, A.; Cuenca, N.; Pinilla, I. Optical Coherence Tomography Angiography in Diabetic Patients: A Systematic Review. *Biomedicines* 2022, 10, 88. https://doi.org/10.3390/biomedicines10010088

Academic Editor: Maria Grau

Received: 8 December 2021
Accepted: 29 December 2021
Published: 31 December 2021

Publisher's Note: MDPI stays neutral with regard to jurisdictional claims in published maps and institutional affiliations.

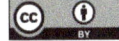

Copyright: © 2021 by the authors. Licensee MDPI, Basel, Switzerland. This article is an open access article distributed under the terms and conditions of the Creative Commons Attribution (CC BY) license (https://creativecommons.org/licenses/by/4.0/).

1. Introduction

Diabetes mellitus (DM) is a metabolic disease caused by an increase in glucose levels due to a diminution of insulin secretion or an increase in resistance to its activity. DM is expected to increase worldwide in a rapid manner, increasing by 25% by 2030 and 51% by 2045 [1].

Diabetic retinopathy (DR) is the most severe and frequent ophthalmic complication [1,2]. DR is the leading cause of legal blindness in the working population in developing countries. Diabetic patients may primarily have a neurodegeneration process in the retina, followed by well-known changes at the microvascular net, with pericyte loss and an increase in thickness of the basal membrane, with a breakdown of the inner blood retinal barrier. Although there is a trend towards a reduction in proliferative DR incidence due to improved control, the prevalence of DR in DM patients is approximately 35% of that in other patients [3–6]. There was a period with no DR signs but neuronal degeneration and microvascular changes, which were not detectable by ordinary examination. Any method that could help to find changes before these changes are evident would be a fundamental tool as a disease biomarker [7].

The Early Treatment Diabetic Retinopathy Study (ETDRS) divided DR into groups: nonproliferative DR (NPDR) and proliferative DR (PDR). NPDR can be divided into mild, moderate, and severe DR [8]. At each level, patients present different changes in their fundus related to either an increase in vessel permeability or a diminution of the vascular supply, including microaneurysms (MAs), exudation or oedema, haemorrhages, intraretinal microvascular abnormalities (IRMAs), vascular changes, and neovascularization (NV) [9].

Clinical examination of diabetic patients was based on ophthalmoscopy under mydriasis, fundus photography, fluorescein angiography (FA), and optical coherence tomography (OCT).

FA has been considered the gold standard to evaluate retinal vascularization [10]. FA can evaluate vascular integrity, the presence of MA, the loss of vascular perfusion, and the increased permeability of the vessels generating oedema and NV. FA is an invasive test that can generate severe adverse effects in a small percentage of patients [11]. Due to its potential secondary effects, it is not usually performed as a screening method.

The development of OCT angiography (OCTA) has been an important tool in the control of DM patients with and without microvascular lesions.

1.1. Morphology of the Retinal and Choroidal Blood Vessels

The central retinal artery, a terminal branch of the ophthalmic artery, divides and forms the different retina plexuses covering the entire retina, excluding the central foveal avascular zone (FAZ) and the most peripheral 1–1.5 mm [12–15]. The number of retinal plexuses varies from one to four depending on the eccentricity [16]. These plexuses are the radial peripapillary capillary network (RPCN), close to the optic nerve head, the superficial capillary plexus (SCP), the intermediate capillary plexus (ICP), and the deep capillary plexus (DCP) [17]. The rest of the central retina is formed by the SCP, ICP, and DCP [17] (Figure 1). For more information about retinal morphology and vascularization, see Supplementary File S1.

1.2. Optical Coherence Tomography Angiography (OCTA)

OCTA is a new non-invasive angiography technique based on OCT technology that can be performed without pupillary dilation. It provides high-resolution images of the retinal capillary plexuses and the choriocapillaris (CC) without using any contrast in a rapid and easy way. Using more advanced hardware and acquisition software, OCTA enables greyscale retinal vascular flow imaging. It can provide perfusion density maps and average perfusion density. OCTA is able to visualise changes in the DR, such as MA, nonperfusion areas, IRMA, or NV. OCTA can demonstrate noncapillary perfusion areas even better than FA, and the image will not have interference from any leakage [18,19]. It is based on the detection of moving blood cells, such as red blood cells. Performing consecutive B-scans in the same location on the retina shows the presence of movement through the blood vessels. The change in contrast over time indicates the vessel location and erythrocyte movement through them [20]. Changes are subsequently processed with different computer algorithms. This technology allows en face images and reconstructions of different retinal layers to be obtained. Image capture in OCTA requires great precision because it is based on differential analysis of the B-scan changes related to erythrocyte micromovements and the high sequential image speeds of the devices [20].

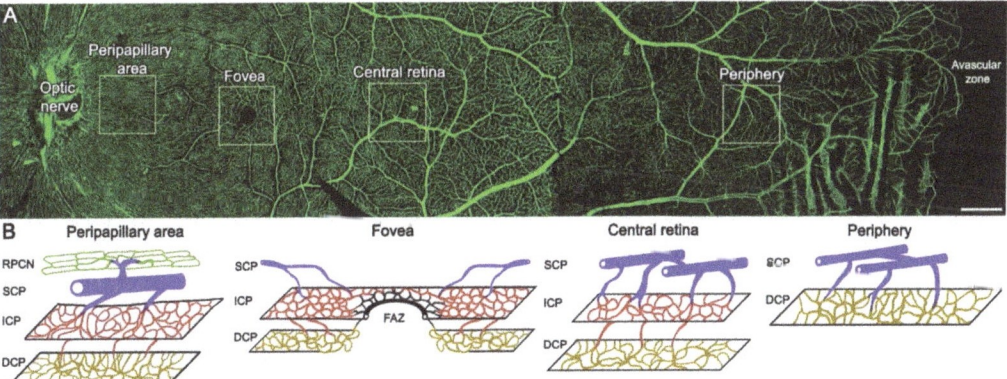

Figure 1. Morphological changes in the vascular plexuses throughout the human retina. (**A**) Whole-mount human retina immunostained with an antibody against collagen type IV showing the vascular network from the optic nerve to *Ora serrata*. (**B**) Drawings of the different plexuses corresponding to the insets in (**A**). Four plexuses can be observed in the peripapillary area (RPCN, SCP, ICP, and DCP) close to the optic nerve. The central retina is composed of three plexuses (SCP, ICP, and DCP), except in the fovea where the foveal avascular zone (FAZ) exists. Only two plexuses (SCP and DCP) are present in the far-periphery area. RPCN, radial peripapillary capillary network; SCP, superficial capillary plexus; ICP, intermediate capillary plexus; DCP, deep capillary plexus. Scale bar: 1 mm.

The maps generated by OCTA are a representation of retinal vascularization over a particular area of interest, in this case the macular area, and according to different anatomically interesting segmentation profiles. In OCTA, the introduction of projection resolved OCTA algorithms and three-dimensional visualisation increased the depth quality of the images. OCTA allows retinal segmentation into different vascular and nonvascular layers: SCP, ICP, DCP, external retina, and CC. The introduction of wild field (WF) OCTA allows better knowledge of the capillary plexuses in both the mid- and far periphery. The in-depth resolution enables visualisation of aneurysmal dilatations in the plexuses, avascular or low perfusion areas, retinal NV or intraretinal shunts, vascular structures in the choroid, or loss of CC vessels.

OCTA provides a dye-free image useful to detect angiographic signs of DR and changes in the capillary network at the macular level, even before onset of the disease. In patients with DR, areas of nonperfusion and their location in the SCP and DCP, as well as irregular capillaries, MA dilatations, and modifications in the CC layer, have been clearly analysed [21,22]. In addition to these qualitative characteristics, OCTA can provide a quantitative analysis of the density and flow of retinal blood vessels in each layer [23].

OCTA disadvantages include the loss of findings in which flow is slow, the inability to see leakage or staining, and difficulty visualising the peripheral retina. OCTA is an effective tool to evaluate DR, but the large amount of data and protocols can generate problems in the most sensitive parameters [24].

In summary, OCTA data acquisition is faster than FA and is three-dimensional and depth-resolved, allowing individual capillary plexuses automatically assessment based on current software algorithm. OCTA allows the visualisation of all plexuses, including the intermediate capillary, detecting pathological features that are not available in traditional dye-based angiography. In addition, as a non-invasive and rapid test, it is adequate for patients who require frequent follow-up exams. Nevertheless, FA is still the gold standard for retinal vessel evaluation, providing some additional findings such as leakage.

The purpose of this review was to provide an actual summary of the different findings assessed by OCTA and the diagnostic value of OCTA in DR patients, which is a great future challenge due to the prevalence of DM and the heavy burden caused by DR.

2. Methods

2.1. Literature Search

A systematic review was performed following the Preferred Reporting Items for Systematic Reviews and Meta-Analyses (PRISMA) guidelines [25] using a PRISMA checklist. It included a comprehensive search of different databases, including PubMed and EMBASE, last run-on 15 April 2021, for the following terms: OCTA OR OCT angiography OR optical coherence tomography angiography AND diabetes OR diabetes mellitus OR diabetic retinopathy OR diabetic maculopathy OR diabetic macular oedema OR diabetic macular ischaemia including MeSH terms and synonyms.

2.2. Inclusion/Exclusion Criteria

The search was performed to identify those studies in which OCTA was used to image diabetes patients with or without any type of DR. The included studies were limited to those published in English and in peer-reviewed journals, excluding case reports, conference proceedings and letters, and studies based on time-domain OCT. No restrictions existed for age, diabetes type or control, or follow-up.

2.3. Literature Review

Using the search criteria described above, a total of 829 results in PubMed and 627 in Embase, a total of 1456 records were found. PRISMA search was performed by three authors. After an initial review of abstracts by two independent reviewers, removal of duplicate studies or those articles that did not meet the selection criteria, 107 articles were selected for a full literature review. Other papers previously cited that were not selected, which appeared to be important to our review, were added supported by a third author, and at the end, a total of 135 studies were included in this qualitative systematic review. OCTA has been used to evaluate any kind of change in DM patients with or without DR. We described selected paper findings in the FAZ, MA, nonperfusion areas, ischaemia, IRMA, NV, and diabetic macular oedema (DME) (Figure 2).

Each of these topics will be discussed in turn, followed by a discussion of OCTA's future directions in DR.

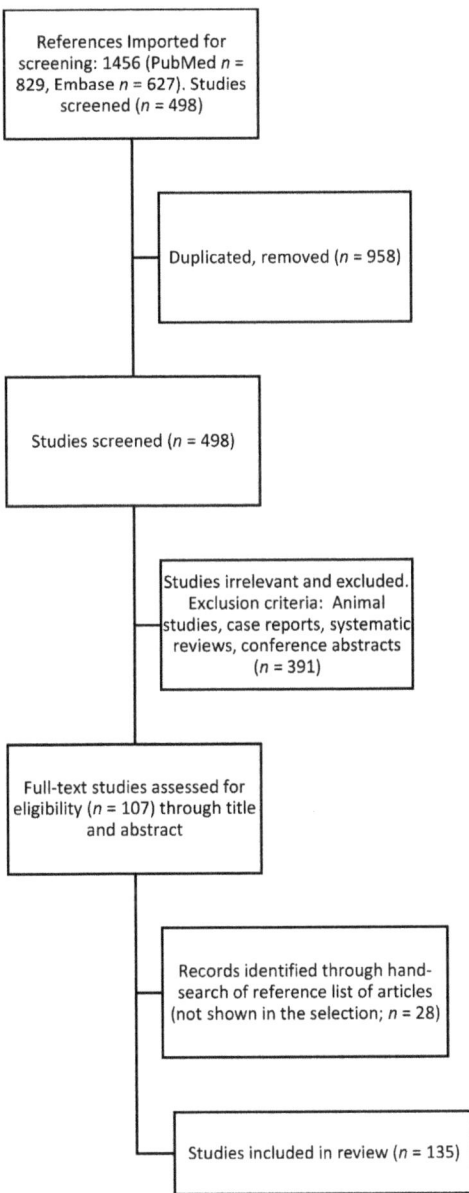

Figure 2. Flow chart explaining the literature selection. A systematic review was performed following PRISMA guidelines. A total of 1456 records were selected (829 in PubMed and 627 in Embase), and after the removal of duplicate studies or articles that did not meet the selection criteria, 107 articles were selected for a full literature review. Ultimately, a total of 135 studies were included after adding important works that were not found in the databases.

3. Results and Discussion

3.1. Foveal Avascular Zone

Different papers have analysed FAZ changes in either diabetes mellitus type 1 (DM1) or diabetes mellitus type 2 (DM2) with or without DR. FAZ has previously been analysed using FA, only evaluating changes at the SCP. FA showed that FAZ increased in DR with retinopathy stage [26] due to loss of the surrounding capillary [27]. Studies have demonstrated that compared with FA, OCTA allows better discrimination of the central and parafoveal macular microvasculature, especially for FAZ disruption and capillary dropout [28] (Figure 3A,B).

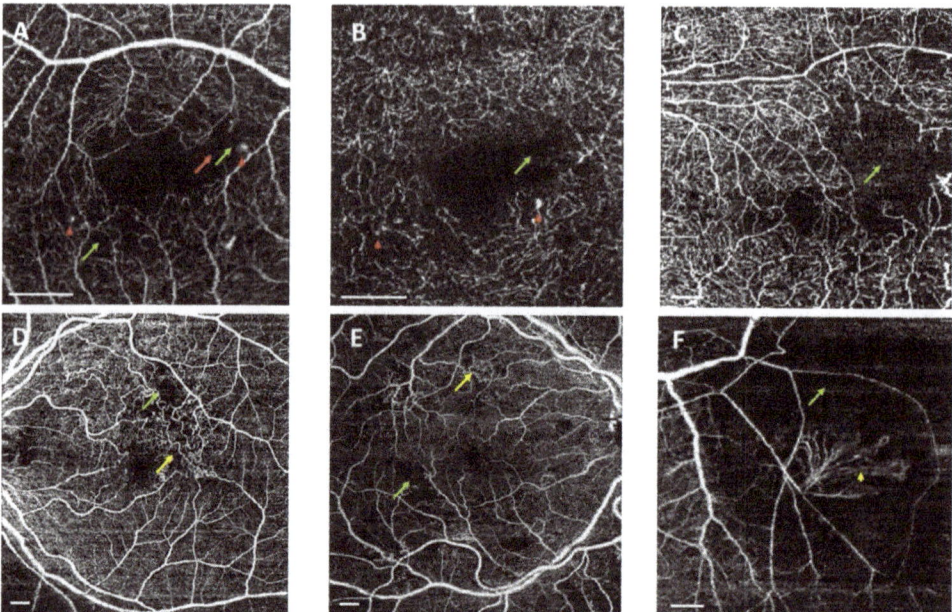

Figure 3. Swept source optical coherence tomography angiography (SS-OCTA) showing representative examples of OCTA findings in diabetic patients. OCTA was acquired using DRI-Triton SS-OCT (Topcon, Tokyo, Japan). (**A,B**) Superficial (SCP) and deep capillary plexuses (DCP) in 3 × 3 mm scans. Figure 3C shows SCP in a 6 × 6 scan. (**D,E**) The SCP in a 9 × 9 scan and 3F SCP in a 6 × 6 scan protocol. (**B**) An irregular foveal avascular zone (red arrows) and microaneurysms (red arrowheads) in the superficial and deep capillary plexuses. (**C**) Nonperfusion areas in the temporal area (green arrows). (**D,E**) Areas of impaired perfusion associated with intraretinal microvascular abnormalities (yellow arrows). (**F**) Retinal neovascularization elsewhere (yellow arrowhead). Scale bar represents 1 mm.

Nevertheless, not all OCTA studies in DM had the same results evaluating the FAZ, and the methodology differed between them, evaluating the plexuses one by one or all in total. Other discrepancies between studies were in the way they dealt with projection artefacts or artefacts caused by vitreous opacities [29].

The first author who analysed OCTA changes in patients with no DR signs was De Carlo [30], who demonstrated that DM without DR showed an increase in the FAZ and areas of capillary nonperfusion (considering both DM1 and DM2 patients). Similarly, Dimitrova and colleagues showed an increase in the FAZ of the SCP in DM patients without DR as well as a decrease in vessel density (VD) in both plexuses [31] (Figure 4).

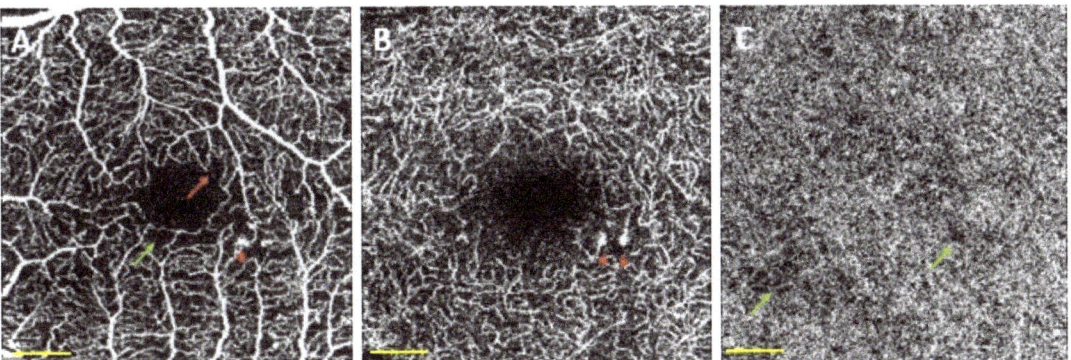

Figure 4. Optical coherence tomography angiography (OCTA) of a diabetic patient without detectable diabetic lesions. OCTA was acquired using DRI-Triton SS-OCT (Topcon, Tokyo, Japan) with a 3 × 3 mm scan protocol. (**A**) Superficial capillary plexus, (**B**) deep capillary plexus, and (**C**) choriocapillaris (CC). Red arrow shows a disruption in the foveal avascular zone (FAZ), red arrowheads correspond to microaneurysms, and green arrows correspond to non-perfusion areas in the CC. Scale bar (in yellow) represents 500 microns.

Takase et al., found an increase in the en face FAZ in all DM patients with or without DR signs [32], and Di et al., described an increase in FAZ in DM patients. They found that patients with more severe retinal damage had a much larger FAZ, with changes in the area and vertical and horizontal radius [33]. An enlarged FAZ associated with a reduction in the VD of the SCP and DCP in the foveal and parafoveal areas has been observed in patients with NPDR [34]. Comparing DM1 patients without DR or with mild NPDR with controls, Simonett et al., suggested that parafoveal capillary nonperfusion in DM1 is an early marker of retinal changes starting in the DCP [35]. Wang et al., as previously described, postulated that FAZ metrics may have a prognostic value in DR progression, DME, and visual acuity (VA), but highlighted that the high variation among normal individuals in FAZ area and perimeter makes them less than ideal biomarkers for staging DR. None of their FAZ metrics differed with the severity of DR, indicating that they may not play an important role in advanced DR, but may have a prognostic role in predicting DR progression, DME, and VA [36].

Parafoveal nonperfusion has been analysed using different strategies to identify a better biomarker for DR severity [23,37–39] and ischaemic index [40]. When the DR appeared, this density changed into a progressive loss of the capillary network. Xu and You [29,41] indicated that FAZ and nonperfusion areas were both significantly larger in the diabetic group, whereas the FAZ circularity was significantly smaller [41]. You et al. also demonstrated that treatment requirements were related to the extrafoveal avascular areas for the baseline DCP [29]. The nonperfusion ratio was studied by Wang et al., who found a significantly lower parafoveal VD in DR patients compared with those without DR, with an increase in VD loss related to DR severity [42]. VD diminished with age and higher HbA1c levels, and patients with DME had a significantly lower average parafoveal VD according to Xie and colleagues [43]. Other authors, such as Rosen, found an increased area of capillary density in DM patients without DR after extracting the noncapillary structures, suggesting an autoregulatory response to an increase in metabolic needs [44], highlighting that OCTA may help identify early-stage DR before retinopathy is apparent. Rosen suggested that perfused capillary density is a more sensitive marker to detect differences between healthy individuals and DM patients than FAZ metrics [44].

In contrast, some studies deny OCTA as the most appropriate tool for detecting preclinical changes in patients with diabetes, suggesting that clinical examinations and glycaemic control should be kept on as the primary clinical parameter during DR screening [45].

Differences in FAZ parameters between DM1 and DM2 patients have been studied. Oliverio et al. found that changes in FAZ parameters were more pronounced in DM1, and these modifications were correlated with the duration of the disease [46]. Vujosevic and Um indicated that the increase in FAZ area, and a decrease in VD, are related to DR progression and are more severe in the DCP than in the SCP in both DM types [47,48].

Changes in the FAZ can be related to visual impairment [49,50], as was demonstrated in Samara's study. They found a negative correlation between logMAR VA and VD in both SCP and DCP, and a positive correlation between logMAR VA and FAZ area in both plexuses [51].

FAZ morphology can be visualised in en face projections. The SCP is formed by large and small capillaries that end at the FAZ as a terminate capillary ring with a centripetally branching pattern. The DCP ends at the macula with lobular patterns with no direction [16]. The acircularity index provides information about the extent to which the FAZ differs from a circle. Krawitz and colleagues found differences in the FAZ shape between controls and all DR patients, but not DM patients with no lesions. The mean acircularity index was 1.32 in both the control and no DR groups, 1.57 in the NPDR group, and 1.78 in the PDR group. There were no differences between NPDR and PDR [52]. They also considered the axis ratio as an index of disease progression and therapeutic interventions. The average axis ratios were 1.17, 1.12, 1.27, and 1.33 in the different stages. A higher acircularity index and axis ratio were associated with a worse stage of DR.

Zahid and colleagues [53], using fractal dimension (FD) analysis, a mathematical method to evaluate the complexity of tissues, found a reduction in the flow in DR, both in SCP and DCP, in the absence of DME. Tang et al. also observed a lower FD associated with DR severity and an increased FAZ area and decreased FAZ circularity [54]. The study performed by Sun et al. evaluated the risk of DR progression and DME development beyond traditional risk factors and related FAZ area, VD, and FD of DCP with DR progression, whereas VD of SCP would predict DME development [55]. Other authors suggested FD-300 analysis (VD of a 300 μm width annulus surrounding the FAZ) was useful for detecting preclinical microvascular alterations in DR screening [56].

In addition, the decrease in FAZ circularity and parafoveal vessel density are postulated to be related to structural retinal neurodegeneration, because they would be highly correlated with ganglion cell layer—inner plexiform layer (GCL-IPL) thinning, regardless of the presence of DR, and would predict microvascular impairment in early DR [57,58].

3.1.1. Microaneurysms

Microaneurysms (MAs) were identified using OCTA (Figure 3A,B). We found saccular dilatation or fusiform capillaries, as described by Ishibazawa et al. [18], in both the SCP and DCP. According to Park and colleagues [59], it is also possible to identify MAs in the ICP. OCTA is able to identify a smaller number of MAs than FA, but it has the ability to detect MAs in both the SCP and DCP (Figure 5).

Salz and colleagues found that compared with FA, OCTA had a sensitivity of 85% (95% CI, 53–97%) and a specificity of 75% (95% CI, 21–98%) in detecting MAs. [60]. These results have been supported by other studies [19,61]. Soares and colleagues compared FA and OCTA AngioVue and AngioPlex, with FA being superior to both for detecting MAs in both the SCP and total retina slab [28]. As already described, MAs were more frequently located in the DCP. MAs were related to ischaemic areas, and they found MAs surrounding nonperfusion areas (NPAs) [19]. Parrulli et al. also found that FA is the best way to detect MAs. OCTA devices can differentiate their detection depending on the number of B-scans, with great variability between devices [62]. Hamada et al. also found discrepancies between FA, OCT B-scan, and OCTA, with the latter being able to overlook MAs in patients with diabetic macular oedema (DME) [63].

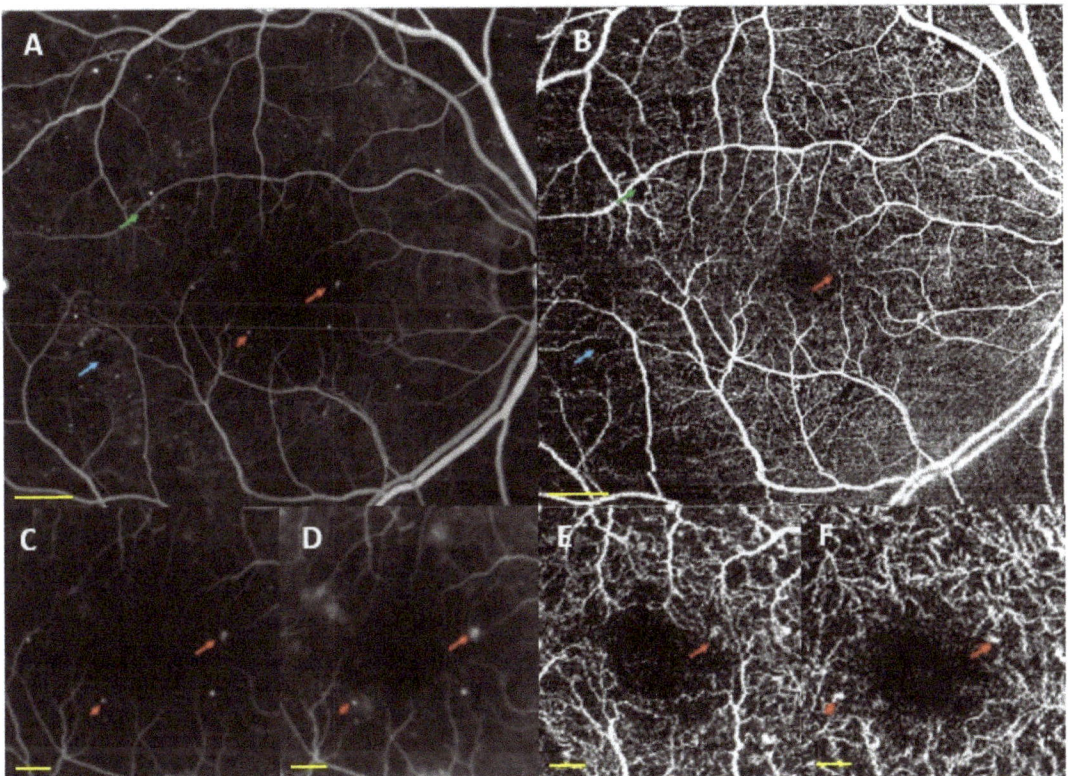

Figure 5. Fluorescein angiography (FA) (**A,C,D**) vs. swept source optical coherence tomography angiography (SS-OCTA) (**B,E,F**) showing microaneurysms (MAs) (red arrow and arrowhead) in diabetic patients. (**A,C,D**) MAs in the superficial and deep capillary plexuses (SCP and DCP) and nonperfusion areas (green and blue arrows) detected by (**A,B,E,F**) show the same MAs in SCP (**E**), DCP (**F**), and nonperfusion areas (**B**), visualised by OCTA. FA was acquired using a Spectralis-HRA (Heidelberg Engineering, Heidelberg, Germany). (**A,C**) Arterial time in the FA and (**D**) tissue times. OCTA was acquired with DRI-Triton SS-OCT (Topcon, Tokyo, Japan). (**B**) 9 × 9 mm OCTA and (**E,F**) 3 × 3 mm OCTA of both SCP and DCP, respectively. Scale bar (in yellow) represents 1 mm in Figure 5A,B and 250 microns in Figure 5C,F.

Park et al. described MAs in all three plexuses [59]. Other authors found a higher number of MAs in the DCP than in the SCP [18,19,64]. Byeon et al. described the deep location of the MA [65] leaking in the outer plexiform layer (OPL). MAs can protrude towards outer layers, such as the outer nuclear layer (ONL).

Some authors have correlated the MAs on structural OCT and OCTA. Parravano studied the correlation between them and their evolution [64,66]. They described two MA patterns based on OCT findings. Hyporeflective lesions on structural OCT were less visualised using OCTA than hyper-reflective or moderate lesions (66.7% vs. 88.9%). They suggested that the hyporeactive lesions could have a lower flow that was not detected with OCTA. Other authors have suggested the possibility of turbulent flow [18], or that MAs are not perfused with luminal fibrosis and lipid infiltration in their histology [67]. Parravano [64,66] also described the different behaviours depending on their OCT reflectivity. MAs that developed over 12 months in extracellular fluid were hyper-reflective (66% vs. 18% of the hyporeactive MAs). The location was also related to fluid development: those located in the DCP were those which leaked after one year. The relationship of DCP MAs with the development of DME has also been described by Hasegawa et al. [68]. In summary, 12 months after their description, MAs with a hyper-reflective pattern persisted on OCTA and were mainly located in the DCP.

Schaal et al., studied the agreement in the detection of DR signs on colour fundus photography (CFP) versus SS-OCTA. In patients with an ETDRS level ≥ CFP, MAs were found in 90% of the cases, close to 91% of which were found with OCTA. They suggested that MAs are more apparent on the 3 × 3 mm scan than on the 12 × 12 scan due to the lower resolution [69]. Following their assessment of WF-OCTA, Tian and colleagues used 12 × 12 mm scanning with different slabs for MAs. They analysed 247 eyes of patients with DM and detected MAs in 60.6% of the eyes using the retinal slab and 59.8% in the SCP slab, with no significant differences between them. No MAs were evaluated in the deep slab because of the poor details. This study provides similar results in relation to IRMAs [70].

Carnevalli and colleagues did not find MAs in their DM1 patients or other anatomical changes. Their population was young (mean age 22 ± 2 years) and had a short disease duration (11 ± 4 years) [71]. They only found rarefaction of the perifoveal capillary network in the SCP in 28% of their series. Park and colleagues evaluated the microvascular changes in the foveal and parafoveal areas in 64 patients with NDR and a mean age of 61.0 ± 9.34 years. They identified MAs in only 9.38% of the cases. They found no association between changes in VD occurring in the different plexuses, disease duration, best corrected visual acuity (BCVA), FAZs, or analytical parameters (HbA1c, serum creatinine or e-GRF) [72].

In 2019, Thompson et al., found MAs in 60% of their patients, a small sample of DM2 with good glycaemic control and without DR signs [73].

3.1.2. Nonperfusion Areas

Loss of vascular perfusion is an indication of ischaemia. OCTA can evaluate both macular and peripheral retinas using WF strategies, including WF-OCTA. Macular ischaemia is related to VA in DM patients. NPAs were evaluated using automated quantification of the VD or the total area of vessel nonperfusion and with the FAZ diameter and changes.

FA shows NPA between the large retinal vessel. OCTA detected NPAs not only in the SCP, but also in the ICP and DCP (Figure 3C–F). OCTA clearly visualised the border between sparse capillary areas and dense capillary areas, with a sensitivity of 98% and specificity of 82%. Therefore, OCTA is a better procedure to detect capillary density than conventional FA [18,19,74]. This capillary density reduction is associated with remodelling and enlargement of the FAZ even before MAs, which are currently believed to be the first clinical sign of DR [75]. De Carlo et al. [30] reported changes in the FAZ (increased FAZ area and the presence of FAZ remodelling) and capillary nonperfusion in patients with DM with no signs of DR.

Loss of perfusion has been described in all plexuses, including the ICP [76]. Onishi et al. suggested a significant increase in NPAs in all three plexuses in the NPDR group compared with controls. Zhang et al., also identified a significant increase in superficial NPAs in DM patients without DR compared with controls [74,76]. The authors emphasise the importance of OCTA segmentation schemes that consider the ICP separately from the SCP and DCP. Simonett et al. [35], studying patients with DM1 and without DR or with mild NPDR, reported a decreased parafoveal VD (similar to parafoveal capillary nonperfusion) only in the DCP, with no changes in the FAZ area in either the SCP or DCP. Dimitrova et al. [31] documented a decreased parafoveal VD in the SCP and DCP and an increased FAZ area in the SCP in patients with DM (mostly in DM2) and no DR compared with control subjects. Choi et al. [77] documented retinal microvascular abnormalities (including capillary dropout, dilated capillary loops, tortuous capillary branches, patches of reduced capillary perfusion, irregular FAZ contours, and/or FAZ enlargement) in all 3 plexuses in 18 of the 51 eyes with DM and no clinical signs of DR (with no specification of DM type). Moreover, these authors reported focal or diffuse CC flow impairment in almost half of the evaluated patients without DR.

DM patients showed a progressive diminution of the capillary density with the severity of the ocular manifestations [28]. Severe NPDRs showed an increase in NPAs [78], enlarged spaces between the large and small vessels in the SCP and DCP with an increased and irregular FAZ. IRMAs and NVCs were more frequently associated with NPAs [79]. Vujosevic et al. indicated that both SCP and DCP are prematurely altered in patients with DM1 and without clinical signs of DR, whereas in patients with DM2, the DCP is the first affected plexus [48].

Although there are different results, NPAs and capillary dilation have been described as more prominent in the SCP, and MA is common in the DCP. Studies have revealed that the severity of vascular changes in the SCP is closely related to abnormalities in the SCP [78].

Nesper et al., described the percentage area of the retina and CC related to NPA. NPA was significantly correlated with disease stage when considering retinal vascular changes, but no significant correlation was found for CC [75,80].

Yasukura et al. studied differences between macular and extramacular NPAs related to arterial distribution [81]. They did not find differences in extramacular NPAs between severe NPDR and PDR. Eyes with PDR had significantly greater NPAs in the macular area than those with severe NPDR. They suggested that the extramacular region between two arteriolar branches is the most vulnerable to DM capillary loss [81].

OCTA demonstrated impaired perfusion within cotton-wool spots [21]. Extramacular cotton-wool spots (or white spots) are mostly associated with NPAs encompassing all retinal layers, in contrast to macular cotton-wool spots that are more associated with NPAs in the superficial layer only [80].

WF-OCTA demonstrates preferential location of NPAs along the main retinal arteries in all stages of DR. Tan et al., using 12 × 12 WF-OCTA, found an increase in capillary dropout in the peripheral annulus that increases with the severity of DR. They suggested that the capillary dropout density in the peripheral subfield is the best parameter to discriminate between mild NPDR and DM patients without DR [82]. Diabetic microangiopathy is a midperipheral disease and firstly affects the temporal quadrants. The midperiphery has a smaller vascular supply (vascular plexuses merged from three to two plexuses), and the nasal quadrants are supplied by the radial peripapillary capillary plexus [83]. Ishibazawa et al. studied NPAs with OCT images and found that NPAs were more frequently adjacent to arterial vessels. They hypothesised that diabetic microangiopathy started near the arterial side, with no regard to the level of DR severity, and then progressed towards the venous side [84].

In addition, more pronounced vascular involvement in the DCP has been described, regardless of the stage of DR, which may be explained by the difference in the perfusion pressure between the SCP and the DCP [85].

Thus, the advantage of OCTA lies in its ability to detect both peripheral retinal non-perfusion and eventual peripheral active NV, which remains difficult to visualise clinically.

3.1.3. Ischaemia

DM patients exhibit a reduction in capillary density. Diabetic macular ischaemia (DMI) is associated with an enlargement and disruption of the FAZ and with retinal capillary dropout in noncontiguous areas of the macula, providing important clinical and prognostic information regarding disease severity and predicting DR progression [52,86–88]. Similar to FA, OCTA is capable of grading and quantifying DMI through several OCTA parameters, such as the perifoveal intercapillary area, total avascular area, or extrafoveal avascular area [89]. OCTA is better at detecting capillary density than conventional FA [18,19]. One of the key advantages of OCTA over FA is the ability to noninvasively detect DMI [90]. OCTA could even identify DMI in eyes with relatively few symptoms. The FAZ area in both the SCP and DCP increased with DR severity, and the FAZ area (at SCP) correlated with retinal sensitivity at baseline [91]. However, it remains unclear whether eyes with DMI detected by OCTA have higher risk of progressive visual loss the OCTA findings continue to deteriorate over time. Loss of perfusion has been described in all plexuses. Authors agree that grading DMI in the three plexuses (SCP, ICP, and DCP) had a higher sensitivity and specificity for determining DR stage and comparing DR versus healthy controls [59] than full retinal angiograms [92]. Changes in the ICP are important to consider [76].

Significant deterioration in OCTA parameters over time in DR patients has been described. Kim et al. [57] recently reported that microvascular impairment is progressive even in early stages of DR. They observed SCP VD loss in 40 eyes with no DR or mild NPDR over a period of two years. However, DCP VD was not studied in this report [57]. Tsai et al. [91] observed a significant deterioration in the DCP parafoveal VD and SCP FAZ area in patients with various severities of DR at baseline over a one-year follow-up period. A larger DCP FAZ area at baseline was associated with a significant worsening of BCVA over one year. Similar to previous studies, Xie et al. [43] and Ragkousis et al. [56] observed a decrease in parafoveal vascular density as the disease progressed. In this sense, in addition to the density of the DCP, other parameters, such as the VD of the extrafoveal avascular area and the vessel length fraction of the DCP, appear to decrease with the severity of the disease [36]. Specifically, the vessel diameter index at the SCP and the VD in the DCP showed the best correlations with the severity of DR [36]. This finding not only provided evidence that OCTA parameters are able to predict visual outcomes in DR, but also suggests the importance of the detection and monitoring of DCP parameters in ischaemic conditions such as DR, as previously described.

Previous cross-sectional studies have correlated central visual loss in diabetic eyes with the degree of parafoveal capillary loss [50,51]. Such relationships are more prominent with alterations in the DCP than in the SCP [93,94]. Changes in the DCP have also been found to correlate better with DR severity than changes in the SCP [76]. These observations are supported by histologic studies that show higher vulnerability of the deep foveal plexus to endothelial injury [95]. Furthermore, there have been many reports highlighting DCP ischaemia, which is an important finding in DR. Scarinci et al. [96] suggested that nonperfusion of the DCP is associated with photoreceptor disruption in DMI. The flow density of CC in patients with severe DR seems to be associated with the severity of the disease because the flow decreases as the disease worsens [97]. Lee et al. [98] showed that a poor response to anti-VEGF agents in DME is associated with DCP damage but not SCP damage. An increase in DCP destruction with DR progression was also reported [99]. Early DCP vascular alterations were found, especially in DM1, which were evident even before the diagnosis of clinically detectable DR [71,100]. Moreover, VD in the fovea, parafovea, and peripapillary area and the flow area in the choroid was also reduced in DM2 patients without signs of DR [101,102]. The FAZ area and VD change more rapidly as DR progresses in the DCP than in the SCP during the progression of DR [47].

Tsai et al. [91] also demonstrated the predictive value of structural OCTA parameters in relation to visual outcomes beyond current established systemic risk factors. Larger baseline FAZ areas in the DPC were associated with worsening visual outcomes, and larger decreases in SCP VD were associated with worsening retinal sensitivity over one year. These associations support the use of OCTA in the early detection and monitoring of DMI. Additionally, it has been demonstrated that OCTA parameters such as larger FAZ areas and lower VD in DCP at baseline increase the likelihood of DR progression within two years [55].

Cao et al. found that OCTA can be a useful way to identify preclinical lesions in DM2 based on capillary perfusion. They found a decreased vessel density in the SCP, DCP, and CC in DM2 patients before having any DR signs, without changes in the FAZ area [103]. When analysing capillary perfusion in SCP, DCP, and CC in the 3 × 3 mm and 6 × 6 mm protocols, diabetic patients had significantly lower perfusion than the control group. Normal subjects had higher capillary perfusion rates than patients diagnosed with mild nonproliferative DR (NPDR) [104,105].

The identification of DCP by OCTA plays an important role in DMI. Minnella et al. studied eyes with DMI and demonstrated significantly increased perifoveal "no flow" areas in both the SCP and DCP compared with controls, and Scarinci et al. found that these areas of DCP nonperfusion corresponded precisely with areas of outer retinal disruption on structural OCT imaging [96,106].

Furthermore, vascular complexity and morphology are evaluated by combining VD, fractal dimension, and vessel diameter and allow to define the state of DR. VD, defined as the ratio of blood vessel area to the total measured area, decreases in both SCP and DCP in patients with DR and in diabetic patients without DR [78,107].

Taewoong et al. [47] showed a deterioration in the FAZ area and VD in the SCP and DCP as DR progressed in both DM1 and DM2, similar to previous reports [23,108]. This deterioration was more prominent in DCP than in SCP, regardless of the diabetic type. However, in DM1, the deterioration of VD was delayed until the DR reached a severe NPDR stage, whereas there was a gradual decline in VD in DM2. This finding may be caused by differences in the pathophysiology of the two types of diabetes and may explain the different clinical manifestations [47].

Compared with eyes with mild and moderate NPDR, eyes with severe NPDR and PDR demonstrated a significant decrease in VD [86,109]. The superficial capillary network supplies the ganglion cell complex and inner nuclear layer; thus, a decreased superficial capillary network and loss of the ganglion cell complex have been detected [110].

Authors such as Wang et al. [111] and Agemy et al. [86] showed statistically significant reductions in VD in diabetic patients compared with controls using different approaches to calculate vascular density as a trend towards reducing vascular density with worsening severity of diabetic disease. Thus, the analysis of vessel density is associated with the degree of disease and risk of DR progression and may be a useful potential predictor of proliferative DR.

On the other hand, FD represents vascular complexity and microvascular morphology related to macular ischaemia in both SCP and DCP. Zahid et al. studied this entity and observed, DR patients showed a decrease in vascular density and increased fractal dimension with a greater average vascular calibre secondary to hypoxic conditions [7,53]. Ting et al. studied the capillary density index and FD in DM2 patients and reported a decrease in both SCP and DCP capillary density with DR progression and an increase in FD in both plexuses [108]. Moreover, receiver operating characteristic (ROC) curve analysis defined skeletonised FD, vessel length density, and vessel diameter index as the most effective parameters to detect glycaemic changes in DM2 patients [105].

FA images use the ETDRS protocols to grade DMI as follows: absent (no FAZ disruption), questionable (FAZ not smooth/oval, but no clear pathology), mild (<half FAZ circumference destroyed), moderate (>half FAZ circumference destroyed), severe (FAZ outline destroyed), or ungradable [10].

Several studies have compared OCT to the FA grading of DMI. Bradley et al., studied the reproducibility of the OCTA-based grading. SCP OCTA images were graded using the ETDRS protocols [88] and compared with FA images, at the DCP, this grading was absent (no disruption of FAZ), questionable (FAZ not smooth/oval, but no clear pathology), mild/moderate (FAZ disrupted in ≤ 2 quadrants), severe (FAZ disrupted in ≥ 3 quadrants), or ungradable (poor image quality, artefact). CC was graded as ischaemia present (loss of speckled hyper-reflectance or dark defects), ischaemia absent, or ungradable, and obtained substantial intergrader agreement in terms of the DMI grade acquired for the SCP, DCP, and CC [86].

3.1.4. Intraretinal Microvascular Abnormalities

OCTA can detect IRMA as intraretinal looping vessels of capillary origin with a larger calibre than the surrounding vessels with a flow that does not cross the internal limiting membrane (ILM), and they are usually located in areas with little or no perfusion [21,112] (Figure 3D,E). In contrast, NVE passes the ILM and protrudes into the vitreous cavity [85]. Matsunaga et al. described an increase in the calibre of the loops compared them to surrounding capillaries [21], and they described one case whose origin was a vessel with a large diameter [21]. Their characteristics make it difficult to detect them in CFP [69]. Schaal and colleagues found that OCTA had a higher detection rate than CFP. They analysed two cohorts of diabetic eyes in a retrospective cross-sectional observational study, one using SS-OCTA grading and the other comparing OCTA and CFP. In patients with ETDRS severity levels over 43, OCTA was able to detect a significantly higher number of IRMAs (85% of the sample) than CFP (detected in only 35%). The inter-device agreement was only fair, with k = 0.2. They suggested that the presence of adjacent areas of capillary dropout helps to identify IRMA detection with OCTA compared with CFP. These researchers also compared three different slabs with 12 × 12 WF-OCTA to detect DR findings. IRMAs were more frequently detected on the retinal slab but with no differences from the SCP slab [70]. Compared with FA, according to Arya et al. [113], OCTA achieved 99% specificity and 92% sensitivity. It might even be more accurate pictures, as it has no dye leakage that appears with FA and its ability to segment layers [112].

Furthermore, Cui et al. published a study [114] showing that ultra-widefield OCTA (UW-OCTA) was superior in the number of IRMAs detected per ultra-widefield CFP (UW-CFP) ($p < 0.001$) and had almost 100% agreement (k = 0.916) with ultra-widefield FA (UW-FA).

Regarding their distribution, Tian et al. [70] found no significant differences between the retinal and SCP slabs, detecting none in the SCP slab using the 12 × 12 mm swept source OCTA (SS-OCTA) protocol.

The utility of OCTA in the follow-up of DR patients with IRMA before and after different therapies has also been evaluated. Sorour et al. [115] used it to study the structural changes in 45 IRMAs after anti-VEGF treatment compared with patients with similar DR who did not receive treatment. At the baseline visit, they characterised different morphologies (dilated trunk, loop, pigtail, sea-fan-shaped, and net-shaped) with higher complexity and more advanced pathology. However, they found no relationship between them, the number of injections and their response to treatment. The quantity of IRMA detected with OCTA has also been related to the severity of DM according to Kaoual et al. [116].

Shimouchi et al. [117] conducted a retrospective study in 46 eyes of 29 patients proposing a classification to standardise the changes after panretinal photocoagulation (PRP). They established five groups: unchanged, tuft regression, repercussion, mixed, and worsening [118]. Those IRMAs that regressed were adjacent to areas of restored perfusion after PRP [117]. Russell et al. [119] also focused on changes after PRP in a prospective study of 20 patients. They found how four IRMAs detected in two different patients by FA, OCTA, and B-scan progressed to NV. The description of IRMAs as precursors of NV, although controversial, has been proposed and described in other investigations [120–122].

3.1.5. Neovascularization

Retinal NV is one of the key signs of PDR responsible for vision loss. Thus, early detection could improve visual prognosis [123]. Fundus eye exam, OCT, and FA have been used to identify NV [121]. FA has always been the gold standard to analyse NV. However, early leakage in FA prevents the exact assessment of NV areas, which can already be seen with OCTA [19,30,124]. OCTA imaging has become a useful tool for NV diagnosis [121]. OCTA can identify NV arising at the optic nerve (NVD) or in other retinal places (NVE). OCTA was also able to estimate NV activity (Figure 3F).

OCTA detects changes prior to the appearance of neovascularization and the presence of NV and assesses its progression, either in active or fibrotic NV. Onishi et al. discussed how the vascular changes "precursors of neovascularization" observed in the superficial plexus (dilatation, telangiectasia with high flows) can lead to a "steal phenomenon" increasing ischaemic phenomena in deeper plexuses [76].

Different authors have classified active NV by evaluating either the morphology of the NV and its origin [121,125] or blood flow and density maps [126]. One of the first descriptions of NV was given by Ishibazawa et al., characterising two different patterns both at the optic nerve and in other retinal places: one included exuberant vascular proliferation with small and irregular new vessels, and the other was described as pruned NVs that did not show leakage at the FA [125]. Elbendary et al. categorised active NVD according to their morphology on OCT, OCTA, and B-scan [126]. Blood flow data and density maps were the main features used to determine NV activity. They defined three different patterns in disk NV depending on the blood flow observed in OCT (vascular, fibrovascular, or fibrous component), and two in NV elsewhere, branching vascular tufts that turned into pruned vessels after treatment, or a flow area associated with a smaller lesion, similar to those that Hwang described similar to MA [127] or to type 1 NVE described by Pan [121]. In 2018, Pan and colleagues studied NVD origins and found that it could originate either from the retinal artery or vein or from the choroid. They provided the most comprehensive classification of NVE types: type 1, the most frequent type, which arises from veins of the superficial plexus, and after reaching the posterior hyaloid, it branches forming a tree-like shape; type 2 is born from capillaries of deep vascular layers and presents as an octopus-like structure at the ILM; type 3 originates from veins located between the inner nuclear layer (INL) and GCL and creates sea-fan-like IRMAs [121]. These NVE types arise from capillary nonperfusion areas or close to them [121]. This venous origin contravenes previous studies where arteries were considered the origin of NVEs using FA [128].

In diabetic patients, OCTA is an effective tool to recognise poorly perfused or ischaemic areas at the margins of which NV is thought to arise both at the level of the optic disc, which has been most studied to date and has been related to a larger area of nonperfused retina, and other locations, despite being more frequent according to some studies [125]. Moreover, although the presence of NV is linked with diabetic retinopathy per se, several demographic factors, such as male sex and black ethnicity, are related to larger areas of NV [129].

OCTA imaging has shown clear advantages over traditional systems for NV. Nevertheless, recent studies have proven that WF-OCTA) detects more NV areas than conventional OCTA [129]. In this sense, it is important to define the best protocol to detect most vascular alterations in retinal areas. Most of these lesions are located at the posterior pole or mid-periphery of the retina, and $12 \times 12°$ scans centred at the fovea and optic nerve and 15×9 scans are the most useful scans to localise NVE [129]. Although no differences were found between these scans, the 15×9 scan showed a greater number of artefacts [129]. Specifically, the detection rate of NV with 15×9 scans was 34.6%, compared with the detection rate of 17.6% using a 6×6 scan [129].

Thus, WF-OCTA has been proposed to be the only test necessary for the diagnosis and follow-up of NV because, taking FA as a reference, it has been demonstrated that fovea-centred WF-OCTA is able to reveal between 99.4% and 99.7% of NV [125]. Hirano and colleagues, using WF-OCTA with vitreoretinal interface segmentation, were able to detect NV in 84% of cases after manual segmentation. Automated segmentation with their devices had a 16% false-positive rate that diminished due to segmentation errors but was able to find nine NVs undetected with FA because of their small size [130]. Papayannis et al., using three new vitreo-retinal segmentation protocols with a Triton device, found a sensitivity and specificity in detecting NVD and NVE of 100% and 96.6%, respectively [124]. They used these new protocols to assess the activity of the NV.

On the other hand, Ishibazawa et al. observed and quantified the vascular changes (vascular density, ischaemia in the different plexuses) in NV and possible changes in the disc but did not confirm a correlated structural alteration [21,55,71]. Other changes in patients with NV were FAZ enlargement in both the SCP and DCP and/or nonperfusion areas [127].

3.1.6. Diabetic Macular Oedema

DME is the main cause of vision loss in patients with DR. Macular cysts are visualised on OCTA as hyporeflective areas devoid of capillaries or flow signals with smooth borders [60,131]. They are located in the deep layers of the neurosensorial retina [131]. Some concerns exist about the reliability of OCTA to visualise DCP in DME. The absence of capillaries in the cysts of both plexuses may be secondary to the displacement of capillaries at the periphery of the cysts or to the preferential development of cysts in nonperfusion areas [19,132]. There are other possible factors related to the vascular changes in DME, such as the fluid attenuating the decorrelation signal from surrounding capillaries, the cyst exerting mechanical pressure on the vessel, or the capillaries being incompetent, leading to DME [23]. De Carlo et al., in 17 eyes, described the differences between cysts, with an oblong shape and smooth borders, devoid of flow and capillary nonperfusion with irregular borders and greyer hue [133].

Eyes with DR and DME are associated with reduced VD in OCTA compared with those with DR without DME [55,57]. They also present lower VD in the SCP and decreased perfusion of the DCP, revealing a more significant effect of oedema on macular perfusion at the level of the DCP and greater macular ischaemia at the deep retinal layers [55,132]. Kim and colleagues found different data depending on the DR grade. Diabetic patients with mild NPDR, with and without DME, showed that those with DME (8/32) had a lower VD, skeletal density, and fractal dimension in both superficial and deep retinal layers (60% of the inner retina vs. 40% of the outer retina) with a higher vessel density index in the deep retina layers [23]. Severe NPDR with DME (13/16) showed only a greater VD index in the deep retina layer, and patients with PDR with and without DME (24/36) showed no differences in the studied parameters [23]. Ting et al. also found a diminution in capillary density index in DM2 patients with DME in both the SCP (0.344 vs. 0.347) and DCP (0.349 vs. 0.357), but these differences did not reach statistical significance [108]. Mane and colleagues, studying 24 eyes with chronic diabetic cystoid macular oedema, described that the cysts were surrounded by capillary dropout areas in 71% and 96% of the cases in the SCP and DCP, respectively, with a diminished VD [134]. Sun et al. studied OCTA biomarkers for the progression of DR or development of DME. Patients with lower VD in the SCP were at higher risk of developing DME [55]. In DME, there is an imbalance between the liquid entering and exiting the retina. The leakage could proceed from the SCP, but the Müller cells and the DCP may be involved in removal. The DCP is the main venous outflow system, and its damage could generate DME [135].

Samara et al. [51] determined a significant enlargement of the FAZ area in diabetic eyes with DME at both the SCP and DCP, compared with the control group, and at the SRL when compared with diabetic eyes without DME. As previous studies, such as that of Balaratnasingam et al. [49], have observed, a significant correlation between FAZ area and VA in diabetic eyes with macular oedema existed with decreased VA in the larger FAZ area at both the superficial and deep retinal plexus [132]. Di et al. also described a larger FAZ in patients with DME than in DM patients without DME [33].

Additionally, VD at the SRL could be a predictive tool for VA in diabetic eyes with DME; a significant negative correlation is observed between VD at the SRL and LogMAR VA [132].

Spaces are surrounded by capillary nonperfusion, which shows no evidence of reperfusion after the resolution of DME [19], suggesting that DME might preferentially develop in areas of ischaemia. Mane and colleagues also described that after DME resolution, capillary density remained almost the same without reperfusion [134]. The same findings were reported by Ghasemi Falavarjani et al., in 13 DME patients after a single intravitreal injection, with no changes in capillary density or FAZ area [136]. Lee and colleagues described the response to anti-VEGF treatment. DM patients who did not respond to anti-VEGF therapy were those with damage to the integrity of the DCP but not the SCP, including lower flow density, larger FAZ, and a higher number of MAs [98]. They discussed the mechanism between the decrease in flow density in the DCP and the resistance to anti-VEGF treatment.

MAs in the DCP are thought to contribute to DME pathogenesis, with correlations between macular volume and MA density of the DCP [68]. They may also contribute to therapy, finding that the greater the MA proportion and the larger the FAZ area in the DCP, the worse the response to anti-VEGF therapy [137].

Some studies, such as Sun et al. [55], postulate that OCTA metrics provide independent risk information on microvasculature and could improve predictive discrimination for both DR progression and DME development compared with traditional, established risk. In their 2-year follow-up study, although they found changes in the DCP VD and FAZ, DME development was related to the VD of the SCP. However, OCTA metrics of the DCP were related to DR progression. They pointed out some limitations in their study but highlighted the role of OCTA metrics.

Further studies are needed to elucidate whether DME vascular changes are secondary to oedema and other OCTA risk biomarkers for DME.

3.1.7. OCTA, DR and Deep Learning

There are significant differences between current multimodal devices and image processing methods, and reference ranges have not been established. Thus, some authors use artificial intelligence (AI), including deep learning (DL), to evaluate OCTA images; this is a machine learning technique which learns representations of data based on computational models with more efficient and precise results, and has already been applied to other ocular conditions [138]. In fact, the combination of AI models using OCT, OCTA and multimodal images appears to be more precise to detect changes in diabetic patients than the OCT AI model [139].

Guo et al., used DL to detect the NPA [140] using a multi-scale feature extraction capability to segment them from OCTA 6×6 m^2 images, with great specificity and sensitivity and excellent performance (F1-score > 80%). This model was valid for different DR severities or image qualities (dice coefficient > 0.87) and was able to detect signal reduction artefacts [141].

Different DL-models assess OCTA image quality assessment [142], object segmentation [143], and quantification [144], with high accuracies. Ryu et al. developed a convolutional neural network (CNN) model classification algorithm with a sensitivity of 86–97%, a specificity of 94–99%, and an accuracy of 91–98% to diagnose DR through OCTA [145]. Le et al.'s DL classifier differentiated among healthy, no DR, and DR eyes with 83.76% sensitivity, 90.82% specificity, and an 87.27% accuracy [146] and Heisler et al. achieved an accuracy of between 90% and 92% [147]. Other DL techniques have shown an AUC of 0.91 to differentiate diabetic patients without DR from those with DR and an AUC of 0.8 to diagnose DR from non-diabetic patients [139]. This AUC was increased up to 92.33% in the DL model of Alam et al. to distinguish controls from DR [148].

Nazir et al.'s DL study was able to identify different severities of the DR based on local tetragonal OCTA patterns [149]. Hwang et al., suggested that the automated quantification of non-perfusion areas using projection-resolved OCTA is able to distinguish levels of DR [87]. Nagasawa and colleagues used a combination of UW fundus ophthalmoscopy and OCTA to stage DR [150]. They obtained a DL algorithm with sensitivities of 78.6% and 80.4% and specificities of 69.8% and 96.8% to distinguish NDR and DR and NPDR from PDR, respectively. These high percentages were, in part, related to Optos accuracy.

Xiong et al. compared commercial software measuring extrafoveal vessel density (EVD) with a DL-based macular extrafoveal avascular area (EAA) on 6×6 mm OCTA and demonstrated a better DR severity diagnostic accuracy; the results seem to be less conditioned by the signal strength and shadow artefacts [151]. Moreover, AI enabled the obtaining of OCTA images with less noise in order to analyse different vascular parameters more correctly, such as vessel density or fractal dimension [152]. Alam et al. also analysed several vascular parameters, and the algorithm that combined all of them reached 94.45% sensitivity, 92.29% specificity, and 92.96% accuracy in identifying mild NPDR with respect to the controls [38]. Among them, the vessel density obtained the best sensitivity to detect DR (with an accuracy of 93.89%) [38]. Otherwise, Detectron2, a new DL model, accurately measured the FAZ in diabetic eyes in a similar way to manual measurements [18].

Classifications of different stages of DR with OCTA DL models have obtained values of AUC of 0.865. Nevertheless, the combination of both OCT and OCTA images, and clinical and demographic data, reached the best AUC (0.96) [148]. The use of this new technique provides the possibility of early detection and may help in DR progression assessments with great accuracy and reliability, evaluating large amounts of data in a short time and reducing human labour, playing a key role in OCTA image analysis of this developing pathology. Multi-ethnic individuals with millions of samples are required to train DL-OCTA devices.

4. Summary and Conclusions

OCTA can provide a large number of findings about the retinal capillary layers and CC in DM patients even without signs of DR. OCTA offers advantages over FA, because it is a non-invasive and faster assessment that can be used as a routine exploration. A variety of metrics can be obtained, including FAZ, acircularity index, axis ratio, VD, NV, and other vascular parameters, such as fractal dimension, vessel tortuosity, or skeleton density, that can be considered markers of the disease and progression. Due to variability between subjects, OCTA results differ from one study to another.

We performed a systematic review of the studies published in this field. We checked for other papers missing after the review process, but some information could have been missed.

Development and improvements in OCTA devices, such as the protocols, the studied field, acquisition speed, and automatically performed measurements including FAZ measurements and irregularity, density, and flow index, and other quantitative features including blood vessel calibre, tortuosity, vessel branching coefficient, and angle, etc., are important clinical benefits in the diagnosis and control of both preclinical and clinical DR. It will offer great advantages in detecting vascular changes, NPA, or NV, not only at the macula, but also at the periphery with WF-OCTA, which could change the diagnosis and disease management.

Several studies have detected potential OCTA biomarkers for DR development or for treatment response. OCTA with multimodal images and systemic biomarkers may guide follow-up and treatment options as well as vascular changes after treatment response. More studies are needed to address the importance of all these factors.

Supplementary Materials: The following supporting information can be downloaded at: https://www.mdpi.com/article/10.3390/biomedicines10010088/s1, File S1: Morphology of the retinal and choroidal blood vessels.

Author Contributions: A.B.-M. and I.P. selected the papers. A.B.-M., H.A.-A., E.O.-H., M.D.D.-B. and I.P. analysed and interpreted the selected data regarding the ophthalmic disease. A.B.-M., H.A.-A., M.D.D.-B., E.O.-H. and I.P. were major contributors in writing the manuscript. A.S.-C., A.F. and N.C. made substantial contributions to the drafting and revision of the work. All authors have read and agreed to the published version of the manuscript.

Funding: Spanish Ministry of Universities (FPU18/02964) and the Health Research Fund Instituto de Salud Carlos III (Fondo de Investigación Sanitaria, Spanish Ministry of Health) PI20/00740.

Institutional Review Board Statement: Not applicable.

Informed Consent Statement: Not applicable.

Data Availability Statement: Not applicable.

Acknowledgments: This research was funded by the Instituto de Salud Carlos III Ocular Pathology National project PI20/00740, the General Council of Aragon (Diputación General de Aragón) Group B08_20R and Fondo Europeo de Desarrollo Regional (FEDER) funds: "Una manera de hacer Europa".

Conflicts of Interest: All authors certify that they have no affiliations with or involvement in any organisation or entity with any financial interest or non-financial interest in the subject matter or materials discussed in this manuscript.

References

1. Saeedi, P.; Petersohn, I.; Salpea, P.; Malanda, B.; Karuranga, S.; Unwin, N.; Colagiuri, S.; Guariguata, L.; Motala, A.A.; Ogurtsova, K.; et al. Global and regional diabetes prevalence estimates for 2019 and projections for 2030 and 2045: Results from the International Diabetes Federation Diabetes Atlas, 9th edition. *Diabetes Res. Clin. Pract.* **2019**, *157*, 107843. [CrossRef] [PubMed]
2. Shaw, J.E.; Sicree, R.A.; Zimmet, P.Z. Global estimates of the prevalence of diabetes for 2010 and 2030. *Diabetes Res. Clin. Pract.* **2010**, *87*, 4–14. [CrossRef]
3. Sabanayagam, C.; Banu, R.; Chee, M.L.; Lee, R.; Wang, Y.X.; Tan, G.; Jonas, J.B.; Lamoureux, E.L.; Cheng, C.-Y.; Klein, B.E.K.; et al. Incidence and progression of diabetic retinopathy: A systematic review. *Lancet Diabetes Endocrinol.* **2019**, *7*, 140–149. [CrossRef]
4. Harding, J.L.; Pavkov, M.E.; Magliano, D.J.; Shaw, J.E.; Gregg, E.W. Global trends in diabetes complications: A review of current evidence. *Diabetologia* **2019**, *62*, 3–16. [CrossRef]
5. Williams, R.; Airey, M.; Baxter, H.; Forrester, J.; Kennedy-Martin, T.; Girach, A. Epidemiology of diabetic retinopathy and macular oedema: A systematic review. *Eye* **2004**, *18*, 963–983. [CrossRef] [PubMed]
6. Fong, D.S.; Aiello, L.P.; Ferris, F.L.; Klein, R. Diabetic retinopathy. *Diabetes Care* **2004**, *27*, 2540–2553. [CrossRef]
7. Safi, H.; Safi, S.; Hafezi-Moghadam, A.; Ahmadieh, H. Early detection of diabetic retinopathy. *Surv. Ophthalmol.* **2018**, *63*, 601–608. [CrossRef]
8. Early Treatment Diabetic Retinopathy Study Research Group. Fundus photographic risk factors for progression of diabetic retinopathy: ETDRS report number 12. *Ophthalmology* **1991**, *98*, 823–833. [CrossRef]
9. Wilkinson, C.; Ferris, F.; Klein, R.; Lee, P.; Agardh, C.D.; Davis, M.; Dills, D.; Kampik, A.; Pararajasegaram, R.; Verdaguer, J.T. Proposed international clinical diabetic retinopathy and diabetic macular edema disease severity scales. *Ophthalmology* **2003**, *110*, 1677–1682. [CrossRef]
10. Early Treatment Diabetic Retinopathy Study Research Group. Classification of diabetic retinopathy from fluorescein angiograms: ETDRS report number 11. *Ophthalmology* **1991**, *98*, 807–822. [CrossRef]
11. Kwan, A.S.L.; Barry, C.; McAllister, I.L.; Constable, I. Fluorescein angiography and adverse drug reactions revisited: The Lions Eye experience. *Clin. Experiment. Ophthalmol.* **2006**, *34*, 33–38. [CrossRef]
12. Hogan, M.J.; Alvarado, J.A.; Weddell, J. Retina. In *Histology of the Human Eye*; Hogan, M.J., Alvarado, J.A., Weddell, J.E., Eds.; Saunders: Philadelphia, PA, USA, 1971; pp. 508–519.
13. Provis, J.M. Development of the primate retinal vasculature. *Prog. Retin. Eye Res.* **2001**, *20*, 799–821. [CrossRef]
14. Snodderly, D.M.; Weinhaus, R.S.; Choi, J.C. Neural-vascular relationships in central retina of macaque monkeys (Macaca fascicularis). *J. Neurosci.* **1992**, *12*, 1169–1193. [CrossRef] [PubMed]
15. Hayreh, S. Phisiological anatomy of the retinal vasculature. In *Immunology, Inflammation and Diseases of the Eye*; Dartt, D., D'Amore, P., Niederkorn, J., Eds.; Elsevier: Amsterdam, The Netherlands, 2010; pp. 207–212.
16. Campbell, J.P.; Zhang, M.; Hwang, T.; Bailey, S.T.; Wilson, D.J.; Jia, Y.; Huang, D. Detailed Vascular Anatomy of the Human Retina by Projection-Resolved Optical Coherence Tomography Angiography. *Sci. Rep.* **2017**, *7*, 1–11. [CrossRef] [PubMed]
17. Cuenca, N.; Ortuño-Lizarán, I.; Sánchez-Sáez, X.; Kutsyr, O.; Albertos-Arranz, H.; Fernández-Sánchez, L.; Gil, N.M.; Noailles, A.; López-Garrido, J.A.; López-Gálvez, M.; et al. Interpretation of OCT and OCTA images from a histological approach: Clinical and experimental implications. *Prog. Retin. Eye Res.* **2020**, *77*, 100828. [CrossRef] [PubMed]
18. Ishibazawa, A.; Nagaoka, T.; Takahashi, A.; Omae, T.; Tani, T.; Sogawa, K.; Yokota, H.; Yoshida, A. Optical coherence tomography angiography in diabetic retinopathy: A prospective pilot study. *Am. J. Ophthalmol.* **2015**, *160*, 35–44.e1. [CrossRef]
19. Couturier, A.; Mané, V.; Bonnin, S.; Erginay, A.; Massin, P.; Gaudric, A.; Tadayoni, R. Capillary plexus anomalies in diabetic retinopathy on optical coherence tomography angiography. *Retina* **2015**, *35*, 2384–2391. [CrossRef]
20. Nghiem-Buffet, S.; Ayrault, A.; Delahaye-Mazza, C.; Grenet, T.; Quentel, G.; Fajnkuchen, F.; Cohen, S.Y. *OCT-Angiography. Neovascularization, Edema, Schema and Degeneration*; Elsevier: Amsterdam, The Netherlands, 2017; pp. 14–15.
21. Matsunaga, D.R.; Yi, J.J.; De Koo, L.O.; Ameri, H.; Puliafito, C.A.; Kashani, A.H. Optical Coherence Tomography Angiography of Diabetic Retinopathy in Human Subjects. *Ophthalmic. Surg. Lasers Imaging. Retin.* **2015**, *46*, 796–805. [CrossRef]
22. Bandello, F.; Corbelli, E.; Carnevali, A.; Pierro, L.; Querques, G. Optical Coherence Tomography Angiography of Diabetic Retinopathy. *Dev. Ophthalmol.* **2016**, *56*, 107–112.
23. Kim, A.Y.; Chu, Z.; Shahidzadeh, A.; Wang, R.K.; Puliafito, C.A.; Kashani, A.H. Quantifying Microvascular Density and Morphology in Diabetic Retinopathy Using Spectral-Domain Optical Coherence Tomography Angiography. *Investig. Ophthalmol. Vis. Sci.* **2016**, *57*, 362–370. [CrossRef] [PubMed]
24. Li, X.; Xie, J.; Zhang, L.; Cui, Y.; Zhang, G.; Chen, X.; Wang, J.; Zhang, A.; Huang, T.; Meng, Q. Identifying microvascular and neural parameters related to the severity of diabetic retinopathy using optical coherence tomography angiography. *Investig. Ophthalmol. Vis. Sci.* **2020**, *61*, 39. [CrossRef] [PubMed]
25. Page, M.J.; McKenzie, J.E.; Bossuyt, P.M.; Boutron, I.; Hoffmann, T.C.; Mulrow, C.D.; Shamseer, L.; Tetzlaff, J.M.; Akl, E.A.; Brennan, S.E.; et al. The PRISMA 2020 statement: An updated guideline for reporting systematic reviews. *BMJ* **2021**, *372*, n71. [CrossRef]
26. Conrath, J.; Giorgi, R.; Raccah, D.; Ridings, B. Foveal avascular zone in diabetic retinopathy: Quantitative vs qualitative assessment. *Eye* **2005**, *19*, 322–326. [CrossRef]
27. Bresnick, G.H.; Condit, R.; Syrjala, S.; Palta, M.; Groo, A.; Korth, K. Abnormalities of the foveal avascular zone in diabetic retinopathy. *Arch. Ophthalmol.* **1984**, *102*, 1286–1293. [CrossRef]

28. Soares, M.; Neves, C.; Marques, I.; Pires, I.; Schwartz, C.; Costa, M.Â.; Santos, T.; Durbin, M.; Cunha-Vaz, J. Comparison of diabetic retinopathy classification using fluorescein angiography and optical coherence tomography angiography. *Br. J. Ophthalmol.* **2017**, *101*, 62–68. [CrossRef] [PubMed]
29. You, Q.S.; Wang, J.; Guo, Y.; Pi, S.; Flaxel, C.J.; Bailey, S.T.; Huang, D.; Jia, Y.; Hwang, T.S. Optical Coherence Tomography Angiography Avascular Area Association With 1-Year Treatment Requirement and Disease Progression in Diabetic Retinopathy. *Am. J. Ophthalmol.* **2020**, *217*, 268–277. [CrossRef]
30. De Carlo, T.E.; Chin, A.T.; Filho, M.A.B.; Adhi, M.; Branchini, L.; Salz, D.A.; Baumal, C.R.; Crawford, C.; Reichel, E.; Witkin, A.J.; et al. Detection of microvascular changes in eyes of patients with diabetes but not clinical diabetic retinopathy using optical coherence tomography angiography. *Retina* **2015**, *35*, 2364–2370. [CrossRef] [PubMed]
31. Dimitrova, G.; Chihara, E.; Takahashi, H.; Amano, H.; Okazaki, K. Quantitative retinal optical coherence tomography angiography in patients with diabetes without diabetic retinopathy. *Investig. Ophthalmol. Vis. Sci.* **2017**, *58*, 190–196. [CrossRef]
32. Takase, N.; Nozaki, M.; Kato, A.; Ozeki, H.; Yoshida, M.; Ogura, Y. Enlargement of foveal avascular zone in diabetic eyes evaluated by en face optical coherence tomography angiography. *Retina* **2015**, *35*, 2377–2383. [CrossRef]
33. Di, G.; Weihong, Y.; Xiao, Z.; Zhikun, Y.; Xuan, Z.; Yi, Q.; Fangtian, D. A morphological study of the foveal avascular zone in patients with diabetes mellitus using optical coherence tomography angiography. *Graefe's Arch. Clin. Exp. Ophthalmol.* **2016**, *254*, 873–879. [CrossRef]
34. Ciloglu, E.; Unal, F.; Sukgen, E.A.; Koçluk, Y. Evaluation of Foveal Avascular Zone and Capillary Plexuses in Diabetic Patients by Optical Coherence Tomography Angiography. *Korean J. Ophthalmol.* **2019**, *33*, 359–365. [CrossRef] [PubMed]
35. Simonett, J.M.; Scarinci, F.; Picconi, F.; Giorno, P.; De Geronimo, D.; Di Renzo, A.; Varano, M.; Frontoni, S.; Parravano, M. Early microvascular retinal changes in optical coherence tomography angiography in patients with type 1 diabetes mellitus. *Acta Ophthalmol.* **2017**, *95*, e751–e755. [CrossRef] [PubMed]
36. Wang, X.; Han, Y.; Sun, G.; Yang, F.; Liu, W.; Luo, J.; Cao, X.; Yin, P.; Myers, F.L.; Zhou, L. Detection of the Microvascular Changes of Diabetic Retinopathy Progression Using Optical Coherence Tomography Angiography. *Transl. Vis. Sci. Technol.* **2021**, *10*, 31. [CrossRef]
37. Krawitz, B.D.; Phillips, E.; Bavier, R.D.; Mo, S.; Carroll, J.; Rosen, R.B.; Chui, T.Y.P. Parafoveal nonperfusion analysis in diabetic retinopathy using optical coherence tomography angiography. *Transl. Vis. Sci. Technol.* **2018**, *7*, 4. [CrossRef] [PubMed]
38. Alam, M.; Zhang, Y.; Lim, J.I.; Chan, R.V.P.; Yang, M.; Yao, X. Quantitative optical coherence tomography angiography features for objective classification and staging of diabetic retinopathy. *Retina* **2020**, *40*, 322–332. [CrossRef] [PubMed]
39. Lu, Y.; Simonett, J.M.; Wang, J.; Zhang, M.; Hwang, T.; Hagag, A.; Huang, D.; Li, D.; Jia, Y. Evaluation of Automatically Quantified Foveal Avascular Zone Metrics for Diagnosis of Diabetic Retinopathy Using Optical Coherence Tomography Angiography. *Investig. Ophthalmol. Vis. Sci.* **2018**, *59*, 2212–2221. [CrossRef]
40. Rabiolo, A.; Cicinelli, M.V.; Corbelli, E.; Baldin, G.; Carnevali, A.; Lattanzio, R.; Querques, L.; Bandello, F.; Querques, G. Correlation Analysis between Foveal Avascular Zone and Peripheral Ischemic Index in Diabetic Retinopathy: A Pilot Study. *Ophthalmol. Retin.* **2018**, *2*, 46–52. [CrossRef]
41. Xu, X.; Chen, C.; Ding, W.; Yang, P.; Lu, H.; Xu, F.; Lei, J. Automated quantification of superficial retinal capillaries and large vessels for diabetic retinopathy on optical coherence tomographic angiography. *J. Biophotonics* **2019**, *12*, e201900103. [CrossRef]
42. Wang, F.; Saraf, S.S.; Zhang, Q.; Wang, R.K.; Rezaei, K.A. Ultra-Widefield Protocol Enhances Automated Classification of Diabetic Retinopathy Severity with OCT Angiography. *Ophthalmol. Retin.* **2020**, *4*, 415–424. [CrossRef]
43. Xie, N.; Tan, Y.; Liu, S.; Xie, Y.; Shuai, S.; Wang, W.; Huang, W. Macular vessel density in diabetes and diabetic retinopathy with swept-source optical coherence tomography angiography. *Graefe's Arch. Clin. Exp. Ophthalmol.* **2020**, *258*, 2671–2679. [CrossRef] [PubMed]
44. Rosen, R.B.; Romo, J.A.; Krawitz, B.D.; Mo, S.; Fawzi, A.; Linderman, R.; Carroll, J.; Pinhas, A.; Chui, T.Y. Earliest Evidence of Preclinical Diabetic Retinopathy Revealed Using Optical Coherence Tomography Angiography Perfused Capillary Density. *Am. J. Ophthalmol.* **2019**, *203*, 103–115. [CrossRef] [PubMed]
45. Agra, C.L.D.M.; Lira, R.P.C.; Pinheiro, F.G.; Sá, L.H.S.E.; Bravo Filho, V.T.F. Optical coherence tomography angiography: Microvascular alterations in diabetic eyes without diabetic retinopathy. *Arq. Bras. Oftalmol.* **2021**, *84*, 149–157. [CrossRef]
46. Oliverio, G.W.; Ceravolo, I.; Bhatti, A.; Trombetta, C.J. Foveal avascular zone analysis by optical coherence tomography angiography in patients with type 1 and 2 diabetes and without clinical signs of diabetic retinopathy. *Int. Ophthalmol.* **2021**, *41*, 649–658. [CrossRef]
47. Um, T.; Seo, E.J.; Kim, Y.J.; Yoon, Y.H. Optical coherence tomography angiography findings of type 1 diabetic patients with diabetic retinopathy, in comparison with type 2 patients. *Graefe's Arch. Clin. Exp. Ophthalmol.* **2020**, *258*, 281–288. [CrossRef]
48. Vujosevic, S.; Muraca, A.; Alkabes, M.; Villani, E.; Cavarzeran, F.; Rossetti, L.; De Cilla', S. Early microvascular and neural changes in patients with type 1 and type 2 diabetes mellitus without clinical signs of diabetic retinopathy. *Retina* **2019**, *39*, 435–445. [CrossRef] [PubMed]
49. Balaratnasingam, C.; Inoue, M.; Ahn, S.; McCann, J.; Dhrami-Gavazi, E.; Yannuzzi, L.A.; Freund, K.B. Visual Acuity Is Correlated with the Area of the Foveal Avascular Zone in Diabetic Retinopathy and Retinal Vein Occlusion. *Ophthalmology* **2016**, *123*, 2352–2367. [CrossRef]
50. DaCosta, J.; Bhatia, D.; Talks, J. The use of optical coherence tomography angiography and optical coherence tomography to predict visual acuity in diabetic retinopathy. *Eye* **2020**, *34*, 942–947. [CrossRef]

51. Samara, W.A.; Shahlaee, A.; Adam, M.; Khan, M.A.; Chiang, A.; Maguire, J.I.; Hsu, J.; Ho, A.C. Quantification of Diabetic Macular Ischemia Using Optical Coherence Tomography Angiography and Its Relationship with Visual Acuity. *Ophthalmology* **2017**, *124*, 235–244. [CrossRef]
52. Krawitz, B.D.; Mo, S.; Geyman, L.S.; Agemy, S.A.; Scripsema, N.K.; Garcia, P.M.; Chui, T.Y.; Rosen, R.B. Acircularity index and axis ratio of the foveal avascular zone in diabetic eyes and healthy controls measured by optical coherence tomography angiography. *Vision Res.* **2017**, *139*, 177–186. [CrossRef]
53. Zahid, S.; Dolz-Marco, R.; Freund, K.B.; Balaratnasingam, C.; Dansingani, K.; Gilani, F.; Mehta, N.; Young, E.; Klifto, M.R.; Chae, B.; et al. Fractal dimensional analysis of optical coherence tomography angiography in eyes with diabetic retinopathy. *Investig. Ophthalmol. Vis. Sci.* **2016**, *57*, 4940–4947. [CrossRef] [PubMed]
54. Tang, F.Y.; Ng, D.S.; Lam, A.; Luk, F.; Wong, R.; Chan, C.; Mohamed, S.; Fong, A.; Lok, J.; Tso, T.; et al. Determinants of Quantitative Optical Coherence Tomography Angiography Metrics in Patients with Diabetes. *Sci Rep.* **2017**, *7*, 2575. [CrossRef]
55. Sun, Z.; Tang, F.; Wong, R.; Lok, J.; Szeto, S.K.H.; Chan, J.C.K.; Chan, C.K.M.; Tham, C.C.; Ng, D.S.; Cheung, C.Y. OCT Angiography Metrics Predict Progression of Diabetic Retinopathy and Development of Diabetic Macular Edema: A Prospective Study. *Ophthalmology* **2019**, *126*, 1675–1684. [CrossRef] [PubMed]
56. Ragkousis, A.; Kozobolis, V.; Kabanarou, S.; Bontzos, G.; Mangouritsas, G.; Heliopoulos, I.; Chatziralli, I. Vessel Density around Foveal Avascular Zone as a Potential Imaging Biomarker for Detecting Preclinical Diabetic Retinopathy: An Optical Coherence Tomography Angiography Study. *Semin. Ophthalmol.* **2020**, *35*, 316–323. [CrossRef]
57. Kim, K.; Kim, E.S.; Kim, D.G.; Yu, S.-Y. Progressive retinal neurodegeneration and microvascular change in diabetic retinopathy: Longitudinal study using OCT angiography. *Acta Diabetol.* **2019**, *56*, 1275–1282. [CrossRef]
58. Kim, K.; Kim, E.S.; Yu, S.-Y. Optical coherence tomography angiography analysis of foveal microvascular changes and inner retinal layer thinning in patients with diabetes. *Br. J. Ophthalmol.* **2018**, *102*, 1226–1231. [CrossRef]
59. Park, J.J.; Soetikno, B.T.; Fawzi, A.A. Characterization of the middle capillary plexus using optical coherence tomography angiography in healthy and diabetic eyes. *Retina* **2016**, *36*, 2039–2050. [CrossRef]
60. Salz, D.A.; De Carlo, T.E.; Adhi, M.; Moult, E.M.; Choi, W.; Baumal, C.R.; Witkin, A.J.; Duker, J.S.; Fujimoto, J.G.; Waheed, N.K. Select Features of Diabetic Retinopathy on Swept-Source Optical Coherence Tomographic Angiography Compared With Fluorescein Angiography and Normal Eyes. *JAMA Ophthalmol.* **2016**, *134*, 644–650. [CrossRef] [PubMed]
61. Stattin, M.; Haas, A.-M.; Ahmed, D.; Stolba, U.; Graf, A.; Krepler, K.; Ansari-Shahrezaei, S. Detection rate of diabetic macular microaneurysms comparing dye-based angiography and optical coherence tomography angiography. *Sci. Rep.* **2020**, *10*, 16274. [CrossRef]
62. Parrulli, S.; Corvi, F.; Cozzi, M.; Monteduro, D.; Zicarelli, F.; Staurenghi, G. Microaneurysms visualisation using five different optical coherence tomography angiography devices compared to fluorescein angiography. *Br. J. Ophthalmol.* **2021**, *105*, 526–530. [CrossRef]
63. Hamada, M.; Ohkoshi, K.; Inagaki, K.; Ebihara, N.; Murakami, A. Visualization of microaneurysms using optical coherence tomography angiography: Comparison of OCTA en face, OCT B-scan, OCT en face, FA, and IA images. *Jpn. J. Ophthalmol.* **2018**, *62*, 168–175. [CrossRef] [PubMed]
64. Parravano, M.; De Geronimo, D.; Scarinci, F.; Querques, L.; Virgili, G.; Simonett, J.M.; Varano, M.; Bandello, F.; Querques, G. Diabetic Microaneurysms Internal Reflectivity on Spectral-Domain Optical Coherence Tomography and Optical Coherence Tomography Angiography Detection. *Am. J. Ophthalmol.* **2017**, *179*, 90–96. [CrossRef] [PubMed]
65. Byeon, S.H.; Chu, Y.K.; Hong, Y.T.; Kim, M.; Kang, H.M.; Kwon, O.W. New insights into the pathoanatomy of diabetic macular edema: Angiographic patterns and optical coherence tomography. *Retina* **2012**, *32*, 1087–1099. [CrossRef] [PubMed]
66. Parravano, M.; De Geronimo, D.; Scarinci, F.; Virgili, G.; Querques, L.; Varano, M.; Bandello, F.; Querques, G. Progression of Diabetic Microaneurysms According to the Internal Reflectivity on Structural Optical Coherence Tomography and Visibility on Optical Coherence Tomography Angiography. *Am. J. Ophthalmol.* **2019**, *198*, 8–16. [CrossRef]
67. Stitt, A.W.; Gardiner, T.A.; Archer, D.B. Histological and ultrastructural investigigation of retinal microaneurysm development in diabetic patients. *Br. J. Ophthalmol.* **1995**, *79*, 362–367. [CrossRef] [PubMed]
68. Hasegawa, N.; Nozaki, M.; Takase, N.; Yoshida, M.; Ogura, Y. New insights into microaneurysms in the deep capillary plexus detected by optical coherence tomography angiography in diabetic macular edema. *Investig. Ophthalmol. Vis. Sci.* **2016**, *57*, 348–355. [CrossRef]
69. Schaal, K.B.; Munk, M.R.; Wyssmueller, I.; Berger, L.E.; Zinkernagel, M.S.; Wolf, S. Vascular abnormalities in diabetic retinopathy assessed with swept-source optical coherence tomography angiography widefield imaging. *Retina* **2019**, *39*, 79–87. [CrossRef]
70. Tian, M.; Wolf, S.; Munk, M.R.; Schaal, K.B. Evaluation of different Swept'Source optical coherence tomography angiography (SS-OCTA) slabs for the detection of features of diabetic retinopathy. *Acta Ophthalmol.* **2020**, *98*, e416–e420. [CrossRef] [PubMed]
71. Carnevali, A.; Sacconi, R.; Corbelli, E.; Tomasso, L.; Querques, L.; Zerbini, G.; Scorcia, V.; Bandello, F.; Querques, G. Optical coherence tomography angiography analysis of retinal vascular plexuses and choriocapillaris in patients with type 1 diabetes without diabetic retinopathy. *Acta Diabetol.* **2017**, *54*, 695–702. [CrossRef]
72. Park, Y.G.; Kim, M.; Roh, Y.J. Evaluation of Foveal and Parafoveal Microvascular Changes Using Optical Coherence Tomography Angiography in Type 2 Diabetes Patients without Clinical Diabetic Retinopathy in South Korea. *J. Diabetes Res.* **2020**, *2020*, 6210865. [CrossRef] [PubMed]

73. Thompson, I.A.; Durrani, A.K.; Patel, S. Optical coherence tomography angiography characteristics in diabetic patients without clinical diabetic retinopathy. *Eye* **2019**, *33*, 648–652. [CrossRef]
74. Zhang, A.; Zhang, Q.; Chen, C.-L.; Wang, R.K. Methods and algorithms for optical coherence tomography-based angiography: A review and comparison. *J. Biomed. Opt.* **2015**, *20*, 100901. [CrossRef]
75. Coscas, G.; Lupidi, M.; Coscas, F.; Chhablani, J.; Cagini, C. Optical Coherence Tomography Angiography in Healthy Subjects and Diabetic Patients. *Ophthalmologica* **2018**, *239*, 61–73. [CrossRef]
76. Onishi, A.C.; Nesper, P.L.; Roberts, P.K.; Moharram, G.A.; Chai, H.; Liu, L.; Jampol, L.M.; Fawzi, A.A. Importance of considering the middle capillary plexus on OCT angiography in diabetic retinopathy. *Investig. Ophthalmol. Vis. Sci.* **2018**, *59*, 2167–2176. [CrossRef]
77. Choi, W.; Waheed, N.K.; Moult, E.M.; Adhi, M.; Lee, B.; De Carlo, T.; Jayaraman, V.; Baumal, C.R.; Duker, J.S.; Fujimoto, J.G. Ultrahigh speed swept source optical coherence tomography angiography of retinal and choriocapillaris alterations in diabetic patients with and without retinopathy. *Retina* **2017**, *37*, 11–21. [CrossRef] [PubMed]
78. You, Q.S.; Freeman, W.R.; Weinreb, R.N.; Zangwill, L.; Manalastas, P.I.C.; Saunders, L.J.; Nudleman, E. Reproducibility of vessel density measurements with optical coherence tomography angiography in eyes without retinopathy. *Retina* **2017**, *37*, 1475–1482. [CrossRef] [PubMed]
79. Vaz-Pereira, S.; Morais-Sarmento, T.; Esteves Marques, R. Optical coherence tomography features of neovascularization in proliferative diabetic retinopathy: A systematic review. *Int. J. Retin. Vitr.* **2020**, *6*, 26. [CrossRef] [PubMed]
80. Nesper, P.L.; Roberts, P.K.; Onishi, A.C.; Chai, H.; Liu, L.; Jampol, L.M.; Fawzi, A.A. Quantifying Microvascular Abnormalities With Increasing Severity of Diabetic Retinopathy Using Optical Coherence Tomography Angiography. *Investig. Ophthalmol. Vis. Sci.* **2017**, *58*, 307–315. [CrossRef]
81. Yasukura, S.; Murakami, T.; Suzuma, K.; Yoshitake, T.; Nakanishi, H.; Fujimoto, M.; Oishi, M.; Tsujikawa, A. Diabetic Nonperfused Areas in Macular and Extramacular Regions on Wide-Field Optical Coherence Tomography Angiography. *Investig. Ophthalmol. Vis. Sci.* **2018**, *59*, 5893–5903. [CrossRef] [PubMed]
82. Tan, B.; Chua, J.; Lin, E.; Cheng, J.; Gan, A.; Yao, X.; Wong, D.W.K.; Sabanayagam, C.; Wong, D.; Chan, C.M.; et al. Quantitative Microvascular Analysis With Wide-Field Optical Coherence Tomography Angiography in Eyes With Diabetic Retinopathy. *JAMA Netw. Open* **2020**, *3*, e1919369. [CrossRef]
83. Silva, P.S.; Cruz, A.J.D.; Ledesma, M.G.; van Hemert, J.; Radwan, A.; Cavallerano, J.; Aiello, L.M.; Sun, J.K. Diabetic Retinopathy Severity and Peripheral Lesions Are Associated with Nonperfusion on Ultrawide Field Angiography. *Ophthalmology* **2015**, *122*, 2465–2472. [CrossRef]
84. Ishibazawa, A.; De Pretto, L.R.; Alibhai, A.Y.; Moult, E.M.; Arya, M.; Sorour, O.; Mehta, N.; Baumal, C.R.; Witkin, A.J.; Yoshida, A.; et al. Retinal Nonperfusion Relationship to Arteries or Veins Observed on Widefield Optical Coherence Tomography Angiography in Diabetic Retinopathy. *Investig. Ophthalmol. Vis. Sci.* **2019**, *60*, 4310–4318. [CrossRef]
85. Amato, A.; Nadin, F.; Borghesan, F.; Cicinelli, M.V.; Chatziralli, I.; Sadiq, S.; Mirza, R.; Bandello, F. Widefield Optical Coherence Tomography Angiography in Diabetic Retinopathy. *J. Diabetes Res.* **2020**, *2020*, 8855709. [CrossRef]
86. Agemy, S.A.; Scripsema, N.K.; Shah, C.M.; Chui, T.; Garcia, P.M.; Lee, J.G.; Gentile, R.C.; Hsiao, Y.-S.; Zhou, Q.; Ko, T.; et al. Retinal vascular perfusion density mapping using optical coherence tomography angiography in normals and diabetic retinopathy patients. *Retina* **2015**, *35*, 2353–2363. [CrossRef]
87. Hwang, T.; Gao, S.; Liu, L.; Lauer, A.K.; Bailey, S.T.; Flaxel, C.J.; Wilson, D.J.; Huang, D.; Jia, Y. Automated Quantification of Capillary Nonperfusion Using Optical Coherence Tomography Angiography in Diabetic Retinopathy. *JAMA Ophthalmol.* **2016**, *134*, 367–373. [CrossRef] [PubMed]
88. Bradley, P.D.; Sim, D.A.; Keane, P.A.; Cardoso, J.N.; Agrawal, R.; Tufail, A.; Egan, C.A. The Evaluation of Diabetic Macular Ischemia Using Optical Coherence Tomography Angiography. *Investig. Ophthalmol. Vis. Sci.* **2016**, *57*, 626–631. [CrossRef]
89. Nesper, P.L.; Soetikno, B.T.; Zhang, H.F.; Fawzi, A.A. OCT angiography and visible-light OCT in diabetic retinopathy. *Vision Res.* **2017**, *139*, 191–203. [CrossRef] [PubMed]
90. Agrawal, R.; Xin, W.; Keane, P.A.; Chhablani, J.; Agarwal, A. Optical coherence tomography angiography: A non-invasive tool to image end-arterial system. *Expert. Rev. Med. Devices* **2016**, *13*, 519–521. [CrossRef] [PubMed]
91. Tsai, A.S.H.; Jordan-Yu, J.M.; Gan, A.T.L.; Teo, K.Y.C.; Tan, G.S.W.; Lee, S.Y.; Chong, V.; Cheung, C.M.G. Diabetic Macular Ischemia: Influence of Optical Coherence Tomography Angiography Parameters on Changes in Functional Outcomes Over One Year. *Investig. Ophthalmol. Vis. Sci.* **2021**, *62*, 9. [CrossRef]
92. Schottenhamml, J.; Moult, E.M.; Ploner, S.; Lee, B.; Novais, E.A.; Cole, E.; Dang, S.; Lu, C.D.; Husvogt, L.; Waheed, N.K.; et al. An automatic, intercapillary area-based algorithm for quantifying diabetes related capillary dropout using optical coherence tomography angiography. *Retina* **2016**, *36*, S93–S101. [CrossRef] [PubMed]
93. Dupas, B.; Minvielle, W.; Bonnin, S.; Couturier, A.; Erginay, A.; Massin, P.; Gaudric, A.; Tadayoni, R. Association Between Vessel Density and Visual Acuity in Patients With Diabetic Retinopathy and Poorly Controlled Type 1 Diabetes. *JAMA Ophthalmol.* **2018**, *136*, 721–728. [CrossRef]
94. Gill, A.; Cole, E.D.; Novais, E.A.; Louzada, R.N.; De Carlo, T.; Duker, J.S.; Waheed, N.K.; Baumal, C.R.; Witkin, A.J. Visualization of changes in the foveal avascular zone in both observed and treated diabetic macular edema using optical coherence tomography angiography. *Int. J. Retin. Vitr.* **2017**, *3*, 19. [CrossRef]

95. Moore, J.; Bagley, S.; Ireland, G.; McLeod, D.; Boulton, M.E. Three dimensional analysis of microaneurysms in the human diabetic retina. *J. Anat.* **1999**, *194*, 89–100. [CrossRef]
96. Scarinci, F.; Nesper, P.L.; Fawzi, A.A. Deep Retinal Capillary Nonperfusion Is Associated With Photoreceptor Disruption in Diabetic Macular Ischemia. *Am. J. Ophthalmol.* **2016**, *168*, 129–138. [CrossRef] [PubMed]
97. Yang, J.; Wang, E.; Zhao, X.; Xia, S.; Yuan, M.; Chen, H.; Zhang, X.; Chen, Y. Optical coherence tomography angiography analysis of the choriocapillary layer in treatment-naïve diabetic eyes. *Graefe's Arch. Clin. Exp. Ophthalmol.* **2019**, *257*, 1393–1399. [CrossRef] [PubMed]
98. Lee, J.; Moon, B.G.; Cho, A.R.; Yoon, Y.H. Optical Coherence Tomography Angiography of DME and Its Association with Anti-VEGF Treatment Response. *Ophthalmology* **2016**, *123*, 2368–2375. [CrossRef]
99. Rodrigues, T.M.; Marques, J.P.; Soares, M.; Simão, S.; Melo, P.; Martins, A.; Figueira, J.; Murta, J.; Silva, R. Macular OCT-angiography parameters to predict the clinical stage of nonproliferative diabetic retinopathy: An exploratory analysis. *Eye* **2019**, *33*, 1240–1247. [CrossRef]
100. Inanc, M.; Tekin, K.; Kiziltoprak, H.; Ozalkak, S.; Doguizi, S.; Aycan, Z. Changes in Retinal Microcirculation Precede the Clinical Onset of Diabetic Retinopathy in Children With Type 1 Diabetes Mellitus. *Am. J. Ophthalmol.* **2019**, *207*, 37–44. [CrossRef]
101. Zeng, Y.; Cao, D.; Yu, H.; Yang, D.; Zhuang, X.; Hu, Y.; Li, J.; Yang, J.; Wu, Q.; Liu, B.; et al. Early retinal neurovascular impairment in patients with diabetes without clinically detectable retinopathy. *Br. J. Ophthalmol.* **2019**, *103*, 1747–1752. [PubMed]
102. Li, L.; Almansoob, S.; Zhang, P.; Zhou, Y.-D.; Tan, Y.; Gao, L. Quantitative analysis of retinal and choroid capillary ischaemia using optical coherence tomography angiography in type 2 diabetes. *Acta Ophthalmol.* **2019**, *97*, 240–246. [CrossRef]
103. Cao, D.; Yang, D.; Huang, Z.; Zeng, Y.; Wang, J.; Hu, Y.; Zhang, L. Optical coherence tomography angiography discerns preclinical diabetic retinopathy in eyes of patients with type 2 diabetes without clinical diabetic retinopathy. *Acta Diabetol.* **2018**, *55*, 469–477. [CrossRef]
104. Markan, A.; Agarwal, A.; Arora, A.; Bazgain, K.; Rana, V.; Gupta, V. Novel imaging biomarkers in diabetic retinopathy and diabetic macular edema. *Ther. Adv. Ophthalmol.* **2020**, *12*, 2515841420950513. [CrossRef]
105. Zhu, T.P.; Li, E.H.; Li, J.Y.; Dai, X.Z.; Na Zhang, H.; Bin Chen, B.; Ye, P.P.; Su, Z.A.; Ye, J. Comparison of projection-resolved optical coherence tomography angiography-based metrics for the early detection of retinal microvascular impairments in diabetes mellitus. *Retina* **2020**, *40*, 1783–1792. [CrossRef]
106. Minnella, A.M.; Savastano, M.C.; Federici, M.; Falsini, B.; Caporossi, A. Superficial and deep vascular structure of the retina in diabetic macular ischaemia: OCT angiography. *Acta Ophthalmol.* **2018**, *96*, e647–e648. [CrossRef] [PubMed]
107. Al-Sheikh, M.; Akil, H.; Pfau, M.; Sadda, S.R. Swept-Source OCT Angiography Imaging of the Foveal Avascular Zone and Macular Capillary Network Density in Diabetic Retinopathy. *Investig. Opthalmol. Vis. Sci.* **2016**, *57*, 3907–3913. [CrossRef] [PubMed]
108. Ting, D.S.W.; Tan, G.S.W.; Agrawal, R.; Yanagi, Y.; Sie, N.M.; Wong, C.W.; San Yeo, I.Y.; Lee, S.Y.; Cheung, C.M.G.; Wong, T.Y. Optical Coherence Tomographic Angiography in Type 2 Diabetes and Diabetic Retinopathy. *JAMA Ophthalmol.* **2017**, *135*, 306–312. [CrossRef]
109. Liu, G.; Xu, D.; Wang, F. New insights into diabetic retinopathy by OCT angiography. *Diabetes Res. Clin. Pract.* **2018**, *142*, 243–253. [CrossRef] [PubMed]
110. Bek, T. Transretinal histopathological changes in capillary-free areas of diabetic retinopathy. *Acta Ophthalmol.* **1994**, *72*, 409–415. [CrossRef]
111. Wang, Q.; Chan, S.; Yang, J.Y.; You, B.; Wang, Y.X.; Jonas, J.B.; Bin Wei, W. Vascular Density in Retina and Choriocapillaris as Measured by Optical Coherence Tomography Angiography. *Am. J. Ophthalmol.* **2016**, *168*, 95–109. [CrossRef]
112. Kaizu, Y.; Nakao, S.; Sekiryu, H.; Wada, I.; Yamaguchi, M.; Hisatomi, T.; Ikeda, Y.; Kishimoto, J.; Sonoda, K.-H. Retinal flow density by optical coherence tomography angiography is useful for detection of nonperfused areas in diabetic retinopathy. *Graefe's Arch. Clin. Exp. Ophthalmol.* **2018**, *256*, 2275–2282. [CrossRef]
113. Arya, M.; Sorour, O.; Chaudhri, J.; Alibhai, Y.; Waheed, N.K.; Duker, J.S.; Baumal, C.R. Distinguishing intraretinal microvascular abnormalities from retinal neovascularization using optical coherence tomography angiography. *Retina* **2020**, *40*, 1686–1695. [CrossRef]
114. Cui, Y.; Zhu, Y.; Wang, J.C.; Lu, Y.; Zeng, R.; Katz, R.; Vingopoulos, F.; Le, R.; Laíns, I.; Wu, D.M.; et al. Comparison of widefield swept-source optical coherence tomography angiography with ultra-widefield colour fundus photography and fluorescein angiography for detection of lesions in diabetic retinopathy. *Br. J. Ophthalmol.* **2021**, *105*, 577–581. [CrossRef]
115. Sorour, O.; Mehta, N.; Baumal, C.R.; Ishibazawa, A.; Liu, K.; Konstantinou, E.K.; Martin, S.; Braun, P.; Alibhai, A.Y.; Arya, M.; et al. Morphological changes in intraretinal microvascular abnormalities after anti-VEGF therapy visualized on optical coherence tomography angiography. *Eye Vis.* **2020**, *7*, 29. [CrossRef]
116. Kaoual, H.; Zhioua Braham, I.; Boukari, M.; Zhioua, R. Evaluation of the effect of the severity of diabetic retinopathy on microvascular abnormalities and vascular density using optical coherence tomography angiography. *Acta Diabetol.* **2021**, *58*, 1683–1688. [CrossRef] [PubMed]
117. Shimouchi, A.; Ishibazawa, A.; Ishiko, S.; Omae, T.; Ro-Mase, T.; Yanagi, Y.; Yoshida, A. A Proposed Classification of Intraretinal Microvascular Abnormalities in Diabetic Retinopathy Following Panretinal Photocoagulation. *Investig. Ophthalmol. Vis. Sci.* **2020**, *61*, 34. [CrossRef] [PubMed]

118. Fossataro, F.; Rispoli, M.; Pece, A. OCTA in macular intraretinal microvascular abnormalities: Retinal vascular density remodeling after panretinal photocoagulation. *Eur. J. Ophthalmol.* **2021**, *31*, 11206721211059014. [CrossRef] [PubMed]
119. Russell, J.F.; Shi, Y.; Scott, N.L.; Gregori, G.; Rosenfeld, P.J. Longitudinal Angiographic Evidence That Intraretinal Microvascular Abnormalities Can Evolve into Neovascularization. *Ophthalmol. Retin.* **2020**, *4*, 1146–1150. [CrossRef]
120. Lee, C.S.; Lee, A.; Sim, D.A.; Keane, P.A.; Mehta, H.; Zarranz-Ventura, J.; Fruttiger, M.; Egan, C.; Tufail, A. Reevaluating the definition of intraretinal microvascular abnormalities and neovascularization elsewhere in diabetic retinopathy using optical coherence tomography and fluorescein angiography. *Am. J. Ophthalmol.* **2015**, *159*, 101–110.e1. [CrossRef]
121. Pan, J.; Chen, D.; Yang, X.; Zou, R.; Zhao, K.; Cheng, D.; Huang, S.; Zhou, T.; Yang, Y.; Chen, F. Characteristics of Neovascularization in Early Stages of Proliferative Diabetic Retinopathy by Optical Coherence Tomography Angiography. *Am. J. Ophthalmol.* **2018**, *192*, 146–156. [CrossRef]
122. DaCosta, J.; Bhatia, D.; Crothers, O.; Talks, J. Utilisation of optical coherence tomography and optical coherence tomography angiography to assess retinal neovascularisation in diabetic retinopathy. *Eye* **2021**, 1–9. [CrossRef] [PubMed]
123. You, Q.S.; Guo, Y.; Wang, J.; Wei, X.; Camino, A.; Zang, P.; Flaxel, C.J.; Bailey, S.T.; Huang, D.; Jia, Y.; et al. Detection of clinically unsuspected retinal neovascularization with wide-field optical coherence tomography angiography. *Retina* **2020**, *40*, 891–897. [CrossRef]
124. Papayannis, A.; Tsamis, E.; Stringa, F.; Iacono, P.; Battaglia Parodi, M.; Stanga, P.E. Swept-source optical coherence tomography angiography vitreo-retinal segmentation in proliferative diabetic retinopathy. *Eur. J. Ophthalmol.* **2021**, *31*, 1925–1932. [CrossRef] [PubMed]
125. Ishibazawa, A.; Nagaoka, T.; Yokota, H.; Takahashi, A.; Omae, T.; Song, Y.; Takahashi, T.; Yoshida, A. Characteristics of retinal neovascularization in proliferative diabetic retinopathy imaged by optical coherence tomography angiography. *Investig. Ophthalmol. Vis. Sci.* **2016**, *57*, 6247–6255. [CrossRef]
126. Elbendary, A.M.; Abouelkheir, H.Y. Bimodal imaging of proliferative diabetic retinopathy vascular features using swept source optical coherence tomography angiography. *Int. J. Ophthalmol.* **2018**, *11*, 1528–1533. [PubMed]
127. Hwang, T.S.; Jia, Y.; Gao, S.S.; Bailey, S.T.; Lauer, A.K.; Flaxel, C.J.; Wilson, D.J.; Huang, D. Optical coherence tomography angiography features of diabetic retinopathy. *Retina* **2015**, *35*, 2371–2376. [CrossRef] [PubMed]
128. Muraoka, K.; Shimizu, K. Intraretinal neovascularization in diabetic retinopathy. *Ophthalmology* **1984**, *91*, 1440–1446. [CrossRef]
129. Zhu, Y.; Cui, Y.; Wang, J.C.; Lu, Y.; Zeng, R.; Katz, R.; Wu, D.M.; Eliott, D.; Vavvas, D.G.; Husain, D.; et al. Different Scan Protocols Affect the Detection Rates of Diabetic Retinopathy Lesions by Wide-Field Swept-Source Optical Coherence Tomography Angiography. *Am. J. Ophthalmol.* **2020**, *215*, 72–80. [CrossRef] [PubMed]
130. Hirano, T.; Hoshiyama, K.; Hirabayashi, K.; Wakabayashi, M.; Toriyama, Y.; Tokimitsu, M.; Murata, T. Vitreoretinal Interface Slab in OCT Angiography for Detecting Diabetic Retinal Neovascularization. *Ophthalmol. Retin.* **2020**, *4*, 588–594. [CrossRef] [PubMed]
131. Stanga, P.E.; Papayannis, A.; Tsamis, E.; Stringa, F.; Cole, T.; D'Souza, Y.; Jalil, A. New Findings in Diabetic Maculopathy and Proliferative Disease by Swept-Source Optical Coherence Tomography Angiography. *Dev. Ophthalmol.* **2016**, *56*, 113–121.
132. AttaAllah, H.R.; Mohamed, A.A.M.; Ali, M.A. Macular vessels density in diabetic retinopathy: Quantitative assessment using optical coherence tomography angiography. *Int. Ophthalmol.* **2019**, *39*, 1845–1859. [CrossRef]
133. De Carlo, T.E.; Chin, A.T.; Joseph, T.; Baumal, C.R.; Witkin, A.J.; Duker, J.S.; Waheed, N.K. Distinguishing Diabetic Macular Edema From Capillary Nonperfusion Using Optical Coherence Tomography Angiography. *Ophthalmic. Surg. Lasers Imaging. Retina* **2016**, *47*, 108–114. [CrossRef] [PubMed]
134. Mané, V.; Dupas, B.; Gaudric, A.; Bonnin, S.; Pedinielli, A.; Bousquet, E.; Erginay, A.; Tadayoni, R.; Couturier, A. Correlation between cystoid spaces in chronic diabetic marular edema and capillary nonperfusion detected by optical coherence tomgraphy angiography. *Retina* **2016**, *36*, S102–S110. [CrossRef]
135. Spaide, R.F. Retinal vascular cystoid edema: Review and New Theory. *Retina* **2016**, *36*, 1823–1842. [CrossRef]
136. Ghasemi Falavarjani, K.; Iafe, N.A.; Hubschman, J.P.; Tsui, I.; Sadda, S.R.; Sarraf, D. Optical coherence tomography angiography analysis of the foveal avascular zone and macular vessel density after anti-VEGF therapy in eyes with diabetic macular edema and retinal vein occlusion. *Investig. Ophthalmol. Vis. Sci.* **2017**, *58*, 30–34. [CrossRef] [PubMed]
137. Balaratnasingam, C.; An, D.; Sakurada, Y.; Lee, C.S.; Lee, A.Y.; McAllister, I.L.; Freund, K.B.; Sarunic, M.; Yu, D.-Y. Comparisons Between Histology and Optical Coherence Tomography Angiography of the Periarterial Capillary-Free Zone. *Am. J. Ophthalmol.* **2018**, *189*, 55–64. [CrossRef] [PubMed]
138. Ting, D.S.W.; Pasquale, L.R.; Peng, L.; Campbell, J.P.; Lee, A.Y.; Raman, R.; Tan, G.S.W.; Schmetterer, L.; Keane, P.A.; Wong, T.Y. Artificial intelligence and deep learning in ophthalmology. *Br. J. Ophthalmol.* **2019**, *103*, 167–175. [CrossRef] [PubMed]
139. Govindaswamy, N.; Ratra, D.; Dalan, D.; Doralli, S.; Tirumalai, A.A.; Nagarajan, R.; Mochi, T.; Shetty, N.; Roy, A.S. Vascular changes precede tomographic changes in diabetic eyes without retinopathy and improve artificial intelligence diagnostics. *J. Biophotonics* **2020**, *13*, e202000107. [CrossRef]
140. Guo, Y.; Camino, A.; Wang, J.; Huang, D.; Hwang, T.S.; Jia, Y. MEDnet, a neural network for automated detection of avascular area in OCT angiography. *Biomed. Opt. Express.* **2018**, *9*, 5147. [CrossRef]
141. Guo, Y.; Hormel, T.T.; Xiong, H.; Wang, B.; Camino, A.; Wang, J.; Huang, D.; Hwang, T.S.; Jia, Y. Development and validation of a deep learning algorithm for distinguishing the nonperfusion area from signal reduction artifacts on OCT angiography. *Biomed. Opt. Express* **2019**, *10*, 3257. [CrossRef] [PubMed]

142. Lauermann, J.L.; Treder, M.; Alnawaiseh, M.; Clemens, C.R.; Eter, N.; Alten, F. Automated OCT angiography image quality assessment using a deep learning algorithm. *Graefes Arch. Clin. Exp. Ophthalmol.* **2019**, *257*, 1641–1648. [CrossRef] [PubMed]
143. Prentašic, P.; Heisler, M.; Mammo, Z.; Lee, S.; Merkur, A.; Navajas, E.; Beg, M.F.; Šarunic, M.; Loncaric, S. Segmentation of the foveal microvasculature using deep learning networks. *J. Biomed. Opt.* **2016**, *21*, 075008. [CrossRef]
144. Guo, M.; Zhao, M.; Cheong, A.M.Y.; Dai, H.; Lam, A.K.C.; Zhou, Y. Automatic quantification of superficial foveal avascular zone in optical coherence tomography angiography implemented with deep learning. *Vis. Comput. Ind. Biomed. Art* **2019**, *2*, 1–9. [CrossRef]
145. Ryu, G.; Lee, K.; Park, D.; Park, S.H.; Sagong, M. A deep learning model for identifying diabetic retinopathy using optical coherence tomography angiography. *Sci. Rep.* **2021**, *11*, 1–9. [CrossRef]
146. Le, D.; Alam, M.; Yao, C.K.; Lim, J.I.; Hsieh, Y.-T.; Chan, R.V.P.; Toslak, D.; Yao, X. Transfer Learning for Automated OCTA Detection of Diabetic Retinopathy. *Transl. Vis. Sci. Technol.* **2020**, *9*, 1–9. [CrossRef] [PubMed]
147. Heisler, M.; Karst, S.; Lo, J.; Mammo, Z.; Yu, T.; Warner, S.; Maberley, D.; Beg, M.F.; Navajas, E.V.; Sarunic, M.V. Ensemble Deep Learning for Diabetic Retinopathy Detection Using Optical Coherence Tomography Angiography. *Transl. Vis. Sci. Technol.* **2020**, *9*, 1–11. [CrossRef] [PubMed]
148. Sandhu, H.S.; Elmogy, M.; Sharafeldeen, A.; Elsharkawy, M.; El-Adawy, N.; Eltanboly, A.; Shalaby, A.; Keynton, R.; El-Baz, A. Automated Diagnosis of Diabetic Retinopathy Using Clinical Biomarkers, Optical Coherence Tomography, and Optical Coherence Tomography Angiography. *Am. J. Ophthalmol.* **2020**, *216*, 201–206. [CrossRef] [PubMed]
149. Nazir, T.; Irtaza, A.; Shabbir, Z.; Javed, A.; Akram, U.; Mahmood, M.T. Diabetic retinopathy detection through novel tetragonal local octa patterns and extreme learning machines. *Artif. Intell. Med.* **2019**, *99*, 101695. [CrossRef] [PubMed]
150. Nagasawa, T.; Tabuchi, H.; Masumoto, H.; Morita, S.; Niki, M.; Ohara, Z.; Yoshizumi, Y.; Mitamura, Y. Accuracy of Diabetic Retinopathy Staging with a Deep Convolutional Neural Network Using Ultra-Wide-Field Fundus Ophthalmoscopy and Optical Coherence Tomography Angiography. *J. Ophthalmol.* **2021**, *2021*, 1–10. [CrossRef] [PubMed]
151. Xiong, H.; You, Q.S.; Guo, Y.; Wang, J.; Wang, B.; Gao, L.; Flaxel, C.J.; Bailey, S.T.; Hwang, T.S.; Jia, Y. Deep learning-based signal-independent assessment of macular avascular area on 6 × 6 mm optical coherence tomography angiogram in diabetic retinopathy: A comparison to instrument-embedded software. *Br. J. Ophthalmol.* **2021**. [CrossRef] [PubMed]
152. Kawai, K.; Uji, A.; Murakami, T.; Kadomoto, S.; Oritani, Y.; Dodo, Y.; Muraoka, Y.; Akagi, T.; Miyata, M.; Tsujikawa, A. Image evaluation of artificial intelligence supported optical coherence tomography imaging using OCT-A1 device in diabetic retinopathy. *Retina* **2021**, *41*, 1730–1738. [CrossRef]

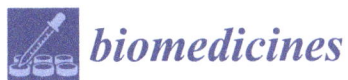

Review

Type 2 Diabetes Mellitus and COVID-19: A Narrative Review

Cristina Rey-Reñones [1,2,3], Sara Martinez-Torres [2], Francisco M. Martín-Luján [1,2,3], Carles Pericas [4], Ana Redondo [5], Carles Vilaplana-Carnerero [4,6], Angela Dominguez [4,7] and María Grau [7,8,9,*]

1. Research Support Unit-Camp de Tarragona, Catalan Institute of Health (ICS), 43005 Tarragona, Spain
2. IDIAP Jordi Gol, Catalan Institute of Health (ICS), USR Camp de Tarragona, 43202 Reus, Spain
3. School of Medicine and Health Sciences, Universitat Rovira i Virgili, 43201 Reus, Spain
4. Department of Medicine, University of Barcelona, 08036 Barcelona, Spain
5. Hospital Universitario Bellvitge, Catalan Institute of Health (ICS), 08907 Barcelona, Spain
6. IDIAP Jordi Gol, Catalan Institute of Health (ICS), 08007 Barcelona, Spain
7. Biomedical Research Consortium in Epidemiology and Public Health (CIBERESP), 28029 Madrid, Spain
8. Serra Hunter Fellow, Department of Medicine, University of Barcelona, 08036 Barcelona, Spain
9. August Pi i Sunyer Biomedical Research Institute (IDIBAPS), 08036 Barcelona, Spain
* Correspondence: mariagrau@ub.edu

Abstract: Type-2 diabetes mellitus (T2DM) is a chronic metabolic disorder. The incidence and prevalence of patients with T2DM are increasing worldwide, even reaching epidemic values in most high- and middle-income countries. T2DM could be a risk factor of developing complications in other diseases. Indeed, some studies suggest a bidirectional interaction between T2DM and COVID-19. A growing body of evidence shows that COVID-19 prognosis in individuals with T2DM is worse compared with those without. Moreover, various studies have reported the emergence of newly diagnosed patients with T2DM after SARS-CoV-2 infection. The most common treatments for T2DM may influence SARS-CoV-2 and their implication in infection is briefly discussed in this review. A better understanding of the link between TD2M and COVID-19 could proactively identify risk factors and, as a result, develop strategies to improve the prognosis for these patients.

Keywords: type-2 diabetes mellitus; epidemiology; COVID-19; bidirectional link; antidiabetic treatment

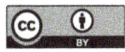

1. Introduction

In the last decades, type-2 diabetes mellitus (T2DM) has become a chronic metabolic disorder caused by the interaction of different genetic and environmental factors. The incidence and prevalence of patients with T2DM are increasing worldwide, even reaching epidemic values in most high- and middle-income countries [1]. The World Health Organization (WHO) estimates that T2DM will be the seventh leading cause of death by 2030 worldwide (Figure 1) [2]. The main reasons for this increase seem the high prevalence of obesity and the unhealthy lifestyles. Uncontrolled and prolonged T2DM can lead to serious complications, some of them being life-threatening [3]. As a result, the healthcare cost of T2DM and the related diseases is growing every year [4]. Strategies to control T2DM include appropriate life-style changes as well as medication intake when necessary [5].

T2DM could be a risk factor for developing complications in other diseases. At the onset of the pandemics, the USA Centers for Disease Control and Prevention (CDC) described that one third of patients infected with COVID-19 had comorbidities. Thus, people with at least one underlying condition account for 78% of admissions to the intensive care unit (ICU) and 94% of deaths. T2DM was the most frequently reported, being the 10.9% of the cases [6]. In addition, a fast-growing evidence reports a bidirectional interplay between T2DM and COVID-19. Clinical data so far suggest that the severe acute respiratory syndrome coronavirus 2 (SARS-CoV-2) infection may result in metabolic dysregulation and in impaired glucose homeostasis [7].

The objective of this review is to provide an overview of the most recent studies that point to T2DM as a risk factor and poor prognosis of COVID-19, as well as, to summarize the potential mechanisms involved in this relationship.

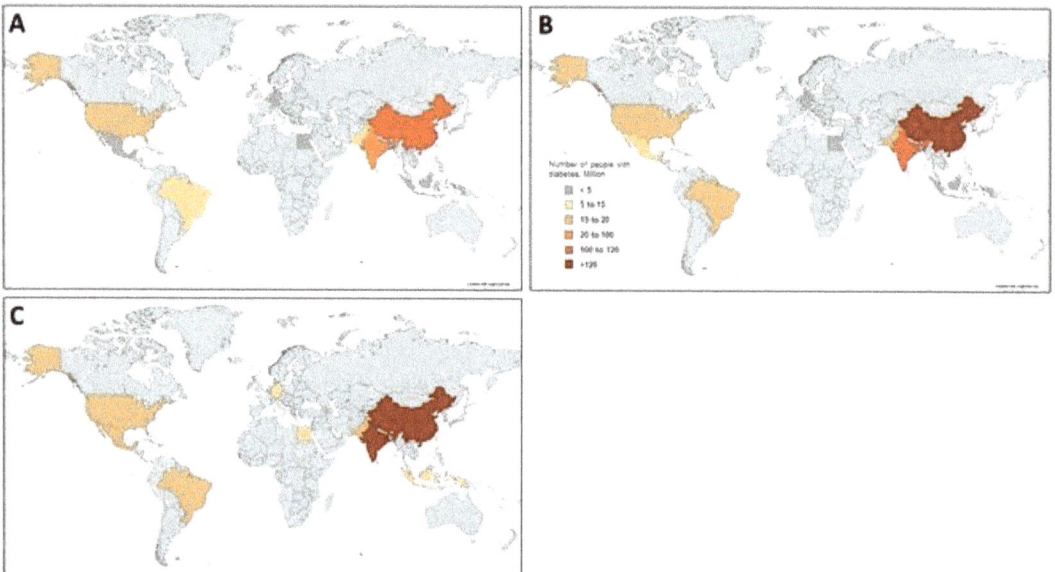

Figure 1. Estimated number of adults with diabetes (20–79 years) in the top 10 countries worldwide in (**A**) 2019, (**B**) 2030 and (**C**) 2045. Data for this figure is obtained from Mathers et al. [2].

2. T2DM as a Risk Factor for the Development and Prognosis of COVID-19

Several risk factors have been associated with an increased risk of SARS-CoV-2 infection and complication. For instance, male sex, older age, deprivation and comorbidities such as cardiopathy, hypertension, chronic obstructive pulmonary disease, immunosuppression or T2DM [8,9]. Thus, 33.8% of 5700 of patients with COVID-19 admitted to 12 hospitals within the Northwell Health system in New York had T2DM [10]. In addition, a random meta-analysis of 18 different studies determined that the risk of severe disease was 2.4-fold higher in patients with T2DM compared with those without [11], whereas another one showed a 2.6-fold higher severity risk by increased fasting blood glucose at admission [12].

2.1. Risk of Death and Complications in T2DM Patients with COVID-19

So far, different studies have shown that people with T2DM have higher risk of COVID-19 mortality compared with non-diabetic individuals [11–19]. Nevertheless, Al-Salameh et al., reported that COVID-19-related death in patients with T2DM was lower than in general population, but the rate of intensive care unit (ICU) admission was increased [20]. As highlighted by Diedisheim et al., the age may play a key role because after age 50 years, diabetes-related risk might be weakened by all other comorbidities or conditions associated with aging [15] (Table 1).

In addition to the increased mortality associated with COVID-19, patients with T2DM also present with more complications from such infection, even requiring admission to the ICU or dying [10,20]. Moreover, uncontrolled hyperglycemia can also be a risk factor for an adverse COVID-19 prognosis. An observational study including more than 1000 patients hospitalized with COVID-19 in USA showed that 40% of patients had diabetes or uncontrolled hyperglycemia at admission, and hospital mortality was four times higher for DM patients. The same study showed that mortality was seven times higher for those without pre-existing T2DM who developed in-hospital hyperglycemia [14]. Similarly, a recent meta-analysis that included 14,502 patients confirmed these findings and showed a nonlinear relationship between fasting blood glucose at admission and severity: every mmol/L enhancement in glucose levels increased the risk of COVID-19 severity by 33% [12].

Table 1. COVID-19 Death in T2DM: Summary of the main results.

	Country	n	Mortality (%)		COVID-19 Death in T2DM
			No T2DM	T2DM	HR (95% CI)
Al-Salameh [20]	France	433	21.5	17.4	0.77 (0.44–1.32)
Barron [13]	UK	61,414,470	0.03	0.26	2.03 (1.97–2.09)
Bode [14]	USA	1122	6.2	28.8	–
De Almeida-Pititto [11]	Meta-analysis	4,305	12.4	29.9	2.50 (1.74–3.59)
Diedisheim [15]	France	6314	22	26	1.81 (1.14–2.87)
Espiritu [16]	Philippines	10,881	12.9	26.4	1.46 (1.28–1.68)
Kim [17]	USA	10,861	–	–	1.20 (1.08–1.32)
Lazarus [12]	Meta-analysis	14,502	–	–	1.81 (1.41–2.33)
Williamson [18]	UK	17,278,392	0.06	0.26	1.95 (1.83–2.08)
Wu [19]	China	44,672	2.3	7.3	–

CI, confidence interval. HR, Hazard Ratio. T2DM, type 2 diabetes mellitus.

2.2. Potential Mechanisms Underlying Unfaborable Clinical Outcomes of COVID-19 in People with Diabetes

Epidemiological studies have determined the severity of COVID-19 due to a number of complications or comorbidities associated with T2DM. Co-occurrence of microvascular and macrovascular T2DM complications, including cardiovascular disease, renal failure, retinopathy and reduced renal function, could be responsible for the increased poor COVID-19 outcomes and mortality after infection [21–23].

T2DM, even in the stages of prediabetes, is characterized by a dysregulation of glucose homeostasis, chronic inflammatory and prothrombotic state accompanied with other affectations, such as metabolic, vascular, immune and hematological abnormalities, which could explain the negative response to infections [24]. Some of these alterations have been proposed to explain T2DM impact on COVID-19 prognosis, including glucotoxicity, endothelial damage, chronic inflammatory state, oxidative stress and abnormal cytokine production [25,26].

Hyperglycemia could directly exacerbate SARS-CoV-2 infection, promoting the expression and activation of, angiotensin-converting enzyme 2 (ACE2) cellular receptor, the main receptor of the SARS-CoV-2, and increasing the expression of the serine protease TMPRSS2, which mediates the cleavage of the viral spike protein [27]. Of note, high glucose levels increase the production of inflammatory cytokines and cellular mediators and pro-thrombotic processes, promoting the development of acute cardiovascular complications [28]. Moreover, chronic hyperglycemia could compromise the innate and humoral immune response inhibiting lymphocyte proliferation, reducing the activity of natural killer cells and affecting the function of monocyte/macrophage and neutrophils [24,29]. According to this, different reports demonstrated that elevated glucose levels in admission is an independent risk factor for critical progression and in-hospital mortality in COVID-19 patients [30–33]. Therefore, uncontrolled hyperglycemia takes part to other COVID-19 complications, such as atherosclerosis, diabetic nephropathy, peripheral arteriosclerosis, and diabetic ketoacidosis [30]. Thus, hyperglycemia management has been proposed to improve clinical COVID-19 outcomes.

Other evidences suggested that chronic endothelial dysfunction predisposes to severe COVID-19 disease. In this regard, hyperglycemia and insulin resistance leads to endothelial dysfunction and glycocalyx damage in patients with T2DM, leading to leucocyte adhesion and promoting procoagulant and antifibrinolytic state [34,35]. A recent study of in-hospital COVID-19 patients from China reported that the COVID-19 severity was correlated with increased blood levels of IL-6 and lactate dehydrogenase (LDH) [36]. Of note, patients with T2DM have a higher inflammatory response, mainly characterized by increased levels of interleukin-6 (IL-6), interleukin-2 (IL-2) and the tumor necrosis factor α (TNF-α) [37]. This fact could explain the rapid COVID-19 progression and severity in patients with T2DM.

Altogether, these alterations could explain why patients with T2DM have a worse prognosis of COVID-19 (Figure 2).

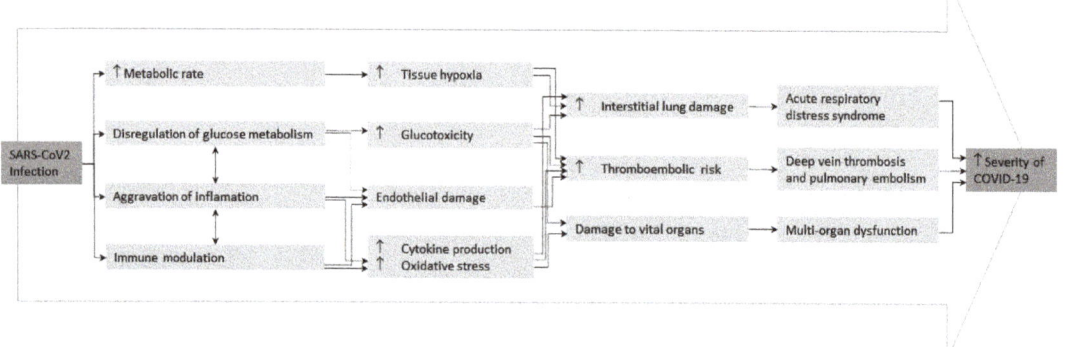

Figure 2. Possible mechanisms behind adverse clinical outcomes of COVID-19 in people with type 2 diabetes mellitus. Adapted from Lim et al. [25].

3. SARS-CoV-2 Infection as a Risk Factor of Morbidity and Mortality: Metabolic Deregulation and Homeostasis Alteration

Infection affects several pathophysiological pathways, during the course of the disease, which eventually leads to late complications. So far, clinical data suggest that SARS-CoV-2 may cause metabolic dysregulation and impairment of glucose homeostasis. A study suggests that infection may be a precipitating factor for acute hyperglycemia, worsening prognosis in poorly controlled T2DM patients [38]. Moreover, some studies focus on the role of glycemic control as a critical factor to reduce complications, severe outcomes and mortality during SARS-CoV-2 infection [39,40].

Other studies identified the endothelium, which expressed both the ACE2 receptor and the serine protease TMPRSS2, as a first key player on the homeostasis alteration. In healthy individuals, endothelium is considered to be major contributor to various physiological processes supporting homeostasis. Lambadiari et al. showed that SARS-CoV-2 can cause endothelial and vascular dysfunction, which was associated with impaired cardiac performance for four months after SARS-CoV-2 infection [41]. After infection, there is an increase of cytokine levels and immune cells, which could induce insulin resistance and hyperglycemia [42]. Similarly, studies about Severe Acute Respiratory Syndrome (SARS) and Middle Eastern Respiratory Syndrome (MERS) point out how inflammatory cells may affect the liver, altering insulin-mediated glucose uptake, resulting in hyperinsulinemia and hyperglycemia [43].

Other studies suggest that there are possible underlying mechanisms that could explain the acute damage of pancreatic islets by SARS-CoV-2 and the consequent loss of insulin secretory capacity [40,44]. The exacerbated immune response through the virus-mediated release of chemokines and cytokines could also damage pancreatic cells and impair their ability to detect glucose and release insulin. Moreover, the immune response of the virus can further affect the ability of the liver and muscles to identify alterations [40,44]. Considering previous experience with inflammatory responses, COVID-19 inflammatory and viral immune responses can affect insulin sensitivity and deregulate glucose metabolism, leading to a vicious cycle of hyperglycemia and inflammatory response that destroys tissue integrity and physiological function during critical stages of infection. Thus, frequently used drugs in the treatment of COVID-19, such as corticosteroids or antiviral agents, can aggravate hyperglycemia and result in lipodystrophy and insulin resistance [45,46].

Regarding glucose homeostasis, severe SARS-CoV-2 infection contributes to insulin resistance and hyperglycemia by increased cytokines and unregulated compensatory hormonal response [21,47]. Moreover, glucotoxicity and the associated consequences, added to the increase of inflammatory cytokines by SARS-CoV-2 infection, oxidative stress, immune dysfunction and endothelial damage, predict an increase in metabolic complications, an increased risk of thromboembolism and multiorgan damage in individuals with T2DM [25,48].

4. Newly Emerging Patients with T2DM Infected with SARS-CoV-2

SARS-CoV-2 infection would have a direct effect of on glucose metabolism. A recent metanalysis have shown 492 cases of newly diagnosed diabetes from eight studies that included 3711 COVID-19 patients with a pooled proportion of 14.4% (95% confidence interval [5.9–25.8%]) [49]. Recent findings suggest a direct effect of SARS-CoV-2 on glucose metabolism resulting in new presentations of T2DM characterized by diabetic ketoacidosis, hyperosmolarity and unusually high insulin requirements to achieve glycemic control [49,50]. Although the evidence of a direct relationship between how SARS-CoV-2 is still sparse, Kazakou et al. described to possible links. First, the SARS-CoV-2 infection could damage B cells in the pancreas through the direct cytolytic effect of the virus. Second, the direct damage to the endocrine system during infection, which could contribute to the development of glucose and metabolic abnormalities in people previous infected (Figure 3) [42]. Understanding the effects of COVID-19 on glucose metabolism and homeostasis is essential to prevent and control complications associated with this infection and to help patients recovery [7].

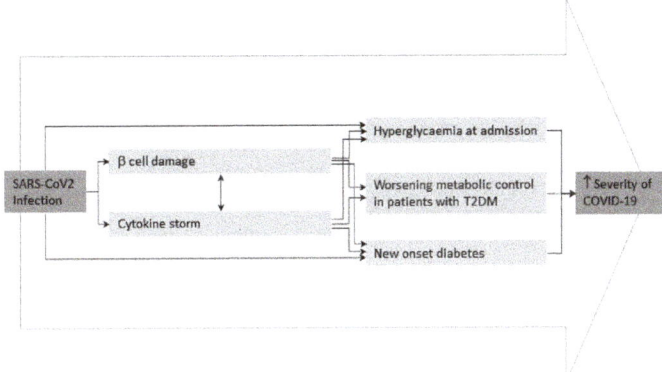

Figure 3. Potential pathogenic mechanisms of SARS-CoV-2 infection underlying metabolic deregulation and homeostasis alteration. Adapted from Apicella et al. [51].

5. How Antidiabetic Treatment Influences SARS-CoV-2 Infection

Blood glucose control may be crucial as a preventive measure for adverse outcomes related to COVID-19 [7]. Table 2 shows the influence of the most common treatments for T2DM on SARS-CoV-2 infection.

5.1. Metformin

As discussed above, inflammatory exacerbation due to increased cytokines levels has been recognized as one of the main keys to poor prognosis in COVID-19. The anti-inflammatory properties of metformin are already known, suggesting a beneficial effect for COVID-19 disease [52]. Despite this, immunomodulatory actions of metformin in the context of COVID-19 remain unclear. Some evidence point out the positive implications of metformin in COVID-19 as reduced insulin resistance and inhibition of virus entry through AMPK activation and phosphorylation of ACE2 [7]. Crouse et al., affirmed that although T2DM is a factor risk for COVID-19-related mortality, the risk is drastically reduced in subjects treated with metformin before the diagnosis of COVID-19, considering that metformin can provide a protective effect in this high-risk population [53]. In addition, a meta-analysis estimated a risk reduction associated with this treatment in individuals with T2DM and SARS-CoV-2 infection (Odds ratio (OR) = −0.37; 95% CI [−0.59; −0.16]) [54].

Table 2. Beneficial and adverse effects and clinical recommendations of antidiabetic treatment for COVID-19.

Anti-Diabetic Treatment	Beneficial Effect	Adverse Effect	Recommendations
Metformin	Anti-inflammatory effect Reduction insulin resistance Inhibition virus entry	Lactic acidosis (kidney damage)	Avoid in dehydrated patients
Insulin	Continuous glycemic control		First treatment
SGLT2 inhibitors	Anti-inflammatory effects		Avoid in severely affected patients with COVID-19 and at risk of dehydration
Sulfonylureas	Anti-inflammatory effects	Risk of hypoglycemia	Avoid in severe COVID-19 disease and combination with chloroquine or hydroxychloroquine treatments
Thiazolidinediones	Insulin resistance improvement Anti-inflammatory and anti-atherosclerotic effects and effects	Weight gain and swelling Heart failure	Not recommended in patients with COVID-19
DPP4 inhibitors	Anti-inflammatory and antifibrotic effects		Mild and severe cases of COVID-19
GLP-1 receptor agonists	Anti-inflammatory effect Reduction cardiac events Control glucose homeostasis	Gastrointestinal side effects	Control of blood glucose levels in ICU hospitalized patients

According to the practical recommendations for the management of T2DM in patients with COVID-19 a treatment cessation with metformin is recommended in dehydrated patients and follow the guidelines according to the infection, because lactic acidosis is likely to appear [55]. The same guide recommends careful surveillance of kidney function because of the high risk of chronic kidney disease or acute kidney damage [27].

5.2. Insulin

Insulin treatment is the first treatment option for controlling hyperglycemia in critical patients. Available evidence suggests that it is also the most appropriate hypoglycemic agent in hospitalized patients with severe T2DM and COVID-19 [56]. Recent studies have shown that severe cases of newly onset or pre-existing T2DM patients with COVID-19, high doses of intravenous insulin infusion are needed to control glycemic levels [42]. According to this, continuous glucose monitoring during hospitalization helps to ensure good control and minimize the risk of hypoglycemia in people on insulin therapy. Thus, insulin treatment results in an improvement in glycemic control in patients hospitalized in the ICU and offers the advantage of remote monitoring [57,58].

Some evidences indicate that patients with T2DM under insulin treatment for COVID-19 present worse clinical outcomes when compared with other antidiabetic drugs in early-stage of the disease. In fact, insulin treatment was associated with increased systemic inflammation and increased damage to vital organs, suggesting that insulin therapy for patients with COVID-19 and T2DM needs to be used with caution (27.2% versus 3.5%; adjusted Hazard Ratio = 5.38; 95% CI [2.75–10.54]) [59]. Thus, insulin treatment reflects a more advanced stage of the disease with associated co-morbidities, indicating the need of studies in this regard [60]. However, insulin remains the star treatment in serious hospitalized patients [27,48].

5.3. SGLT2 (Sodium-Glucose Cotransporter-2) Inhibitors

SGLT2 inhibitors are a type of oral medication indicated to reduce blood glucose in adults with T2DM. Patients treated with SGLT2 inhibitors have an increased risk of dehydration and euglycemic diabetic ketoacidosis in case of acute illness, especially if the disease accompanies anorexia and vomiting [61]. Some studies suggest that SGLT2 inhibitors may reduce viral load due to increased lactate concentrations and decreased intracellular pH. In addition to the already known anti-inflammatory properties, primarily on endothelial function, SGLT2 inhibitors therapy could play a protective role in COVID-19-related organ failure [25]. The meta-analysis performed by Nguyen et al. showed a significant mortality reduction in individuals with T2DM treated with SGLT2 inhibitors previous to hospital admission (OR = 0.60 [0.40–0.88]) [62]. Nevertheless, a double-blind, placebo-controlled clinical trial with dapagliflozin in COVID-19 hospitalized patients with one or more cardiometabolic risk factors did not show a significant reduction in organ dysfunction or death, or in clinical recovery [63]. The recommendations for the practice in the management of T2DM in patients with COVID-19 suggest the discontinuation of treatment with SGLT2 inhibitors in severely affected patients with COVID-19 and at risk of dehydration [27].

5.4. Sulfonylureas

Sulfonylureas are the oldest oral type of antidiabetic drugs. Sulfonylureas bind to the ATP-sensitive potassium channels on the pancreatic β-cells, resulting in membrane depolarization and, therefore, stimulating insulin secretion [64]. On the one side, a systematic review and meta-analysis highlight the potential for sulfonylurea treatment to reduce the risk of mortality in T2DM patients with COVID-19 (OR = 0.80; 95% CI [0.66; 0.96]) [54]. On the other side, as Drucker's review points out, patients with T2DM and severe COVID-19 disease should avoid treatment with sulfonylureas and discontinue treatment in case of hospitalization due to the risk of hypoglycemia, especially in situations of low oral food intake or in combination with chloroquine or hydroxychloroquine treatments [48].

5.5. Thiazolidinediones

These drugs act as partial or selective agonists of the peroxisome activated by proliferator-γ (PPAR-γ) receptor, a nuclear receptor that regulates the transcription of several genes involved in glucose and lipid metabolism. Thiazolidinediones have shown to improve insulin resistance and have anti-inflammatory properties and anti-atherosclerotic effects, having the potential to mediate the protective effects of the cardiovascular system [25]. This treatment has been associated with weight gain and swelling, which has also led to an increase in heart failure. Therefore, its use is not recommended in patients with COVID-19, although the literature suggests that more clinical trials are needed to maximize the risk-benefit relationship of thiazolidinediones use in patients with COVID-19 [65].

5.6. Dipeptidyl Peptidase-4 (DPP4) Inhibitors

DPP4 is a transmembrane glycoprotein expressed in the spleen, lung, liver, kidneys, and immune cells or soluble circulating in the bloodstream. DPP4 has a crucial role in glucose homeostasis. DPP4 inhibitors in patients with DM2 have been used for a long time since 2006, with good tolerance and few adverse reactions reported [66]. The role of DPP-4 inhibition as an inflammation mitigator and potent antifibrotic agent is supported by several experimental studies [67].

Recent studies suggest that DPP4 inhibitors could benefit the treatment of mild or even severe cases of COVID-19. A metanalysis including 10 observational studies found that DDP-4 inhibitors reduce the risk for COVID-19-related mortality by 50% [67]. Other metanalysis also support the hypothesis that DDP-4 inhibitors could have a protective effect on COVID-19 (OR = 0.58; 95% CI [0.34–0.99]) [68]. Finally, the reduction in mortality was marginally significant in the metanalysis performed by Kan et al. (OR = 0.72; 95% CI [0.51–1.01]) [54]. Thus, further research is necessary to evaluate the role of DPP4 inhibitors in patients with T2DM and COVID-19 [69].

5.7. Glucagon-Like Peptide 1 (GLP-1) Receptor Agonist

GLP-1 is an incretine hormone responsible of blood glucose reduction through its receptor that reduce blood. Beyond controlling glycemia, GLP-1 receptor agonist has great potential for treating hyperglycemia [70]. Indeed, a review concluded that GLP-1 receptor agonist was able to reduce blood glucose levels and in turn, the administration of insulin without increasing the incidence of hypoglycemia. A recent Bayesian Network Metanalysis GLP-1 receptor agonist treatment was liked to a decrease in COVID-19-related mortality in T2DM individuals compared to non-users (OR = 0.91; 95% CI [0.84; 0.98]) [71]. However, there is not sufficient evidence to recommend GLP-1 receptor agonist for critical patients with T2DM and COVID-19 [72]. Regarding the adverse effects, this treatment can trigger gastrointestinal side effects such as nausea and vomiting, and consequently, aspiration in this type of patients. For this reason, GLP-1 receptor agonists are not recommended for patients with mild or moderate COVID-19 [27]. Among the most outstanding findings about GLP-1 receptor agonists is the reduction of major cardiac events in patients with T2DM, and its anti-inflammatory action under conditions of low-grade inflammation such as atherosclerosis and non-alcoholic fatty liver disease [73,74].

6. Summary

This review provides the latest insights into the interaction between COVID-19 and T2DM, which is considered a major risk factor for COVID-19 disease. Furthermore, new data have identified hyperglycemia and insulin resistance in patients after SARS-CoV-2 infection, leading to an emerging form of T2DM. The pathophysiological effects of both diseases (e.g. inflammation, immune response, endothelial damage and glucotoxicity) have been proposed as the main potential mechanisms behind this bidirectional interplay. Moreover, research works have identified the interaction between several T2DM treatments and the prognosis of COVID-19, leading to more specific recommendations for the treatment of hyperglycemia during COVID-19. A better understanding of the link between TD2M and COVID-19 could proactively identify risk factors and, as a result, develop strategies to improve the prognosis for these patients.

Author Contributions: Conceptualization, M.G. and F.M.M.-L.; methodology, C.R.-R., S.M.-T. and M.G.; investigation, C.R.-R., S.M.-T. and M.G.; writing—original draft preparation, C.R.-R., S.M.-T., C.P., A.R. and M.G.; writing—review and editing, C.R.-R., S.M.-T., F.M.M.-L., A.R., C.P., C.V.-C., A.D. and M.G. All authors have read and agreed to the published version of the manuscript.

Funding: This research received no external funding.

Institutional Review Board Statement: Not applicable.

Informed Consent Statement: Not applicable.

Data Availability Statement: Data sharing not applicable.

Conflicts of Interest: The authors declare no conflict of interest.

References

1. International Diabetes Federation. *IDF Diabetes Atlas*, 10th ed.; International Diabetes Federation: Brussels, Belgium; Available online: https://www.diabetesatlas.org (accessed on 24 June 2022).
2. Mathers, C.D.; Loncar, D. Projections of global mortality and burden of disease from 2002 to 2030. *PLoS Med.* **2006**, *3*, e442. [CrossRef] [PubMed]
3. Baena-Díez, J.M.; Peñafiel, J.; Subirana, I.; Ramos, R.; Elosua, R.; Marín-Ibañez, A.; Guembe, M.J.; Rigo, F.; Tormo-Díaz, M.J.; Moreno-Iribas, C.; et al. Risk of cause-specific death in individuals with diabetes: A competing risks analysis. *Diabetes Care* **2016**, *39*, 1987–1995. [CrossRef] [PubMed]
4. Bommer, C.; Sagalova, V.; Heesemann, E.; Manne-Goehler, J.; Atun, R.; Bärnighausen, T.; Davies, J.; Vollmer, S. Global economic burden of diabetes in adults: Projections from 2015 to 2030. *Diabetes Care* **2018**, *41*, 963–970. [CrossRef]
5. Alam, S.; Hasan, K.; Neaz, S.; Hussain, N.; Hossain, F.; Rahman, T. Diabetes mellitus: Insights from epidemiology, biochemistry, risk factors, diagnosis, complications and comprehensive management. *Diabetology* **2021**, *2*, 36–50. [CrossRef]
6. Chow, N.; Fleming-Dutra, K.; Gierke, R.; Hall, A.; Hughes, M.; Pilishvili, T.; Ritchey, M.; Roguski, K.; Skoff, T.; Ussery, E. Preliminary estimates of the prevalence of selected underlying health conditions among patients with coronavirus disease 2019—United States, February 12–March 28, 2020. *MMWR. Morb. Mortal. Wkly. Rep.* **2020**, *69*, 382–386. [CrossRef]
7. Kazakou, P.; Lambadiari, V.; Ikonomidis, I.; Kountouri, A.; Panagopoulos, G.; Athanasopoulos, S.; Korompoki, E.; Kalomenidis, I.; Dimopoulos, M.A.; Mitrakou, A. Diabetes and COVID-19: A bidirectional interplay. *Front. Endocrinol.* **2022**, *13*, 780663. [CrossRef] [PubMed]
8. Baena-Díez, J.M.; Barroso, M.; Cordeiro-Coelho, S.I.; Díaz, J.L.; Grau, M. Impact of COVID-19 outbreak by income: Hitting hardest the most deprived. *J. Public Health* **2020**, *42*, 698–703. [CrossRef]
9. Baena-Díez, J.M.; Gonzalez-Casafont, I.; Cordeiro-Coelho, S.; Fernández-González, S.; Rodríguez-Jorge, M.; Pérez-Torres, C.U.F.; Larrañaga-Cabrera, A.; García-Lareo, M.; de la Arada-Acebes, A.; Martín-Jiménez, E.; et al. Effectiveness of telephone monitoring in primary care to detect pneumonia and associated risk factors in patients with SARS-CoV-2. *Healthcare* **2021**, *9*, 1548. [CrossRef]
10. Richardson, S.; Hirsch, J.S.; Narasimhan, M.; Crawford, J.M.; McGinn, T.; Davidson, K.W.; the Northwell COVID-19 Research Consortium. Presenting characteristics, comorbidities, and outcomes among 5700 patients hospitalized with COVID-19 in the New York City area. *JAMA* **2020**, *323*, 2052–2059. [CrossRef]
11. de Almeida-Pitito, B.; Dualib, P.M.; Zajdenverg, L.; Dantas, J.R.; de Souza, F.D.; Rodacki, M.; Bertoluci, M.C.; Brazilian Diabetes Society Study Group (SBD). Severity and mortality of COVID 19 in patients with diabetes, hypertension and cardiovascular disease: A meta-analysis. *Diabetol. Metab. Syndr.* **2020**, *12*, 1–12. [CrossRef]
12. Lazarus, G.; Audrey, J.; Wangsaputra, V.K.; Tamara, A.; Tahapary, D.L. High admission blood glucose independently predicts poor prognosis in COVID-19 patients: A systematic review and dose-response meta-analysis. *Diabetes Res. Clin. Pract.* **2020**, *171*, 108561. [CrossRef] [PubMed]
13. Barron, E.; Bakhai, C.; Kar, P.; Weaver, A.; Bradley, D.; Ismail, H.; Knighton, P.; Holman, N.; Khunti, K.; Sattar, N.; et al. Associations of type 1 and type 2 diabetes with COVID-19-related mortality in England: A whole-population study. *Lancet Diabetes Endocrinol.* **2020**, *8*, 813–822. [CrossRef]
14. Bode, B.; Garrett, V.; Messler, J.; McFarland, R.; Crowe, J.; Booth, R.; Klonoff, D.C. Glycemic characteristics and clinical outcomes of COVID-19 patients hospitalized in the United States. *J. Diabetes Sci. Technol.* **2020**, *14*, 813–821. [CrossRef] [PubMed]
15. Diedisheim, M.; Dancoisne, E.; Gautier, J.-F.; Larger, E.; Cosson, E.; Fève, B.; Chanson, P.; Czernichow, S.; Tatulashvili, S.; Raffin-Sanson, M.-L.; et al. Diabetes increases severe COVID-19 outcomes primarily in younger adults. *J. Clin. Endocrinol. Metab.* **2021**, *106*, e3364–e3368. [CrossRef] [PubMed]
16. Espiritu, A.I.; Chiu, H.H.C.; Sy, M.C.C.; Anlacan, V.M.M.; Macalintal, C.M.S.A.; Robles, J.B.; Cataniag, P.L.; Flores, M.K.C.; Tangcuangco-Trinidad, N.J.C.; Juangco, D.N.A.; et al. The outcomes of patients with diabetes mellitus in The Philippine CORONA Study. *Sci. Rep.* **2021**, *11*, 1–10. [CrossRef]
17. Kim, T.S.; Roslin, M.; Wang, J.J.; Kane, J.; Hirsch, J.S.; Kim, E.J.; the Northwell Health COVID-19 Research Consortium. BMI as a Risk factor for clinical outcomes in patients hospitalized with COVID-19 in New York. *Obesity* **2020**, *29*, 279–284. [CrossRef]
18. Williamson, E.J.; Walker, A.J.; Bhaskaran, K.; Bacon, S.; Bates, C.; Morton, C.E.; Curtis, H.J.; Mehrkar, A.; Evans, D.; Inglesby, P.; et al. Factors associated with COVID-19-related death using Open SAFELY. *Nature* **2020**, *584*, 430–436. [CrossRef]
19. Wu, Z.; McGoogan, J.M. Characteristics of and Important Lessons From the Coronavirus Disease 2019 (COVID-19) Outbreak in China: Summary of a report of 72,314 cases from the Chinese Center for Disease Control and Prevention. *JAMA* **2020**, *323*, 1239–1242. [CrossRef]
20. Al-Salameh, A.; Lanoix, J.; Bennis, Y.; Andrejak, C.; Brochot, E.; Deschasse, G.; Dupont, H.; Goeb, V.; Jaureguy, M.; Lion, S.; et al. Characteristics and outcomes of COVID-19 in hospitalized patients with and without diabetes. *Diabetes/Metab. Res. Rev.* **2020**, *37*, e3388. [CrossRef]
21. Holman, N.; Knighton, P.; Kar, P.; O'Keefe, J.; Curley, M.; Weaver, A.; Barron, E.; Bakhai, C.; Khunti, K.; Wareham, N.J.; et al. Risk factors for COVID-19-related mortality in people with type 1 and type 2 diabetes in England: A population-based cohort study. *Lancet Diabetes Endocrinol.* **2020**, *8*, 823–833. [CrossRef]
22. Cariou, B.; Pichelin, M.; Goronflot, T.; Gonfroy, C.; Marre, M.; Raffaitin-Cardin, C.; Thivolet, C.; Wargny, M.; Hadjadj, S.; Gourdy, P. Phenotypic characteristics and prognosis of newly diagnosed diabetes in hospitalized patients with COVID-19: Results from the CORONADO study. *Diabetes Res. Clin. Pract.* **2021**, *175*, 108695. [CrossRef] [PubMed]

23. McGurnaghan, S.J.; Weir, A.; Bishop, J.; Kennedy, S.; Blackbourn, L.A.K.; McAllister, D.A.; Hutchinson, S.; Caparrotta, T.M.; Mellor, J.; Jeyam, A.; et al. Risks of and risk factors for COVID-19 disease in people with diabetes: A cohort study of the total population of Scotland. *Lancet Diabetes Endocrinol.* **2020**, *9*, 82–93. [CrossRef]
24. Knapp, S. Diabetes and infection: Is there a link?—A mini-Review. *Gerontology* **2012**, *59*, 99–104. [CrossRef] [PubMed]
25. Lim, S.; Bae, J.H.; Kwon, H.-S.; Nauck, M.A. COVID-19 and diabetes mellitus: From pathophysiology to clinical management. *Nat. Rev. Endocrinol.* **2020**, *17*, 11–30. [CrossRef]
26. Roberts, J.; Pritchard, A.L.; Treweeke, A.T.; Rossi, A.G.; Brace, N.; Cahill, P.; MacRury, S.M.; Wei, J.; Megson, I.L. Why Is COVID-19 More Severe in Patients With Diabetes? The role of angiotensin-converting enzyme 2, endothelial dysfunction and the immunoinflammatory system. *Front. Cardiovasc. Med.* **2021**, *7*, 629933. [CrossRef]
27. Bornstein, S.R.; Rubino, F.; Khunti, K.; Mingrone, G.; Hopkins, D.; Birkenfeld, A.L.; Boehm, B.; Amiel, S.; Holt, R.I.; Skyler, J.S.; et al. Practical recommendations for the management of diabetes in patients with COVID-19. *Lancet Diabetes Endocrinol.* **2020**, *8*, 546–550. [CrossRef]
28. Sardu, C.; D'Onofrio, N.; Balestrieri, M.L.; Barbieri, M.; Rizzo, M.R.; Messina, V.; Maggi, P.; Coppola, N.; Paolisso, G.; Marfella, R. Hyperglycaemia on admission to hospital and COVID-19. *Diabetologia* **2020**, *63*, 2486–2487. [CrossRef]
29. Alves, C.; Casqueiro, J.; Casqueiro, J. Infections in patients with diabetes mellitus: A review of pathogenesis. *Indian J. Endocrinol. Metab.* **2012**, *16*, S27–S36. [CrossRef]
30. Cummings, M.J.; Baldwin, M.R.; Abrams, D.; Jacobson, S.D.; Meyer, B.J.; Balough, E.M.; Aaron, J.G.; Claassen, J.; Rabbani, L.E.; Hastie, J.; et al. Epidemiology, clinical course, and outcomes of critically ill adults with COVID-19 in New York City: A prospective cohort study. *Lancet* **2020**, *395*, 1763–1770. [CrossRef]
31. Zhou, F.; Yu, T.; Du, R.; Fan, G.; Liu, Y.; Liu, Z.; Xiang, J.; Wang, Y.; Song, B.; Gu, X.; et al. Clinical course and risk factors for mortality of adult inpatients with COVID-19 in Wuhan, China: A retrospective cohort study. *Lancet* **2020**, *395*, 1054–1062. [CrossRef]
32. Wu, C.; Chen, X.; Cai, Y.; Xia, J.; Zhou, X.; Xu, S.; Huang, H.; Zhang, L.; Zhou, X.; Du, C.; et al. Risk factors associated with acute respiratory distress syndrome and death in patients with coronavirus disease 2019 pneumonia in Wuhan, China. *JAMA Intern. Med.* **2020**, *180*, 934–943. [CrossRef] [PubMed]
33. Wang, S.; Ma, P.; Zhang, S.; Song, S.; Wang, Z.; Ma, Y.; Xu, J.; Wu, F.; Duan, L.; Yin, Z.; et al. Fasting blood glucose at admission is an independent predictor for 28-day mortality in patients with COVID-19 without previous diagnosis of diabetes: A multi-centre retrospective study. *Diabetologia* **2020**, *63*, 2102–2111. [CrossRef] [PubMed]
34. Ikonomidis, I.; Pavlidis, G.; Lambadiari, V.; Kousathana, F.; Varoudi, M.; Spanoudi, F.; Maratou, E.; Parissis, J.; Triantafyllidi, H.; Dimitriadis, G.; et al. Early detection of left ventricular dysfunction in first-degree relatives of diabetic patients by myocardial deformation imaging: The role of endothelial glycocalyx damage. *Int. J. Cardiol.* **2017**, *233*, 105–112. [CrossRef] [PubMed]
35. Lambadiari, V.; Pavlidis, G.; Kousathana, F.; Maratou, E.; Georgiou, D.; Andreadou, I.; Kountouri, A.; Varoudi, M.; Balampanis, K.; Parissis, J.; et al. Effects of different antidiabetic medications on endothelial glycocalyx, myocardial function, and vascular function in type 2 diabetic patients: One year follow–up study. *J. Clin. Med.* **2019**, *8*, 983. [CrossRef]
36. Zeng, Z.; Yu, H.; Chen, H.; Qi, W.; Chen, L.; Chen, G.; Yan, W.; Chen, T.; Ning, Q.; Han, M.; et al. Longitudinal changes of inflammatory parameters and their correlation with disease severity and outcomes in patients with COVID-19 from Wuhan, China. *Crit. Care* **2020**, *24*, 1–12. [CrossRef] [PubMed]
37. Chen, G.; Wu, D.; Guo, W.; Cao, Y.; Huang, D.; Wang, H.; Wang, T.; Zhang, X.; Chen, H.; Yu, H.; et al. Clinical and immunological features of severe and moderate coronavirus disease 2019. *J. Clin. Investig.* **2020**, *130*, 2620–2629. [CrossRef]
38. Kim, N.-Y.; Ha, E.; Moon, J.S.; Lee, Y.-H.; Choi, E.Y. Acute hyperglycemic crises with coronavirus disease-19: Case reports. *Diabetes Metab. J.* **2020**, *44*, 349–353. [CrossRef]
39. Zhu, L.; She, Z.-G.; Cheng, X.; Qin, J.-J.; Zhang, X.-J.; Cai, J.; Lei, F.; Wang, H.; Xie, J.; Wang, W.; et al. Association of blood glucose control and outcomes in patients with COVID-19 and pre-existing type 2 diabetes. *Cell Metab.* **2020**, *31*, 1068–1077. [CrossRef]
40. Rubino, F.; Amiel, S.A.; Zimmet, P.; Alberti, G.; Bornstein, S.; Eckel, R.H.; Mingrone, G.; Boehm, B.; Cooper, M.E.; Chai, Z.; et al. New-onset diabetes in Covid-19. *N. Engl. J. Med.* **2020**, *383*, 789–790. [CrossRef]
41. Lambadiari, V.; Mitrakou, A.; Kountouri, A.; Thymis, J.; Katogiannis, K.; Korakas, E.; Varlamos, C.; Andreadou, I.; Tsoumani, M.; Triantafyllidi, H.; et al. Association of COVID-19 with impaired endothelial glycocalyx, vascular function and myocardial deformation 4 months after infection. *Eur. J. Hear. Fail.* **2021**, *23*, 1916–1926. [CrossRef]
42. Kazakou, P.; Paschou, S.A.; Psaltopoulou, T.; Gavriatopoulou, M.; Korompoki, E.; Stefanaki, K.; Kanouta, F.; Kassi, G.N.; Dimopoulos, M.-A.; Mitrakou, A. Early and late endocrine complications of COVID-19. *Endocr. Connect.* **2021**, *10*, R229–R239. [CrossRef] [PubMed]
43. Channappanavar, R.; Perlman, S. Pathogenic human coronavirus infections: Causes and consequences of cytokine storm and immunopathology. *Semin. Immunopathol.* **2017**, *39*, 529–539. [CrossRef] [PubMed]
44. Li, M.-Y.; Li, L.; Zhang, Y.; Wang, X.-S. Expression of the SARS-CoV-2 cell receptor gene ACE2 in a wide variety of human tissues. *Infect. Dis. Poverty* **2020**, *9*, 1–7. [CrossRef] [PubMed]
45. Pal, R.; Banerjee, M. COVID-19 and the endocrine system: Exploring the unexplored. *J. Endocrinol. Investig.* **2020**, *43*, 1027–1031. [CrossRef] [PubMed]

46. Korytkowski, M.; Antinori-Lent, K.; Drincic, A.; Hirsch, I.B.; McDonnell, M.E.; Rushakoff, R.; Muniyappa, R. A pragmatic approach to inpatient diabetes management during the COVID-19 pandemic. *J. Clin. Endocrinol. Metab.* **2020**, *105*, dgaa342. [CrossRef]
47. Mifsud, S.; Schembri, E.L.; Gruppetta, M. Stress-induced hyperglycaemia. *Br. J. Hosp. Med.* **2018**, *79*, 634–639. [CrossRef]
48. Drucker, D.J. Coronavirus infections and type 2 diabetes—Shared pathways with therapeutic implications. *Endocr. Rev.* **2020**, *41*, 457–470. [CrossRef]
49. Sathish, T.; Kapoor, N.; Cao, Y.; Tapp, R.J.; Zimmet, P. Proportion of newly diagnosed diabetes in COVID-19 patients: A systematic review and meta-analysis. *Diabetes Obes. Metab.* **2020**, *23*, 870–874. [CrossRef]
50. Joshi, S.C.; Pozzilli, P. COVID-19 induced diabetes: A novel presentation. *Diabetes Res. Clin. Pract.* **2022**, *191*, 110034. [CrossRef]
51. Apicella, M.; Campopiano, M.C.; Mantuano, M.; Mazoni, L.; Coppelli, A.; Del Prato, S. COVID-19 in people with diabetes: Understanding the reasons for worse outcomes. *Lancet Diabetes Endocrinol.* **2020**, *8*, 782–792. [CrossRef]
52. Rey-Reñones, C.; Baena-Díez, J.M.; Aguilar-Palacio, I.; Miquel, C.; Grau, M. Type 2 diabetes mellitus and cancer: Epidemiology, physiopathology and prevention. *Biomedicines* **2021**, *9*, 1429. [CrossRef] [PubMed]
53. Crouse, A.B.; Grimes, T.; Li, P.; Might, M.; Ovalle, F.; Shalev, A. Metformin use is associated with reduced mortality in a diverse population with COVID-19 and diabetes. *Front. Endocrinol.* **2021**, *11*, 600439. [CrossRef] [PubMed]
54. Kan, C.; Zhang, Y.; Han, F.; Xu, Q.; Ye, T.; Hou, N.; Sun, X. Mortality risk of antidiabetic agents for type 2 diabetes with COVID-19: A systematic review and meta-analysis. *Front. Endocrinol.* **2021**, *12*, 708494. [CrossRef] [PubMed]
55. Takayama, K.; Obata, Y.; Maruo, Y.; Yamaguchi, T.; Kosugi, M.; Irie, Y.; Hazama, Y.; Yasuda, T. Metformin-associated lactic acidosis with hypoglycemia during the COVID-19 pandemic. *Intern. Med.* **2022**, *61*, 2333–2337. [CrossRef]
56. Sardu, C.; D'Onofrio, N.; Balestrieri, M.L.; Barbieri, M.; Rizzo, M.R.; Messina, V.; Maggi, P.; Coppola, N.; Paolisso, G.; Marfella, R. Outcomes in patients with hyperglycemia affected by COVID-19: Can we do more on glycemic control? *Diabetes Care* **2020**, *43*, 1408–1415. [CrossRef]
57. Galindo, R.J.; Aleppo, G.; Klonoff, D.C.; Spanakis, E.K.; Agarwal, S.; Vellanki, P.; Olson, D.E.; Umpierrez, G.E.; Davis, G.M.; Pasquel, F.J. Implementation of continuous glucose monitoring in the hospital: Emergent considerations for remote glucose monitoring during the COVID-19 pandemic. *J. Diabetes Sci. Technol.* **2020**, *14*, 822–832. [CrossRef]
58. Davis, G.M.; Faulds, E.; Walker, T.; Vigliotti, D.; Rabinovich, M.; Hester, J.; Peng, L.; McLean, B.; Hannon, P.; Poindexter, N.; et al. Remote continuous glucose monitoring with a computerized insulin infusion protocol for critically ill patients in a COVID-19 medical ICU: Proof of concept. *Diabetes Care* **2021**, *44*, 1055–1058. [CrossRef]
59. Yu, B.; Li, C.; Sun, Y.; Wang, D.W. Insulin treatment is associated with increased mortality in patients with COVID-19 and type 2 diabetes. *Cell Metab.* **2020**, *33*, 65–77. [CrossRef]
60. Chen, Y.; Yang, D.; Cheng, B.; Chen, J.; Peng, A.; Yang, C.; Liu, C.; Xiong, M.; Deng, A.; Zhang, Y.; et al. Clinical characteristics and outcomes of patients with diabetes and COVID-19 in association with glucose-lowering medication. *Diabetes Care* **2020**, *43*, 1399–1407. [CrossRef]
61. Hahn, K.; Ejaz, A.A.; Kanbay, M.; Lanaspa, M.A.; Johnson, R.J. Acute kidney injury from SGLT2 inhibitors: Potential mechanisms. *Nat. Rev. Nephrol.* **2016**, *12*, 711–712. [CrossRef]
62. Nguyen, N.N.; Ho, D.S.; Nguyen, H.S.; Ho, D.K.N.; Li, H.-Y.; Lin, C.-Y.; Chiu, H.-Y.; Chen, Y.-C. Preadmission use of antidiabetic medications and mortality among patients with COVID-19 having type 2 diabetes: A meta-analysis. *Metabolism* **2022**, *131*, 155196. [CrossRef]
63. Kosiborod, M.N.; Esterline, R.; Furtado, R.H.M.; Oscarsson, J.; Gasparyan, S.B.; Koch, G.G.; Martinez, F.; Mukhtar, O.; Verma, S.; Chopra, V.; et al. Dapagliflozin in patients with cardiometabolic risk factors hospitalised with COVID-19 (DARE-19): A randomised, double-blind, placebo-controlled, phase 3 trial. *Lancet Diabetes Endocrinol.* **2021**, *9*, 586–594. [CrossRef]
64. Lv, W.; Wang, X.; Xu, Q.; Lu, W. Mechanisms and characteristics of sulfonylureas and glinides. *Curr. Top. Med. Chem.* **2020**, *20*, 37–56. [CrossRef] [PubMed]
65. Yki-Järvinen, H. Thiazolidinediones. *N. Engl. J. Med.* **2004**, *351*, 1106–1118. [CrossRef] [PubMed]
66. Mulvihill, E.E. Dipeptidyl peptidase inhibitor therapy in type 2 diabetes: Control of the incretin axis and regulation of postprandial glucose and lipid metabolism. *Peptides* **2018**, *100*, 158–164. [CrossRef]
67. Patoulias, D.; Doumas, M. Dipeptidyl peptidase-4 inhibitors and COVID-19-related deaths among patients with type 2 diabetes mellitus: A meta-analysis of observational studies. *Endocrinol. Metab.* **2021**, *36*, 904–908. [CrossRef]
68. Yang, Y.; Cai, Z.; Zhang, J. DPP-4 inhibitors may improve the mortality of coronavirus disease 2019: A meta-analysis. *PLoS ONE* **2021**, *16*, e0251916. [CrossRef]
69. Iacobellis, G. COVID-19 and diabetes: Can DPP4 inhibition play a role? *Diabetes Res. Clin. Pract.* **2020**, *162*, 108125. [CrossRef]
70. Campbell, J.E.; Drucker, D.J. Pharmacology, physiology, and mechanisms of incretin hormone action. *Cell Metab.* **2013**, *17*, 819–837. [CrossRef]
71. Chen, Y.; Lv, X.; Lin, S.; Arshad, M.; Dai, M. The association between antidiabetic agents and clinical outcomes of COVID-19 patients with diabetes: A bayesian network meta-analysis. *Front. Endocrinol.* **2022**, *13*, 895458. [CrossRef]
72. Hulst, A.H.; Plummer, M.P.; Hollmann, M.W.; DeVries, J.H.; Preckel, B.; Deane, A.M.; Hermanides, J. Systematic review of incretin therapy during peri-operative and intensive care. *Crit. Care* **2018**, *22*, 299. [CrossRef] [PubMed]

73. Lim, S.; Lee, G.Y.; Park, H.S.; Lee, D.-H.; Jung, O.T.; Min, K.K.; Kim, Y.-B.; Jun, H.-S.; Chul, J.H.; Park, K.S. Attenuation of carotid neointimal formation after direct delivery of a recombinant adenovirus expressing glucagon-like peptide-1 in diabetic rats. *Cardiovasc. Res.* **2016**, *113*, 183–194. [CrossRef] [PubMed]
74. Lim, S.; Oh, T.J.; Dawson, J.; Sattar, N. Diabetes drugs and stroke risk: Intensive versus conventional glucose-lowering strategies, and implications of recent cardiovascular outcome trials. *Diabetes Obes. Metab.* **2019**, *22*, 6–15. [CrossRef] [PubMed]

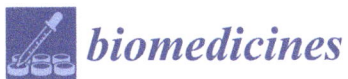

Article

Clinical Interest of Serum Alpha-2 Macroglobulin, Apolipoprotein A1, and Haptoglobin in Patients with Non-Alcoholic Fatty Liver Disease, with and without Type 2 Diabetes, before or during COVID-19

Olivier Deckmyn [1,†], Thierry Poynard [2,3,*,†], Pierre Bedossa [4], Valérie Paradis [4], Valentina Peta [1,3], Raluca Pais [2,3], Vlad Ratziu [2,3], Dominique Thabut [2,3], Angelique Brzustowski [5,6], Jean-François Gautier [6,7], Patrice Cacoub [8,9,10,†] and Dominique Valla [5,6,†,‡] on behalf of the QUID-NASH, FLIP and PROCOP Research Groups

1. BioPredictive, 75007 Paris, France; olivier.deckmyn@biopredictive.com (O.D.); valentina.peta@biopredictive.com (V.P.)
2. Assistance Publique-Hôpitaux de Paris (AP-HP), Department of Hepato-Gastroenterology, Pitié-Salpêtrière Hospital, 75013 Paris, France; raluca.pais@aphp.fr (R.P.); vlad.ratziu@inserm.fr (V.R.); dominique.thabut@aphp.fr (D.T.)
3. Sorbonne Université, INSERM, Centre de Recherche Saint-Antoine (CRSA), Institute of Cardiometabolism and Nutrition (ICAN), 75013 Paris, France
4. Department of Pathology, Physiology and Imaging, Beaujon Hospital APHP Diderot University, 75006 Paris, France; pierre.bedossa@inserm.fr (P.B.); valerie.paradis@aphp.fr (V.P.)
5. Assistance Publique-Hôpitaux de Paris (AP-HP), Department of Hepatology, Beaujon Hospital, 92110 Clichy, France; angelique.brzustowski@inserm.fr (A.B.); dominique.valla@aphp.fr (D.V.)
6. Inserm U1149, Centre de Recherche sur l' Inflammation CRI, 92110 Clichy, France; jean-francois.gautier@aphp.fr
7. Department of Diabetes and Endocrinology, Lariboisière Hospital APHP, Université de Paris, 75007 Paris, France
8. Assistance Publique-Hôpitaux de Paris (AP-HP), Department of Internal Medicine and Clinical Immunology, Pitié-Salpêtrière Hospital, 75013 Paris, France; patrice.cacoub@aphp.fr
9. Département Hospitalo-Universitaire I2B, Sorbonne Université, 75006 Paris, France
10. UMR 7211 (UPMC/CNRS), UMR S-959 (INSERM), 75006 Paris, France
* Correspondence: thierry@poynard.com
† The two first authors and the two last authors share these places.
‡ Coauthors of the Research Groups are listed in Supplementary File S1.

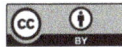

Abstract: In patients with non-alcoholic fatty liver disease (NAFLD) with or without type 2 diabetes mellitus (T2DM), alpha-2 macroglobulin (A2M), apolipoprotein A1 (ApoA1), and haptoglobin are associated with the risk of liver fibrosis, inflammation (NASH), and COVID-19. We assessed if these associations were worsened by T2DM after adjustment by age, sex, obesity, and COVID-19. Three datasets were used: the "Control Population", which enabled standardization of protein serum levels according to age and sex (N = 27,382); the "NAFLD-Biopsy" cohort for associations with liver features (N = 926); and the USA "NAFLD-Serum" cohort for protein kinetics before and during COVID-19 (N = 421,021). The impact of T2DM was assessed by comparing regression curves adjusted by age, sex, and obesity for the liver features in "NAFLD-Biopsy", and before and during COVID-19 pandemic peaks in "NAFLD-Serum". Patients with NAFLD without T2DM, compared with the values of controls, had increased A2M, decreased ApoA1, and increased haptoglobin serum levels. In patients with both NAFLD and T2DM, these significant mean differences were magnified, and even more during the COVID-19 pandemic in comparison with the year 2019 (all $p < 0.001$), with a maximum ApoA1 decrease of 0.21 g/L in women, and a maximum haptoglobin increase of 0.17 g/L in men. In conclusion, T2DM is associated with abnormal levels of A2M, ApoA1, and haptoglobin independently of NAFLD, age, sex, obesity, and COVID-19.

Keywords: alpha-2 macroglobulin; apolipoprotein A1; haptoglobin; type 2 diabetes; non-alcoholic fatty liver disease NAFLD; non-alcoholic steatohepatitis NASH; SAF-scoring system; liver fibrosis; steatosis; COVID-19

1. Introduction

For more than a century, diabetes has been associated with liver disease and severe pneumonia [1]. Recently, the COVID-19 pandemic revealed that patients with type 2 diabetes (T2DM), non-alcoholic fatty liver disease (NAFLD), or metabolic liver disease were at higher risk of being infected with and hospitalized for moderate-to-severe COVID-19 complications than control patients without T2DM or NAFLD [2–6]. However, the causal relationship between COVID-19 susceptibility/severity and NAFLD remains unclear because of confounders such as age, sex, obesity, T2DM, stage of fibrosis, and grade of inflammation, also called non-alcoholic steatohepatitis (NASH) [6–8].

Three ubiquitous serum proteins that are involved in cell repair and immunity, alpha-2 macroglobulin (A2M) [9–12], apolipoprotein A1 (ApoA1) [9,10,13,14], and haptoglobin [9,10,15–18], which are mainly synthetized by the liver, are associated with the risk of being infected with COVID-19 and are associated with the severity of its complications compared with controls without diabetes nor NAFLD [9–18]. These proteins are also associated with liver fibrosis and inflammatory activity in the most frequent liver diseases, including NAFLD [19–61].

These serum proteins are easy to assess and could be used as biomarkers of the risk of SARS-CoV-2 infection, particularly in patients with T2DM and NAFLD, a large part of the global population that has a higher risk of SARS-CoV-2 infection [9,10].

The epidemiological purpose of this work was to assess the impact of T2DM on the concentrations of these proteins in the blood according to the main confounders of age, sex, and obesity, and the severity of three liver features, fibrosis, NASH inflammatory activity, and steatosis.

The clinical purpose of this work was to prevent misinterpretation and false positives and negatives of the serum levels of such major proteins observed in patients with metabolic liver disease who express T2DM with or without SARS-CoV-2 infection. Increasing numbers of new or known proteins were included in multivariate diagnostic/prognostic tests and analyzed. In simple terms, a serum level of 3.8 g/L A2M can be observed in an asymptomatic 18-year-old girl or in an obese 60-year-old man with cirrhosis, but should not be interpreted similarly.

Because of their highly conserved evolutionary ubiquitous properties, it is logical that these three proteins are associated with three global human diseases, T2DM, COVID-19, and liver fibrosis [20–23].

A2M, a glycoprotein of 720 kDa mass, is a major component in the circulation of vertebrates. It belongs to a family of extracellular matrix regulators. As well as the rapid inhibition of proteinases released during inflammation, A2M has many functions [19,23]. As stated by Rehman et al.: "This multipurpose antiproteinase is not "fail safe" and could be damaged by reactive species generated endogenously or exogenously, leading to various pathophysiological conditions" [19]. Indeed, in children and adults younger than 25 years old, A2M expression is significantly higher than in older healthy adults [24] and is associated with a lower risk of several severe diseases such as severe COVID-19, *Trypanosoma cruzi* infection (Chagas disease) [25], and intervertebral disc degeneration [26].

In COVID-19, a possible protective role of elevated native A2M in children was recently identified and deserves more in-depth scientific exploration [12].

In T2DM, increased A2M was first described in 1967 [27], both in adults and children with very early T2DM [27,28], suggesting very early damage by the protein [19,27].

In chronic liver disease, increased A2M has been described since 1963 and is associated with liver fibrosis, [29,30]. A2M has been successfully included in multivariate analyses of fibrosis biomarkers, mostly combined with ApoA1 and haptoglobin, for the surveillance of chronic viral hepatitis C and B, alcoholic liver disease, and various metabolic liver diseases including dyslipidemia, NAFLD with and without T2DM [31,32], sole T2DM [27,28,32–37], steatosis [33], and non-alcoholic steatohepatitis (NASH) [34–37], and has been associated with severe obesity [39], patients with bariatric surgery [39], obstructive sleep apnea [40], and the general population [31].

ApoA1, a 45.4 kDa mass protein, is mostly found in association with the high-density cholesterol (HDL) moiety. In addition to its role in regulating cholesterol and protecting against cardiovascular disease, ApoA1 has many functions in inflammatory and immune responses. ApoA1 inhibits apoptosis and pro-oxidative and proinflammatory processes in endothelial cells, induces vasodilation, inhibits the activation of platelets, and contributes to innate immunity [41].

In severe pneumonia, the association between low HDL and severe pneumonia has been well established for more than a century [9], and the lowest levels have been observed in patients with moderate and severe COVID-19 with significant prognostic value [9,10,42–49]. There is a causal association for subjects with low ApoA1 and, 10 years later, low levels were correlated with the risk of COVID-19 [13].

In T2DM, decreased ApoA1 was first described in 1982 [46]. Downregulated ApoA1 in T2DM could be related to damage of the protein and loss of the protective functions of the native protein including three post translational modifications: oxidation, carbamylation, and glycation [46–49].

In chronic liver disease, the decrease in ApoA1 according to the progression of liver fibrosis was first described in 1986 [50,51], and has been successively included in multivariate biomarkers, mostly combined with A2M and haptoglobin, for the surveillance of chronic liver diseases including NAFLD and NASH with or without T2DM [32–38,52]. In a large cohort of patients at risk of NAFLD in the USA, the "NAFLD-Serum" cohort, there was a significant decrease in ApoA1 during the first wave of the 2020 pandemic compared with the respective months in 2019 [9]. ApoA1 is mainly synthetized in the liver and intestine. In liver fibrosis, decreased serum ApoA1 is observed without hepatic insufficiency, the ApoA1 being trapped by the collagenization of the endothelial cells [51] before advanced fibrosis and before the hepatic insufficiency. In patients with cirrhosis, ApoA1 and HDL3 levels were significantly lower in patients who developed severe infection [53]. This sensitivity of ApoA1 is an advantage for its inclusion in multivariate biomarkers because of its prognostic value.

Another possible source of major ApoA1 variability is that enterically derived HDL restrains liver injury through the portal vein, with ApoA1 inhibiting the bacterial lipopolysaccharide (LPS) source of inflammation [53]. The biogenesis of HDL requires ApoA1 and the cholesterol transporter ABCA1. Although the liver generates most of the HDL in the blood, HDL synthesis also occurs in the small intestine. The intestine produces the small form of HDL called HDL3 that it is enriched in lipopolysaccharide (LPS)-binding protein (LBP). In complexes with LBP, HDL3 prevented LPS-binding and the inflammatory activation of liver macrophages [53]. Indeed, ApoA1 and HDL3 have strong translational potential in the understanding of T2DM, NASH, and severe infection.

Haptoglobin is synthesized predominantly in hepatocytes as a single 45 kDa polypeptide that rapidly forms dimers through disulfide bond formation [54]. The α-chain of haptoglobin is then proteolytically cleaved, resulting in the final tetrameric form, Hp 1-1. One of the most striking effects of the haptoglobin polymorphism resides in its structural heterogeneity, with the existence of haptoglobin in different oligomeric states depending on its genotype: Hp1-1, Hp2-1, or Hp2-2. Haptoglobin has a significant role in clearing toxic hemoglobin (Hb) through high-affinity binding to the macrophage scavenger receptor CD163. In addition to this antioxidant function, haptoglobin has a role in the immune response and during the acute phase response. In healthy subjects, haptoglobin concentrations in the circulation are very low. Haptoglobin reduces the loss of free Hb through glomerular filtration, controlling heme detoxification and promoting iron recycling.

Haptoglobin can act either as an anti-inflammatory modulator or as a pro-inflammatory activator suppressing T cell proliferation and regulating the balance between T helper cells Th1 and Th2. Hp1-1:Hb complexes induce Th2 cell-dependent pathways that allow healing and repair. Conversely, macrophages activated by Hp2-2:Hb stimulate the Th1 response that promotes pro-inflammatory cytokines. Haptoglobin is a marker of inflammation, its level increasing during infections, injuries, and malignancies. The functional properties of haptoglobin reflect the different phenotypes Hp1-1, Hp2-1, and Hp2-2. Hp2-2 is the less active form of haptoglobin, and patients with this phenotype show a significantly higher risk of cardiovascular, neurological, and infectious complications compared with Hp1-1 and Hp2-1 individuals [15,55].

In patients with COVID-19, haptoglobin phenotypes (Hp1 and Hp2 alleles) were not associated with mortality [56]. Regardless of the phenotype, serum haptoglobin in humans and non-human primates is elevated very early, at 2 days after SARS-CoV-2 infection, and for a longer time than C-reactive protein (CRP) [9,10].

Patients with T2DM and Hp2-2 phenotypes are at a significantly higher risk of microvascular and macrovascular complications via obesity effects in the Mexican population [56,57]. To date, a direct causal association between haptoglobin phenotypes and the occurrence of T2DM has not been established [56–58]. In the progression of asymptomatic obesity to a T2DM status, the increased influx of immune cells, especially macrophages, into visceral adipose tissue is mediated by adipocyte-derived chemokines, and this influx is accompanied by inflammatory cytokines such as tumor necrosis factor α (TNFα) and interleukin 6 (IL6) [59,60]. Haptoglobin related protein (HPR) mRNA expression is significantly increased when comparing healthy obese individuals with impaired glucose fasting obese patients and obese patients with T2DM [15].

In patients at risk of NAFLD, haptoglobin is increased in obese patients with T2DM but decreased in patients who progress to advanced fibrosis [61]. No study thus far has assessed the respective impacts of elementary histological features (steatosis, NASH inflammatory activity, and fibrosis) adjusted according to T2DM and obesity on serum haptoglobin.

Here, the aim was first to standardize the three protein values according to age and sex, two major confounding factors, using published normal values from a healthy general population in the USA, called here the "Control Population" cohort.

Second, we assessed the impact of T2DM on these proteins according to the main metabolic liver features of fibrosis and inflammation (NASH) and steatosis without inflammation, stratified by obesity. We used NAFLD patients with liver biopsies who were centralized and analyzed using the validated scoring systems (SAF), called the "NAFLD-Biopsy" cohort.

Third, we assessed the impact of T2DM on these proteins in "NAFLD-Serum" patients followed before and during the COVID-19 pandemic, adjusted according to the confounders of age, sex, and obesity.

We found that in patients at risk of NAFLD, the impact of T2DM on these three proteins should be studied not only after standardization according to age and sex, but also after stratification by obesity. In the two cohorts, the three proteins levels were significantly different than the normal values. In patients at risk of NAFLD without T2DM, A2M was increased, ApoA1 was decreased, and haptoglobin was increased. In patients with both NAFLD and T2DM, these significant differences were magnified. During SARS-CoV-2 infection, this population acquire a third factor of decreased ApoA1 and increased haptoglobin. These results were in line with the independent diagnostic and prognostic values of ApoA1 in COVID-19.

2. Materials and Methods

2.1. Study Participants and Design

This retrospective non-interventional epidemiological study had three co-primary aims (Figure 1).

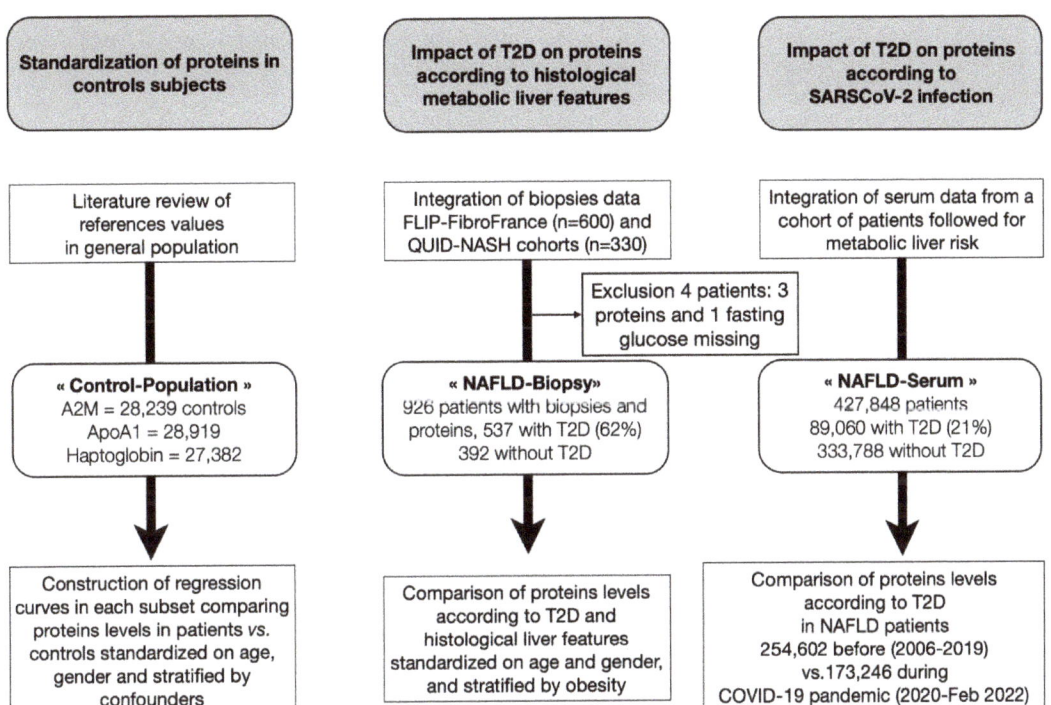

Figure 1. Study design.

2.2. Standardization of Protein Values

To standardize the three protein values, we used the reference values of studies based on the "Control Population" cohort of 40,420 Caucasian individuals from northern New England. Sera were assessed between 1994 and 2000. Measurements were standardized against Certified Reference Material for Proteins in Human Serum (RPPHS), and the results were analyzed using a previously described statistical approach. Individuals with unequivocal laboratory evidence of inflammation, CRP > 10 mg/L defining significant acute phase reactant (APR), were excluded in one leg of the study and included in the other, confirming that A2M does not respond to acute phase drive in humans [24]. Most samples were sent for study by physicians because of a suspected diagnosis or symptom. Computer processing of over 28,000 unique diagnostic strings required that they be classified into 93 categories representing related conditions. Diagnostic codes containing individuals with conditions expected to have a direct effect on serum protein levels, for example multiple myeloma, cirrhosis, hepatitis, infection, lung disease, leukemia, renal failure, rheumatic disease, and immunodeficiency, were excluded. Outliers were identified in this way among the diagnostic group parameters associated with codes not expected to alter serum protein values. A logarithmic transformation of the variance was corrected for skewness. The resulting trimmed mean value, ±1.96 standard deviation for both the multiples of the median (MoM) and the log variance, defined the limits of acceptability. Measurements from any diagnostic group falling within the limits were considered reference values, and those falling outside were not.

Statistical Analysis

Here, we applied the methodology previously published by Ritchie et al. [24,62–64]. For studying proteins, 28,239, 28,919, and 27,382 cases were available without significant APR for A2M [24], ApoA1 [63], and haptoglobin [64], respectively. In this "Control Population", there were 225 cases with a diagnosis of T2DM and no APR, and 95 with APR, and both were outside the reference range for log MoM and log variance. The proposed method of converting laboratory results to multiples of the age- and sex-specific MoMs has several advantages. Conversion permits each analyte to fit a logarithmic Gaussian distribution reasonably well, allowing each MoM level to be assigned a centile. Thus, a laboratory measurement can not only be reported in mass units but also through conversion to MoM, the associated centile based on that individual's age and sex. The regression models and coefficients for median proteins measurements by age and sex have been described previously [24,63,64].

2.3. Impact of T2DM on Proteins According to Histological Metabolic Liver Features

2.3.1. Patients

Two previously published datasets that validated the diagnostic performances of blood biomarkers were retrospectively integrated in the present "NAFLD-Biopsy" cohort [37,52] (Figure 1). One was the construction and internal validation performed in the fatty liver inhibition of progression (FLIP) and FibroFrance cohorts [52], and the other was the external validation in the QUIDNASH prospective cohort [37]. Details were provided in each publication and summarized in Supplementary File S1 with the list of participants and the projects' summaries. All these clinical non-interventional studies were approved by the ethics committee at each participating institution and were performed according to good clinical practice and the Declaration of Helsinki, and all patients provided written informed consent.

The FLIP project is supported by the European Community's Seventh Framework Program (FP7/2007-2013) under grant agreement number HEALTH-F2-2009-241762. FibroFrance is supported by the National Clinical Research (CPP-IDF-VI, 10-1996-DR-964, DR-2012-222) and declared in the Clinical Registry (number: NCT01927133).

The QUIDNASH study, NCT03634098, was approved by the Research Ethics Committee (#18.021-2018-A00311-54). In patients with T2DM, the diagnostic accuracy of FibroTest, NashTest-2, and SteatoTest-2 was assessed using liver histology as the reference to evaluate liver fibrosis, NASH, and steatosis, and is detailed elsewhere [39]. Briefly, NAFLD was suspected on the basis of the presence of abnormal liver enzymes as well as an ultrasound scan showing a bright liver echo pattern in patients with T2DM diagnosed at a diabetology outpatient clinic. Consecutive patients were prospectively recruited between October 2018 and 2020 at four outpatient diabetology clinics in the Assistance-Publique-Hopitaux-de-Paris. All patients gave written informed consent. The study was performed in accordance with the Declaration of Helsinki. All authors had access to the study data and reviewed and approved the final manuscript. The chosen same sample size of n = 300 for the primary aim of the study was the same as that used for the internal validation of SteatoTest-2 and for validation of the original SteatoTest. To increase the power of the present study, we added 57 T2DM cases who shared the same inclusion criteria as the QUIDNASH non-interventional cohort after the end of the validation study to the original 272 cases [39].

2.3.2. Blood Tests

A2M, ApoA1, haptoglobin, and fasting glucose were assessed in fresh samples from FibroFrance and QUIDNASH patients. For FLIP patients, serum stored at −80 °C was sent to the reference center, the Biochemistry Department at Pitié-Salpêtrière Hospital, Paris, France.

2.3.3. Histological Reference

The SAF activity scoring system was considered as the simplified histological reference for NASH without the requirements used for NASH-CRN and the FLIP algorithm definition [65–67]. The histological references for significant metabolic liver disease (NAFLD) were those defined by the SAF scoring system, fibrosis stage ≥ 2 and activity grade ≥ 2 [66,67].

The goal of the SAF score was to identify a compromise between the development of a simple, easily applied system to make a firm diagnosis in individual patients, even when applied by non-specialists, and of a more reliable and discriminating system for therapeutic trials or for the assessment of biomarker diagnostic performance. A FLIP Histopathology Consortium of eight members developed the FLIP algorithm, a diagnostic tool for the diagnosis and staging of severe forms of NAFLD according to the combination of each semi-quantification of the three elementary features of NAFLD using the SAF score for steatosis SAF-S, inflammatory activity SAF-A, and fibrosis SAF-F. The use of the SAF-A score leads to the selection of patients with more severe disease activity and fibrosis, as observed in a recent trial in NASH [68] in which 76% of patients had significant (F2) or advanced (F3) fibrosis even though no inclusion criterion, with respect to fibrosis stage, was set except for the exclusion of patients with cirrhosis. The use of the SAF-A score enriched the trial, with patients more likely to benefit from pharmacological treatment. As for the other histological end points, the validity of the SAF-A score to define the primary end point as a surrogate for long term outcomes warrants further study [67]. The steatosis score (S) assesses the quantities of large-sized or medium-sized lipid droplets, with the exception of foamy microvesicles, and rates them from 0 to 3 (S0: <5%; S1: 5–33%, mild; S2: 34–66%, moderate; S3: and >66%, marked). Activity (NASH) grade (A, from 0 to 4) is the unweighted addition of hepatocyte ballooning (0–2) and lobular inflammation (0–2). Patients with A0 (A = 0) had no activity; patients with A1 (A = 1) had mild activity; patients with A2 (A = 2) had moderate activity; patients with A3 (A = 3) had severe activity; and patients with A4 (A = 4) had very severe activity. Fibrosis stage (F) was assessed using the following scoring system: stage 0 (F0), none; stage 1 (F1), 1a or 1b perisinusoidal zone 3 or 1c portal fibrosis; stage 2 (F2), perisinusoidal and periportal fibrosis without bridging; stage 3 (F3), bridging fibrosis; and stage 4 (F4), cirrhosis. To reduce interobserver variability and homogenize the reading using the SAF-FLIP histological classification, we used only reports reviewed by members of the FLIP Pathology Consortium (DT and PB for FLIP and FC for the FibroFrance subset), and VP, PB, and BT for the QUIDNASH subset.

2.3.4. Statistical Analysis

We compared the levels of each protein in patients with or without T2DM, defined as fasting glucose ≥ 7 mmol/L [69], versus their expected values in the general population [24,62–64] to test the hypothesis that early low levels of A2M and ApoA1 before the onset of T2DM and NAFLD could explain an intrinsic fragility. To account for obesity, these curves were also compared in patients with or without obesity (Figure 1) according to the possible histological confounders, each of them grouped into three classes, fibrosis F2F3F4, NASH A2A3, and steatosis S2S3. For each protein, the curves were assessed by regression according to age separately for women and men, one in patients and one in their expected normal controls. The Loess method was used with 95% confidence intervals and comparisons between curves used the unpaired t-test.

Univariate correlation matrices were used to assess the correlation between the three proteins and the four confounders in four subsets, with and without obesity, in women and men, called here "sex/obesity" (female/non-obese, male/non-obese, female/obese, and male/obese). A significant association was defined as $p < 0.05$ adjusted by the number of covariables according to the Holm method [70].

Independent associations between the presence of T2DM and the three proteins were assessed by logistic regression analysis in the four subsets, including the three histological features of the SAF scoring system, the five stages of fibrosis (F0 to F4), the four grades of NASH (A0 to A3), and the four grades of steatosis (S0 to S3). This analysis allowed adjustment of the association between T2DM and each protein, independently of the two other proteins of interest after taking into account age and the SAF classes of each feature in each of the four sex/obesity subsets. According to significant correlations between the three features, it seemed fair to perform these regressions separately for each feature. R software was used for the analyses.

2.4. Impact of T2DM on the Serum Proteins Levels According to Obesity

2.4.1. Patients

We used both the "NAFLD-Biopsy" cohort and the "NAFLD-Serum" cohort, a large laboratory US cohort from anonymous subjects at risk of liver fibrosis, followed by FibroTest (also known as FibroSure in USA) [9,71].

2.4.2. Blood Tests

A2M, ApoA1, haptoglobin, and fasting glucose were assessed in fresh samples, and all laboratories used the methods of the manufacturer of FibroTest [31].

2.4.3. Statistical Analysis

The same statistical methods were used as those assessing the impact of T2DM on histological features. Thanks to the sample size, we focused on the impact of T2DM on the three proteins in the four confounder subsets of sex/obesity.

First, we analyzed the impact of T2DM on proteins stratified by obesity and sex in the "NAFLD-Serum" cohort. Second, we analyzed the univariate correlations between proteins and histological features inside the four sex/obesity subsets. Third, we analyzed the multivariate correlations by logistic regression between proteins and histological features inside the four sex/obesity subsets. Fourth, we analyzed to correlation between the serum level for each protein with BMI, using 5 groups according to WHO definition (18.5, 25, 30, 35 and above 40 kg/m^2) in all patients and stratified by age in 2 groups (below and equal or above 50 years old).

2.5. Impact of T2DM on the Three Proteins According to SARS-CoV-2 Infection

2.5.1. Patients

The "NAFLD-Serum" cohort [9,71] was used.

2.5.2. Blood Tests

A2M, ApoA1, haptoglobin, and fasting glucose were assessed in fresh samples according to the recommendations of the manufacturer of FibroTest [31].

2.5.3. Statistical Analysis

Three methods were used. First, the comparison of proteins levels was performed before and during the COVID-19 pandemic according to T2DM, standardized by age and sex and stratified by obesity. Second, for each patient, the difference between the observed value of the three proteins and the expected normal value adjusted for age and sex were observed. The observed 7-day rolling mean of these differences were compared between 2019 (before the pandemic) and the pandemic period from January 2020 to February 2022.

A figure was built using both the "NAFLD-Serum" dataset and the public data from John Hopkins University (JHU) [72]. The curves of the protein values from January 2019 to 30 January 2022 of the "NAFLD-Serum" dataset, stratified by sex, were graphically compared with those of the JHU dataset regarding mortality and the hospitalization rate, which were only available since March 2020 and August 2020, respectively, and without sex stratification available.

3. Results

3.1. Standardization of Proteins Values in the Studied Cohorts Using the "Control Population"

For each age group, the mean difference (%95CI) between the patient protein value and the expected normal value (for the respective age and sex), with its significant *p*-value is displayed at top of each figure. The significance between non-T2DM vs. T2DM patients is displayed in color between the two panels. Characteristics of all "NAFLD-Biopsy" and "NAFLD-Serum" are shown in Table 1, and the subsets according to T2DM, obesity, sex, and age <50 years or ≥50 years are shown in Tables 2–5.

Table 1. Characteristics of "NAFLD-Biopsy" and NAFLD subsets according to diabetes and obesity. * = Significant vs. No-T2DM and Non-Obese subset.

	No-T2DM and Non-Obese	T2DM and Non-Obese	No-T2DM and Obese	T2DM and Obese	All
NAFLD-Biopsy					
N	270	161	194	301	926
Male %	187 (69.3%)	72 (44.7%) *	119 (61.3%)	123 (40.9%) *	501 (54.1%)
Age year (IQR)	49.9 (39.8–58.9)	60.0 (52.5–67.0) *	51.5 (40.7–60.8)	59.0 (51.0–64.0) *	55 (46–63) *
A2M g/L	1.67 (1.29–2.13)	2.16 (1.53–2.83) *	1.79 (1.34–3.07)	2.03 (1.56–2.74) *	1.86 (1.39–2.57)
ApoA1 g/L	1.41 (1.23–1.61)	1.33 (1.17–1.50) *	1.37 (1.21–1.55)	1.34 (1.22–1.49)	1.37 (1.21–1.55)
Hapto g/L	1.13 (0.80–1.46)	1.35 (1.00–1.76) *	1.30 (0.86–1.68) *	1.49 (1.11–1.92) *	1.31 (0.92–2.12)
Advanced fibrosis	98 (36.3%)	85 (52.8%) *	116 (59.8%) *	173 (57.5%) *	472 (51.0%)
Advanced NASH	184 (68.2%)	93 (57.8%)	157 (80.9%) *	205 (68.1%)	639 (69.0%)
Advanced steatosis	153 (56.7%)	130 (90.8%) *	134 (69.1%) *	276 (91.7%) *	693 (74.8%)
NAFLD-Serum					
N	160,136	29,439	178,652	59,621	427,848
Male %	75,519 (47.2)	14,779 (50.2)	78,302 (43.8)	26,363 (44.2)	194,963 (45.6)
Age year (IQR)	57.4 (46.2–66.4)	62.8 (54.7–70.3)	54.3 (43.4–63.3)	58.9 (50.5–66.9)	56.8 (46.2–65.6)
A2M g/L	1.91 (1.52–2.53)	2.29 (1.69–3.02)	1.83 (1.44–2.42)	2.17 (1.63–2.81)	1.93 (1.50–2.57)
ApoA1 g/L	1.44 (1.25–1.68)	1.37 (1.19–1.58)	1.37 (1.21–1.57)	1.34 (1.18–1.52)	1.39 (1.22–1.60)
Hapto g/L	1.19 (0.82–1.59)	1.31 (0.87–1.76)	1.42 (1.01–1.85)	1.51 (1.06–1.99)	1.34 (0.92–1.78)

Table 2. Characteristics and median protein levels in women <50 years of age according to T2DM and obese status.

	No-T2DM and Non-Obese	T2DM and Non-Obese	No-T2DM and Obese	T2DM and Obese
N	23,007	1983	35,303	7891
Age year (IQR)	40.1 (32.6–45.8)	43.7 (37.9–47.4)	40.3 (33.1–45.8)	43.11 (37.3–47.2)
A2M g/L	1.89 (1.57–2.29)	1.95 (1.55–2.42)	1.76 (1.46–2.16)	1.92 (1.53–2.37)
ApoA1 g/L	1.47 (1.29–1.69)	1.39 (1.21–1.60)	1.38 (1.23–1.57)	1.35 (1.20–1.53)
Hapto g/L	1.21 (0.86–1.58)	1.43 (0.99–1.86)	1.61 (1.22–2.03)	1.74 (1.31–2.22)

Table 3. Characteristics and median protein levels in women ≥50 years of age according to T2DM and obese status.

	No-T2DM and Non-Obese	T2DM and Non-Obese	No-T2DM and Obese	T2DM and Obese
N	61,610	12,677	65,047	25,367
Age year (IQR)	63.0 (57.0–69.9)	65.3 (58.9–71.8)	61.3 (55.8–67.6)	62.5 (56.7–68.9)
A2M g/L	2.02 (1.65–2.63)	2.32 (1.76–3.01)	1.95 (1.57–2.54)	2.20 (1.70–2.81)
ApoA1 g/L	1.57 (1.37–1.80)	1.45 (1.27–1.65)	1.49 (1.32–1.68)	1.43 (1.26–1.61)
Hapto g/L	1.27 (0.89–1.66)	1.35 (0.93–1.80)	1.49 (1.08–1.92)	1.57 (1.11–2.05)

Table 4. Characteristics and median protein levels in men <50 years of age according to T2DM and obese status.

	No-T2DM and Non-Obese	T2DM and Non-Obese	No-T2DM and Obese	T2DM and Obese
N	27,744	2467	33,759	6303
Age year (IQR)	39.3 (32.4–45.0)	43.5 (38.1–47.1)	39.7 (32.7–45.3)	43.3 (37.9–47.2)
A2M g/L	1.53 (1.26–1.96)	1.69 (1.29–2.35)	1.47 (1.20–1.92)	1.70 (1.28–2.29)
ApoA1 g/L	1.31 (1.16–1.48)	1.27 (1.12–1.46)	1.25 (1.12–1.40)	1.25 (1.11–1.40)
Hapto g/L	1.06 (0.72–1.44)	1.22 (0.80–1.65)	1.28 (0.91–1.68)	1.40 (0.98–1.87)

Table 5. Characteristics and median protein levels in men ≥50 years of age according to T2DM and obese status.

	No-T2DM and Non-Obese	T2DM and Non-Obese	No-T2DM and Obese	T2DM and Obese
N	47,775	12,312	44,543	20,006
Age year (IQR)	62.9 (56.9–69.5)	64.8 (58.4–71.2)	60.9 (55.5–67.3)	62.5 (56.8–68.6)
A2M g/L	2.04 (1.52–2.88)	2.48 (1.77–3.20)	2.07 (1.49–2.82)	2.44 (1.76–3.09)
ApoA1 g/L	1.36 (1.19–1.57)	1.30 (1.13–1.49)	1.30 (1.15–1.47)	1.27 (1.13–1.43)
Hapto g/L	1.16 (0.77–1.59)	1.26 (0.81–1.73)	1.29 (0.88–1.71)	1.38 (0.95–1.85)

For haptoglobin, in the "NAFLD-Serum" cohort, there was a cut-off effect for the lower values due to the lowest value being adjusted to 0.06 g/L.

In the NAFLD-Biopsy subset, for subjects with T2DM, with or without obesity, all characteristics were different vs. subjects without T2DM and non-obese (controls), except for ApoA1 level and NASH prevalence. In subject with T2DM and non-obesity ApoA1 was lower. In subjects with no-T2DM and obese the advanced NASH prevalence was higher. In the NAFLD-Serum subset, all comparisons showed p-value < 0.001.

3.1.1. A2M Normal Values

Variations of A2M were wider in men than in women, normal values of A2M were much higher before 40 years of age, and normal values of A2M increased slowly after 50 years of age.

3.1.2. ApoA1 Normal Values

ApoA1 in men was very stable from 10 to 70 years of age and was much lower than in women. ApoA1 in women increased from birth to 60 years of age, with a slow decrease thereafter.

3.1.3. Hapto Normal Values

Haptoglobin decreased from birth to 10 years of age, and then re-increased slowly up to 70 years of age in women and up to 50 years of age in men.

3.2. Impact of T2DM on Proteins According to Histological Metabolic Liver
3.2.1. A2M Values

Type 2 diabetes was associated with a significant and earlier increase in A2M (Figure 2). In male patients with T2DM, the mean levels of A2M were significantly higher than in patients without T2DM (all p-values ≤ 0.05), whatever the histological confounder subset. In females with T2DM, A2M was higher than in non-T2DM but only in subsets with significant NASH or significant steatosis grades and in subsets stratified by obesity. A2M was higher than the normal values in all subsets except for women without T2DM and with stage F0F1 (n = 85), with an unexpected significant decrease in A2M versus normal values up to 65 of age, by −0.14 g/L. A2M was associated with clinically significant fibrosis (Figure 3) and NASH (Supplementary Figure S1). As expected, the increase in A2M after 50 years of age was the highest in patients with significant fibrosis stage F2F3F4 (more than 0.70 g/L in men and more than 0.45 g/L in women) and significant NASH grade A2A3 (more than 0.68 g/L in men and more than 0.46 g/L in women) versus non-significant features. A2M levels were decreased in comparison with normal values in patients with significant steatosis, S2S3, before the age of 50 years and with no T2DM (Figure 4).

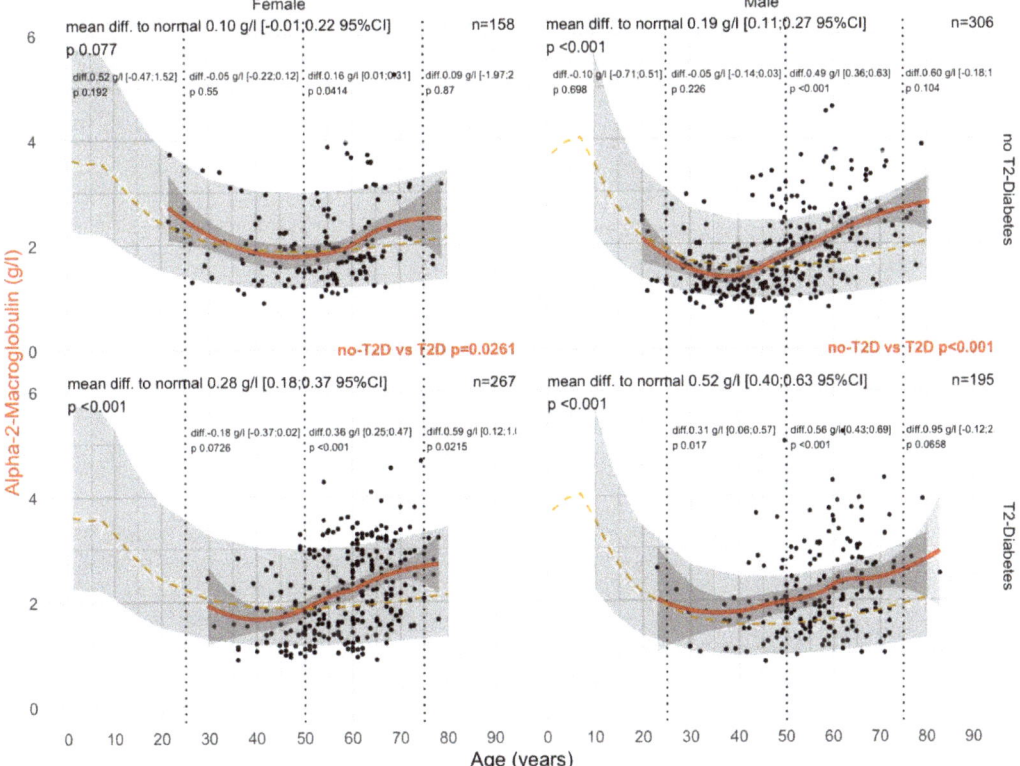

Figure 2. A2M levels in all "NAFLD-Biopsy" patients. Impact of T2DM on A2M concentration in all "NAFLD-Biopsy" patients (n = 926). Normal serum mean values according to age and sex (dashed–orange lines), with 95% confidence intervals (light-gray ribbon). Three vertical dotted lines mark the four age groups (before 25 years, between 25 and 50 years, between 50 and 75 years, and above 75 years old). Each point is a patient's protein value. The red curve is a Loess regression of the median A2M value, along with its 95% confidence interval (darker gray). For each age group, the mean difference (%95CI) between the patient protein value and the expected normal value (for age and sex) with its significant p-value is displayed at the top of the figure. The significance between the non-T2DM and T2DM patients is displayed in red between the two panels.

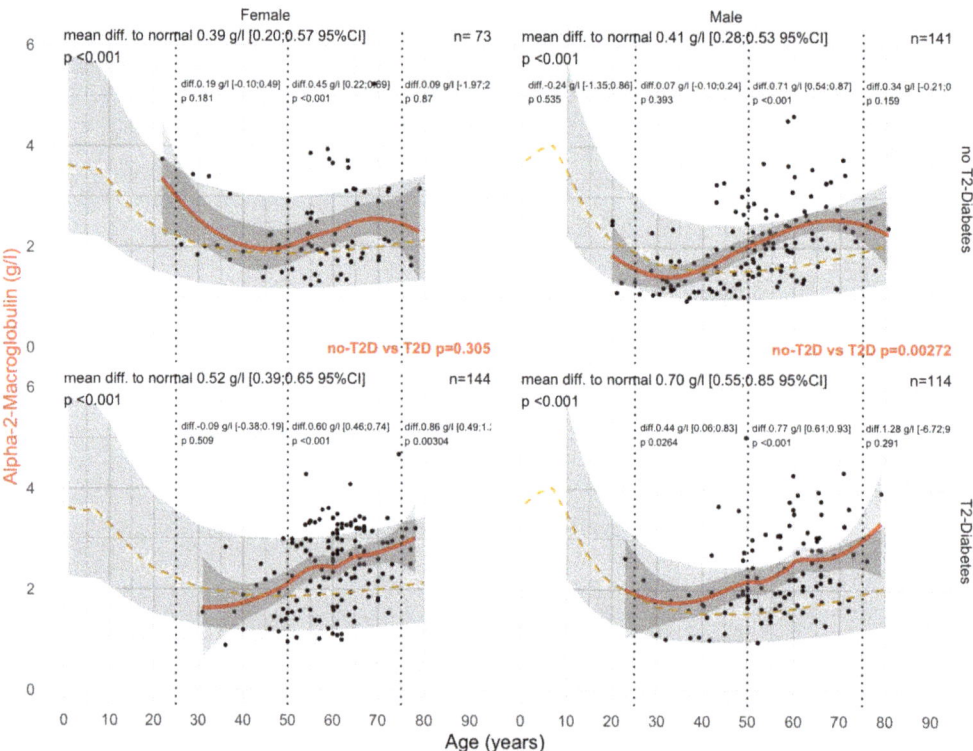

Figure 3. A2M levels in "NAFLD-Biopsy" patients with significant fibrosis stages F2F3F4. Impact of T2DM on A2M concentration in NAFLD-biopsied patients with clinically significant fibrosis F2F3F4 (n = 472). Normal serum means values according to age and sex (dashed–orange lines), with 95% confidence intervals (light-gray ribbon). Three vertical–dotted lines mark the four age groups (before 25, between 25 and 50, between 50 and 75, and above 75 years old). Each point is a patient's protein value. The red curve is a Loess regression of the median A2M values, along with its 95% confidence interval (darker gray). For each age group, the mean difference (%95CI) between the patient protein value and the expected normal value (for age and sex) with its significance p-value is displayed at the top of the figure. The significance between the non-T2DM and T2DM patients is displayed in red between the 2 panels.

Regarding A2M versus normal values in women, patients with significant steatosis S2S3 started with T2DM at 50 years of age, 10 years earlier than in non-T2DM, and in men at 40 years of age. Interestingly, A2M levels were lower than normal in women before the age of 50 years, both without T2DM (−0.07 g/L) and with T2DM (−0.19 g/L). The significant increases above the normal levels started after 50 years of age, ranging from −019 to +0.38 in T2DM, and from −0.07 to +0.16 g/L in non T2DM (Figure 4).

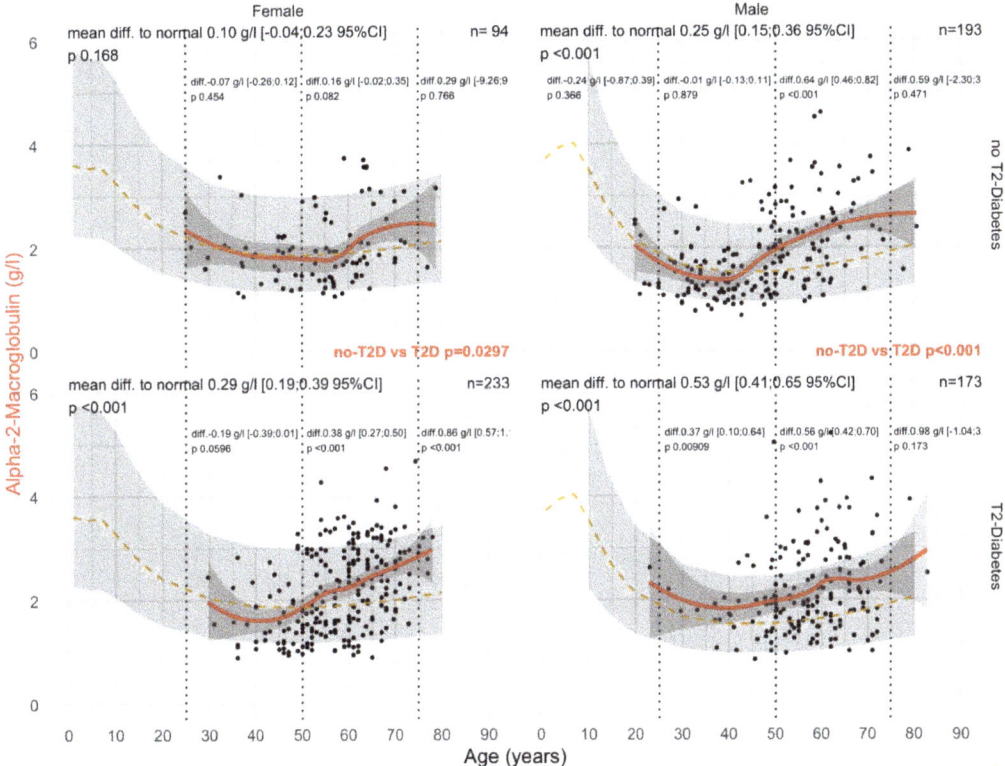

Figure 4. A2M levels in "NAFLD-Biopsy" patients with significant steatosis stages S2S3. Impact of T2DM on A2M concentration in NAFD-biopsied patients with significant steatosis S2S3 (n = 693). Normal serum means values according to age and sex (dashed–orange lines), with 95% confidence intervals (light-gray ribbon). Three vertical–dotted lines mark the four age groups (before 25, between 25 and 50, between 50 and 75, and above 75 years old). Each point is a patient's protein value. The red curve is a Loess regression of the median of A2M values, along with its 95% confidence interval (darker gray). For each age group, the mean difference (%95CI) between patient protein value and the expected normal value (for age and sex) with its significance p-value is displayed at the top of the figure. The significance between the non-T2DM and T2DM patients is displayed in red between the 2 panels.

3.2.2. ApoA1 Values

ApoA1 levels were significantly decreased in women with T2DM compared with those without T2DM from the age of 30 years, whatever the confounders. In women and men with T2DM, ApoA1 values before the age of 50 years were already significantly lower than in patients without T2DM, at −0.25 g/L and −0.09 g/L, respectively (Figure 5). T2DM was associated with lower ApoA1 ($p < 0.001$) in women with significant NASH A2A3 (Supplementary Figure S2). T2DM was also associated with lower ApoA1 ($p = 0.002$) in men and women with significant steatosis S2S3 (Supplementary Figure S3). Furthermore, T2DM was associated with lower ApoA1 ($p = 0.04$) in obese men (Supplementary Figure S4).

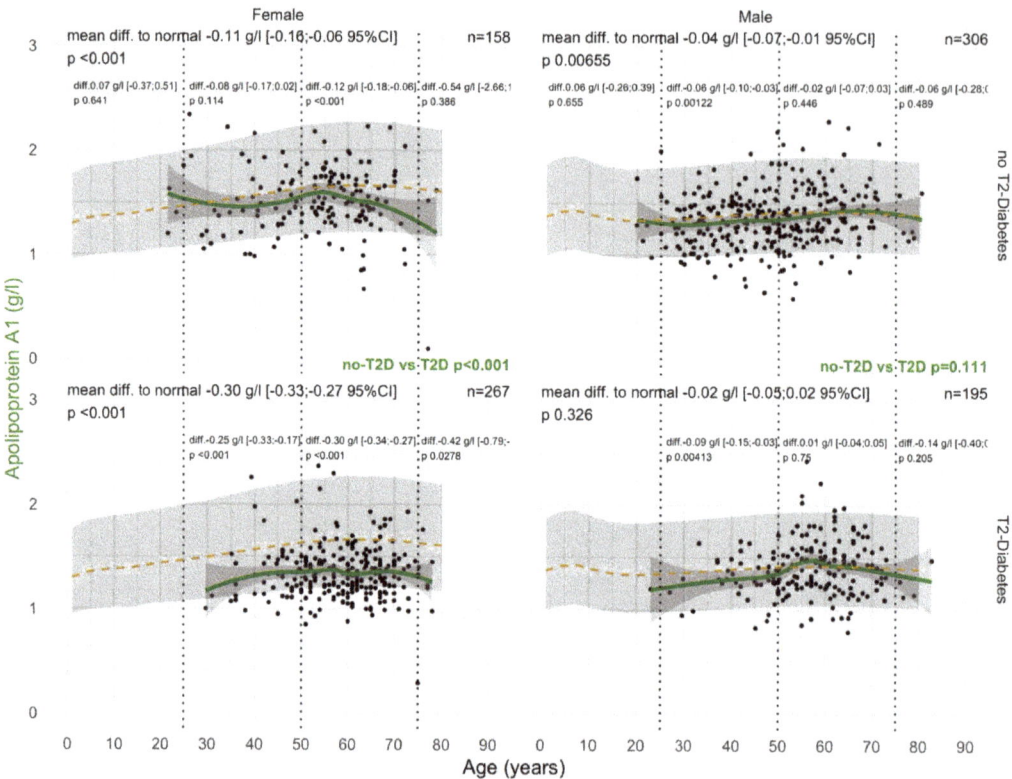

Figure 5. ApoA1 levels in all "NAFLD-Biopsy" patients. Impact of T2DM on ApoA1 concentration in all NAFD-biopsied patients (n = 926). Normal serum means according to age and sex (dashed–orange lines), with 95% confidence intervals (light-gray ribbon). Three vertical–dotted lines mark the four age groups (before 25, between 25 and 50, between 50 and 75, and above 75 years old). Each point is a patient's protein value. The green curve is a Loess regression of the median of ApoA1 values, along with its 95% confidence interval (darker gray). For each age group, the mean difference (%95CI) between the patient protein value and the expected normal value (for age and sex) with its significance p–value is displayed at the top of the figure. The significance between the non-T2DM and T2DM patients is displayed in green between the 2 panels.

3.2.3. Hapto Values

T2DM was associated with a significant increase in haptoglobin levels (+0.23 g/L) versus non-T2DM (−0.11 g/L) in men (Figure 6). This association persisted in men whatever the confounders. In women, the only significant variability was an increase in haptoglobin in patients without T2DM 0.26 g/L; $p = 0.01$ (Figure 6).

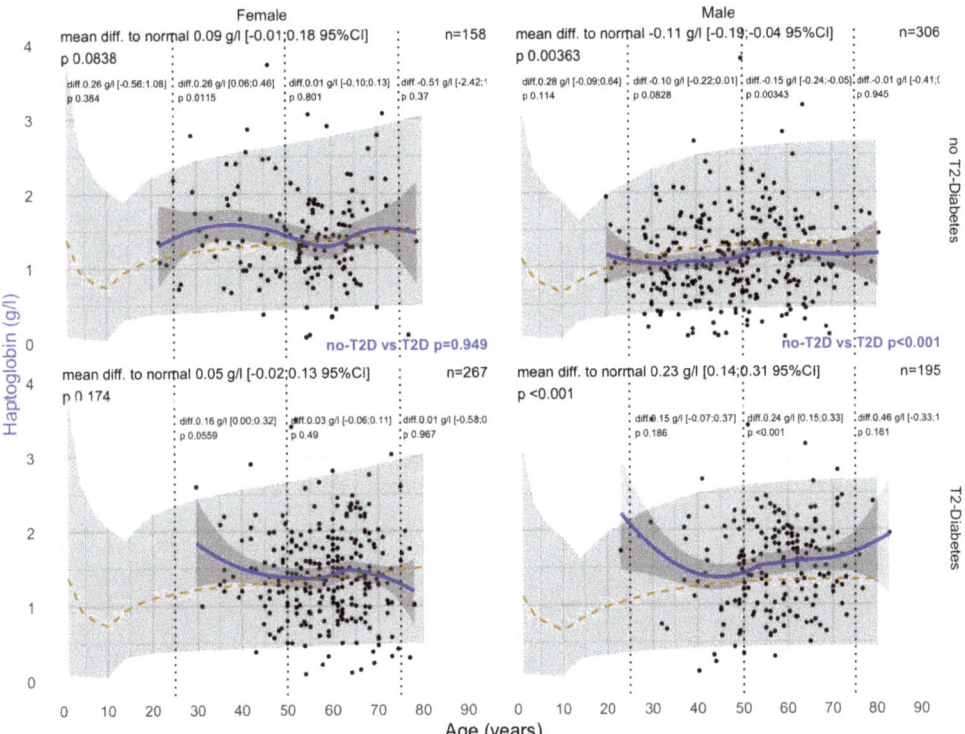

Figure 6. Haptoglobin levels in all "NAFD-Biopsy" patients. Impact of T2DM on Hapto concentration in all NAFD-biopsied patients (n = 926). Normal serum means values according to age and sex (dashed–orange lines), with 95% confidence intervals (light-gray ribbon). Three vertical–dotted lines mark the four age groups (before 25, between 25 and 50, between 50 and 75, and above 75 years old). Each point is a patient's protein value. The green curve is a Loess regression of the median of Hapto values, along with its 95% confidence interval (darker gray). For each age group, the mean difference (%95CI) between the patient protein value and the expected normal value (for age and sex) with its significance p-value is displayed at the top of the figure. The significance between the non-T2DM and T2DM patients is displayed in blue between the 2 panels.

3.3. Impact of T2DM on Serum Protein Levels According to Obesity

3.3.1. A2M

A2M levels were higher in patients with T2DM versus non T2DM regardless of the presence of obesity (all $p = 0.04$). In obese women with T2DM, A2M was decreased before the age of 50 years (-0.15 g/L) and increased after 50 years of age ($+0.30$ g/L) compared with normal values (Figure 7). In non-obese females without T2DM, A2M was also increased after the age of 50 years, (0.25 g/L) compared with normal values. In non-obese individuals, A2M differences versus normal value ranged from 0.15 g/L in women without T2DM (Supplementary Figure S5) to 0.48 g/L in obese men with T2DM (Supplementary Figure S6).

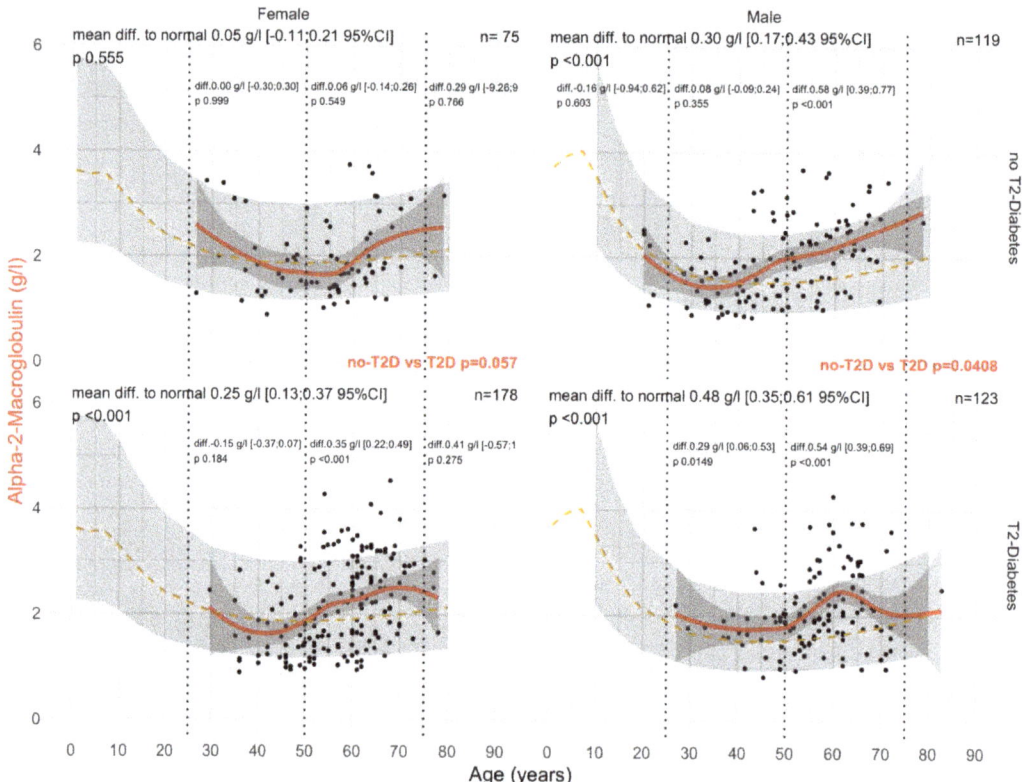

Figure 7. A2M levels in "NAFLD-Biopsy" patients with obesity. Impact of T2DM on A2M concentration in NAFD-biopsied patients according to obesity (n = 495). Normal serum means values according to age and sex (dashed–orange lines), with 95% confidence intervals (light-gray ribbon). Three vertical–dotted lines mark the four age groups (before 25, between 25 and 50, between 50 and 75, and above 75 years old). Each point is a patient's protein value. The red curve is a Loess regression of the median of A2M values, along with its 95% confidence interval (darker gray). For each age group, the mean difference (%95CI) between the patient protein value and the expected normal value (for age and sex) with its significance p-value is displayed at the top of the figure. The significance between the non-T2DM and T2DM patients is displayed in red between the 2 panels.

3.3.2. ApoA1

In non-obese (Supplementary Figure S7) and obese (Supplementary Figure S4) individuals, decreased ApoA1 levels were associated with T2DM in women but not in men.

3.3.3. Hapto

In non-obese (Supplementary Figure S8) and obese (Supplementary Figure S9) individuals, reduced haptoglobin levels were associated with T2DM ($p = 0.003$) in men but not in women. Haptoglobin levels in men, in comparison with normal values, ranged from −0.18 g/L in non-obese individuals without T2DM to +0.26 g/L in obese men with T2DM.

3.3.4. Univariate Correlations between Proteins and between Histological Features

There was no significant association between the three proteins within the four sex/obesity subsets (Supplementary Figures S10 and S11). Among the three histological features, fibrosis stage was associated positively, as expected, with NASH grades in the four sex/obesity subsets. There was an unexpected association with steatosis grades in non-obese men. Fibrosis stage was associated with age in the four sex/obesity subsets with the exception of non-obese women (Supplementary Figure S11). Both NASH and steatosis grades were not significantly associated with age. Steatosis grade was significantly and positively associated with NASH and fibrosis only in non-obese women (Supplementary Figure S10). A2M level, as expected, was significantly ($p < 0.05$) and positively associated with age, fibrosis stage, and NASH grade in the four sex/obesity subsets. ApoA1 level was only associated positively with age in obese men (Supplementary Figure S10). Haptoglobin was associated positively with age only in non-obese men and surprisingly positively associated with the grade of steatosis both in obese and non-obese men (Supplementary Figure S10).

3.3.5. Multivariate Regression

This analysis permitted adjustment of the association between T2DM and each protein, independently of the two other proteins of interest after taking into account age and the SAF class of each feature in each of the four sex/obesity subsets.

T2DM Multivariate Association with Proteins and Fibrosis (Supplementary Table S1).

A2M was not associated with the presence of T2DM in the four sex/obesity subsets. ApoA1 was significantly and negatively associated with T2DM in women with or without obesity. Haptoglobin was significantly and positively associated with T2DM in men with or without obesity.

T2DM Multivariate Association with Proteins and NASH (Supplementary Table S2).

A2M was only associated with the presence of T2DM in non-obese men. ApoA1 was significantly and negatively associated with T2DM in women with or without obesity. Haptoglobin was significantly and positively associated with T2DM in men with or without obesity.

T2DM Multivariate Association with Proteins and Steatosis (Supplementary Table S3)

A2M was not associated with the presence of T2DM in the four sex/obesity subsets. ApoA1 was significantly and negatively associated with T2DM in women without obesity. Haptoglobin was significantly and positively associated with T2DM in men without obesity.

3.3.6. Impact of BMI on Serum Level Proteins

Impact of BMI on A2M Serum Level in the "NAFLD-Serum" Cohort

In diabetic patients, there was a higher level of A2M according to BMI vs non-diabetic patients, both in males and females, in patients above 25 kg/m^2 (Figure 8).

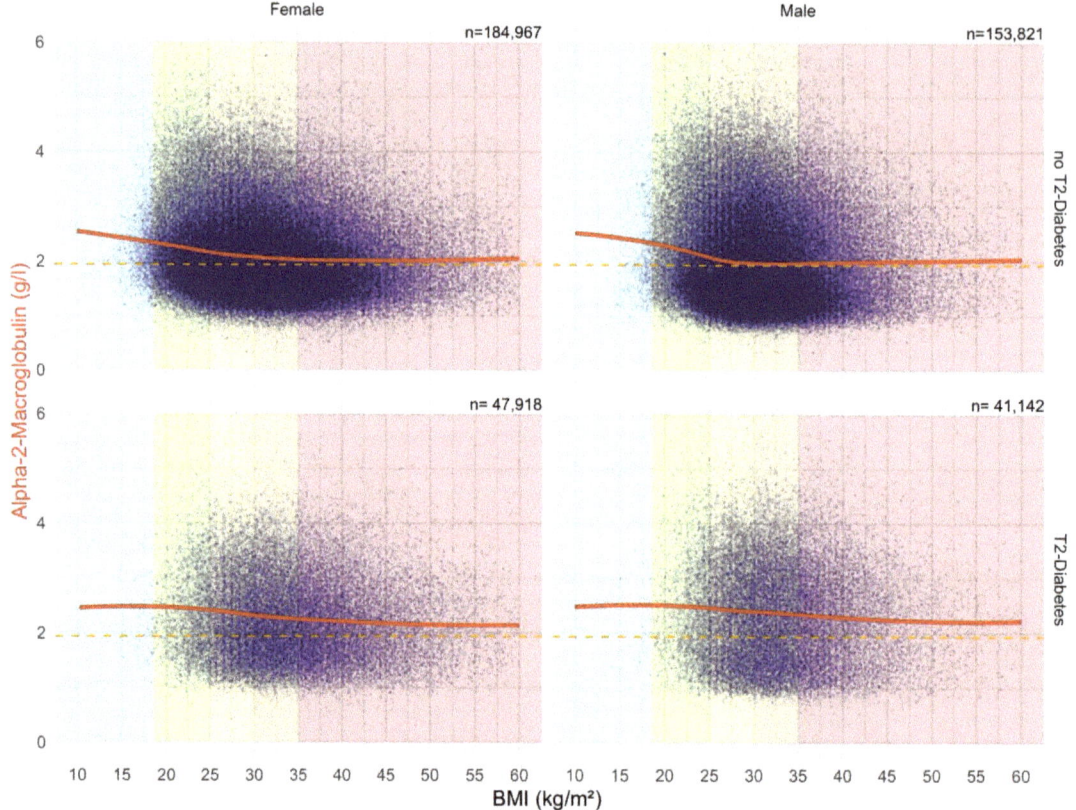

Figure 8. Impact of BMI on the A2M concentrations in "NAFD–Serum" cohort. Median value is the horizontal orange–dashed line. Five vertical zones mark the 5 BMI groups (WHO definition cut-offs: 18.5, 25, 30, 35 and above 40 kg/m^2). Each blue point is a protein patient value with its BMI. The red curve is a Loess regression of the median of A2M values.

Impact of BMI on ApoA1 Serum Level in the "NAFLD-Serum" Cohort

In all patients, there was a negative correlation between ApoA1 and BMI (Figure 9).

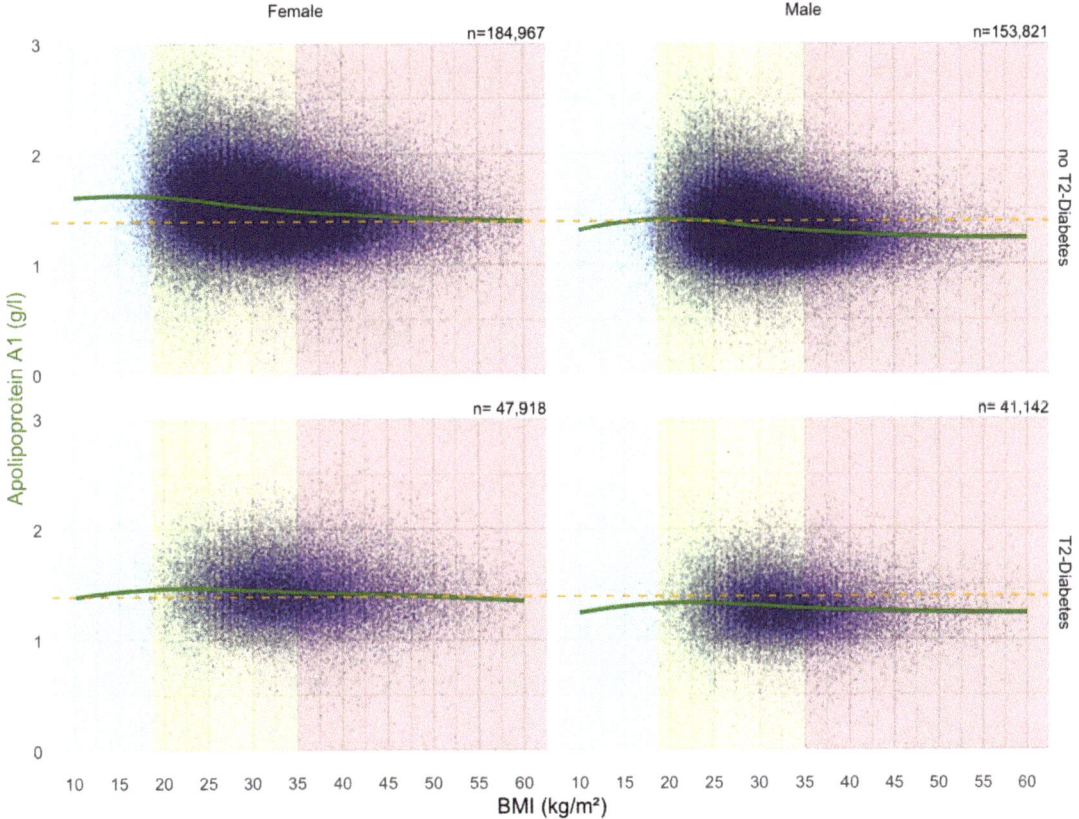

Figure 9. Impact of BMI on the ApoA1 concentrations in "NAFD–Serum" cohort. Median value is the horizontal orange–dashed line. Five vertical zones mark the 5 BMI groups (WHO definition cut-offs: 18.5, 25, 30, 35 and above 40 kg/m^2). Each blue point is a protein patient value with its BMI. The green curve is a Loess regression of the median of ApoA1 values.

Impact of BMI on Haptoglobin Serum Level in the "NAFLD-Serum" Cohort

There was a strong positive correlation between Haptoglobin serum level and BMI, particularly in females (Figure 10).

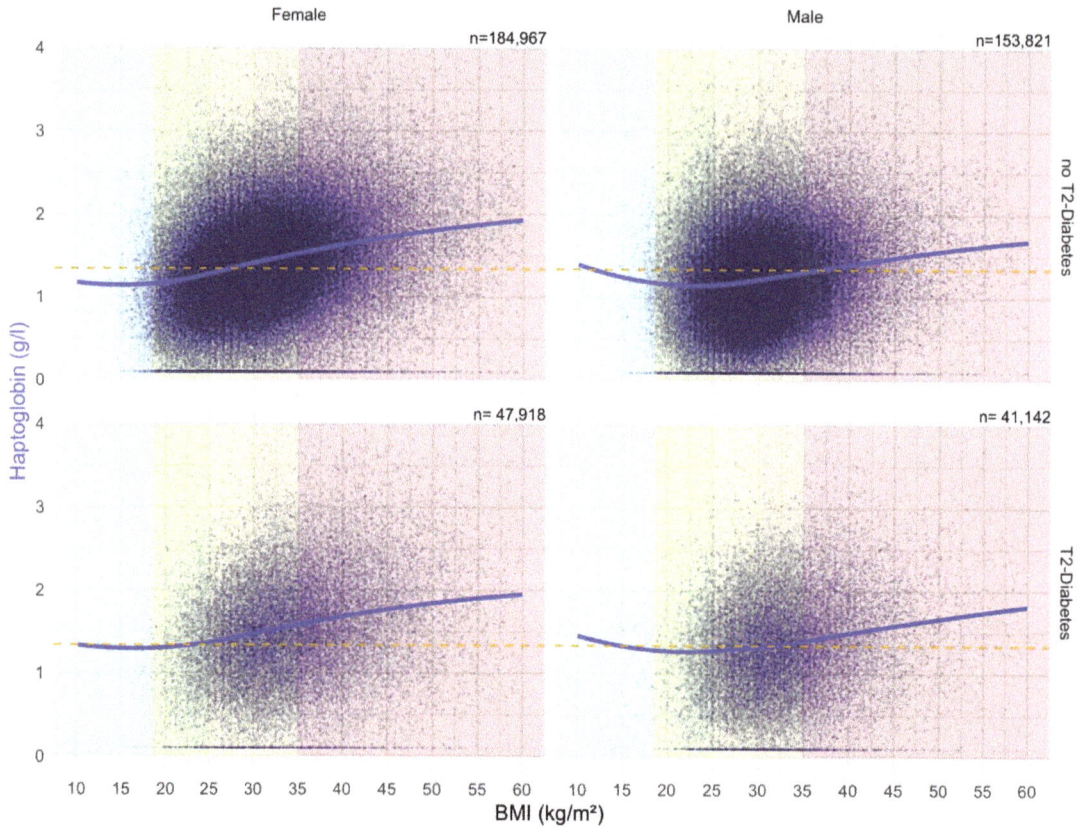

Figure 10. Impact of BMI on the Haptoglobin concentrations in "NAFD–Serum" cohort. Median value is the horizontal orange–dashed line. Five vertical zones mark the 5 BMI groups (WHO definition cut-offs: 18.5, 25, 30, 35 and above 40 kg/m^2). Each blue point is a protein patient value with its BMI. The blue curve is a Loess regression of the median of Haptoglobin values.

3.4. Impact of T2DM on the Three Proteins According to SARS-CoV-2 Infection

Before COVID-19, the means of A2M were higher and ApoA1 lower than normal expected values. The means of haptoglobin were higher than normal expected values only in obese patients (Figure 11).

During COVID-19, the means of ApoA1 were even lower than before COVID-19. The means of haptoglobin were higher than the normal expected value only in obese patients. The means of haptoglobin were even higher than before COVID-19 only in obese patients (Figure 11).

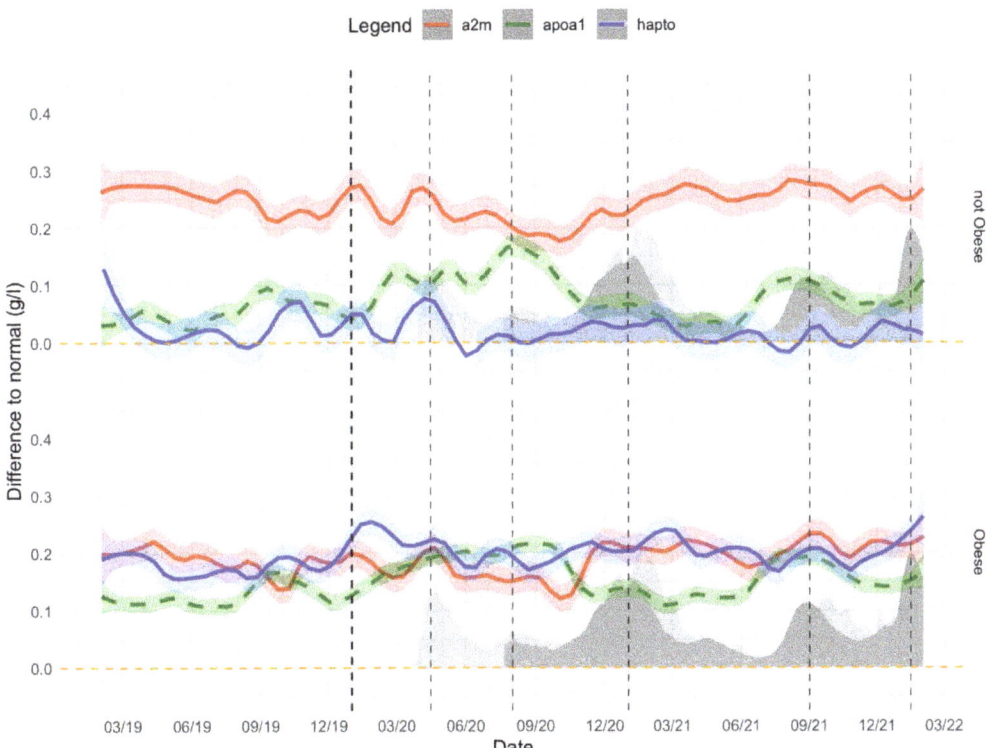

Figure 11. A2M, ApoA1, and haptoglobin levels before and during the COVID-19 pandemic. Impact of COVID-19 waves on A2M, ApoA1 and haptoglobin level differences with normal values before and during COVID-19 pandemic in obese and non-obese "NAFLD-Serum" subjects followed for metabolic liver risk (n = 135,911). X-axis is time, between January 2019 and February 2022. Dashed–vertical black lines show the different COVID-19 waves. In light gray and dark gray are the standardized COVID-19-related death and hospitalization rates, respectively, in the USA. The red line, blue line, and dashed–green line are the 7-day rolling mean difference and %95CI between the observed A2M, haptoglobin, and negative Apoa1 concentration, respectively, and the expected normal values for these subjects adjusted by their age and gender.

3.4.1. A2M

Before COVID-19, T2DM was associated with a significant and very early increase in A2M before 30 years of age compared with non-T2DM, both in men and women (Figure 12). In women with T2DM, A2M levels were increased by 0.38 g/L compared with 0.19 g/L without T2DM, and in men by 0.76 g/L compared with 0.42 g/L without T2DM (all $p < 0.001$). During COVID-19, T2DM was associated with different A2M kinetics compared with those prior to COVID-19. The levels decreased below the normal values under the age of 20 years and increased 15 years later (45 years of age) compared with 30 years before COVID-19 (Figure 13). A2M increases were also lower during COVID-19 than before. In women with T2DM, A2M levels were increased by 28 g/L compared with 6 g/L without T2DM, and in men by 0.61 g/L compared with 0.26 g/L without T2DM (all $p < 0.001$).

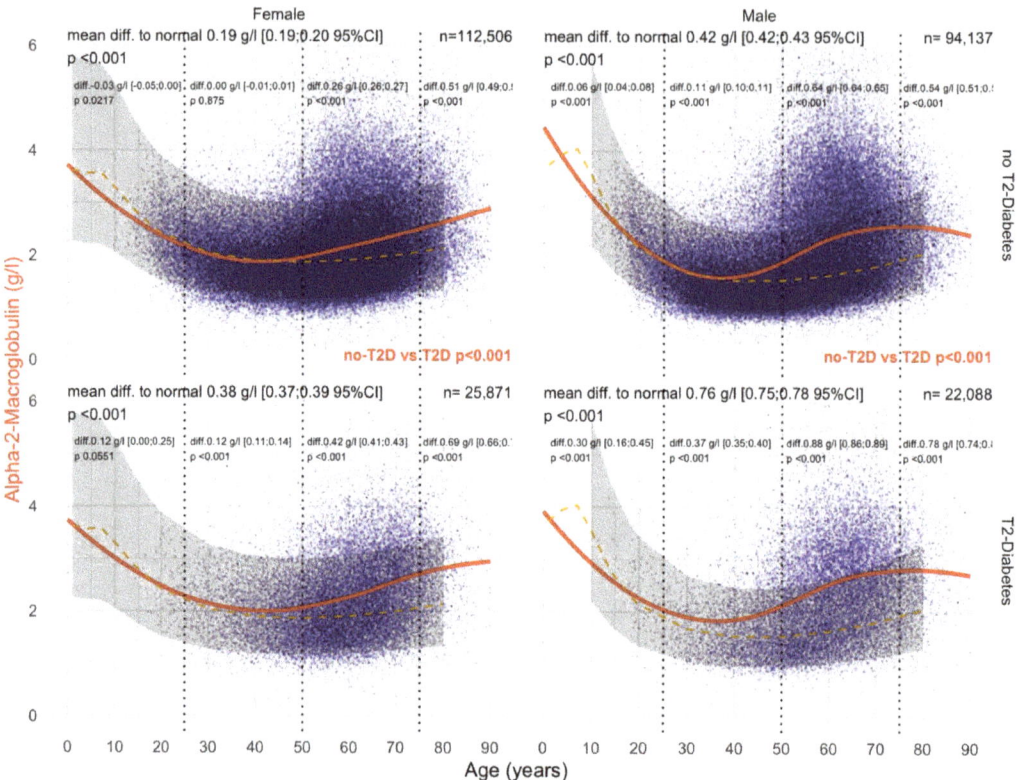

Figure 12. A2M levels before the COVID-19 pandemic. Impact of T2DM on A2M concentration before SARS-CoV-2 pandemic in "NAFLD-Serum" patients followed for metabolic liver risk (n = 254,602). Normal serum mean values according to age and sex (dashed–orange lines), with 95% confidence intervals (gray ribbon). Three vertical–dotted lines mark the four age groups (before 25, between 25 and 50, between 50 and 75, and above 75 years old). The red curve is a Loess regression of the median of A2M values. For each age group, the mean difference (%95CI) between the patient protein value and the expected normal value (for age and sex) with its significance p-value is displayed at the top of the figure. The significance between the non-T2DM and T2DM patients is displayed in red between the 2 panels.

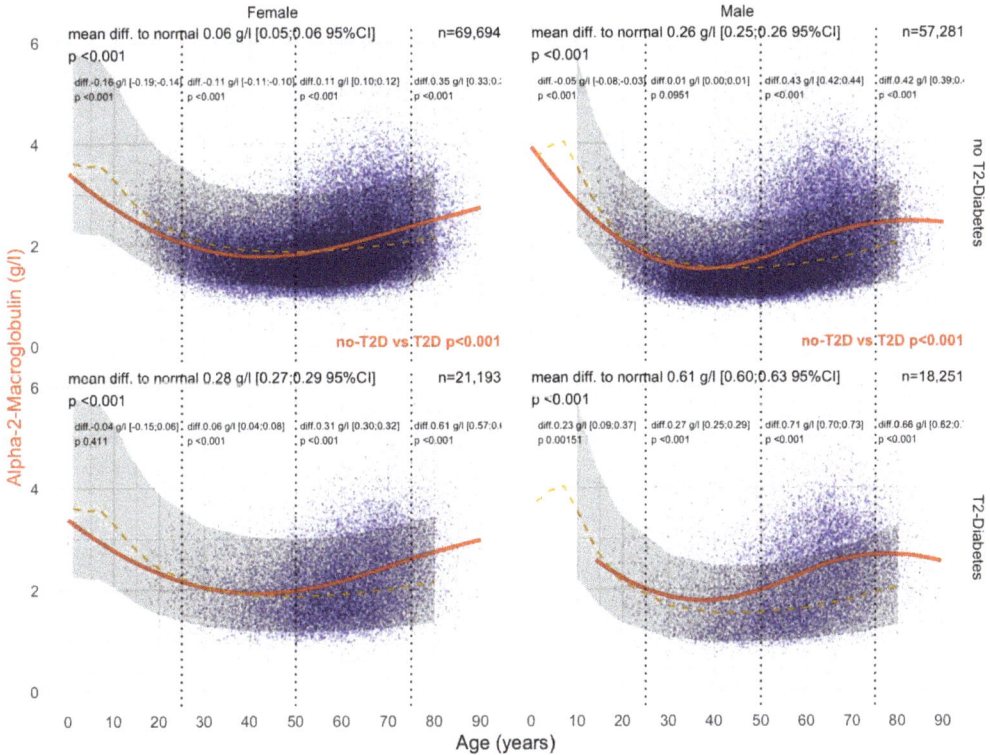

Figure 13. A2M levels during the COVID-19 pandemic. Impact of T2DM on A2M concentration during SARS-CoV-2 pandemic in "NAFLD-Serum" patients followed for metabolic liver risk (n = 173,246). Normal serum means values according to age and sex (dashed–orange lines), with 95% confidence intervals (gray ribbon). Three vertical–dotted lines mark the four age groups (before 25, between 25 and 50, between 50 and 75, and above 75 years old). The red curve is a Loess regression of the median of A2M values. For each age group, the mean difference (%95CI) between the patient protein value and the expected normal (for age and sex) with its significance p-value is displayed at the top of the figure. The significance between the non-T2DM and T2DM patients is displayed in red between the 2 panels.

3.4.2. ApoA1

Before COVID-19, T2DM was associated with a significant and very early decrease in ApoA1 in patients younger than 20 years of age compared with non-T2DM patients, in both in men and women (Figure 14). In women with T2DM, ApoA1 levels were decreased by −0.18 g/L compared with −0.09 g/L in those without T2DM, and in men by −0.10 g/L compared with −0.06 g/L without T2DM (all $p < 0.001$). During COVID-19, T2DM was associated with a significant and very early decrease in ApoA1 in patients younger than 20 years of age compared with non-T2DM patients, both in men and women (Figure 15). In women with T2DM, ApoA1 levels were −0.22 g/L compared with −0.12 g/L without T2DM, and in men by −0.13 g/L compared with −0.08 g/L without T2DM (all $p < 0.001$).

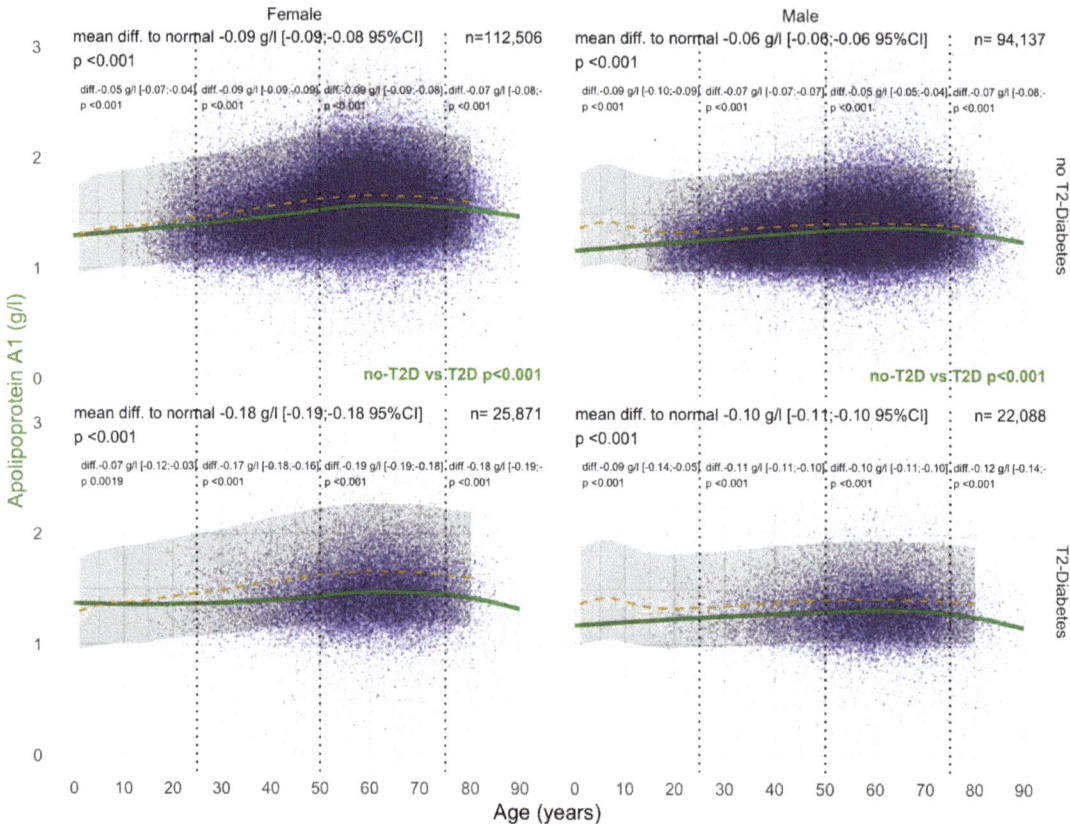

Figure 14. ApoA1 levels before the COVID-19 pandemic. Impact of T2DM on ApoA1 concentration before SARS-CoV-2 pandemic in "NAFLD-Serum" patients followed for metabolic liver risk (n = 254,602). Normal serum means values according to age and sex (dashed–orange lines), with 95% confidence intervals (gray ribbon). Three vertical–dotted lines mark the four age groups (before 25, between 25 and 50, between 50 and 75 and above 75 years old). The green curve is a Loess regression of the median of ApoA1 values. For each age group, the mean difference (%95CI) between the patient protein value and the expected normal value (for age and sex) with its significance *p*-value is displayed at the top of the figure. The significance between the non-T2DM and T2DM patients is displayed in green between the 2 panels.

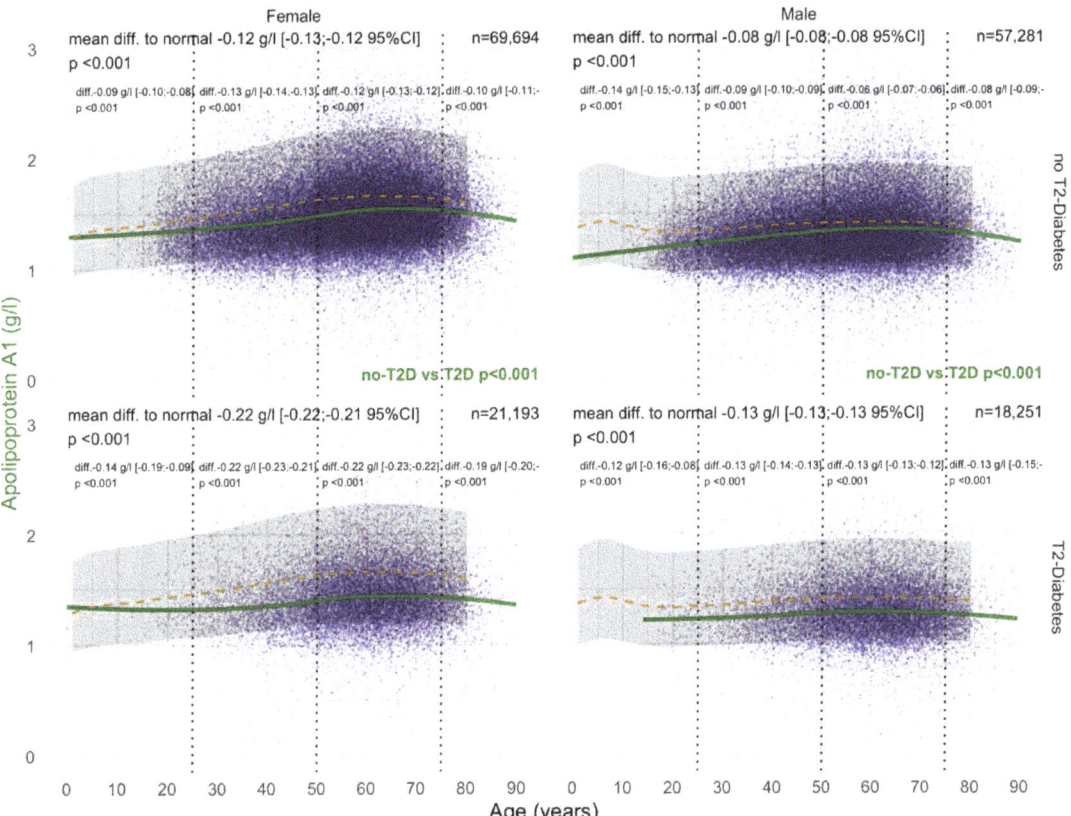

Figure 15. ApoA1 levels during the COVID-19 pandemic. Impact of T2DM on ApoA1 concentration during SARS-CoV-2 pandemic in "NAFLD-Serum" patients followed for metabolic liver risk (n = 173,246). Normal serum means values according to age and sex (dashed–orange lines), with 95% confidence intervals (gray ribbon). Three vertical–dotted lines mark the four age groups (before 25, between 25 and 50, between 50 and 75, and above 75 years old). The green curve is a Loess regression of the median of ApoA1 values. For each age group, the mean difference (%95CI) between the patient protein value and the expected normal value (for age and sex) with its significance p-value is displayed on top of figure. The significance between the non-T2DM and T2DM patients is displayed in green between the 2 panels.

3.4.3. Haptoglobin

Before COVID-19, T2DM was associated with a significant and very early increase in haptoglobin in patients younger than 20 years of age compared with non-T2DM patients, both in men and women (Figure 16). In women with T2DM, ApoA1 levels were increased by 0.16 g/L compared with 0.06 g/L without T2DM, and in men by 0.05 g/L compared with 0.06 g/L without T2DM (all $p < 0.001$). During COVID-19, T2DM was associated with a significant and very early increase in haptoglobin in patients younger than 20 years of age compared with non-T2DM patients, both in women (0.25 g/L vs 0.12 g/L) and men (0.14 g/L vs 0.02 g/L) (Figure 17).

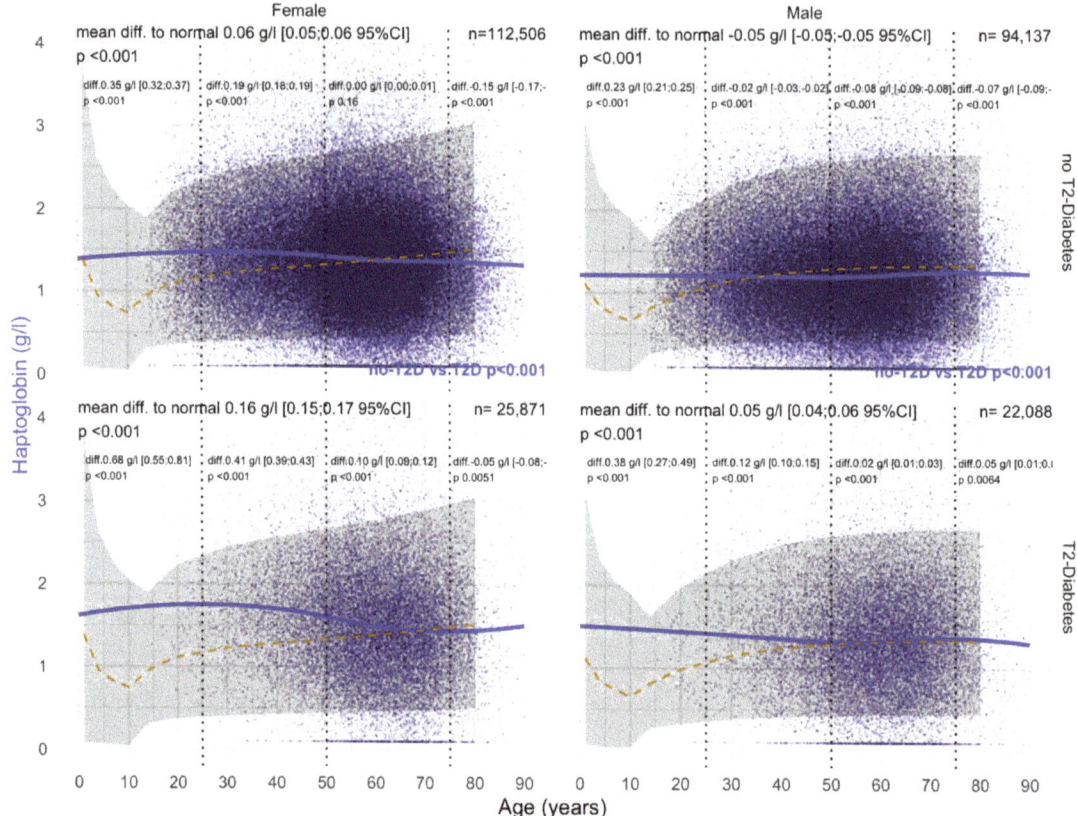

Figure 16. Haptoglobin levels before the COVID-19 pandemic. Impact of T2DM on Hapto concentration before SARS-CoV-2 pandemic in "NAFLD-Serum" patients followed for metabolic liver risk (n = 254,602). Normal serum means values according to age and sex (dashed–orange lines), with 95% confidence intervals (gray ribbon). Three vertical–dotted lines mark the four age groups (before 25, between 25 and 50, between 50 and 75, and above 75 years old). The blue curve is a Loess regression of the median of Hapto values. For each age group, the mean difference (%95CI) between the patient protein value and the expected normal value (for age and sex) with its significance *p*-value is displayed at the top of the figure. The significance between the non-T2DM and T2DM patients is displayed in blue between the 2 panels.

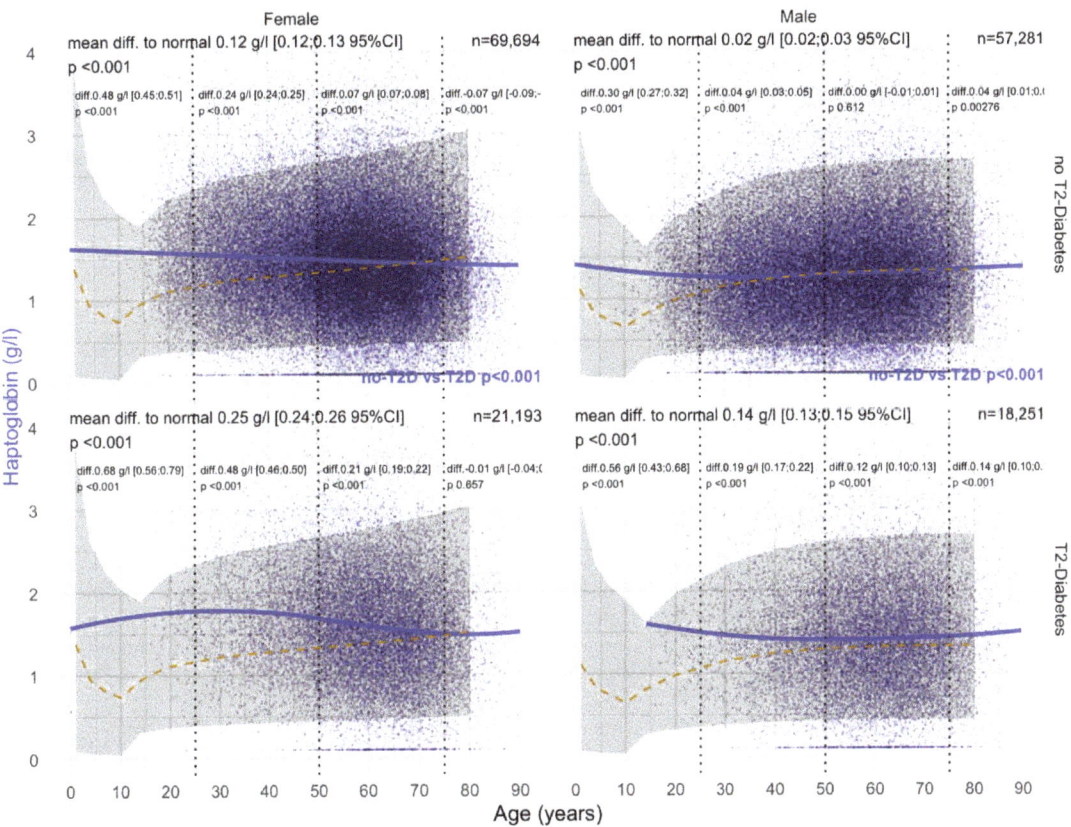

Figure 17. Haptoglobin levels during the COVID-19 pandemic. Impact of T2DM on Hapto concentration during SARS-CoV-2 pandemic in "NAFLD-Serum" patients followed for metabolic liver risk (n = 173,246). Normal serum means values according to age and sex (dashed–orange lines), with 95% confidence intervals (gray ribbon). Three vertical–dotted lines mark the four age groups (before 25, between 25 and 50, between 50 and 75, and above 75 years old). The blue curve is a Loess regression of the median of Hapto values. For each age group, the mean difference (%95CI) between the patient protein value and the expected normal value (for age and sex) with its significance p-value is displayed at the top of the figure. The significance between the non-T2DM and T2DM patients is displayed in blue between the 2 panels.

4. Discussion

Here, the impact of T2DM on the serum levels of three proteins in patients at risk of NAFLD was assessed according to eight major confounding factors: age, sex, obesity, NAFLD histological liver features (fibrosis, NASH steatosis), and SARS-CoV-2 infection. Such a study has never been performed before, despite the rationale and evidence base of such correlations [1–61].

Overall, we found that the levels of the three proteins were significantly different than normal values in patients at risk of NAFLD without T2DM, with increased A2M, decreased ApoA1, and increased haptoglobin. In patients with both NAFLD and T2DM, these significant differences were magnified. Furthermore, in cases of SARS-CoV-2 infection, this population had a third factor of decreased ApoA1 and increased haptoglobin. These results are in line with the independent diagnostic and prognostic values of ApoA1 and haptoglobin combined with A2M in COVID-19 [9,10].

In patients at risk of NAFLD, several multivariate tests used at least one of these three proteins for the non-invasive diagnosis or prognosis of liver features [73,74], as follows: A2M (FibroTest/FibroSure [35,37,75], FibroMeter V2G and V3G [73,74], Hepascore [73,74], and NIS4 [76]), ApoA1 (FibroTest/FibroSure, Chunming score, Shukla score) [35,37,77,78], and haptoglobin (FibroTest/FibroSure Fuc–Hpt–Mac2bp) [35,37,79].

The recent increase in the knowledge of these proteins, as well as their inclusion in multivariate biomarkers, deserves discussion regarding their clinical interest and limitations, including their respective risks of false positives and false negatives.

4.1. A2M Variability in Patients at Risk of NAFLD

4.1.1. Strengths

The variability of A2M according to age, in comparison with expected USA normal values, was retrieved in both the "NAFLD-Biopsy" and "NAFLD-Serum" cohorts.

The normal values were highly different according to the four age periods, decreasing rapidly between 5 to 25 years of age, almost stable between 25 to 50, and re-increasing slowly up to more than 75 years of age. These results support both the hypothesis of a preventive role of A2M in SARS-CoV-2 infection in children up to the age of 25 years, and also the aging damage role of A2M after the age of 50 years.

Here, A2M in T2DM was significantly increased at an earlier time point (Figures 2 and 9) than in non-T2DM. This is in line not only with the role of A2M as a regulator of the extracellular matrix [19,23,26] and the well-known positive association of A2M in the extracellular matrix of liver fibrosis (Supplementary Table S1) [19,23,30,32–38], but also with the early damage of proteins associated with the very early presence of T2DM [19,27–29,80]. In men with T2DM of the "NAFLD-Serum" cohort, A2M increased as soon as the age of 40 years, reaching a mean increase of 0.88 g/L between 50 to 75 years of age (Figure 9).

4.1.2. Limitations

In the "NAFLD-Biopsy" cohort, the sample size was too small to assess the kinetics before the age of 25 years, and therefore to assess the association with liver features. However, thanks to the large sample size of the "NAFLD-Serum" cohort, the sample size of patients at risk before the age of 25 years was sufficient to compare curves of A2M in patients with T2DM2 vs. normal expected values, at least in USA NAFLD patients. Here, thanks to the large sample size, we observed a decrease in the mean A2M in obese patients at risk of NAFLD, with or without T2DM, when compared with normal USA values adjusted for age and sex, as described in other contexts of use.

A2M is a candidate biomarker mirroring key metabolic steps for health and disease. It gains insight into the interaction of anabolism with catabolism [81]. The results of several studies in Thai adults in Bangkok showed different associations between A2M serum levels compared with normal Thai individuals, with lower levels than in the USA. In hardworking male construction laborers, a negative correlation was found for the variables age, weight, height, BMI, and HDL, with A2M as the dependent variable [82]. A2M of female construction workers did relate to any of the variables investigated. A dietary survey conducted with apparently health Thai farmers found a statistically significant negative correlation of A2M with energy, protein, fat, and carbohydrate intake [83]. Tobacco smoking could be a confounding factor [84,85]. All these results obtained from the variety of different studies seem indeed to be in accordance with the assumption that A2M supports homeostasis in situations of a "challenged" nutritional status [83].

In the "NAFLD-Biopsy" cohort, A2M levels were decreased in comparison with normal values in patients with significant steatosis S2S3 before the age of 50 years and without T2DM (Figure 4). Such an unexpected result requires confirmation and further physio–pathological evidence. Degradations of the proteins could be an explanation [86].

During SARS-CoV-2 studies in non-human primates, we recently observed an unexpected very early decrease in serum A2M 2 days post-infection at the peak of nasopharyngeal viral loads, with a return to baseline values at the seventh day [10]. Similar kinetics of A2M were observed in hospitalized patients with COVID-19 not requiring intensive care [9,10]. If confirmed, this kinetic could be associated with the rapid consumption or degradation of native A2M during the peak of the acute phase response. Similar early kinetics of A2M levels were observed in hemodialysis patients, with lower levels during COVID-19 vs. healthy controls, and vs. hemodialysis patients without COVID-19 [11].

4.1.3. Causal Relationships with Clinical Endpoints

In patients with T2DM, the predominant circulating form of A2M is degraded [86]. In nephrotic syndrome, serum A2M levels start to rise when a trace amount of albumin is excreted. Hepatic synthesis of A2M is enhanced significantly to replace lost liver-derived proteins in experimental animals and humans, resulting in a net increase in its serum levels [87–89]. Because of this risk of the confounding factors, we checked the absence of correlations (logistic regression) between the presence of obesity and kidney function assessed by CKD index and A2M levels adjusted by age and sex in the T2DM cohort post–hoc. There was no significant association between A2M and kidney function (Supplementary Table S2).

In the plasma proteomic profile of T2DM patients submitted to bariatric surgery, A2M significantly increased in individuals whose diabetes persisted or remitted after weight loss, using non-diabetic but similarly obese persons as controls [90]. Therefore, in this context, A2M could be a prognostic marker.

4.2. ApoA1

4.2.1. Strengths

Our epidemiological results support the causal relationship between low ApoA1 as an independent risk factor of infection by SARS-CoV-2 in NAFLD patients with additive risks of T2DM and obesity [2–10,13,91].

In the "NAFLD-Biopsy" cohort, ApoA1 levels were already significantly decreased (-0.30 g/L) in women with T2DM compared with non-T2DM patients from the age of 30 years (Figure 5), whatever the confounders (Supplementary Figures S2–S4). This early decrease in patients with biopsy was retrieved in the "NAFLD-Serum" cohort with a mean decrease of 0.20 g/L (Figure 5). In men, the ApoA1 decrease compared with normal values was also significant, but much less than in women where the levels increased significantly from birth to 60 years of age.

The association of T2DM with lower ApoA1 ($p < 0.001$) in women with histologically significant NASH, grades A2A3, is original and in line with other more severe liver diseases with high grades of necro-inflammatory inflammation, such as severe alcoholic hepatitis, which was described in previous studies.

We used the "NAFLD-Serum" cohort to confirm the previous findings [9]: that before (Figure 14) and during (Figure 15) COVID-19, T2DM was associated with a decrease in ApoA1 compared with non-T2DM patients, in both in men and women. For the first time, to the best of our knowledge, we observed that this decrease in ApoA1 was lower in obese vs. non-obese, both before and during COVID-19 (Figure 11).

4.2.2. Limitations

The present results were limited by the absence of adjustments on confounding factors associated with serum ApoA1 levels, such as dietary folate, physical exercise, and vitamin C [92] and alcohol intake both before [93] and during [94] COVID-19.

4.2.3. Causal Relationships with Clinical Endpoints

Recent phase 2 randomized trials in patients with NAFLD used serum ApoA1 as secondary endpoints for assessing the drug's benefit [68,95].

Lanifibranor is a pan-PPAR (peroxisome proliferator-activated receptor) agonist that modulates key metabolic, inflammatory, and fibrogenic pathways in the pathogenesis of NASH [68].

Pegbelfermin (PGBF) is a hormone that can reduce bile acids (BA) that have previously been shown to have toxic effects on the liver. 7a-hydroxy-4-cholesten-3-one (C4), a biomarker of primary BA synthesis in the liver, was measured in plasma of the patients with NASH together with ApoA1. After PGBF treatment, C4 and ApoA1 were increased vs. control, and associated with decreases in the LDL/HDL ratio, suggesting that PGBF-associated changes in BA metabolism may contribute to an improvement in lipoprotein profiles that could possibly lead to a reduction in cardiovascular risk in patients with NASH [96,97].

Numerous experimental results explained how ApoA1 may lose its functionality in many inflammatory and pathological conditions, including T2DM, liver diseases, obesity and COVID-19 [41]. ApoA1 is secreted by the liver (about 70%) and the intestine (about 30%). This lipid free ApoA1 interacts with the ATP-binding cassette transporter A1 (ABCA1) on peripheral cells, leading to the transfer of cholesterol and cellular phospholipids from the cell membrane to ApoA1. T2DM, liver diseases, obesity and COVID-19 can impair the biogenesis of ApoA1, as well as its post-translational modifications, including oxidation, carbamylating, and glycation.

Several recent studies separating the roles of the main HDL components, such as HDL2, HDL3, and ApoA1 (or according to the HDL size), have suggested that the causal relationships between serum levels of ApoA1 with clinical endpoints such as cardiovascular events [13], risk of severe COVID-19 [14], or glycosylated hemoglobin [96] were easier to prove than using the HDL overall levels.

Finally, a recent work demonstrating a new source of ApoA1 for the liver through the portal vein directly from the intestine opens up many possible causal mechanisms with the risks of T2DM, liver diseases, obesity, and COVID-19 [53]. HDL3 produced by the intestine protects the liver from the inflammation and fibrosis observed in a variety of mouse models of liver injury that parallel clinically relevant conditions in humans, including surgical resection of the small bowel, alcohol consumption, or high-fat diets.

4.3. Haptoglobin

4.3.1. Strengths

The present results underline the performance of haptoglobin as a sensitive biomarker of inflammation in chronic liver disease. Thus far, the clinical utility of serum haptoglobin is its prognostic value in multivariate blood tests when its level is decreased, which has been observed mostly in advanced fibrosis stages.

Here, in patients at risk of NAFLD, haptoglobin levels were positively associated with male sex, T2DM, and obesity, and surprisingly with the grade of steatosis in non–obese men, in univariate and multivariate analyses. These associations are in line with a chronic inflammation profile in these patients before the onset of histological NASH [54–61].

During SARS-CoV-2 studies in non-human primates, we recently observed that haptoglobin levels, in comparison with CRP, had the same early increase 2 days after infection, but remained more consistently elevated for at least 10 days post-infection [10]. Recent human studies underlined the clinical interest in haptoglobin in SARS-CoV-2 infection [16–18], including one that described the normal distribution of haptoglobin versus the bimodal distribution of CRP [16].

Finally, for the first time, in patients at risk of NAFLD, the correlation between haptoglobin serum level and BMI was demonstrated, probably due to a chronic inflammation.

4.3.2. Limitations

The present results were limited by the absence of adjustments on confounding factors associated with serum haptoglobin levels, such as haptoglobin polymorphism, inflammatory bowel disease, hemolysis, iron deficiency, and exercise [98–100]. Several studies found associations between haptoglobin 2-2 and liver fibrosis, but the causality has not been validated thus far [16].

4.3.3. Causal Relationships with Clinical Endpoints

Haptoglobin increase is a validated direct early consequence of the acute phase reaction. However, as for ApoA1, serum haptoglobin variability observed in T2DM, obesity, and COVID-19 could also be directly due to the intestine, such as changes in endothelial permeability. Higher serum levels of haptoglobin were observed in obese patients with increased jejunal permeability revealed by lipid challenge and linked to inflammation and T2DM [101]. After a lipid load, haptoglobin was two-fold higher in obese patients compared to non-obese controls and correlated with systemic and intestinal inflammation. Lipid-induced permeability was associated with the presence of T2DM and obesity. In such correlations, the mechanisms explaining the variability of serum haptoglobin could be both genetic defects (such as Gata6 gene and a decrease in zonulin—the pre-haptoglobin protein), and specific environmental factors (such as high-fat diet, alcohol, fiber-deprived diet, bacterial or viral infection, and medication exposure) known to contribute to break the intestinal barrier balance and promote gut dysbiosis [102].

In mice, exercise before a polyunsaturated fatty acid-based (PUFA) diets upregulates haptoglobin fourfold and eightfold according to isocaloric or ad libitum diets, respectively [103]. In both humans and mice, haptoglobin has been shown to increase in plasma because of increased secretion both by the liver and adipose tissue, and is increased by many factors including tumor necrosis factor–alpha and interleukin–6. These cytokines are known to be increased in their abundance when animals are placed on a high PUFA diet [104]. A consequence of a haptoglobin increase is increased plasma abundance on an HFD, which may include increased risk for cardiovascular disease [105].

4.4. Methodological Limitations

The main limitations of the present study are those of the epidemiological study in the non-interventional cohort, which identified significant associations but with multiple tests, many confounding factors, several risks of collinearity, and few direct proofs of causality.

Furthermore, the impact of T2DM on the three proteins according to SARS-CoV-2 infection was indirectly estimated in a large population at risk of NAFLD, but without direct virological markers. We retrieved the same kinetics of decreased ApoA1 during the successive waves of SARS-CoV-2 infection in comparison with those in 2019, but new confounders appeared such as decreased physical exercise and increased tobacco and/or alcohol consumption [93,94]. However, concerning ApoA1, an increase in alcohol consumption would have been associated with an increase in ApoA1 [50,51] in the "NAFLD-Serum" cohort, which included 78% of subjects without advanced fibrosis [9]. The body weight means were also similar (88.5 kg) in 2019 and 2020 [9].

In epidemiological studies of patients with T2DM, several variable and bias factors remained possible candidates, such as the definition of T2DM (clinical definition by diabetologists or fasting glucose) and the number of treatments of protein levels [69]. In the meantime, these variable factors should be discussed in the context of the use of such blood test components. Here, the results of the "Control Population" were derived from a relatively homogeneous Caucasian population, and the findings may not be applicable to other ethnic groups. The "NAFLD-Biopsy" cohort was limited by the selection of patients who accepted a liver biopsy in tertiary centers and their enrollment according to abnormal ALT or the presence of steatosis at ultrasonography. The "NAFLD-Serum" cohort was limited by the absence of ethnic origin information and the few available clinical characteristics, including age, sex, BMI, ApoA1, A2M, haptoglobin, liver function tests, fasting glucose, total cholesterol, and triglycerides.

Finally, forty years ago, clinicians were not using A2M, ApoA1 was interesting for predicting cardiovascular diseases, and haptoglobin was mostly used for the diagnosis of hemolysis. Nowadays, these proteins are widely prescribed in multivariate noninvasive tests for the diagnosis of liver diseases. However, these three proteins—without collinearity between them but with ubiquitous functions now better understood—should permit the construction of better multivariate tests in metabolic diseases for cumulating the risk of liver diseases and the risk of severe infections such as T2DM, NAFLD, and COVID-19.

Supplementary Materials: The following supporting information can be downloaded at: please add https://www.mdpi.com/article/10.3390/biomedicines10030699/s1. Figure S1: A2M in NAFLD-Biopsied patients with NASH; Figure S2: ApoA1 NAFLD-Biopsied patients with significant NASH; Figure S3: ApoA1 NAFLD-Biopsied patients with significant steatosis; Figure S4: ApoA1 in NAFLD-Biopsied patients with obesity; Figure S5: A2M in NAFLD-Biopsied patients without obesity; Figure S6: A2M in NAFLD-Biopsied patients with obesity; Figure S7: ApoA1 in NAFLD-Biopsied patients without obesity; Figure S8: Hapto NAFLD-Biopsied patients without obesity; Figure S9: Hapto in NAFLD-Biopsied patients with obesity; Figure S10: Univariate correlations between three proteins and histological features in not-obese et obese male; Figure S11: Univariate correlations between three proteins and histological features in not-obese et obese female; Figure S12: Variation of the serum protein levels according to BMI for patients <50 years old; Figure S13: Variation of the serum protein levels according to BMI for patients >=50 years old; Table S1: T2D multivariate association with proteins and fibrosis; Table S2. T2D multivariate association with proteins and NASH; Table S3. T2D multivariate association with proteins and steatosis.

Author Contributions: Conceptualization, O.D., T.P., D.V., P.C., and J.-F.G.; methodology O.D., and T.P.; software, O.D., and T.P.; validation, O.D., T.P., D.V., P.C., and J.-F.G.; formal analysis, O.D., T.P., D.V., P.B., and V.P. (Valérie Paradis); investigation, O.D., T.P., D.V., P.C., V.P., V.R. and J.-F.G.; resources, O.D., T.P., D.V., P.C., A.B., D.T. and J.-F.G.; data curation, O.D., T.P., D.V., P.C., and V.P (Valentina Peta).; writing—original draft preparation, O.D., T.P., D.V., R.P. and P.C.; writing—review and editing, O.D., T.P., D.V., P.C., R.P and V.P. (Valentina Peta); visualization, O.D., T.P., D.V., and P.C.; supervision, O.D., T.P., D.V., and P.C.; project administration, O.D., T.P., D.V., P.C., A.B., D.T. and J.-F.G.; funding acquisition, O.D., T.P., D.V., P.C., A.B., D.T. and J.-F.G. All authors have read and agreed to the published version of the manuscript.

Funding: The RHU QUID-NASH Project, funded by Agence Nationale de la Recherche programe Investissements d'Avenir, (Reference ANR-17-T171105J-RHUS-0009 to DV), Agence Nationale de la Recherche, is carried out by Institut National de la Recherche Medicale, Paris Descartes University, Paris Diderot University, Centre National de la Recherche Scientifique, Centre de l'Energie Atomique, Servier, Biopredictive, and Assistance Publique-Hôpitaux de Paris under the coordination of Prof. Dominique Valla and project leader Angélique Brzustowski. The FLIP project was supported by the European Community's Seventh Framework Program (FP7/2007-2013) under grant agreement number HEALTH-F2-2009-241762. FibroFrance is supported by the National Clinical Research (CPP-IDF-VI, 10-1996-DR-964, DR-2012-222) and declared in the Clinical Registry (number: NCT01927133).

Institutional Review Board Statement: The QUIDNASH study, NCT03634098, was approved by the Research Ethics Committee (#18.021-2018-A00311-54). All these clinical non-interventional studies were approved by the ethics committee at each participating institution and were performed according to good clinical practice and the Declaration of Helsinki.

Informed Consent Statement: In the "NAFLD-Biopsy" Cohort all patients provided written informed consent. The "NAFLD-Serum" cohort was anonymous.

Data Availability Statement: Almost all data and all results were available in the manuscript and in supplementary files. Contact olivier@biopredictive.com for more information.

Acknowledgments: We thank H. Nikki March, from Edanz (https://www.edanz.com/ac, accessed on 1 March 2022) for editing a draft of this manuscript.

Conflicts of Interest: TP is the inventor of FibroTest (FibroSure in USA) and NASH-FibroTest, and the co-founder of BioPredictive. The patents belong to French public organizations Assistance Publique Hôpitaux de Paris and Sorbonne University. OD is cofounder BioPredictive. OD and VP are full employee of BioPredictive. The other coauthors declare no conflict of interest.

References

1. Fremont, V. Diabetes. In *Thesis French Academy of Medicine*; Masson, G., Ed.; Paris, France, 1891; p. 51.
2. Bornstein, S.R.; Rubino, F.; Khunti, K.; Mingrone, G.; Hopkins, D.; Birkenfeld, A.L.; Boehm, B.; Amiel, S.; Holt, R.; Skyler, J.S.; et al. Practical recommendations for the management of diabetes in patients with COVID-19. *Lancet Diabetes Endocrinol.* **2020**, *8*, 546–550. [CrossRef]
3. Ramon, J.; Llauradó, G.; Güerri, R.; Climent, E.; Ballesta, S.; Benaiges, D.; López-Montesinos, I.; Navarro, H.; Fernández, N.; Carrera, M.J.; et al. Acute-to-chronic glycemic ratio as a predictor of COVID-19 severity and mortality. *Diabetes Care* **2021**, *45*, 255–258. [CrossRef] [PubMed]
4. Stefan, N.; Birkenfeld, A.L.; Schulze, M.B. Global pandemics interconnected—obesity, impaired metabolic health and COVID-19. *Nat. Rev. Endocrinol.* **2021**, *17*, 135–149. [CrossRef]
5. Wu, S.; Zhou, K.; Misra-Hebert, A.; Bena, J.; Kashyap, S.R. Impact of metabolic syndrome on severity of COVID-19 illness. In *Metabolic Syndrome and Related Disorders*; Mary Ann Liebert, Inc.: New York, NY, USA, 2022. [CrossRef]
6. Martinez, M.A.; Franco, S. Impact of COVID-19 in liver disease progression. *Hepatol. Commun.* **2021**, *5*, 1138–1150. [CrossRef] [PubMed]
7. Ando, W.; Horii, T.; Uematsu, T.; Hanaki, H.; Atsuda, K.; Otori, K. Impact of overlapping risks of type 2 diabetes and obesity on coronavirus disease severity in the United States. *Sci. Rep.* **2021**, *11*, 17968. [CrossRef] [PubMed]
8. Mallet, V.; Parlati, L.; Martinino, A.; Pereira, J.P.S.; Jimenez, C.N.; Sakka, M.; Bouam, S.; Retbi, A.; Krasteva, D.; Meritet, J.-F.; et al. Burden of liver disease progression in hospitalized patients with type 2 diabetes mellitus. *J. Hepatol.* **2021**, *76*, 265–274. [CrossRef]
9. Poynard, T.; Deckmyn, O.; Rudler, M.; Peta, V.; Ngo, Y.; Vautier, M.; Akhavan, S.; Calvez, V.; Franc, C.; Castille, J.M.; et al. Performance of serum apolipoprotein-A1 as a sentinel of Covid-19. *PLoS ONE* **2020**, *15*, e0242306. [CrossRef]
10. Maisonnasse, P.; Poynard, T.; Sakka, M.; Akhavan, S.; Marlin, R.; Peta, V.; Deckmyn, O.; Ghedira, N.; Ngo, Y.; Rudler, M.; et al. Validation of the performance of A1HPV6, a triage blood test for the early diagnosis and prognosis of SARS-CoV-2 infection. *Gastro Hep Adv.* **2022**, in press.
11. Medjeral-Thomas, N.R.; Troldborg, A.; Hansen, A.G.; Pihl, R.; Clarke, C.L.; Peters, J.E.; Thomas, D.C.; Willicombe, M.; Palarasah, Y.; Botto, M.; et al. Protease inhibitor plasma concentrations associate with COVID-19 infection. *Oxf. Open Immunol.* **2021**, *2*, 014. [CrossRef]
12. Seitz, R.; Gürtler, L.; Schramm, W. Thromboinflammation in COVID-19: Can α 2 -macroglobulin help to control the fire? *J. Thromb. Haemost.* **2021**, *19*, 351–354. [CrossRef]
13. Scalsky, R.J.; Chen, Y.-J.; Desai, K.; O'Connell, J.R.; Perry, J.A.; Hong, C.C. Baseline cardiometabolic profiles and SARS-CoV-2 infection in the UK Biobank. *PLoS ONE* **2021**, *16*, e0248602. [CrossRef] [PubMed]
14. Hilser, J.R.; Han, Y.; Biswas, S.; Gukasyan, J.; Cai, Z.; Zhu, R.; Tang, W.W.; Deb, A.; Lusis, A.J.; Hartiala, J.A.; et al. Association of serum HDL-cholesterol and apolipoprotein A1 levels with risk of severe SARS-CoV-2 infection. *J. Lipid Res.* **2021**, *62*, 100061. [CrossRef] [PubMed]
15. Van Bilsen, J.H.M.; Brink, W.V.D.; Hoek, A.M.V.D.; Dulos, R.; Caspers, M.P.M.; Kleemann, R.; Wopereis, S.; Verschuren, L. Mechanism-based biomarker prediction for low-grade inflammation in liver and adipose tissue. *Front. Physiol.* **2021**, *12*, 703370. [CrossRef] [PubMed]
16. Kumar, N.P.; Venkataraman, A.; Hanna, L.E.; Putlibai, S.; Karthick, M.; Rajamanikam, A.; Sadasivam, K.; Sundaram, B.; Babu, S. Systemic inflammation and microbial translocation are characteristic features of SARS-CoV-2-related multisystem inflammatory syndrome in children. *Open Forum Infect. Dis.* **2021**, *8*, ofab279. [CrossRef] [PubMed]
17. Yağcı, S.; Serin, E.; Acicbe, Ö.; Zeren, M.I.; Odabaşı, M.S. The relationship between serum erythropoietin, hepcidin, and haptoglobin levels with disease severity and other biochemical values in patients with COVID-19. *Int. J. Lab. Hematol.* **2021**, *43*, 142–151. [CrossRef] [PubMed]
18. Naryzny, S.N.; Legina, O.K. Haptoglobin as a biomarker. *Biochem. Moscow Suppl. Ser. B* **2021**, *15*, 184–198. [CrossRef]
19. Rehman, A.A.; Ahsan, H.; Khan, F.H. Alpha-2-macroglobulin: A physiological guardian. *J. Cell. Physiol.* **2013**, *228*, 1665–1675. [CrossRef]
20. Swarnakar, S.; Asokan, R.; Quigley, J.P.; Armstrong, P.B. Binding of alpha2-macroglobulin and limulin: Regulation of the plasma haemolytic system of the American horseshoe crab, Limulus. *Biochem. J.* **2000**, *347*, 679–685. [CrossRef]
21. Puppione, D.L.; Tran, D.P.; Zenaidee, M.A.; Charugundla, S.; Whitelegge, J.P.; Buffenstein, R. Naked mole-rat, a rodent with an apolipoprotein A-I dimer. *Lipids* **2021**, *56*, 269–278. [CrossRef]
22. Nevo, E.; Ben-Shlomo, R.; Maeda, N. Haptoglobin DNA polymorphism in subterranean mole rats of the Spalax ehrenbergi superspecies in Israel. *Heredity* **1989**, *62*, 85–90. [CrossRef]
23. Vandooren, J.; Itoh, Y. Alpha-2-macroglobulin in inflammation, immunity and infections. *Front. Immunol.* **2021**, *12*, 803244. [CrossRef] [PubMed]
24. Ritchie, R.F.; Palomaki, G.E.; Neveux, L.M.; Navolotskaia, O. Reference distributions for 2-macroglobulin: A comparison of a large cohort to the world's literature. *J. Clin. Lab. Anal.* **2004**, *18*, 148–152. [CrossRef] [PubMed]
25. Medrano, N.M.; Luz, M.R.M.P.; Cabello, P.H.; Tapia, G.T.; Van Leuven, F.; Araujo-Jorge, T.C. Acute chagas' disease: Plasma levels of alpha-2-macroglobulin and C-reactive protein in children under 13 years in a high endemic area of Bolivia. *J. Trop. Pediatr.* **1996**, *42*, 68–74. [CrossRef] [PubMed]

26. Tam, V.; Chen, P.; Yee, A.; Solis, N.; Klein, T.; Kudelko, M.; Sharma, R.; Chan, W.C.; Overall, C.M.; Haglund, L.; et al. DIPPER, a spatiotemporal proteomics atlas of human intervertebral discs for exploring ageing and degeneration dynamics. *eLife* **2020**, *9*, e64940. [CrossRef]
27. Ganrot, P.O.; Gydell, K.; Ekelund, H. Serum concentration of α2-macroglobulin, haptoglobin and α1-antitrypsin in diabetes mellitus. *Eur. J. Endocrinol.* **1967**, *55*, 537–544. [CrossRef]
28. James, K.; Merriman, J.; Gray, R.S.; Duncan, L.J.; Herd, R. Serum alpha 2-macroglobulin levels in diabetes. *J. Clin. Pathol.* **1980**, *33*, 163–166. [CrossRef]
29. Hartmann, L.; Viallet, A.; Fauvert, R. The effect of macroglobulins on flocculation tests. *Clin. Chim. Acta* **1963**, *8*, 872–883. [CrossRef]
30. Naveau, S.; Poynard, T.; Benattar, C.; Bedossa, P.; Chaput, J.-C. Alpha-2-macroglobulin and hepatic fibrosis: Diagnostic interest. *Am. J. Dig. Dis.* **1994**, *39*, 2426–2432. [CrossRef]
31. Poynard, T.; Munteanu, M.; Deckmyn, O.; Ngo, Y.; Drane, F.; Messous, D.; Castille, J.M.; Housset, C.; Ratziu, V.; Imbert-Bismut, F. Applicability and precautions of use of liver injury biomarker FibroTest. A reappraisal at 7 years of age. *BMC Gastroenterol.* **2011**, *11*, 39. [CrossRef]
32. Jacqueminet, S.; Lebray, P.; Morra, R.; Munteanu, M.; Devers, L.; Messous, D.; Bernard, M.; Hartemann-Heurtier, A.; Imbert-Bismut, F.; Ratziu, V. Screening for liver fibrosis by using a noninvasive biomarker in patients with diabetes. *Clin. Gastroenterol. Hepatol.* **2008**, *6*, 828–831. [CrossRef]
33. De Lédinghen, V.; Vergniol, J.; Gonzalez, C.; Foucher, J.; Maury, E.; Chemineau, L.; Villars, S.; Gin, H.; Rigalleau, V. Screening for liver fibrosis by using FibroScan® and fibrotest in patients with diabetes. *Dig. Liver Dis.* **2012**, *44*, 413–418. [CrossRef] [PubMed]
34. Perazzo, H.; Munteanu, M.; Ngo, Y.; Lebray, P.; Seurat, N.; Rutka, F.; Couteau, M.; Jacqueminet, S.; Giral, P.; Monneret, D.; et al. Prognostic value of liver fibrosis and steatosis biomarkers in type-2 diabetes and dyslipidaemia. *Aliment. Pharmacol. Ther.* **2014**, *40*, 1081–1093. [CrossRef] [PubMed]
35. Poynard, T.; Peta, V.; Deckmyn, O.; Pais, R.; Ngo, Y.; Charlotte, F.; Ngo, A.; Munteanu, M.; Imbert-Bismut, F.; Monneret, D.; et al. Performance of liver biomarkers, in patients at risk of nonalcoholic steato-hepatitis, according to presence of type-2 diabetes. *Eur. J. Gastroenterol. Hepatol.* **2019**, *32*, 998–1007. [CrossRef] [PubMed]
36. Bril, F.; McPhaul, M.J.; Caulfield, M.P.; Clark, V.C.; Soldevilla-Pico, C.; Firpi-Morell, R.J.; Lai, J.; Shiffman, D.; Rowland, C.M.; Cusi, K. Performance of plasma biomarkers and diagnostic panels for nonalcoholic steatohepatitis and advanced fibrosis in patients with type 2 diabetes. *Diabetes Care* **2019**, *43*, 290–297. [CrossRef]
37. Poynard, T.; Paradis, V.; Mullaert, J.; Deckmyn, O.; Gault, N.; Marcault, E.; Manchon, P.; Mohammed, N.S.; Parfait, B.; Ibberson, M.; et al. Prospective external validation of a new non-invasive test for the diagnosis of non-alcoholic steatohepatitis in patients with type 2 diabetes. *Aliment. Pharmacol. Ther.* **2021**, *54*, 952–966. [CrossRef]
38. Younossi, Z.M.; Anstee, Q.M.; Wong, V.W.-S.; Trauner, M.; Lawitz, E.J.; Harrison, S.A.; Camargo, M.; Kersey, K.; Subramanian, G.M.; Myers, R.P.; et al. The association of histologic and noninvasive tests with adverse clinical and patient-reported outcomes in patients with advanced fibrosis due to nonalcoholic steatohepatitis. *Gastroenterology* **2021**, *160*, 1608–1619.e13. [CrossRef] [PubMed]
39. Netanel, C.; Goitein, D.; Rubin, M.; Kleinbaum, Y.; Katsherginsky, S.; Hermon, H.; Tsaraf, K.; Tachlytski, I.; Herman, A.; Safran, M.; et al. The impact of bariatric surgery on nonalcoholic fatty liver disease as measured using non-invasive tests. *Am. J. Surg.* **2021**, *222*, 214–219. [CrossRef]
40. Jullian-Desayes, I.; Trzepizur, W.; Boursier, J.; Joyeux-Faure, M.; Bailly, S.; Benmerad, M.; Le Vaillant, M.; Jaffre, S.; Pigeanne, T.; Bizieux-Thaminy, A.; et al. Obstructive sleep apnea, chronic obstructive pulmonary disease and NAFLD: An individual participant data meta-analysis. *Sleep Med.* **2021**, *77*, 357–364. [CrossRef]
41. Nazir, S.; Jankowski, V.; Bender, G.; Zewinger, S.; Rye, K.-A.; van der Vorst, E.P. Interaction between high-density lipoproteins and inflammation: Function matters more than concentration! *Adv. Drug Deliv. Rev.* **2020**, *159*, 94–119. [CrossRef]
42. Ulloque-Badaracco, J.R.; Hernandez-Bustamante, E.A.; Herrera-Añazco, P.; Benites-Zapata, V.A. Prognostic value of apolipoproteins in COVID-19 patients: A systematic review and meta-analysis. *Travel Med. Infect. Dis.* **2021**, *44*, 102200. [CrossRef]
43. Begue, F.; Tanaka, S.; Mouktadi, Z.; Rondeau, P.; Veeren, B.; Diotel, N.; Tran-Dinh, A.; Robert, T.; Vélia, E.; Mavingui, P.; et al. Altered high-density lipoprotein composition and functions during severe COVID-19. *Sci. Rep.* **2021**, *11*, 2291. [CrossRef] [PubMed]
44. Geyer, P.E.; Arend, F.M.; Doll, S.; Louiset, M.; Winter, S.V.; Müller-Reif, J.B.; Torun, F.M.; Weigand, M.; Eichhorn, P.; Bruegel, M.; et al. High-resolution serum proteome trajectories in COVID-19 reveal patient-specific seroconversion. *EMBO Mol. Med.* **2021**, *13*, e14167. [CrossRef] [PubMed]
45. Pushkarev, V.V.; Sokolova, L.K.; Chervyakova, S.A.; Belchina, Y.B.; Kovzun, O.I.; Pushkarev, V.M.; Tronko, M.D. Plasma apolipoproteins A1/B and OxLDL levels in patients with COVID-19 as possible markers of the disease. *Cytol. Genet.* **2021**, *55*, 519–523. [CrossRef] [PubMed]
46. Billingham, M.S.; Leatherdale, B.A.; Hall, R.A.; Bailey, C.J. High density lipoprotein cholesterol and apolipoprotein a-1 concentrations in non-insulin dependent diabetics treated by diet and chlorpropamide. *Diabete Metab.* **1982**, *8*, 229–233.
47. Lapolla, A.; Brioschi, M.; Banfi, C.; Tremoli, E.; Bonfante, L.; Cristoni, S.; Seraglia, R.; Traldi, P. On the search for glycated lipoprotein ApoA-I in the plasma of diabetic and nephropathic patients. *Biol. Mass Spectrom.* **2007**, *43*, 74–81. [CrossRef]

48. Song, F.; Zhou, Y.; Zhang, K.; Liang, Y.-F.; He, X.; Li, L. The role of the plasma glycosylated hemoglobin A1c/Apolipoprotein A-l ratio in predicting cardiovascular outcomes in acute coronary syndrome. *Nutr. Metab. Cardiovasc. Dis.* **2021**, *31*, 570–578. [CrossRef]
49. Trieb, M.; Rainer, F.; Stadlbauer, V.; Douschan, P.; Horvath, A.; Binder, L.; Trakaki, A.; Knuplez, E.; Scharnagl, H.; Stojakovic, T.; et al. HDL-related biomarkers are robust predictors of survival in patients with chronic liver failure. *J. Hepatol.* **2020**, *73*, 113–120. [CrossRef]
50. Poynard, T.; Abella, A.; Pignon, J.-P.; Naveau, S.; Leluc, R.; Chaput, J.-C. Apolipoprotein AI and alcoholic liver disease. *Hepatology* **1986**, *6*, 1391–1395. [CrossRef]
51. Poynard, T.; Bedossa, P.; Mathurin, P.; Ratziu, V.; Paradis, V. Apolipoprotein A1 and hepatic fibrosis. *J. Hepatol.* **1995**, *22*, 107–110.
52. Munteanu, M.; Pais, R.; Peta, V.; Deckmyn, O.; Moussalli, J.; Ngo, Y.; Rudler, M.; Lebray, P.; Charlotte, F.; Thibault, V.; et al. Long-term prognostic value of the FibroTest in patients with non-alcoholic fatty liver disease, compared to chronic hepatitis C, B, and alcoholic liver disease. *Aliment. Pharmacol. Ther.* **2018**, *48*, 1117–1127. [CrossRef]
53. Han, Y.-H.; Onufer, E.J.; Huang, L.-H.; Sprung, R.W.; Davidson, W.S.; Czepielewski, R.S.; Wohltmann, M.; Sorci-Thomas, M.G.; Warner, B.W.; Randolph, G.J. Enterically derived high-density lipoprotein restrains liver injury through the portal vein. *Science* **2021**, *373*, 6729. [CrossRef] [PubMed]
54. Tamara, S.; Franc, V.; Heck, A.J.R. A wealth of genotype-specific proteoforms fine-tunes hemoglobin scavenging by haptoglobin. *Proc. Natl. Acad. Sci. USA* **2020**, *117*, 15554–15564. [CrossRef] [PubMed]
55. Delanghe, J.R.; De Buyzere, M.L.; Speeckaert, M.M. Genetic Polymorphisms in the host and COVID-19 infection. In *Coronavirus Disease-COVID-19*; Rezaei, N., Ed.; Advances in Experimental Medicine and Biology; Springer International Publishing: Cham, Switzerland, 2021; Volume 1318, pp. 109–118. ISBN 978-3-030-63760-6.
56. Vázquez-Moreno, M.; Locia-Morales, D.; Perez-Herrera, A.; Gomez-Diaz, R.A.; Gonzalez-Dzib, R.; Valdez-González, A.L.; Flores-Alfaro, E.; Corona-Salazar, P.; Suarez-Sanchez, F.; Gomez-Zamudio, J.; et al. Causal association of haptoglobin with obesity in Mexican children: A mendelian randomization study. *J. Clin. Endocrinol. Metab.* **2020**, *105*, e2501–e2510. [CrossRef] [PubMed]
57. Vázquez-Moreno, M.; Locia-Morales, D.; Valladares-Salgado, A.; Sharma, T.; Perez-Herrera, A.; Gonzalez-Dzib, R.; Rodríguez-Ruíz, F.; Wacher-Rodarte, N.; Cruz, M.; Meyre, D. The MC4R p.Ile269Asn mutation confers a high risk for type 2 diabetes in the Mexican population via obesity dependent and independent effects. *Sci. Rep.* **2021**, *11*, 3097. [CrossRef] [PubMed]
58. Wang, S.; Zhang, R.; Wang, T.; Jiang, F.; Hu, C.; Jia, W. Association of the genetic variant rs2000999 with haptoglobin and diabetic macrovascular diseases in Chinese patients with type 2 diabetes. *J. Diabetes Its Complicat.* **2018**, *33*, 178–181. [CrossRef]
59. Klooster, J.P.T.; Sotiriou, A.; Boeren, S.; Vaessen, S.; Vervoort, J.; Pieters, R. Type 2 diabetes-related proteins derived from an in vitro model of inflamed fat tissue. *Arch. Biochem. Biophys.* **2018**, *644*, 81–92. [CrossRef]
60. Fain, J.N.; Bahouth, S.W.; Madan, A.K. Haptoglobin release by human adipose tissue in primary culture. *J. Lipid Res.* **2004**, *45*, 536–542. [CrossRef]
61. Anisonyan, A.V.; Sandler, Y.G.; Khaimenova, T.Y.; Keyan, V.A.; Saliev, K.G.; Sbikina, E.S.; Vinnitskaya, E.V. Non-alcoholic fatty liver disease and type 2 diabetes mellitus: Issues of the liver fibrosis diagnostics. *Ter. Arkhiv* **2020**, *92*, 73–78. [CrossRef]
62. Whicher, J.T.; Ritchie, R.F.; Johnson, A.M.; Baudner, S.; Bienvenu, J.; Blirup-Jensen, S.; Carlstrom, A.; Dati, F.; Ward, A.M.; Svendsen, P.J. New international reference preparation for proteins in human serum (RPPHS). *Clin. Chem.* **1994**, *40*, 934–938. [CrossRef]
63. Ritchie, R.F.; Palomaki, G.E.; Neveux, L.M.; Ledue, T.B.; Craig, W.Y.; Marcovina, S.; Navolotskaia, O. Reference distributions for apolipoproteins AI and B and the apolipoprotein B/AI ratios: A practical and clinically relevant approach in a large cohort. *J. Clin. Lab. Anal.* **2006**, *20*, 209–217. [CrossRef]
64. Ritchie, R.F.; Palomaki, G.E.; Neveux, L.M.; Navolotskaia, O.; Ledue, T.B.; Craig, W.Y. Reference distributions for the positive acute phase serum proteins, alpha1-acid glycoprotein (orosomucoid), alpha1-antitrypsin, and haptoglobin: A practical, simple, and clinically relevant approach in a large cohort. *J. Clin. Lab. Anal.* **2000**, *14*, 284–292. [CrossRef]
65. Kleiner, D.E.; Brunt, E.M.; Van Natta, M.; Behling, C.; Contos, M.J.; Cummings, O.W.; Ferrell, L.D.; Liu, Y.-C.; Torbenson, M.S.; Unalp-Arida, A.; et al. Design and validation of a histological scoring system for nonalcoholic fatty liver disease. *Hepatology* **2005**, *41*, 1313–1321. [CrossRef] [PubMed]
66. Bedossa, P.; Poitou, C.; Veyrie, N.; Bouillot, J.-L.; Basdevant, A.; Paradis, V.; Tordjman, J.; Clement, K. Histopathological algorithm and scoring system for evaluation of liver lesions in morbidly obese patients. *Hepatology* **2012**, *56*, 1751–1759. [CrossRef] [PubMed]
67. Bedossa, P.; The FLIP Pathology. Consortium Utility and appropriateness of the fatty liver inhibition of progression (FLIP) algorithm and steatosis, activity, and fibrosis (SAF) score in the evaluation of biopsies of nonalcoholic fatty liver disease. *Hepatology* **2014**, *60*, 565–575. [CrossRef]
68. Francque, S.M.; Bedossa, P.; Ratziu, V.; Anstee, Q.M.; Bugianesi, E.; Sanyal, A.J.; Loomba, R.; Harrison, S.A.; Balabanska, R.; Mateva, L.; et al. A randomized, controlled trial of the Pan-PPAR agonist lanifibranor in NASH. *N. Engl. J. Med.* **2021**, *385*, 1547–1558. [CrossRef]
69. Danaei, G.; Fahimi, S.; Lu, Y.; Zhou, B.; Hajifathalian, K.; Di Cesare, M.; Lo, W.; Reis-Santos, B.; Cowan, M.; Shaw, J.; et al. Effects of diabetes definition on global surveillance of diabetes prevalence and diagnosis: A pooled analysis of 96 population-based studies with 331 288 participants. *Lancet Diabetes Endocrinol.* **2015**, *3*, 624–637. [CrossRef]
70. Holm, S. A Simple sequentially rejective multiple test procedure. *Scand. J. Stat.* **1979**, *6*, 65–70.

71. Poynard, T.; Deckmyn, O.; Munteanu, M.; Ngo, Y.; Drane, F.; Castille, J.M.; Housset, C.; Ratziu, V. Awareness of the severity of liver disease re-examined using software-combined biomarkers of liver fibrosis and necroinflammatory activity. *BMJ Open* **2015**, *5*, e010017. [CrossRef]
72. Dong, E.; Du, H.; Gardner, L. An interactive web-based dashboard to track COVID-19 in real time. *Lancet Infect. Dis.* **2020**, *20*, 533–534. [CrossRef]
73. Younossi, Z.M.; Stepanova, M.; Lam, B.; Cable, R.; Felix, S.; Jeffers, T.; Younossi, E.; Pham, H.; Srishord, M.; Austin, P.; et al. Independent predictors of mortality among patients with NAFLD hospitalized with COVID-19 infection. *Hepatol. Commun.* **2021**. [CrossRef]
74. Vilar-Gomez, E.; Chalasani, N. Non-invasive assessment of non-alcoholic fatty liver disease: Clinical prediction rules and blood-based biomarkers. *J. Hepatol.* **2018**, *68*, 305–315. [CrossRef] [PubMed]
75. Loomba, R.; Jain, A.; Diehl, A.M.; Guy, C.D.; Portenier, D.; Sudan, R.; Singh, S.; Faulkner, C.; Richards, L.; Hester, K.D.; et al. Validation of serum test for advanced liver fibrosis in patients with nonalcoholic steatohepatitis. *Clin. Gastroenterol. Hepatol.* **2019**, *17*, 1867–1876.e3. [CrossRef] [PubMed]
76. Harrison, S.A.; Ratziu, V.; Boursier, J.; Francque, S.; Bedossa, P.; Majd, Z.; Cordonnier, G.; Ben Sudrik, F.; Darteil, R.; Liebe, R.; et al. A blood-based biomarker panel (NIS4) for non-invasive diagnosis of non-alcoholic steatohepatitis and liver fibrosis: A prospective derivation and global validation study. *Lancet Gastroenterol. Hepatol.* **2020**, *5*, 970–985. [CrossRef]
77. Chunming, L.; Jianhui, S.; Hongguang, Z.; Chunwu, Q.; Xiaoyun, H.; Lijun, Y.; Xuejun, Y. The development of a clinical score for the prediction of nonalcoholic steatohepatitis in patients with nonalcoholic fatty liver disease using routine parameters. *Turk. J. Gastroenterol.* **2015**, *26*, 408–416. [CrossRef] [PubMed]
78. Shukla, A.; Kapileswar, S.; Gogtay, N.; Joshi, A.; Dhore, P.; Shah, C.; Abraham, P.; Bhatia, S. Simple biochemical parameters and a novel score correlate with absence of fibrosis in patients with nonalcoholic fatty liver disease. *Indian J. Gastroenterol.* **2015**, *34*, 281–285. [CrossRef] [PubMed]
79. Kamada, Y.; Ono, M.; Hyogo, H.; Fujii, H.; Sumida, Y.; Mori, K.; Tanaka, S.; Yamada, M.; Akita, M.; Mizutani, K.; et al. A novel noninvasive diagnostic method for nonalcoholic steatohepatitis using two glycobiomarkers. *Hepatology* **2015**, *62*, 1433–1443. [CrossRef] [PubMed]
80. Turecký, L.; Kupcová, V.; Szántová, M. Alpha 2-macroglobulin in the blood of patients with diabetes mellitus. *Bratisl. Lek. List.* **1999**, *100*, 25–27.
81. Schelp, F.P.; Kraiklang, R.; Muktabhant, B.; Chupanit, P.; Sanchaisuriya, P. Public health research needs for molecular epidemiology and to emphasize homeostasis-could the omnipotent endopeptidase inhibitor α-2-macroglobulin be a meaningful biomarker? *F1000Research* **2019**, *8*, 1025. [CrossRef]
82. Tungtrongchitr, R.; Pongpaew, P.; Vudhivai, N.; Changbumrung, S.; Tungtrongchitr, A.; Phonrat, B.; Viroonudomphol, D.; Pooudong, S.; Schelp, F.P. Relationship between alpha-2-macroglobulin, anthropometric parameters and lipid profiles in Thai overweight and obese in Bangkok. *Nutr. Res.* **2003**, *23*, 1143–1152. [CrossRef]
83. Chang, C.-Y.; Tung, Y.-T.; Lin, Y.-K.; Liao, C.-C.; Chiu, C.-F.; Tung, T.-H.; Shabrina, A.; Huang, S.-Y. Effects of caloric restriction with protein supplementation on plasma protein profiles in middle-aged women with metabolic syndrome—A preliminary open study. *J. Clin. Med.* **2019**, *8*, 195. [CrossRef]
84. Suriyaprom, K.; Harnroongroj, T.; Namjuntra, P.; Chantaranipapong, Y.; Tungtrongchitr, R. Effects of tobacco smoking on alpha-2-macroglobulin and some biochemical parameters in Thai males. *Southeast Asian J. Trop. Med. Public Health* **2007**, *38*, 918–926. [PubMed]
85. Von Reibnitz, D.; Yorke, E.D.; Oh, J.H.; Apte, A.P.; Yang, J.; Pham, H.; Thor, M.; Wu, A.J.; Fleisher, M.; Gelb, E.; et al. Predictive modeling of thoracic radiotherapy toxicity and the potential role of serum alpha-2-macroglobulin. *Front. Oncol.* **2020**, *10*, 1395. [CrossRef] [PubMed]
86. Yoshino, S.; Fujimoto, K.; Takada, T.; Kawamura, S.; Ogawa, J.; Kamata, Y.; Kodera, Y.; Shichiri, M. Molecular form and concentration of serum α2-macroglobulin in diabetes. *Sci. Rep.* **2019**, *9*, 12927. [CrossRef] [PubMed]
87. Stevenson, F.T.; Greene, S.; Kaysen, G.A. Serum α2-macroglobulin and α1-inhibitor 3 concentrations are increased in hypoalbuminemia by post-transcriptional mechanisms. *Kidney Int.* **1998**, *53*, 67–75. [CrossRef] [PubMed]
88. Velden, M.G.D.S.-V.D.; de Meer, K.; Kulik, W.; Melissant, C.F.; Rabelink, T.J.; Berger, R.; Kaysen, G.A. Nephrotic proteinuria has no net effect on total body protein synthesis: Measurements with 13C valine. *Am. J. Kidney Dis.* **2000**, *35*, 1149–1154. [CrossRef]
89. Seo, D.H.; Suh, Y.J.; Cho, Y.; Ahn, S.H.; Seo, S.; Hong, S.; Lee, Y.-H.; Choi, Y.J.; Lee, E.; Kim, S.H. Advanced liver fibrosis is associated with chronic kidney disease in patients with type 2 diabetes mellitus and nonalcoholic fatty liver disease. *Diabetes Metab. J.* **2022**. [CrossRef]
90. Insenser, M.; Vilarrasa, N.; Vendrell, J.; Escobar-Morreale, H.F. Remission of diabetes following bariatric surgery: Plasma proteomic profiles. *J. Clin. Med.* **2021**, *10*, 3879. [CrossRef]
91. Manolis, A.S.; Manolis, A.A.; Manolis, T.A.; Apostolaki, N.E.; Melita, H. COVID-19 infection and body weight: A deleterious liaison in a J-curve relationship. *Obes. Res. Clin. Pr.* **2021**, *15*, 523–535. [CrossRef]
92. Kim, D.S.; Burt, A.A.; Ranchalis, J.E.; Jarvik, L.E.; Eintracht, J.F.; Furlong, C.E.; Jarvik, G.P. Effects of dietary components on high-density lipoprotein measures in a cohort of 1,566 participants. *Nutr. Metab.* **2014**, *11*, 44. [CrossRef]
93. Dai, X.-J.; Tan, L.; Ren, L.; Shao, Y.; Tao, W.; Wang, Y. COVID-19 risk appears to vary across different alcoholic beverages. *Front. Nutr.* **2022**, *8*, 772700. [CrossRef]

94. Lee, B.P.; Dodge, M.J.L.; Leventhal, A.; Terrault, N.A. Retail alcohol and tobacco sales during COVID-19. *Ann. Intern. Med.* **2021**, *174*, 1027–1029. [CrossRef] [PubMed]
95. Dong, H.; Ni, W.; Bai, Y.; Yuan, X.; Zhang, Y.; Zhang, H.; Sun, Y.; Xu, J. Cross-sectional and longitudinal associations of apolipoprotein A1 and B with glycosylated hemoglobin in Chinese adults. *Sci. Rep.* **2022**, *12*, 2751. [CrossRef] [PubMed]
96. Luo, Y.; Decato, B.E.; Charles, E.D.; Shevell, D.E.; McNaney, C.; Shipkova, P.; Apfel, A.; Tirucherai, G.S.; Sanyal, A.J. Pegbelfermin selectively reduces secondary bile acid concentrations in patients with non-alcoholic steatohepatitis. *JHEP Rep.* **2021**, *4*, 100392. [CrossRef] [PubMed]
97. Appleby, R.; Moghul, I.; Khan, S.; Yee, M.; Manousou, P.; Neal, T.D.; Walters, J.R.F. Non-alcoholic fatty liver disease is associated with dysregulated bile acid synthesis and diarrhea: A prospective observational study. *PLoS ONE* **2019**, *14*, e0211348. [CrossRef]
98. Zou, H.; Ge, Y.; Lei, Q.; Ung, C.O.L.; Ruan, Z.; Lai, Y.; Yao, D.; Hu, H. Epidemiology and disease burden of non-alcoholic steatohepatitis in greater China: A systematic review. *Hepatol. Int.* **2022**, *16*, 27–37. [CrossRef]
99. Yuan, J.-H.; Xie, Q.-S.; Chen, G.-C.; Huang, C.-L.; Yu, T.; Chen, Q.-K.; Li, J.-Y. Impaired intestinal barrier function in type 2 diabetic patients measured by serum LPS, Zonulin, and IFABP. *J. Diabetes Complicat.* **2021**, *35*, 107766. [CrossRef]
100. Vanuytsel, T.; Vermeire, S.; Cleynen, I. The role of Haptoglobin and its related protein, Zonulin, in inflammatory bowel disease. *Tissue Barriers* **2013**, *1*, e27321. [CrossRef]
101. Genser, L.; Aguanno, D.; Soula, H.A.; Dong, L.; Trystram, L.; Assmann, K.; Salem, J.-E.; Vaillant, J.-C.; Oppert, J.-M.; Laugerette, F.; et al. Increased jejunal permeability in human obesity is revealed by a lipid challenge and is linked to inflammation and type 2 diabetes: Jejunal permeability in human obesity. *J. Pathol.* **2018**, *246*, 217–230. [CrossRef]
102. Stolfi, C.; Maresca, C.; Monteleone, G.; Laudisi, F. Implication of intestinal barrier dysfunction in gut dysbiosis and diseases. *Biomedicines* **2022**, *10*, 289. [CrossRef]
103. Martinez-Huenchullan, S.F.; Shipsey, I.; Hatchwell, L.; Min, D.; Twigg, S.M.; Larance, M. Blockade of High-Fat Diet Proteomic phenotypes using exercise as prevention or treatment. *Mol. Cell. Proteom.* **2021**, *20*, 100027. [CrossRef]
104. Hardardottir, I.; Kinsella, J.E. Tumor necrosis factor production by murine resident peritoneal macrophages is enhanced by dietary n−3 polyunsaturated fatty acids. *Biochim. Biophys. Acta (BBA)-Mol. Cell Res.* **1991**, *1095*, 187–195. [CrossRef]
105. Holme, I.; Aastveit, A.H.; Hammar, N.; Jungner, I.; Walldius, G. Haptoglobin and risk of myocardial infarction, stroke, and congestive heart failure in 342,125 men and women in the Apolipoprotein Mortality Risk study (AMORIS). *Ann. Med.* **2009**, *41*, 522–532. [CrossRef] [PubMed]

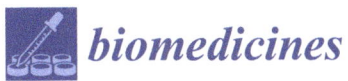

Article

Lipotoxicity in a Vicious Cycle of Pancreatic Beta Cell Exhaustion

Vladimir Grubelnik [1], Jan Zmazek [2], Matej Završnik [3] and Marko Marhl [2,4,5,*]

1. Institute of Mathematics and Physics, Faculty of Electrical Engineering and Computer Science, University of Maribor, 2000 Maribor, Slovenia; vlado.grubelnik@um.si
2. Department of Physics, Faculty of Natural Sciences and Mathematics, University of Maribor, 2000 Maribor, Slovenia; jan.zmazek@um.si
3. Department of Endocrinology and Diabetology, University Medical Center Maribor, Ljubljanska ulica 5, 2000 Maribor, Slovenia; matej.zavrsnik1@gmail.com
4. Department of Elementary Education, Faculty of Education, University of Maribor, 2000 Maribor, Slovenia
5. Department of Biophysics, Faculty of Medicine, University of Maribor, 2000 Maribor, Slovenia
* Correspondence: marko.marhl@um.si

Abstract: Hyperlipidemia is a common metabolic disorder in modern society and may precede hyperglycemia and diabetes by several years. Exactly how disorders of lipid and glucose metabolism are related is still a mystery in many respects. We analyze the effects of hyperlipidemia, particularly free fatty acids, on pancreatic beta cells and insulin secretion. We have developed a computational model to quantitatively estimate the effects of specific metabolic pathways on insulin secretion and to assess the effects of short- and long-term exposure of beta cells to elevated concentrations of free fatty acids. We show that the major trigger for insulin secretion is the anaplerotic pathway via the phosphoenolpyruvate cycle, which is affected by free fatty acids via uncoupling protein 2 and proton leak and is particularly destructive in long-term chronic exposure to free fatty acids, leading to increased insulin secretion at low blood glucose and inadequate insulin secretion at high blood glucose. This results in beta cells remaining highly active in the "resting" state at low glucose and being unable to respond to anaplerotic signals at high pyruvate levels, as is the case with high blood glucose. The observed fatty-acid-induced disruption of anaplerotic pathways makes sense in the context of the physiological role of insulin as one of the major anabolic hormones.

Keywords: diabetes; insulin secretion; lipids; PEP cycle; uncoupling proteins; mitochondrial dysfunction

1. Introduction

Metabolic syndrome is a burdensome public health problem in modern society and is closely related to type 2 diabetes mellitus (T2DM). Obesity and physical inactivity are the two most important risk factors for the development of metabolic syndrome, which is composed of a set of conditions that include high fasting blood glucose and abnormal cholesterol and triglyceride levels, in addition to hypertension and central obesity [1]. Dyslipidemias involving hypertriglyceridemia and low high-density lipoprotein levels are the major phenotypes associated with T2DM [2]. The influence of lipids on glucose metabolism, particularly the role of ectopic lipid accumulation, requires a systemic approach in a complex circuit of the endocrine pancreas and its hormone-targeted tissues, especially the liver and muscle [3,4]. We and others have shown that hyperlipidemia may statistically precede hyperglycemia by several years [5,6], indicating that it is predictive of reduced glucose tolerance in certain individuals. In addition, insulin resistance and prediabetes, conditions closely associated with metabolic syndrome, are thought to be caused by disturbances in energy utilization and storage, which certainly include impaired lipid utilization. While fasting hyperinsulinemia predates hyperglycemia in most cases, suggesting that insulin resistance likely precedes beta cell dysfunction, it is unclear whether fasting insulin hypersecretion is a primary driver of insulin resistance or a consequence in the form of a compensatory whole-body response to insulin resistance [7]. It was also shown that primary insensitivity to insulin does not appear to be fundamental to the pathogenesis of hyperlipidemia in familial dysbetalipoproteinemia [8]. Therefore, it is of great research interest to clarify whether high blood lipids contribute to dysfunctional glucose-stimulated insulin secretion (GSIS).

Several studies have revealed the mechanisms of lipotoxicity on beta cell function in association with T2DM [9–11]. Besides their involvement in tissue inflammation and the development of insulin resistance in peripheral tissues, free fatty acids (FFAs), particularly long-chain (Lc-FFAs) and saturated FFAs, might contribute to abnormal insulin response at several stages of their metabolism. These stages include FFA entry, mitochondrial metabolism, degradation [12], or even the triggering of ER stress-induced apoptosis [13]. Palmitate, the most common saturated FFA found in the human body, plays an important role in the lipotoxicity. It represents 20–30% of total FFAs in membrane phospholipids and adipose tissue triacylglycerols (TAGs) [14], and can be obtained in the diet [15] or synthesized endogenously [11]. In contrast, unsaturated FFAs have been assigned protective roles against the lipotoxic effects of saturated FFAs, such as preventing beta-cell apoptosis, regulating plasma glucose concentrations, and enhancing insulin sensitivity [11,16]. Oleic acid is the most abundant unsaturated FFA in human adipose tissue [17], promoting neutral lipid accumulation and insulin secretion. On the other hand, palmitic acid is poorly incorporated into triglycerides and, at physiological glucose concentrations, does not promote insulin secretion from human pancreatic islets [18].

Beta cells express the FFA transporter cluster of differentiation 36 (CD36), also known as fatty acid translocase (FAT) [19], and FFA receptors (FFAR1, FFAR2, and FFAR3). Short-chain FFAs (Sc-FFAs), produced by gut microbiota, target FFAR2 and FFAR3, but their role in beta cell function is unclear [20]. On the other hand, Lc-FFAs primarily stimulate CD36 and FFAR1 transporters. The latter induce basal hypersecretion of insulin secretion [9] by the activation of inositol triphosphate (IP3) and diacylglycerol (DAG) pathways and increasing cytosolic calcium concentration. At the mitochondrial level, FFAs decrease glutamine levels by the deterioration of anaplerosis (by promoting the formation of glutamate from glutamine). Chronic elevation of FFAs contributes to mitochondrial dysfunction and cellular senescence via signaling pathways and increased oxidative stress levels [12]. Moreover, several studies have linked chronically elevated FFAs levels to increased uncoupling protein 2 (UCP2) expression [21–24], typically observed in T2DM patients. The role of UCP2 in insulin secretion has also been recently reviewed [25], describing studies linking UCP2 to obesity that focus on the inflammatory process associated with ROS. The physiological significance of high UCP2 expression is unclear, but it might represent a signal for beta cells to prefer FFA and amino acid oxidation instead of glucose [24,26–30]. Lastly, the degradation of FFAs leads to ceramide accumulation and ceramide-associated beta-cell dysfunction [31].

In general, acute exposure of beta cells to FFAs has been recognized as beneficial for GSIS. In contrast, chronic increases in plasma FFA concentrations led to disruptions in the regulation of lipid metabolism and impaired beta-cell function due to lipotoxic effects [10]. Moreover, the adaptive signaling pathways induced to counteract lipotoxic stress have secondary adverse effects, as antilipotoxic signaling cascades may contribute to beta cell failure [32]. Experimental results from a recent study suggest a novel non-esterified FFA–stimulated pathway that selectively drives pancreatic islet non-glucose-stimulated insulin secretion (NGSIS) [7]. At low glucose levels reflecting a fasting state, FFAs affect NGSIS by inducing an H^+ leak at the inner mitochondrial membrane that drives tricarboxylic acid (TCA) flux to maintain mitochondrial membrane potential. Combining this knowledge with the recent discovery about the role of the phosphoenolpyruvate (PEP) cycle in beta cells and insulin secretion [33], the increased TCA cycle flux corresponds to the increased PEP cycle and NGSIS. The effect of the PEP cycle on insulin secretion has been recently reviewed [34], summarizing advances in understanding the metabolic mechanisms involved in insulin secretion.

Here we present a computational model including the anaplerotic and cataplerotic pathways of GSIS, which aims to explain the effects of acutely and chronically elevated FFAs on GSIS. Anaplerosis has been recognized as an essential pathway implicated in beta-cell activation by glucose already in early studies employing NMR carbon isotope tracing [35], which was later recognized as one of the significant pathways promoting insulin secretion [36]. Recently, a new conceptual framework for GSIS has been proposed based on the specific role of mitochondrial metabolism and the PEP cycle [33], disrupting the established "consensus model" [37]. The PEP cycle assumes the upregulation of anaplerotic pathways induced by the high expression of the pyruvate carboxylase (PC) enzyme in beta cells [38]. Instead of entering the oxidative metabolism by conversion to acetyl-CoA via pyruvate dehydrogenase (PDH), pyruvate flux is diverted to the production of oxaloacetate (OAA), an intermediate of the TCA cycle. OAA is converted to PEP, which leaves the mitochondria, diffuses, and accumulates locally at the plasma membrane. The conversion of PEP to pyruvate catalyzed by membrane-bound pyruvate kinase (PK) increases the cytosolic ATP/ADP ratio to the level required to inhibit the K_{ATP} channel [33,39]. The vital signaling role of anaplerosis and the PEP cycle for glucose sensing and insulin secretion is confirmed by several experimental studies. PC expression in beta cells is higher than in other tissues [35], and the anaplerotic flux from pyruvate to OAA via PC is strongly responsive to changes in extracellular glucose [40]. In fact, a study on the rat INS-1 insulinoma cell line showed a stronger correlation of GSIS with anaplerotic than with oxidative metabolism of pyruvate [41]. In this context, we also discuss the role of UCP2, which blocks the oxidation of pyruvate and paves the way for its anaplerotic fate [42]. The importance of the PEP-cycle in GSIS is further supported by the results showing that an enhanced TCA-cycle-derived mitochondrial GTP (mGTP) turnover amplifies insulin secretion by increasing insulin content, granule docking, and mitochondrial mass [43,44]. In addition, pyruvate kinase activators (PKa) amplify insulin release via the PEP cycle in preclinical T2DM models [45].

In the following sections, we first present a model of beta cell function, followed by the results in terms of model predictions for insulin secretion at low and high glucose levels. The model predictions agree well with the known mechanisms of dysregulations of insulin secretion, i.e., excessively high fasting levels and inadequate postprandial insulin secretion caused by the pathophysiological conditions of hyperlipidemia, and contribute to a better understanding of the general dysregulations of insulin signaling in obesity and T2DM.

2. Materials and Methods

The model considers the major metabolic pathways of glucose and FFAs that trigger insulin exocytosis. The metabolic pathways of glucose, the metabolism of FFA, and the mechanism of insulin secretion are shown schematically in Figure 1. The importance of the TCA and PEP cycles in mitochondria is particularly emphasized. The PEP cycle and transport of metabolites to microdomains at the plasma membrane cause an increase in ATP concentration near K_{ATP} channels, triggering insulin secretion. Glucose and FFAs enter the cell via glucose transporters (GLUTs) and FFA transporters (e.g., CD36), where they are first metabolized by glycolytic and beta-oxidation pathways, respectively. Glucose-derived pyruvate enters either the cataplerotic direction of the TCA cycle (by conversion to acetyl-CoA) or the anaplerotic direction (by conversion to OAA). Beta-oxidation-derived acetyl-CoA can only enter the cataplerotic metabolism and accelerate the TCA cycle. The increased citrate concentrations induce the formation of malonyl-CoA (MaCoA) in the cytosol and inhibit the entry of fatty acyl-coenzyme A (FA-CoA) via carnitine palmitoyltransferase 1 (CPT1). The mGTP and PEP cycles, which occur concurrently with the TCA cycle, convert OAA to PEP, which is exported from mitochondria and converted back to pyruvate in the cytosol, resulting in ATP production in the K_{ATP} channel microdomains (indicated by the red dashed line in Figure 1). This microdomain ATP concentration also depends on the "classical" energy generation pathway, which consists of the glucose and FFA oxidation pathways. NAD(P)H and FADH$_2$ are oxidized by the electron transport chain (ETC), generating ATP molecules and increasing the global cytosolic ATP concentration (ATP$_{cyt}$) that can diffuse into/from microdomains. The ATP-dependent closure of K$_{ATP}$ channels leads to membrane potential oscillations and the influx of Ca^{2+} ions through voltage-gated calcium channels (VGCC). Increased Ca^{2+} concentrations induce the Ca^{2+}-dependent exocytosis of insulin granules. The mathematical modeling of the processes is described in detail in the following subsections.

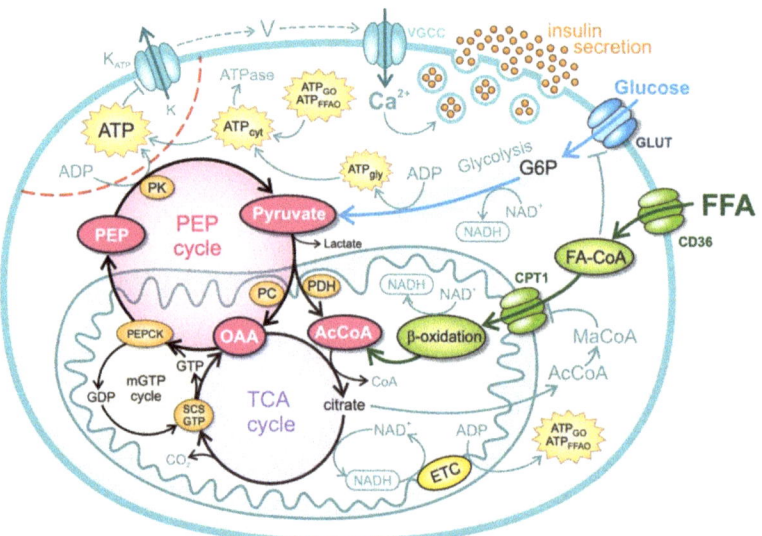

Figure 1. Schematic representation of a mathematical model. ATP—ATP concentration near K$_{ATP}$ channels, ATP$_{cyt}$—cytosolic ATP concentration, ATP$_{gly}$—net glycolytic ATP production, ATP$_{FFAO}$—total ATP production by FFA metabolism, ATP$_{GO}$—ATP production by oxidation of pyruvate and reducing equivalents from glycolysis, AcCoA—acetyl-coenzyme A, CD36—transmembrane FFA transport protein (FFA translocase), CPT1—carnitine palmitoyltransferase 1, ETC—electron transfer chain, FA-CoA—fatty-acyl-coenzyme A, GLUT—glucose transporter, G6P—glucose 6-phosphatase, MaCoA—malonyl-coenzyme A, OAA—oxaloacetate, PC—pyruvate carboxylase, PDH—pyruvate dehydrogenase, PEP—phosphoenolpyruvate, PEPCK—phosphoenolpyruvate carboxykinase, PK—pyruvate kinase, SCS-GTP—GTP-specific succinyl-CoA synthetase.

2.1. Glucose Metabolism

Glucose is first transported into the intracellular space and phosphorylated to glucose-6-phosphate (G6P) during the first priming reaction of glycolysis. This process is considered the rate-limiting step of glycolysis and regulates the glycolytic flux. The uptake of glucose and its phosphorylation are modeled by Michaelis-Menten kinetics (see [46]):

$$J_{G6P} = J_{max}(1 - k_{FFA}f_{FFA})\frac{G^2}{K_m^2 + G^2} \quad (1)$$

The parameters $J_{max} = 8\ \mu M/s$ and $K_m = 3.8\ mM$ were chosen based on experimental data for glucose concentrations G at 1 mM and 10 mM [35]. Equation (1) also considers the inhibition of glycolytic flux caused by FFAs, where the parameter f_{FFA} represents the exposure to FFA. Based on the experimental results of Roden [47], it is assumed that acyl-CoA blocks glucose phosphorylation. The value of $k_{FFA} = 0.08$ is chosen such that J_{G6P} decreases by about 20% when f_{FFA} is increased from 0 to 2.5. This is consistent with the results of Roden, who found that glycolytic flux can be decreased by more than 20% when the plasma concentration of FFA is doubled [47].

In the fourth step of glycolysis, the 6-carbon molecule splits into two 3-carbon molecules, so the glycolytic flux is doubled, which is modeled as follows:

$$J_{gly} = 2\, J_{G6P}. \tag{2}$$

The final products of glycolysis are two molecules of pyruvate. Considering the preparatory and final phases, glycolysis yields a net total of 2 molecules of ATP:

$$J_{ATP,gly} = 2\, J_{G6P}, \tag{3}$$

where $J_{ATP,gly}$ is the net glycolytic ATP production flux. Glycolysis also yields 2 molecules of NADH. Depending on the amount of LDH expressed in the cell, a portion of pyruvate is reduced to lactate in the reaction in which 1 NADH molecule is oxidized to NAD$^+$. We model this effect by introducing a parameter p_L:

$$J_{lac} = p_L\, J_{gly}. \tag{4}$$

Considering that beta cells express very low levels of LDH, we set the parameter to $p_L = 0.05$ [46]. Thus, the NADH flux generated by glycolysis is:

$$J_{NADH,gly} = (1 - p_L)\, J_{gly}. \tag{5}$$

To the same extent, a fraction of pyruvate generated by glycolysis that is not reduced to lactate enters the mitochondria:

$$J_{pyr} = (1 - p_L)\, J_{gly}. \tag{6}$$

The transport of pyruvate into the mitochondria (J_{pyr}), the oxidation of pyruvate to acetyl-CoA, and the production of reducing equivalents in the TCA cycle are modeled by the following equation:

$$J_{pyr,TCA} = (1 - f_{ANA}) J_{pyr}. \tag{7}$$

A portion of pyruvate (f_{ANA}) is used for anaplerotic reactions, which represents an important part of beta cell metabolism related to insulin secretion. In this process, FFAs play an important role by additionally diverting pyruvate flux to anaplerosis. This is particularly important in long-term and chronic hyperlipidemia and may be related, at least in part, to the increase in UCP2, which serves as a metabolic switch that prevents pyruvate oxidation and saves it for anabolic purposes [24,26–30]. This effect of FFAs is modeled by:

$$f_{ANA} = k_{ANA,0} + k_{ANA}\, f_{FFA}. \tag{8}$$

Previous experimental data suggest that anaplerosis in beta cells is relatively important, but there is a large discrepancy between the quantitative results of experimental studies [35,48,49]. We set the basal rate of anaplerosis (in the absence of FFAs) to 40% ($k_{ANA,0} = 0.4$), which is consistent with the above studies, indicating that approximately 60% of pyruvate is directly oxidized via PDH, while the remaining 40% is carboxylated by PC. The value of $k_{ANA} = 0.08$, which corresponds to the FFA-dependent increase of anaplerosis that is set to mirror a 20% elevation of anaplerosis during full exposure to FFAs (at $f_{FFA} = 2.5$). The maximal anaplerotic flux of 60% was used in a previous study which did not consider variation in FFA exposure [46].

The combined PDH and TCA cycle reactions yield 4 NADH ($J_{NADH,pyr,TCA} = 4 J_{pyr,TCA}$), 1 FADH$_2$ ($J_{FADH_2,pyr,TCA} = J_{pyr,TCA}$), and 1 GTP ($J_{GTP,pyr,TCA} = J_{pyr,TCA}$) molecule. As described, mitochondrial PEPCK hydrolyzes GTP to produce PEP (see Figure 1). Consequently, the GTP produced by TCA cycle does not contribute to the overall energy production, since it is coupled to the PEP cycle. The coupling of GTP and PEP cycles is modeled in the continuation.

It is generally accepted that oxidation of 1 FADH$_2$ by the ETC yields 1.5 ATP, while oxidation of 1 NADH yields 2.5 ATP, commonly referred to as the P/O ratio:

$$J_{ATP,pyr,ox} = (2.5\, J_{NADH,\,pyr,TCA} + 1.5\, J_{FADH_2,\,pyr,TCA})(1 - f_{p,leak})(1 - k_{md}). \quad (9)$$

Similarly, the glycolysis-produced NADH molecules (Equation (5)) enter mitochondria and the ETC via glycerol-phosphate and malate-aspartate shuttles [50,51], contributing to aerobic ATP production. While the malate-aspartate shuttle transfers NADH molecules directly, the glycerol-phosphate shuttle transports electrons from NADH (by regenerating NAD$^+$) to glycerol-3-phosphate dehydrogenase 2, reducing enzyme-bound FAD to FADH$_2$. Since beta cells' GSIS depends on the glycerol-phosphate shuttle [52], we assume the P/O ratio of 1.5. Accordingly, the rate of ATP production from the glycolysis-produced NADH molecules is given by:

$$J_{ATP,NADH,gly,ox} = 1.5\, J_{NADH,gly}(1 - f_{p,leak})(1 - k_{md}). \quad (10)$$

Thus, the total production of ATP by glucose metabolism is:

$$J_{ATP,G} = J_{ATP,gly} + J_{ATP,GO} = J_{ATP,gly} + J_{ATP,pyr,ox} + J_{ATP,NADH,gly,ox}. \quad (11)$$

In Equations (9) and (10), we also consider decreasing ATP production due to increased mitochondrial proton leak ($f_{p,leak}$) and mitochondrial dysfunction (k_{md}). Insulin secretion has been shown to be associated with increased UCP2 expression and decreased glucose-stimulated ATP/ADP ratio due to increased mitochondrial proton leak [53,54]. Several studies have linked chronic hyperlipidemia to increased UCP2 levels [23,24], which are typically observed in T2DM patients. Mathematical models have also been created to account for an increase in proton leak due to uncoupling protein (UCP) activation by ROS [55]. In response to FFAs, proton leak may also be enhanced by mitochondrial permeability transition pores (mPTP) [7]. In view of these observations, mitochondrial proton leak is modeled as follows:

$$f_{p,leak} = k_{p,leak}(J_{pyr,TCA} + J_{FFA,TCA}). \quad (12)$$

UCP expression has been shown to alter the ratio of proton leak and proton efflux, leading to a reduction in ATP production of approximately 20% at high glucose concentrations (higher mitochondrial membrane potential) [55]. In Equation (12), this corresponds to the value of the parameter $k_{p,leak} = 0.1$ s/µM.

Mitochondrial dysfunction, commonly observed in T2DM and insulin-resistant individuals [56], is taken into account in the model by changing the k_{md} parameter in Equations (9) and (10), as has been modeled previously [57,58]. In pancreatic tissue, mitochondrial dysfunction has been identified as one of the major causes for impaired secretory response of β-cells to glucose [59,60]. In T2DM, β-cells contain swollen mitochondria with disrupted cristae [53,54,61] and impaired stimulus-secretion coupling. Mitochondrial oxidative phosphorylation has been shown to decrease by 20–40% in insulin-resistant individuals [56,62].

2.2. FFA Metabolism

In the model we focus on Lc-FFAs, which serve as an energy source via beta-oxidation. Food is the major source of lipids and more specifically of poly-unsaturated FFAs. TAGs are split to Lc-FFAs by lipases of the digestive juices releasing, among others, palmitate (C16:0, saturated), oleate (C18:1, mono-unsaturated), and linoleate (C18:2, poly-unsaturated) [20]. Beta cell exposure to Lc-FFAs activates CD36 FFA receptors in the cell membrane which play an important role in the uptake of FFAs and have multiple biological functions that may be important in inflammation and in the development of metabolic diseases, including diabetes [19]. The upregulation of the CD36 transporter in beta-cells increases the uptake of FFAs, resulting in enhanced GSIS and impaired oxidative metabolism [63–65]. We model FFA exposure by introducing a parameter f_{FFA} in Equation (13). It should be noted that an increase in blood glucose level blocks beta oxidation. A rise in blood glucose levels increases glucose-derived pyruvate and the activity of the TCA cycle ($J_{pyr,TCA}$). This results in the production of citrate that escapes the mitochondria and activates the acetyl-CoA carboxylase to generate cytosolic malonyl-CoA. In turn, malonyl-CoA inhibits the CPT1, blocking the entry of acyl-CoA into mitochondria and disabling beta-oxidation [20]. We model this effect with

$$J_{FFA,\beta} = J_{FFA,TCA,0}\left(1 - \frac{J_{pyr,TCA}}{k_{m,CPT} + J_{pyr,TCA}}\right) f_{FFA,p,leak}\, f_{FFA}. \tag{13}$$

Experimental results from a recent study also suggest that elevated circulating FFAs increase proton leak in the mitochondria of beta cells, which drives TCA cycle flux to maintain mitochondrial membrane potential [7,46]. To model this effect, the parameter $f_{FFA,p,leak}$ in Equation (13) accounts for the increase in $J_{FFA,\beta}$ due to the increased mitochondrial proton leak:

$$f_{FFA,p,leak} = \left(1 + k_{l,FFA} k_{p,leak}\right). \tag{14}$$

The constants $J_{FFA,TCA,0} = 0.25\ \mu M/s$, $k_{m,CPT} = 8\ \mu M/s$, and $k_{l,FFA} = 4\ \mu M/s$ are determined by qualitatively obtaining the same ATP production at $f_{FFA} = 1$ as in the previous study in which FFA oxidation was determined from oxygen consumption [46].

Once FFAs enter the mitochondrial matrix, they are repeatedly cleaved during the beta-oxidation pathway, producing acetyl-CoA molecules. Calculations of fluxes in the continuation are performed for 18-carbon oleic acid, the most abundant FFA in human adipose tissue [17]. Beta oxidation of oleic acid requires eight consecutive reactions, yielding nine molecules of acetyl-CoA. Each acetyl-CoA is then converted to succinyl-CoA by carboxylation reaction, yielding four net ATP molecules (due to oxidation of 1 NADH and 1 FADH$_2$), yielding a net total of 32 ATP molecules. However, two ATP molecules are lost during the activation of each FFA. Therefore, the ATP yield during beta-oxidation can be given as follows:

$$J_{ATP,FFA,\beta,ox} = 30\, J_{FFA,\beta}\left(1 - f_{p,leak}\right)(1 - k_{md}). \tag{15}$$

Due to the breakdown of oleic acid into nine molecules of acetyl-CoA during the beta-oxidation pathway, the acetyl-CoA flux into mitochondria is multiplied:

$$J_{FFA,TCA} = 9\, J_{FFA,\beta}. \tag{16}$$

The TCA cycle yields three molecules of NADH ($J_{NADH,FFA,TCA} = 3 J_{FFA,TCA}$), one molecule of FADH$_2$ ($J_{FADH_2,FFA,TCA} = J_{FFA,TCA}$), and one molecule of GTP ($J_{GTP,FFA,TCA} = J_{FFA,TCA}$). The latter is in turn directly consumed (as in Equation (10)) by the PEP cycle, yielding the following:

$$J_{ATP,FFA,TCA,ox} = \left(2.5\, J_{NADH,\,FFA,TCA} + 1.5\, J_{FADH_2,\,FFA,TCA}\right)\left(1 - f_{p,leak}\right)(1 - k_{md}) \tag{17}$$

Thus, the total production of ATP by FFA metabolism is:

$$J_{ATP,FFAO} = J_{ATP,FFA,\beta,ox} + J_{ATP,FFA,TCA,ox}. \tag{18}$$

The decrease in ATP production due to increase in proton leak ($f_{p,leak}$) and mitochondrial dysfunction (k_{md}) in Equations (15) and (17) are modeled identically as in Equation (10).

2.3. Anaplerotic Pathway and PEP Cycle

The PEP cycle with the net flux of PEP (J_{PEP}) is coupled to the mitochondrial GTP cycle, which is modeled as follows:

$$J_{PEP} = \frac{f_{ANA}}{f_{ANA,0}} \left(J_{GTP,pyr,TCA} + J_{GTP,FFA,TCA} \right)(1 - k_{md}). \tag{19}$$

The ratio $\frac{f_{ANA}}{f_{ANA,0}}$ determines the FFA-dependent increase in J_{PEP} (see Equation (8)). Since 1 GTP is consumed during the formation of 1 PEP, the consumption of GTP in mitochondria is also increased by this ratio. This is possible if we have a sufficient concentration of GTP molecules in the mitochondria. Because mammalian mitochondria lack a GTP transporter, GTP is effectively trapped in the mitochondrial matrix [66,67]. PEP diffuses to the plasma membrane, where it is converted to pyruvate by PK. This reaction is coupled by the non-oxidative phosphorylation of ATP that accumulates near K_{ATP} channels [33,39,46,68]. Consequently, the flux of PEP is equal to PEP-cycle-dependent ATP generation ($J_{ATP,PEP} = J_{PEP}$).

2.4. Mechanisms of Insulin Secretion

K_{ATP} channels play a central role in the regulation of insulin secretion. ATP directly inhibits the K_{ATP} channels by binding to Kir6.2 subunits, while ATP and ADP activate the channel by interacting with the NBFs of SUR [68]. A higher ATP/ADP ratio decreases K_{ATP} channel activity, resulting in increased Ca^{2+} concentration and exocytosis of insulin. Previously, we described in detail the role of K_{ATP} channels as a coupling step between the metabolic and electrical activities of beta cells [46]. The phenomenological relationship between K_{ATP}-channel conductance and hormone secretion was modeled by fitting the results of the electrophysiological model of Pedersen et al. [69]. The same equations linking K_{ATP} channel conductance to the insulin secretion rate are also used in this model. The K_{ATP}-channel conductance is modeled according to the proposal of Magnus & Keizer [70].

The concentration of cytosolic ATP, which affects K_{ATP} channel conductance, is determined by the balance between ATP production and consumption. ATP is produced by glucose metabolism and by FFA metabolism. The rate of the ATP production is given by:

$$J_{ATP,cyt} = J_{ATP,G} + J_{ATP,FFA} \tag{20}$$

In general, ATP hydrolysis is assumed to increase with the energy state of the cell, and the kinetics is often modeled according to Michaelis-Menten kinetics (e.g., [71]). The rate of ATP hydrolysis is described by:

$$J_{ATPase} = k_{ATPase} \frac{ATP_{cyt}^2}{K_{m,ATPase}^2 + ATP_{cyt}^2} . \# \tag{21}$$

where $k_{ATPase} = 350\ \mu M/s$ and $K_{m,ATPase} = 2000\ \mu M/s$. The concentration of ATP_{cyt} in the steady-state approximation when the ATP production rate, $J_{ATP,cyt}$, is in equilibrium with the ATP hydrolysis rate J_{ATPase} is given by:

$$ATP_{cyt} = k_{m,ATPase} \left(\frac{J_{ATP,cyt}}{k_{ATPase} - J_{ATP,cyt}} \right)^{\frac{1}{2}}. \tag{22}$$

Considering the accumulation of ATP near the cell membrane due to the PEP cycle, the ATP concentration is modeled by:

$$\frac{dATP}{dt} = k_{ATP,1} J_{PEP} - k_{ATP,2}(ATP - ATP_{cyt}). \tag{23}$$

Consequently, the ATP concentration at steady state is given by:

$$ATP = ATP_{cyt} + \frac{k_{ATP,1}}{k_{ATP,2}} J_{PEP}. \qquad (24)$$

The ratio $\frac{k_{ATP,1}}{k_{ATP,2}} = 200$ is chosen so that the ATP concentration range coupled to the K_{ATP} conductance [70] is consistent with experimental data [72].

3. Results

Using the mathematical model presented in Section 2, we investigate the mechanisms of GSIS and the role of FFA exposure in modulating the physiological beta cell response to plasma glucose. Although it is clear that acute and chronic exposure to FFAs is involved in both altered metabolic and signaling pathways, we are mainly interested in the effects of FFAs from a bioenergetic perspective. In particular, model results reveal the extent to which high lipid levels induce changes in energy production (ATP), which allows us to understand changes in insulin secretion due to cell exposure to FFAs. Furthermore, independent of the analysis of the oxidative pathways of glucose and FFAs, we highlight the essential role of anaplerotic pathways in GSIS. We focus on the PEP cycle as an important anaplerotic pathway in the beta cell that provides an additional mechanism to influence the conductance of K_{ATP} channels and the resulting insulin secretion.

Figure 2 shows the metabolic fluxes that contribute to ATP production. The increase in plasma lipids and the resulting higher exposure of beta cells to FFA is modeled by increasing the parameter f_{FFA}. Figure 2A shows the effects related to the oxidative metabolic pathways. An increase in plasma glucose concentration (G) increases the glucose oxidation pathway ($J_{ATP,GO}$), whereas the FFA oxidation pathway ($J_{ATP,FFAO}$) decreases. High glucose levels inhibit FFA oxidation by blocking the uptake of acyl-CoA into mitochondria (see Equation (13)). Increasing the parameter f_{FFA} has the opposite effect on the glucose and FFA oxidation pathways—as FFAs become the preferred metabolic fuel, glucose oxidation decreases at all glucose concentrations. The FFA-mediated decrease in glucose oxidation results from the reduced glycolytic flux $J_{ATP,gly}$ (see Equation (1)), as shown in Figure 2B. In addition, pyruvate is diverted to the anaplerotic pathway (see Equation (8)), resulting in increased ATP production via the PEP cycle ($J_{ATP,PEP}$), as shown in Figure 2B. The increase in $J_{ATP,PEP}$ (Equation (19)) results from the acceleration of the mGTP cycle due to the increased entry of FFA into the TCA cycle. In addition, the availability of OAA increases with higher PC-catalyzed flux (see Figure 1).

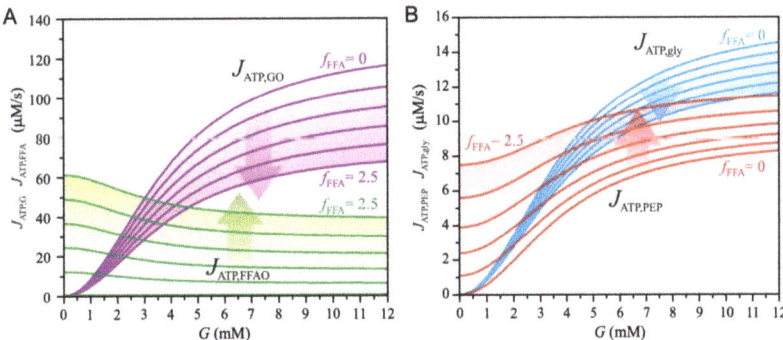

Figure 2. Glucose-dependent metabolic fluxes of ATP production and the effects of beta cell exposure to FFA (f_{FFA}). The parameter f_{FFA} is varied between 0 and 2.5 with a step size of 0.5. (**A**) ATP production due to glucose oxidation ($J_{ATP,GO}$) and ATP production due to FFA oxidation ($J_{ATP,FFAO}$). (**B**) ATP production due to the PEP cycle ($J_{ATP,PEP}$) and due to glycolysis ($J_{ATP,gly}$).

Changes in ATP fluxes, as shown in Figure 2, result in changes in subplasmalemmal ATP concentration near K_{ATP} channels (see Equation (24)). Acute exposure of a healthy beta cell to FFAs results in increased intracellular ATP concentrations which are more pronounced at low plasma glucose concentrations, as shown in Figure 3A. Higher ATP levels at low glucose concentrations result from increased basal FFA oxidation and increased accelerated PEP cycles, as shown in Figure 2. The PEP cycle essentially produces a flux of TCA-cycle-derived GTP to energetically equivalent subplasmalemmal ATP. Both effects contribute to altered insulin secretion, as shown in Figure 3B. Basal relative insulin secretion (RIS) increases as a result of both plasma glucose concentration and increased FFA exposure.

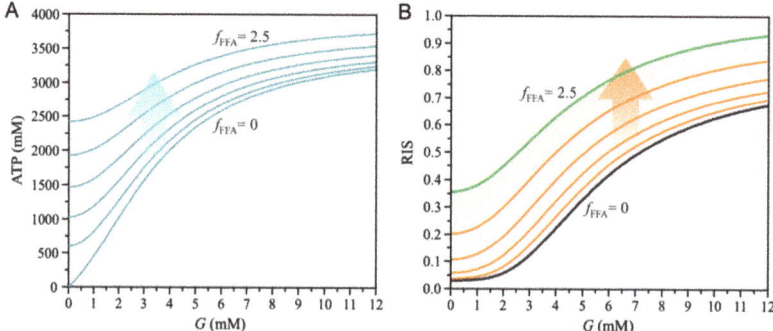

Figure 3. Effect of FFAs (f_{FFA}) on ATP concentration near K_{ATP} channels. The value of parameter f_{FFA} increases from 0 to 2.5 with a step size of 0.5. (**A**) Glucose-dependent ATP concentration. Exposure to FFA increases basal ATP concentration, especially at low glucose levels, which consequently decreases glucose dependence. (**B**) Glucose-dependent relative insulin secretion (RIS). The FFA exposure increases basal RIS.

We further address the changes in insulin secretion that result from chronic exposure of beta cells to FFAs (see Figure 4). First, we note that the increase in mitochondrial proton leak ($k_{p,leak}$) through the inner mitochondrial membrane reduces glucose oxidation (Equations (9) and (10)) and FFA oxidation (Equations (15) and (17)), as shown in Figure 4A. However, increased proton flux promotes the entry of FFA into the TCA cycle (Equations (13) and (14)), which accelerates mGTP and PEP cycles (Equation (19)). As shown in Figure 4B, increased proton leak increases ATP production derived from the PEP cycle.

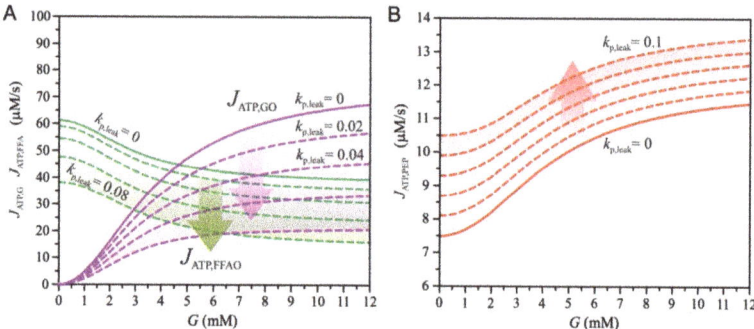

Figure 4. The effects of increased mitochondrial proton leak ($k_{p,leak}$) on energy metabolism ($f_{FFA} = 2.5$ (see Figure 1)). The value of parameter $k_{p,leak}$ increases with a step size of 0.02. (**A**) Glucose-dependent ATP production due to glucose oxidation ($J_{ATP,GO}$) and FFA oxidation ($J_{ATP,FFAO}$). Increased mitochondrial proton leak reduces glucose and FFA oxidation. (**B**) Glucose-dependent PEP-cycle-derived ATP production. Increased mitochondrial leak increases ATP production.

Changes in ATP production due to increased mitochondrial proton leak ($k_{p,leak}$), as shown in Figure 4, lead to changes in insulin secretion (Figure 5). As shown in Figure 5A, mitochondrial proton leak leads to a slight increase in basal insulin secretion, whereas insulin secretion is significantly reduced at high glucose levels. The increase in basal insulin secretion results from the increased subplasmalemmal ATP levels near the K_{ATP} channels. Whereas ATP production decreases due to decreased glucose ($J_{ATP,GO}$) and FFA ($J_{ATP,FFAO}$) oxidation, acceleration of the PEP cycle ($J_{ATP,PEP}$) leads to an increase in ATP flux into the subplasmalemmal space. However, at high glucose concentrations, the increase in $J_{ATP,PEP}$ cannot compensate for the loss that results from reduced metabolite oxidation, leading to decreased insulin secretion.

For long-term exposure of beta cells to FFAs, we also consider mitochondrial dysfunction, modeled by the parameter k_{md}. Figure 5B shows the effects of mitochondrial dysfunction on insulin secretion. Because of a decrease in all fluxes ($J_{ATP,GO}$, $J_{ATP,FFAO}$, $J_{ATP,PEP}$), which are conditioned by mitochondrial function, RIS decreases.

The combination of each effect on RIS is shown in Figure 6. Short-term exposure of beta cells to FFAs, when the decrease in mitochondrial function is not yet present, increases both basal insulin secretion and GSIS (curve b). When mitochondrial proton leak is enhanced, basal insulin secretion increases slightly, whereas it decreases at high glucose (curve c). Because to mitochondrial dysfunction, insulin secretion is further reduced at all glucose concentrations (curve d), and the cell secretes approximately the same amount of insulin regardless of plasma glucose concentration, which is physiologically undesirable and can be observed in T2DM patients.

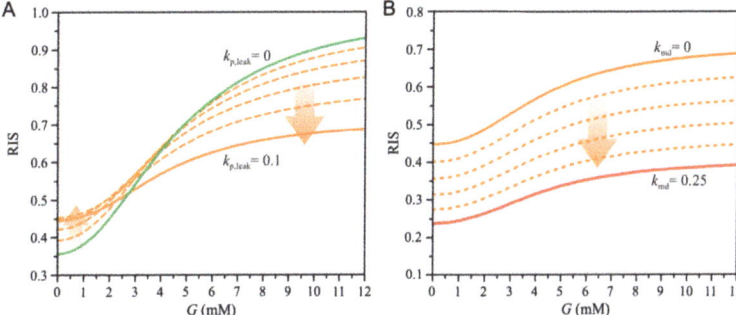

Figure 5. Effects of chronic lipid exposure on relative insulin secretion (RIS). (**A**) Effects of proton leak on glucose-dependent RIS. Increased proton leak flattens the glucose-dependent RIS curve, increases RIS at low glucose concentrations, and decreases RIS at high glucose concentrations. The value of parameter $k_{p,leak}$ increases from 0 to 0.1 with a step size of 0.02. (**B**) The effects of mitochondrial dysfunction on glucose-dependent RIS. Increased mitochondrial dysfunction reduces RIS at all glucose concentrations. The value of parameter k_{md} increases from 0 to 0.25 with a step size of 0.05.

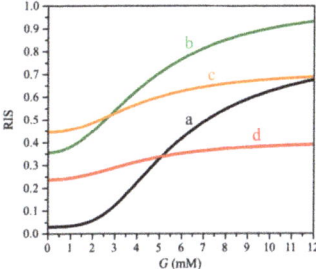

Figure 6. Influence of individual factors on glucose-dependent relative insulin secretion (RIS). (**a**) Absence of FFAs ($f_{FFA} = 0$, $k_{p,leak} = 0$, $k_{md} = 0$). A response of a healthy beta cell under physiological

conditions. (**b**) The presence of FFAs, without increase in mitochondrial proton leak and mitochondrial dysfunction ($f_{FFA} = 2.5$, $k_{p,leak} = 0$, $k_{md} = 0$). RIS is increased at all glucose concentrations. (**c**) Presence of FFAs and increased proton flux, without mitochondrial dysfunction ($f_{FFA} = 2.5$, $k_{p,leak} = 0.1$, $k_{md} = 0$). The RIS curve is flattened. (**d**) Presence of FFAs with increased mitochondrial proton leak and mitochondrial dysfunction ($f_{FFA} = 2.5$, $k_{p,leak} = 0.1$, $k_{md} = 0.25$). RIS is reduced at all glucose concentrations.

4. Discussion

This study provides insight into the major cellular mechanisms involved in insulin secretion. It devotes the simplistic understanding of the beta cell as the sole glucose sensor to the notion of much broader machinery for sensing glucose and other metabolites, particularly FFAs. In the model, the acute exposure of beta cells to FFAs increases insulin secretion due to increased FFA oxidation and an accelerated PEP cycle. This is consistent with experiments showing that after only 4 h, an increase in CPT 1 activity measured in isolated mitochondria leads to increased FFA oxidation, resulting in two-to-three-fold higher FFA oxidation in cells exposed to FFAs measured at low glucose compared to control [73]. Moreover, the interplay of FFA metabolism and its role in modulating the PEP cycle is consistent with a 30% increase in PC mRNA expression and thus a 2.5-fold increase in insulin secretion at 3.3 mM and a 40% increase at 27 mM during an 8-h exposure to 250 µM palmitate [74]. The same study showed that GLUT-2 mRNA expression was reduced by approximately 30% in 48 h in islet cultures with 250 µM palmitate. Furthermore, GK mRNA expression was also reduced by approximately 30%. Other studies have also shown that a high-fat diet (HFD) reduces mRNA expression of GLUT-2 and GK, diminishing glucose oxidation [75,76]. These experimental findings are consistent with our model predictions, showing reduced glycolytic flux and consequently reduced glucose oxidation during exposure to FFAs.

In contrast to acute FFA administration, chronic exposure to FFAs inhibits insulin release under glucotoxic conditions [10]. This is supported by studies showing that glucose-induced insulin release was increased in islets cultured with palmitate for 8 h, whereas glucose-induced insulin release was significantly impaired by the simultaneous presence of palmitate when the culture time was extended to 48 h [74]. There are several reasons for this. The effect of FFAs on insulin release has been associated with FFA metabolism [10,77,78] and signaling via the G protein-coupled receptor FFAR1/GPR40 [10,79–81]. While we are aware of their importance and impact on insulin secretion, the latter were not included in our model since they would not qualitatively influence our results but would rather amplify the individual effects. It has been shown that FFAR1 in the pancreatic beta cell plays an essential role not only in the acute potentiation of GSIS by palmitate but also in the negative long-term effects of palmitate on GSIS and insulin content [81]. Recently published research has also focused on the glycerolipid/NEFA cycle, which provides lipid signals through its lipolysis arm [20,82]. Moreover, mitochondrial dysfunction in the beta cells included in our model has been recognized as one of the most critical consequences of the chronic elevation of FFA, caused mainly by impaired peroxisome proliferator-activated receptor signaling, increased oxidative stress levels, and lipotoxic modulation of the PI3K/Akt and MAPK/ERK pathways [12].

Chronic exposure to FFAs is one of the main problems in beta cell reprogramming. In particular, the detour of oxidative processes from glucose to FFA, sparing pyruvate for anaplerotic purposes, may be one of the leading pathophysiological pathways to inappropriate energy metabolism and beta cell dysfunction, often resulting in beta cell death. The increased basal anaplerosis via the PEP cycle leads to increased basal insulin secretion and beta cell exhaustion with an inappropriate response to high glucose concentrations. The increased basal insulin secretion under lipotoxic conditions shown by our results is consistent with research showing that FFAs increase insulin secretion at fasting glucose concentrations and that improved mitochondrial metabolism is critical for this effect, which is further enhanced by FFAR1 [9]. Research has shown that insulin secretion increases approximately two-fold and continues to increase after a few days. Some studies have demonstrated increased insulin secretion at low glucose levels [83–85], while others have also shown a decreased insulin secretion at higher glucose concentrations [84,85], which is consistent with our findings. In particular, clonal beta cells exposed to oleate for 72 h exhibited impaired GSIS and decreased cellular ATP [84], which is consistent with our results, suggesting that the decreased insulin secretion results from lower ATP concentration due to decreased glucose oxidation and mitochondrial dysfunction. The same study also showed that mitochondria of oleate-exposed cells exhibit increased depolarization caused by acute oleate treatment, which is due to the increase in FFA transport function of UCP2. According to our results, the increased proton leak indeed increases basal insulin secretion and, most importantly, decreases GSI, indicating that chronic exposure to FFA with excessive oxidation of FFAs is a pathway to beta cell exhaustion with too high NGSIS and too low GSIS. The elevated FFAs also block the glucose entry [47], and in a vicious cycle with glucolipotoxicity, beta cells cannot efficiently sense glucose [86,87]. This is one of the most prominent pathways to the pathologies of metabolic syndrome and T2DM associated with obesity and hyperlipidemia, which are statistically observable [6] and represent an even greater problem in modern societies.

In conclusion, the computational model presented here, which incorporates all the basic anaplerotic and cataplerotic mechanisms in beta cells responsible for insulin secretion, provides quantitative estimates of the effects of short- and long-term exposure of beta cells to elevated concentrations of FFA. The results indicate that the major trigger for insulin secretion is the anaplerotic pathway via the phosphoenolpyruvate cycle, which is impaired by FFA and is particularly destructive during long-term chronic exposure to FFA, resulting in increased insulin secretion at low blood glucose and inadequate insulin secretion at high blood glucose. The observed FFA-induced disruption of anaplerotic pathways is consistent with the physiological role of insulin as one of the major anabolic hormones. Future studies could extend the model to include additional signaling pathways and the role of amino acids as metabolites and signaling molecules in the mechanisms of beta cell function and insulin secretion.

Author Contributions: Conceptualization: M.M. and V.G.; software: V.G. and J.Z.; original draft preparation: V.G., J.Z. and M.M.; reviewing and editing, V.G., J.Z., M.Z., M.M.; visualization: V.G.; supervision, M.M. All authors have read and agreed to the published version of the manuscript.

Funding: This research was supported by Javna Agencija za Raziskovalno Dejavnost RS, grant numbers P1-0055, J3-3077.

Institutional Review Board Statement: Not applicable.

Informed Consent Statement: Not applicable.

Data Availability Statement: Not applicable.

Conflicts of Interest: The authors declare that they have no conflicts of interest.

References

1. Eckel, R.H.; Grundy, S.M.; Zimmet, P.Z. The metabolic syndrome. *Lancet* **2005**, *365*, 1415–1428. [CrossRef]
2. Kane, J.P.; Pullinger, C.R.; Goldfine, I.D.; Malloy, M.J. Dyslipidemia and diabetes mellitus: Role of lipoprotein species and interrelated pathways of lipid metabolism in diabetes mellitus. *Curr. Opin. Pharmacol.* **2021**, *61*, 21–27. [CrossRef] [PubMed]
3. Samuel, V.T.; Shulman, G.I. The pathogenesis of insulin resistance: Integrating signaling pathways and substrate flux. *J. Clin. Investig.* **2016**, *126*, 12–22. [CrossRef] [PubMed]
4. Roden, M.; Shulman, G.I. The integrative biology of type 2 diabetes. *Nature* **2019**, *576*, 51–60. [CrossRef]
5. Adiels, M.; Olofsson, S.-O.; Taskinen, M.-R.; Borén, J. Diabetic dyslipidaemia. *Curr. Opin. Lipidol.* **2006**, *17*, 238–246. [CrossRef]
6. Markovič, R.; Grubelnik, V.; Vošner, H.B.; Kokol, P.; Završnik, M.; Janša, K.; Zupet, M.; Završnik, J.; Marhl, M. Age-Related Changes in Lipid and Glucose Levels Associated with Drug Use and Mortality: An Observational Study. *J. Pers. Med.* **2022**, *12*, 280. [CrossRef]

7. Taddeo, E.P.; Alsabeeh, N.; Baghdasarian, S.; Wikstrom, J.D.; Ritou, E.; Sereda, S.; Erion, K.; Li, J.; Stiles, L.; Abdulla, M.; et al. Mitochondrial Proton Leak Regulated by Cyclophilin D Elevates Insulin Secretion in Islets at Nonstimulatory Glucose Levels. *Diabetes* **2019**, *69*, 131–145. [CrossRef]
8. Tan, M.; Havel, R.; Gerich, J.; Soeldner, J.; Kane, J. Pancreatic Alpha and Beta Cell Function in Familial Dysbetalipoproteinemia. *Horm. Metab. Res.* **1980**, *12*, 421–425. [CrossRef]
9. Kristinsson, H.; Sargsyan, E.; Manell, H.; Smith, D.M.; Göpel, S.O.; Bergsten, P. Basal hypersecretion of glucagon and insulin from palmitate-exposed human islets depends on FFAR1 but not decreased somatostatin secretion. *Sci. Rep.* **2017**, *7*, 4657. [CrossRef]
10. Oh, Y.S.; Bae, G.D.; Baek, D.J.; Park, E.-Y.; Jun, H.-S. Fatty Acid-Induced Lipotoxicity in Pancreatic Beta-Cells During Development of Type 2 Diabetes. *Front. Endocrinol.* **2018**, *9*, 384. [CrossRef]
11. Acosta-Montaño, P.; García-González, V. Effects of Dietary Fatty Acids in Pancreatic Beta Cell Metabolism, Implications in Homeostasis. *Nutrients* **2018**, *10*, 393. [CrossRef]
12. Römer, A.; Linn, T.; Petry, S. Lipotoxic Impairment of Mitochondrial Function in β-Cells: A Review. *Antioxidants* **2021**, *10*, 293. [CrossRef]
13. Cnop, M.; Ladrière, L.; Igoillo-Esteve, M.; Moura, R.F.; Cunha, D.A. Causes and cures for endoplasmic reticulum stress in lipotoxic β-cell dysfunction. *Diabetes Obes. Metab.* **2010**, *12*, 76–82. [CrossRef]
14. Carta, G.; Murru, E.; Lisai, S.; Sirigu, A.; Piras, A.; Collu, M.; Batetta, B.; Gambelli, L.; Banni, S. Dietary Triacylglycerols with Palmitic Acid in the sn-2 Position Modulate Levels of N-Acylethanolamides in Rat Tissues. *PLoS ONE* **2015**, *10*, e0120424. [CrossRef]
15. Carta, G.; Murru, E.; Banni, S.; Manca, C. Palmitic Acid: Physiological Role, Metabolism and Nutritional Implications. *Front. Physiol.* **2017**, *8*, 902. [CrossRef]
16. Sargsyan, E.; Artemenko, K.; Manukyan, L.; Bergquist, J.; Bergsten, P. Oleate protects beta-cells from the toxic effect of palmitate by activating pro-survival pathways of the ER stress response. *Biochim. Biophys. Acta (BBA) Mol. Cell Biol. Lipids* **2016**, *1861*, 1151–1160. [CrossRef]
17. Kokatnur, M.G.; Oalmann, M.C.; Johnson, W.D.; Malcom, G.T.; Strong, J.P. Fatty acid composition of human adipose tissue from two anatomical sites in a biracial community. *Am. J. Clin. Nutr.* **1979**, *32*, 2198–2205. [CrossRef]
18. Nemecz, M.; Constantin, A.; Dumitrescu, M.; Alexandru, N.; Filippi, A.; Tanko, G.; Georgescu, A. The Distinct Effects of Palmitic and Oleic Acid on Pancreatic Beta Cell Function: The Elucidation of Associated Mechanisms and Effector Molecules. *Front. Pharmacol.* **2019**, *9*, 1554. [CrossRef]
19. Karunakaran, U.; Elumalai, S.; Moon, J.-S.; Won, K.-C. CD36 Signal Transduction in Metabolic Diseases: Novel Insights and Therapeutic Targeting. *Cells* **2021**, *10*, 1833. [CrossRef]
20. Oberhauser, L.; Maechler, P. Lipid-Induced Adaptations of the Pancreatic Beta-Cell to Glucotoxic Conditions Sustain Insulin Secretion. *Int. J. Mol. Sci.* **2021**, *23*, 324. [CrossRef]
21. Reilly, J.M.; Thompson, M.P. Dietary Fatty Acids Up-Regulate the Expression of UCP2 in 3T3-L1 Preadipocytes. *Biochem. Biophys. Res. Commun.* **2000**, *277*, 541–545. [CrossRef] [PubMed]
22. Joseph, J.W.; Koshkin, V.; Saleh, M.C.; Sivitz, W.I.; Zhang, C.-Y.; Lowell, B.B.; Chan, C.B.; Wheeler, M.B. Free Fatty Acid-induced β-Cell Defects Are Dependent on Uncoupling Protein 2 Expression. *J. Biol. Chem.* **2004**, *279*, 51049–51056. [CrossRef] [PubMed]
23. Sreedhar, A.; Zhao, Y. Uncoupling protein 2 and metabolic diseases. *Mitochondrion* **2017**, *34*, 135–140. [CrossRef] [PubMed]
24. Jaswal, J.; Ussher, J. Myocardial fatty acid utilization as a determinant of cardiac efficiency and function. *Clin. Lipidol.* **2009**, *4*, 379–389. [CrossRef]
25. Sara, M.; Yaser, K.-B.; Maedeh, A.; Mohamadreza, A.; Beitullah, A. The review of the relationship between UCP2 and obesity: Focusing on inflammatory-obesity. *New Insights Obes. Genet. Beyond* **2021**, *5*, 001–013. [CrossRef]
26. Yang, K.; Xu, X.; Nie, L.; Xiao, T.; Guan, X.; He, T.; Yu, Y.; Liu, L.; Huang, Y.; Zhang, J.; et al. Indoxyl sulfate induces oxidative stress and hypertrophy in cardiomyocytes by inhibiting the AMPK/UCP2 signaling pathway. *Toxicol. Lett.* **2015**, *234*, 110–119. [CrossRef]
27. Baffy, G. Mitochondrial uncoupling in cancer cells: Liabilities and opportunities. *Biochim. Biophys. Acta Bioenerg.* **2017**, *1858*, 655–664. [CrossRef]
28. Emre, Y.; Nübel, T. Uncoupling protein UCP2: When mitochondrial activity meets immunity. *FEBS Lett.* **2010**, *584*, 1437–1442. [CrossRef]
29. Bouillaud, F. UCP2, not a physiologically relevant uncoupler but a glucose sparing switch impacting ROS production and glucose sensing. *Biochim. Biophys. Acta Bioenerg.* **2009**, *1787*, 377–383. [CrossRef]
30. Rupprecht, A.; Moldzio, R.; Mödl, B.; Pohl, E.E. Glutamine regulates mitochondrial uncoupling protein 2 to promote glutaminolysis in neuroblastoma cells. *Biochim. Biophys. Acta Bioenerg.* **2019**, *1860*, 391–401. [CrossRef]
31. Manukyan, L.; Ubhayasekera, S.J.K.A.; Bergquist, J.; Sargsyan, E.; Bergsten, P. Palmitate-Induced Impairments of β-Cell Function Are Linked with Generation of Specific Ceramide Species via Acylation of Sphingosine. *Endocrinology* **2015**, *156*, 802–812. [CrossRef]
32. Ye, R.; Onodera, T.; Scherer, P.E. Lipotoxicity and β Cell Maintenance in Obesity and Type 2 Diabetes. *J. Endocr. Soc.* **2019**, *3*, 617–631. [CrossRef]
33. Lewandowski, S.L.; Cardone, R.L.; Foster, H.R.; Ho, T.; Potapenko, E.; Poudel, C.; Van Deusen, H.R.; Sdao, S.M.; Alves, T.C.; Zhao, X.; et al. Pyruvate Kinase Controls Signal Strength in the Insulin Secretory Pathway. *Cell Metab.* **2020**, *32*, 736–750.e5. [CrossRef]

34. Ishihara, H. Metabolism-secretion coupling in glucose-stimulated insulin secretion. *Diabetol. Int.* **2022**, *13*, 463–470. [CrossRef]
35. Schuit, F.; De Vos, A.; Farfari, S.; Moens, K.; Pipeleers, D.; Brun, T.; Prentki, M. Metabolic Fate of Glucose in Purified Islet Cells. *J. Biol. Chem.* **1997**, *272*, 18572–18579. [CrossRef]
36. Prentki, M.; Matschinsky, F.M.; Madiraju, S.M. Metabolic Signaling in Fuel-Induced Insulin Secretion. *Cell Metab.* **2013**, *18*, 162–185. [CrossRef]
37. Rorsman, P.; Braun, M.; Zhang, Q. Regulation of calcium in pancreatic α- and β-cells in health and disease. *Cell Calcium* **2012**, *51*, 300–308. [CrossRef]
38. Sugden, M.C.; Holness, M.J. The pyruvate carboxylase-pyruvate dehydrogenase axis in islet pyruvate metabolism: Going round in circles? *Islets* **2011**, *3*, 302–319. [CrossRef]
39. Corkey, B.E. Targeting Pyruvate Kinase PEPs Up Insulin Secretion and Improves Glucose Homeostasis. *Cell Metab.* **2020**, *32*, 693–694. [CrossRef]
40. Lu, D.; Mulder, H.; Zhao, P.; Burgess, S.C.; Jensen, M.V.; Kamzolova, S.; Newgard, C.B.; Sherry, A.D. ^{13}C NMR isotopomer analysis reveals a connection between pyruvate cycling and glucose-stimulated insulin secretion (GSIS). *Proc. Natl. Acad. Sci. USA* **2002**, *99*, 2708–2713. [CrossRef]
41. Hohmeier, H.E.; Mulder, H.; Chen, G.; Henkel-Rieger, R.; Prentki, M.; Newgard, C.B. Isolation of INS-1-derived cell lines with robust ATP-sensitive K+ channel-dependent and -independent glucose-stimulated insulin secretion. *Diabetes* **2000**, *49*, 424–430. [CrossRef] [PubMed]
42. Sreedhar, A.; Cassell, T.; Smith, P.; Lu, D.; Nam, H.W.; Lane, A.N.; Zhao, Y. UCP2 Overexpression Redirects Glucose into Anabolic Metabolic Pathways. *Proteomics* **2018**, *19*, e1800353. [CrossRef] [PubMed]
43. Jesinkey, S.R.; Madiraju, A.K.; Alves, T.C.; Yarborough, O.H.; Cardone, R.L.; Zhao, X.; Parsaei, Y.; Nasiri, A.R.; Butrico, G.; Liu, X.; et al. Mitochondrial GTP Links Nutrient Sensing to β Cell Health, Mitochondrial Morphology, and Insulin Secretion Independent of OxPhos. *Cell Rep.* **2019**, *28*, 759–772.e10. [CrossRef] [PubMed]
44. Stark, R.; Kibbey, R.G. The mitochondrial isoform of phosphoenolpyruvate carboxykinase (PEPCK-M) and glucose homeostasis: Has it been overlooked? *Biochim. Biophys. Acta (BBA) Gen. Subj.* **2013**, *1840*, 1313–1330. [CrossRef]
45. Abulizi, A.; Cardone, R.L.; Stark, R.; Lewandowski, S.L.; Zhao, X.; Hillion, J.; Ma, L.; Sehgal, R.; Alves, T.C.; Thomas, C.; et al. Multi-Tissue Acceleration of the Mitochondrial Phosphoenolpyruvate Cycle Improves Whole-Body Metabolic Health. *Cell Metab.* **2020**, *32*, 751–766.e11. [CrossRef]
46. Grubelnik, V.; Zmazek, J.; Markovič, R.; Gosak, M.; Marhl, M. Modelling of energy-driven switch for glucagon and insulin secretion. *J. Theor. Biol.* **2020**, *493*, 110213. [CrossRef]
47. Roden, M. How Free Fatty Acids Inhibit Glucose Utilization in Human Skeletal Muscle. *Physiology* **2004**, *19*, 92–96. [CrossRef]
48. Doliba, N.M.; Fenner, D.; Zelent, B.; Bass, J.; Sarabu, R.; Matschinsky, F.M. Repair of diverse diabetic defects of β-cells in man and mouse by pharmacological glucokinase activation. *Diabetes Obes. Metab.* **2012**, *14*, 109–119. [CrossRef]
49. Liang, Y.; Bai, G.; Doliba, N.; Buettger, C.; Wang, L.; Berner, D.K.; Matschinsky, F.M. Glucose metabolism and insulin release in mouse beta HC9 cells, as model for wild-type pancreatic beta-cells. *Am. J. Physiol. Metab.* **1996**, *270*, E846–E857. [CrossRef]
50. MacDonald, M.J. Feasibility of a Mitochondrial Pyruvate Malate Shuttle in Pancreatic Islets. *J. Biol. Chem.* **1995**, *270*, 20051–20058. [CrossRef]
51. MacDonald, M.J.; Tang, J.; Polonsky, K.S. Low Mitochondrial Glycerol Phosphate Dehydrogenase and Pyruvate Carboxylase in Pancreatic Islets of Zucker Diabetic Fatty Rats. *Diabetes* **1996**, *45*, 1626–1630. [CrossRef]
52. Tan, C.; Tuch, B.E.; Tu, J.; Brown, S.A. Role of NADH Shuttles in Glucose-Induced Insulin Secretion from Fetal β-Cells. *Diabetes* **2002**, *51*, 2989–2996. [CrossRef]
53. Anello, M.; Lupi, R.; Spampinato, D.; Piro, S.; Masini, M.; Boggi, U.; Del Prato, S.; Rabuazzo, A.M.; Purrello, F.; Marchetti, P. Functional and morphological alterations of mitochondria in pancreatic beta cells from type 2 diabetic patients. *Diabetologia* **2005**, *48*, 282–289. [CrossRef]
54. Lu, H.; Koshkin, V.; Allister, E.M.; Gyulkhandanyan, A.V.; Wheeler, M.B. Molecular and Metabolic Evidence for Mitochondrial Defects Associated With β-Cell Dysfunction in a Mouse Model of Type 2 Diabetes. *Diabetes* **2009**, *59*, 448–459. [CrossRef]
55. Heuett, W.J.; Periwal, V. Autoregulation of Free Radicals via Uncoupling Protein Control in Pancreatic β-Cell Mitochondria. *Biophys. J.* **2010**, *98*, 207–217. [CrossRef]
56. Petersen, K.F.; Dufour, S.; Befroy, D.; Garcia, R.; Shulman, G.I. Impaired Mitochondrial Activity in the Insulin-Resistant Offspring of Patients with Type 2 Diabetes. *N. Engl. J. Med.* **2004**, *350*, 664–671. [CrossRef]
57. Grubelnik, V.; Markovič, R.; Lipovšek, S.; Leitinger, G.; Gosak, M.; Dolenšek, J.; Valladolid-Acebes, I.; Berggren, P.-O.; Stožer, A.; Perc, M.; et al. Modelling of dysregulated glucagon secretion in type 2 diabetes by considering mitochondrial alterations in pancreatic α-cells. *R. Soc. Open Sci.* **2020**, *7*, 191171. [CrossRef]
58. Grubelnik, V.; Zmazek, J.; Markovič, R.; Gosak, M.; Marhl, M. Mitochondrial Dysfunction in Pancreatic Alpha and Beta Cells Associated with Type 2 Diabetes Mellitus. *Life* **2020**, *10*, 348. [CrossRef]
59. Maechler, P.; Wollheim, C.B. Mitochondrial function in normal and diabetic β-cells. *Nature* **2001**, *414*, 807–812. [CrossRef]
60. Nunemaker, C.S.; Zhang, M.; Satin, L.S. Insulin Feedback Alters Mitochondrial Activity Through an ATP-sensitive K+ Channel–Dependent Pathway in Mouse Islets and β-Cells. *Diabetes* **2004**, *53*, 1765–1772. [CrossRef]
61. Sivitz, W.I.; Yorek, M.A. Mitochondrial Dysfunction in Diabetes: From Molecular Mechanisms to Functional Significance and Therapeutic Opportunities. *Antioxid. Redox Signal.* **2010**, *12*, 537–577. [CrossRef] [PubMed]

62. Patti, M.-E.; Corvera, S. The Role of Mitochondria in the Pathogenesis of Type 2 Diabetes. *Endocr. Rev.* **2010**, *31*, 364–395. [CrossRef] [PubMed]
63. Wallin, T.; Ma, Z.; Ogata, H.; Jørgensen, I.H.; Iezzi, M.; Wang, H.; Wollheim, C.B.; Björklund, A. Facilitation of fatty acid uptake by CD36 in insulin-producing cells reduces fatty-acid-induced insulin secretion and glucose regulation of fatty acid oxidation. *Biochim. Biophys. Acta (BBA) Mol. Cell Biol. Lipids* **2010**, *1801*, 191–197. [CrossRef] [PubMed]
64. Nagao, M.; Esguerra, J.L.; Asai, A.; Ofori, J.K.; Edlund, A.; Wendt, A.; Sugihara, H.; Wollheim, C.B.; Oikawa, S.; Eliasson, L. Potential Protection Against Type 2 Diabetes in Obesity Through Lower CD36 Expression and Improved Exocytosis in β-Cells. *Diabetes* **2020**, *69*, 1193–1205. [CrossRef]
65. Moon, J.S.; Karunakaran, U.; Suma, E.; Chung, S.M.; Won, K.C. The Role of CD36 in Type 2 Diabetes Mellitus: β-Cell Dysfunction and Beyond. *Diabetes Metab. J.* **2020**, *44*, 222–233. [CrossRef]
66. McKee, E.E.; Bentley, A.T.; Smith, R.M.; Kraas, J.R.; Ciaccio, C.E. Guanine nucleotide transport by atractyloside-sensitive and -insensitive carriers in isolated heart mitochondria. *Am. J. Physiol. Physiol.* **2000**, *279*, C1870–C1879. [CrossRef]
67. Vozza, A.; Blanco, E.; Palmieri, L.; Palmieri, F. Identification of the Mitochondrial GTP/GDP Transporter in Saccharomyces cerevisiae. *J. Biol. Chem.* **2004**, *279*, 20850–20857. [CrossRef]
68. Nicholls, D.G. The Pancreatic β-Cell: A Bioenergetic Perspective. *Physiol. Rev.* **2016**, *96*, 1385–1447. [CrossRef]
69. Pedersen, M.G.; Bertram, R.; Sherman, A. Intra- and Inter-Islet Synchronization of Metabolically Driven Insulin Secretion. *Biophys. J.* **2005**, *89*, 107–119. [CrossRef]
70. Magnus, G.; Keizer, J. Model of β-cell mitochondrial calcium handling and electrical activity. I. Cytoplasmic variables. *Am. J. Physiol. Physiol.* **1998**, *274*, C1158–C1173. [CrossRef]
71. Bertram, R.; Sherman, A. A calcium-based phantom bursting model for pancreatic islets. *Bull. Math. Biol.* **2004**, *66*, 1313–1344. [CrossRef]
72. Rorsman, P.; Ramracheya, R.; Rorsman, N.J.G.; Zhang, Q. ATP-regulated potassium channels and voltage-gated calcium channels in pancreatic alpha and beta cells: Similar functions but reciprocal effects on secretion. *Diabetologia* **2014**, *57*, 1749–1761. [CrossRef]
73. Assimacopoulos-Jeannet, F.; Thumelin, S.; Roche, E.; Esser, V.; McGarry, J.D.; Prentki, M. Fatty Acids Rapidly Induce the Carnitine Palmitoyltransferase I Gene in the Pancreatic β-Cell Line INS-1. *J. Biol. Chem.* **1997**, *272*, 1659–1664. [CrossRef]
74. Yoshikawa, H.; Tajiri, Y.; Sako, Y.; Hashimoto, T.; Umeda, F.; Nawata, H. Effects of free fatty acids on β-cell functions: A possible involvement of peroxisome proliferator-activated receptors α or pancreatic/duodenal homeobox. *Metabolism* **2001**, *50*, 613–618. [CrossRef]
75. Lu, B.; Kurmi, K.; Munoz-Gomez, M.; Ambuludi, E.J.J.; Tonne, J.M.; Rakshit, K.; Hitosugi, T.; Kudva, Y.C.; Matveyenko, A.V.; Ikeda, Y. Impaired β-cell glucokinase as an underlying mechanism in diet-induced diabetes. *Dis. Models Mech.* **2018**, *11*, dmm033316. [CrossRef]
76. Del Guerra, S.; Lupi, R.; Marselli, L.; Masini, M.; Bugliani, M.; Sbrana, S.; Torri, S.; Pollera, M.; Boggi, U.; Mosca, F.; et al. Functional and Molecular Defects of Pancreatic Islets in Human Type 2 Diabetes. *Diabetes* **2005**, *54*, 727–735. [CrossRef]
77. Yaney, G.C.; Corkey, B.E. Fatty acid metabolism and insulin secretion in pancreatic beta cells. *Diabetologia* **2003**, *46*, 1297–1312. [CrossRef]
78. Cen, J.; Sargsyan, E.; Bergsten, P. Fatty acids stimulate insulin secretion from human pancreatic islets at fasting glucose concentrations via mitochondria-dependent and -independent mechanisms. *Nutr. Metab.* **2016**, *13*, 59. [CrossRef]
79. Itoh, Y.; Kawamata, Y.; Harada, M.; Kobayashi, M.; Fujii, R.; Fukusumi, S.; Ogi, K.; Hosoya, M.; Tanaka, Y.; Uejima, H.; et al. Free fatty acids regulate insulin secretion from pancreatic β cells through GPR40. *Nature* **2003**, *422*, 173–176. [CrossRef]
80. Nolan, C.J.; Madiraju, M.S.; Delghingaro-Augusto, V.; Peyot, M.-L.; Prentki, M. Fatty Acid Signaling in the β-Cell and Insulin Secretion. *Diabetes* **2006**, *55*, S16–S23. [CrossRef]
81. Kristinsson, H.; Smith, D.M.; Bergsten, P.; Sargsyan, E. FFAR1 Is Involved in Both the Acute and Chronic Effects of Palmitate on Insulin Secretion. *Endocrinology* **2013**, *154*, 4078–4088. [CrossRef] [PubMed]
82. Prentki, M.; Corkey, B.E.; Madiraju, S.R.M. Lipid-associated metabolic signalling networks in pancreatic beta cell function. *Diabetologia* **2019**, *63*, 10–20. [CrossRef]
83. Busch, A.K.; Cordery, D.; Denyer, G.S.; Biden, T.J. Expression Profiling of Palmitate- and Oleate-Regulated Genes Provides Novel Insights into the Effects of Chronic Lipid Exposure on Pancreatic β-Cell Function. *Diabetes* **2002**, *51*, 977–987. [CrossRef] [PubMed]
84. Koshkin, V.; Wang, X.; Scherer, P.E.; Chan, C.; Wheeler, M.B. Mitochondrial Functional State in Clonal Pancreatic β-Cells Exposed to Free Fatty Acids. *J. Biol. Chem.* **2003**, *278*, 19709–19715. [CrossRef] [PubMed]
85. Erion, K.; Corkey, B.E. β-Cell Failure or β-Cell Abuse? *Front. Endocrinol.* **2018**, *9*, 532. [CrossRef] [PubMed]
86. Kim-Muller, J.Y.; Kim, Y.; Fan, J.; Zhao, S.; Banks, A.; Prentki, M.; Accili, D. FoxO1 Deacetylation Decreases Fatty Acid Oxidation in β-Cells and Sustains Insulin Secretion in Diabetes. *J. Biol. Chem.* **2016**, *291*, 10162–10172. [CrossRef] [PubMed]
87. Accili, D.; Talchai, S.C.; Kim-Muller, J.Y.; Cinti, F.; Ishida, E.; Ordelheide, A.M.; Kuo, T.; Fan, J.; Son, J. When β-cells fail: Lessons from dedifferentiation. *Diabetes Obes. Metab.* **2016**, *18* (Suppl. S1), 117–122. [CrossRef]

MDPI
St. Alban-Anlage 66
4052 Basel
Switzerland
Tel. +41 61 683 77 34
Fax +41 61 302 89 18
www.mdpi.com

Biomedicines Editorial Office
E-mail: biomedicines@mdpi.com
www.mdpi.com/journal/biomedicines

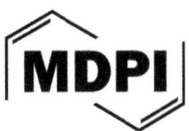

www.ingramcontent.com/pod-product-compliance
Lightning Source LLC
LaVergne TN
LVHW070450100526
838202LV00014B/1699